# Serous Effusions

Ben Davidson  •  Pınar Fırat  •  Claire W. Michael
Editors

# Serous Effusions

## Etiology, Diagnosis, Prognosis and Therapy

Second Edition

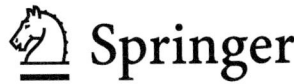 Springer

*Editors*

Ben Davidson
Department of Pathology
The Norwegian Radium Hospital
Oslo University Hospital
Oslo
Norway

Faculty of Medicine
Institute of Clinical Medicine
University of Oslo
Oslo
Norway

Claire W. Michael
UH Cleveland Medical Center
Case Western Reserve University
UH Cleveland Medical Center
Cleveland
Ohio
USA

Pınar Fırat
Department of Pathology
School of Medicine
Koç University
Istanbul
Turkey

Department of Pathology
Istanbul Faculty of Medicine
Istanbul University
Istanbul
Turkey

ISBN 978-3-030-09498-0     ISBN 978-3-319-76478-8   (eBook)
https://doi.org/10.1007/978-3-319-76478-8

# Preface: Second Edition

The 6 years that have passed since the publication of the first edition of this book have seen considerable activity focused at improving effusion diagnosis and at expanding our understanding of the biology of cancer cells in effusions, as well as studies focusing on the role of targeted therapy in this clinical setting. However, activity has not been equally distributed across the different malignancies that commonly affect the serosal cavities. Research of malignant mesothelioma has mostly focused on improved diagnosis, including a set of guidelines published in several journals. Lung carcinoma research has focused on molecular diagnostics that are relevant for targeted therapy, where effusions are now integral part of patient work-up. Studies of ovarian carcinoma have predominantly, though not exclusively focused on research aspects, with several large studies including effusion specimens within the wider context of recurrent disease. Next generation sequencing has been applied in analyses of both lung and ovarian carcinoma. In contrast, breast and gastrointestinal carcinomas have been studied to a lesser extent. Nevertheless, in a medical reality in which liquid biopsies are increasingly regarded as central to the management and follow-up of cancer patients, it is very likely that effusions will become still more relevant in clinical practice. This new edition incorporates research performed in recent years at the diagnostic, therapeutic and experimental avenues. We hope that readers will become as engaged as we are in understanding serous effusions.

With best wishes,
Ben Davidson, Pınar Fırat and Claire Michael

# Contents

# Part I

# Diagnosis

# Benign Effusions

1

## Pınar Fırat

## Introduction

The serous cavities of the body—the peritoneal cavity, the pericardial cavity, and the two pleural cavities—are closed spaces covered by the parietal and visceral layers of serous membranes. Under physiologic conditions, the two layers of the serous membranes are in close apposition, and only a small amount of fluid is present within the cavities, acting as a lubricant between the parietal and visceral layers to prevent friction. Accumulation of fluid in the serous cavities is called effusion. Any serous effusion is considered to be pathologic irrespective of the cause and the content of the accumulated fluid [1, 2]. The serous cavities are lined by a monolayer of mesothelial cells supported by fibrous tissue rich in capillaries and lymphatics. The mechanism underlying serous effusions is basically an alteration in fluid homeostasis. The fluid in the serous cavities is not static; it is constantly being formed and removed [2]. The amount of fluid in the serous cavities is controlled by several factors: the hydrostatic and oncotic pressure in the circulation, negative pressure in the serous cavity, permeability of the capillaries in the membrane, and the capacity of lymphatic absorption. Disturbances in the microcirculation, congestion in the vessels, vasodilation, increased vascular permeability, and blockage of the lymphatic drainage may lead to fluid extravasation into the serous cavity [1].

Serous effusion is a common finding in patients with systemic disease; it may also be a sign of a local disorder. Annually, 1.5 million individuals develop pleural effusions in the USA [3]. Most of the clinically detected effusions, both in adults and children, are associated with reactive conditions [3, 4]. Involvement of more than one cavity is common in systemic disorders. Most common causes show some

variations according to the cavity involved. Congestive heart failure is one of the leading causes of pleural and pericardial effusions. In cirrhosis or pancreatitis, effusions are usually peritoneal. Bilateral pleural effusions generally occur in systemic diseases, whereas unilateral pleural effusions reflect regional pathologies, such as pneumonias. Right-sided pleural effusions may develop secondary to peritoneal effusions and may be the result of subdiaphragmatic and hepatic abscesses or as part of Meigs syndrome (characterized by ascites, pleural effusion, and a benign ovarian tumor, usually fibroma). On the other hand, pancreatic disease, esophageal rupture, splenic abscess, and infarction tend to produce left-sided pleural effusions [1, 2, 5].

## Etiologic Factors and Types of Effusions

According to the properties of the fluid accumulated, effusions are divided into transudates, exudates, and chylous effusions.

Transudates are defined as plasma ultrafiltrates. They have a low cell and protein content and generally occur due to increased hydrostatic pressure or decreased plasma oncotic pressure. Exudates are hypercellular fluids rich in protein; increased vascular and/or membrane permeability and blockage of lymphatic vessels are the major mechanisms underlying exudates. Chylous effusions are characterized by a lipid-rich content and almost always reflect leakage from a major lymphatic duct into the serous cavity [6–8].

As the etiologic factors differ (Table 1.1), to identify whether an effusion is a transudate or an exudate is an important step in the clinical management [3, 7, 9]. Classically, transudates are described as fluids with a specific gravity ≤1.015 (measured by a hydrometer) and a protein level < 3.0 g/dL, whereas exudates are defined as fluids with a specific gravity >1.015 and a total protein level ≥ 3.0 g/dL.

In clinical practice, there are several tests other than protein content used in the evaluation of serous effusions (Table 1.2) [1, 3, 10]. Measuring lactate dehydrogenase

P. Fırat, M.D.
Department of Pathology, School of Medicine, Koc University, Istanbul, Turkey

[*Previously*] Department of Pathology, Istanbul Faculty of Medicine, Istanbul University, Istanbul, Turkey
e-mail: pfirat@kuh.ku.edu.tr; pfirat@istanbul.edu.tr

© Springer International Publishing AG, part of Springer Nature 2018
B. Davidson et al. (eds.), *Serous Effusions*, https://doi.org/10.1007/978-3-319-76478-8_1

**Table 1.1** Etiologic factors underlying different types of serous effusions

| Transudates | Exudates | Chylous effusions |
|---|---|---|
| Congestive heart failure | Infections | Trauma |
| Cirrhosis of the liver | Collagen vascular diseases | Neoplastic infiltration |
| Nephrotic syndrome | Embolism/infarction | |
| Peritoneal dialysis | Hemorrhage | |
| Malnutrition | Uremia | |
| Vena cava obstruction | Pancreatitis | |
| Constrictive pericarditis | Fistulas/perforations | |
| | Malignant neoplasms | |
| | Idiopathic | |

**Table 1.2** The differences between transudates and exudates

| | Transudates | Exudates |
|---|---|---|
| Fluid protein | <3 g/dL | ≥3 g/dL |
| Fluid-to-serum protein ratio | <0.5 | >0.5 |
| Fluid LDH | <200 U/L | >200 U/L |
| Fluid-to-serum LDH ratio | <0.6 | >0.6 |
| Fluid cholesterol | <45–55 mg/dL | >45–55 mg/dL |
| Fluid cholesterol-to-serum cholesterol | <0.3 | >0.3 |
| Albumin gradient | >1.2 g/dL | ≤1.2 g/dL |

(LDH) level is an important adjunct to the diagnosis. There are three commonly used criteria to identify exudates, known as "Light's criteria," described for pleural fluids [11]:

Pleural fluid- to- serum protein ratio > 0.5.

Pleural fluid- to- serum LDH ratio > 0.6.

Pleural fluid LDH concentration > two-thirds of the upper limit of normal serum level.

If at least one of these three criteria is present, the fluid is an exudate with a sensitivity of 95–98% and a specificity of 81–89% [6, 10]. Light's criteria should be applied cautiously to patients with congestive heart failure who are treated with diuretics, as the latter may change the protein and LDH levels in the pleural fluid. Albumin gradient was found to be more reliable in identifying transudates in these patients [12]. High serum or pleural fluid levels of NT-proBNP exceeding 1500 pg/mL are another useful finding in the diagnosis of effusions due to heart failure [6, 9, 13].

In addition to protein and LDH levels, increased cholesterol level (>45–55 mg/dL) is also a sign of an exudate [7, 10, 14]. In physiologic conditions, the glucose concentration and pH of the effusions are nearly equivalent to serum values. In inflammatory diseases such as empyema and rheumatoid arthritis, the effusion fluid is characterized by acidosis and low glucose levels [3].

Adenosine deaminase (ADA) activity is another widely used test in the evaluation of serous effusions: ADA level above 40 U/L is a strong indicator of tuberculosis [15].

However, extremely high levels of ADA are generally associated with empyema or lymphoproliferative diseases [6, 16]. The finding of amylase concentration in the effusion that is higher than plasma level is highly suspicious for pancreatic disease, esophageal rupture, or malignancy [17–19].

Transudates present as clear or straw-colored fluids, though not always, as nearly 10% may appear bloody or turbid [20]. The most common etiologic factors for transudates are congestive heart failure, renal failure, and liver cirrhosis [3, 6, 7, 21].

Exudates appear cloudy, turbid, or bloody. Major causes of exudative serous effusions are inflammation, either regional or systemic, and malignant neoplasms. Effusions due to cancer are almost always exudates. An effusion is considered bloody when it is homogeneously dark red or brown, contains hemosiderin pigment, or has a hematocrit level which is at least 10% of blood hematocrit. Hemorrhagic effusions are commonly associated with malignancy, but only 11% of malignant effusions are bloody [20]. Trauma, infections, and infarcts are nonneoplastic causes of hemorrhagic effusions [1, 6, 8].

Chylous effusions are rarely encountered. They occur due to either trauma or neoplastic infiltration of the major lymphatic ducts. The triglyceride concentration of the fluid (>110 mg/dL) and the presence of chylomicrons are important in the diagnosis of chylous effusions [14]. They generally present as milky fluids and contain many lymphocytes [2]. However, in a series of patients with chylothorax, it was shown that only 45% of the cases had milky effusions [22]. A second type of lipidic effusion is cholesterol effusion. It has the same appearance as chylous effusion, but it contains cholesterol instead of triglycerides, and has a different pathogenesis. A cholesterol effusion is typically the result of long-standing pleurisy; most cases are attributed to tuberculosis or rheumatoid arthritis [14]. Cholesterol crystals can be seen in cytological preparations from these effusions [3].

Differentiating transudates from exudates and chylous effusions is important since malignancy is not an expected finding in transudates. Light's criteria seem to be the best method to differentiate transudates from exudates, providing valuable insight into the etiology and risk of malignancy in patients with effusion [6, 10]. In a literature search done by Wilcox et al., fluid cholesterol levels >55 mg/dL, fluid-to-serum cholesterol ratio > 0.3, and fluid LDH level > 200 U/L were found to be highly sensitive and specific tests, in addition to Light's criteria, to differentiate exudative pleural effusions from transudates [10].

Several biomarkers such as mesothelin, fibulin-3, CEA, CA125, and CA15-3 have also been studied in serous effusions with some success for the detection of malignancy. A considerable amount of research based on genomics, proteomics, and immunomics is going on to identify new markers [9, 13, 23, 24]. The developing area of biomarkers is promising; even though for today they have a limited role in the evaluation of serous effusions, they may be more useful in the future in solving the clinician's main dilemma whether an effusion is benign or malignant.

The malignancy rates for pleural effusions in different series are reported to be 20–27% [25, 26]. The unpublished data from the author's institution is also within the same range, being 25% for pleural, and overall 26% for all samples from different cavities sent for cytologic examination.

## Morphology

The cytomorphologic features of serous effusions do not differ due to the cavity involved and disorders involving different serous cavities present with the same cytomorphologic features. The only exception may be the presence of florid reactive changes in mesothelial cells of the pericardium, caused by the beating heart, which may mimic malignancy [27].

Effusions contain a variety of cells depending on the underlying pathology. Mesothelial cells, as the local elements, are almost always present in the effusions. The other nonneoplastic cells that are frequently encountered in effusion cytology are macrophages and blood-borne cells. Some incidental cellular and noncellular elements may also be observed.

## Mesothelial Cells

Mesothelial cells are mesodermally derived epithelial cells lining the serosal cavities. In the physiological state, they form a flat monolayer. When serous membranes are injured, mesothelial cells proliferate. The cells become cuboidal and larger and may pile up and form papillary projections.

When mesothelial cells exfoliate into the fluid, they round up. They show a wide size variation but usually measure 15–30 μm in diameter [1]. They may present as single cells or form small clusters (Figs. 1.1 and 1.2).

Mesothelial cells are characterized by centrally or paracentrally located nuclei which are round to oval in shape [5, 28] (Figs. 1.3 and 1.4). The nucleus may occasionally be placed eccentrically, but even in this situation, a thin layer of cytoplasm can be seen between the nucleus and the cell border [1] (Fig. 1.4). In contrast, the eccentric nuclei of adenocarcinoma cells contact the cytoplasmic border [28]. The chromatin pattern is finely granular in mesothelial cells, with varying degrees of chromasia (Figs. 1.4 and 1.5). However, as the nucleus gets hyperchromatic, the cytoplasm also stains darker [5, 27]. The nuclear membrane is usually prominent and smooth (Fig. 1.5). Nucleoli may be distinct, but the presence of macronucleoli is not an expected finding [27, 28] (Figs. 1.2 and 1.5). Rarely nuclear pseudoinclusions are seen.

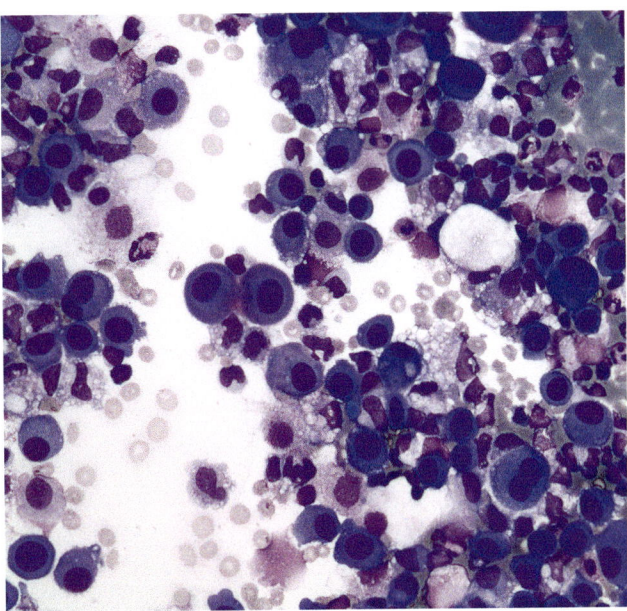

**Fig. 1.1** Single-lying, variably sized mesothelial cells; MGG

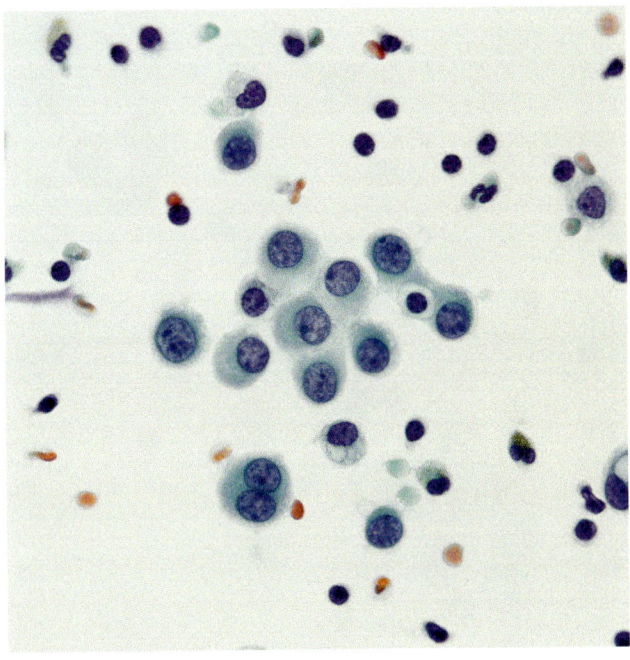

**Fig. 1.2** Mesothelial cells forming loose clusters; PAP

The nuclear-to-cytoplasmic (N/C) ratio of mesothelial cells varies. Small cells with higher N/C ratio and larger cells with lower N/C ratio may be found together (Fig. 1.1). Binucleation is a common feature of mesothelial cells (Figs. 1.2 and 1.6); multinucleated forms may also occur in reactive mesothelial proliferations [5, 27, 29] (Figs. 1.7 and 1.8).

Mesothelial cells have a rather characteristic cytoplasm which is basically dense and shows different staining zones. In Papanicolaou-stained smears, the perinuclear area which

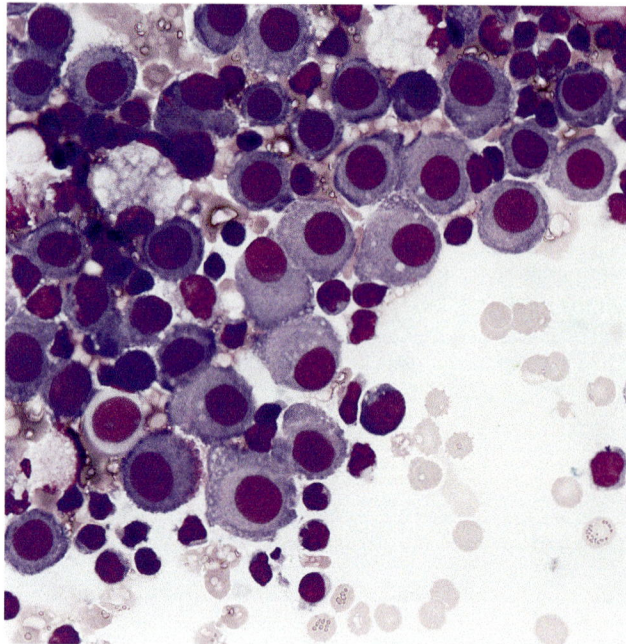

**Fig. 1.3** Centrally or paracentrally located, round to oval nuclei of mesothelial cells; MGG

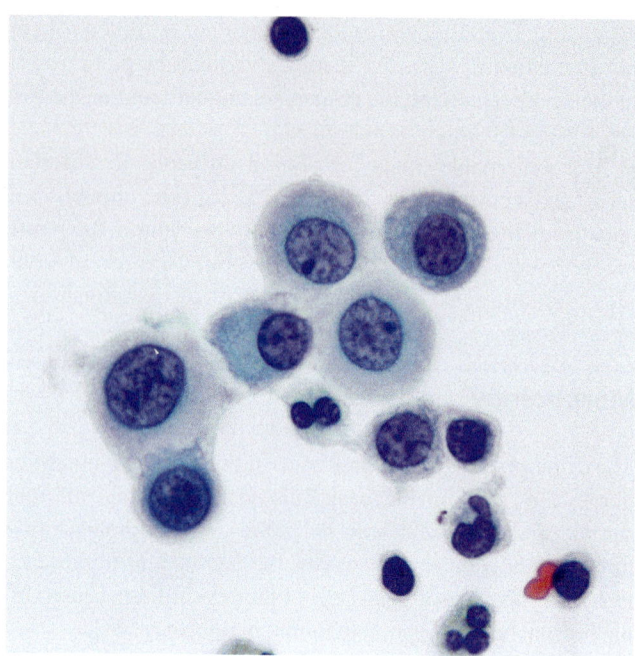

**Fig. 1.5** Mesothelial cells with smooth prominent nuclear membrane, finely granular chromatin, and small nucleoli; PAP

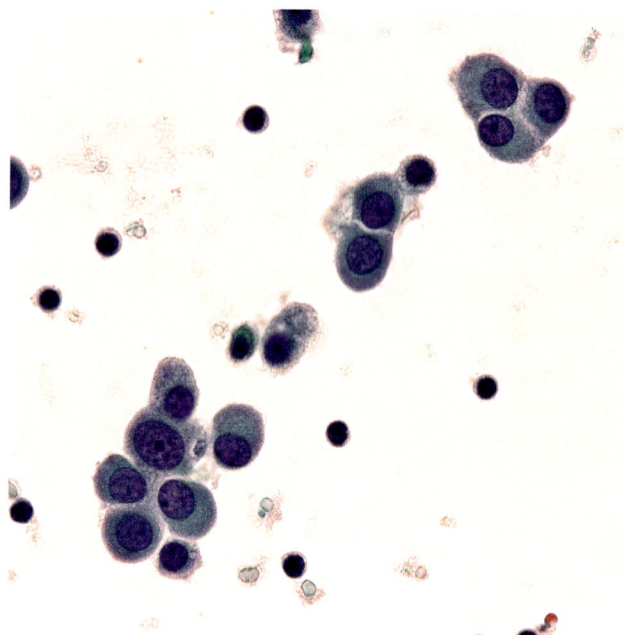

**Fig. 1.4** Mesothelial cells with occasional eccentric nuclei. A thin layer of cytoplasm can be seen between the nuclear and the cytoplasmic borders; PAP

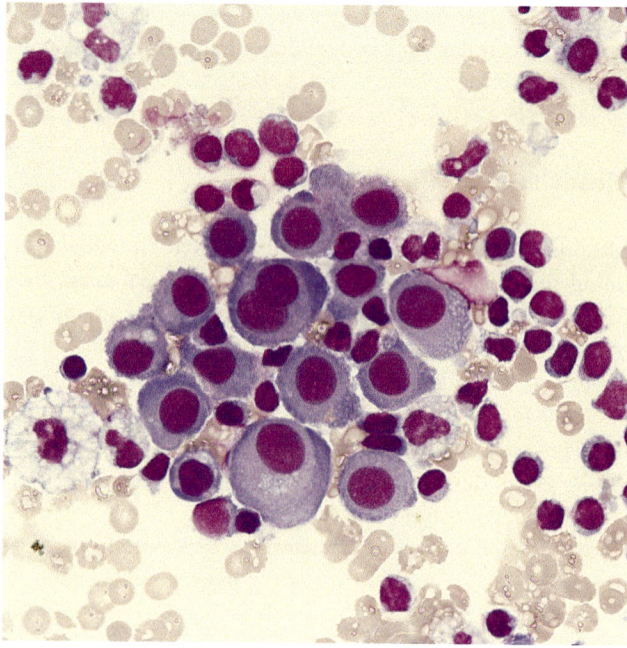

**Fig. 1.6** Binucleation in mesothelial cells; MGG

is rich in intermediate filaments shows denser staining, in contrast to the periphery of the cytoplasm which looks lacy due to the presence of microvilli (Fig. 1.9). This is called endoplasmic/ectoplasmic demarcation. On the other hand, in Romanowsky stains, the inner perinuclear zone is generally stained paler and the outer zone denser (Fig. 1.10).

Cytoplasmic blebs are seen on the surface [1, 27, 28] (Figs. 1.10 and 1.11).

The cytoplasm of mesothelial cells may be vacuolated. They may contain multiple small fat vacuoles around the nucleus or glycogen vacuoles at the periphery (Fig. 1.12), but usually multiple or single degenerative/hydropic vacuoles are

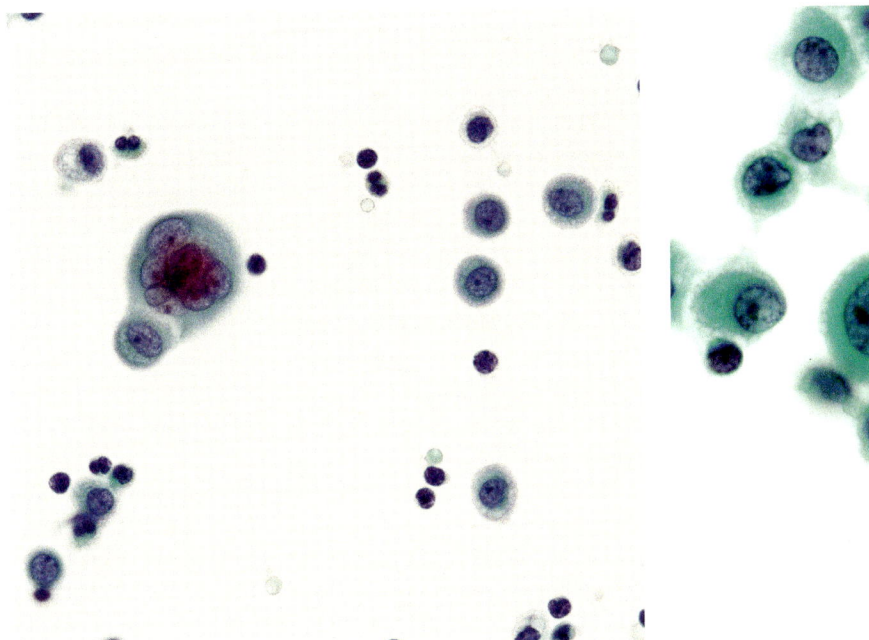

**Fig. 1.7** A multinucleated mesothelial cell; PAP

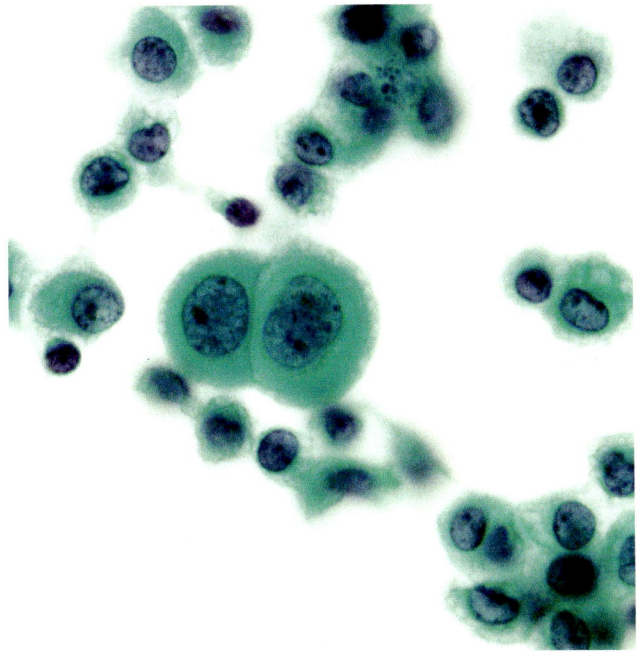

**Fig. 1.9** The cytoplasm of the mesothelial cells looks dense in the perinuclear area and lacy at the periphery, creating an endoplasmic/ectoplasmic demarcation (PAP)

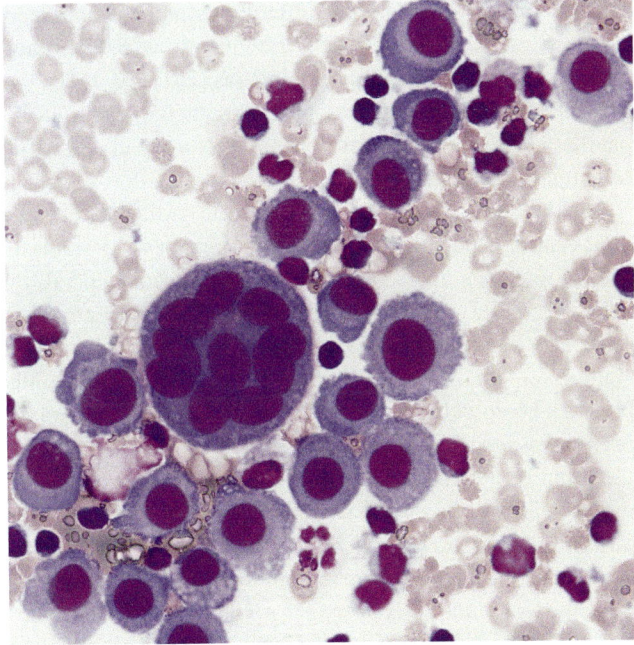

**Fig. 1.8** Multinucleation is a common feature of reactive mesothelial cells; MGG

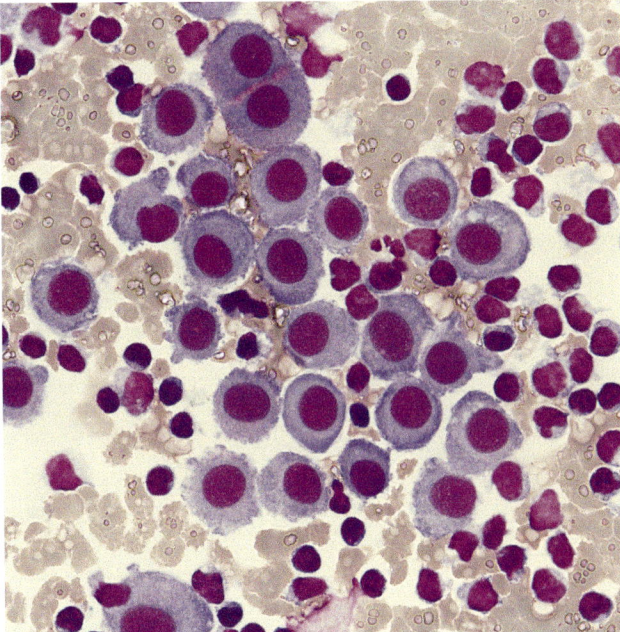

**Fig. 1.10** Two-tone staining in mesothelial cells with Romanowsky stains—inner zone is paler, outer zone is darker—MGG

observed [5, 27]. If a single large hydropic vacuole occurs in the cytoplasm, it displaces the nucleus toward the edge, mimicking a signet ring cell (Fig. 1.13a–c). The nuclear features should be the clue for correct interpretation. Even if pushed aside, the nuclei of mesothelial cells are not indented by the vacuole. The nucleus is wrapped around by the hydropic vac-

uole, creating an overlapping appearance under light microscopy, as the edge of the vacuole overlaps with the edge of the nucleus [29] (Fig. 1.13c). The mesothelial nuclei preserve their characteristics and look bland in comparison to malignant nuclei. In contrast, the nuclei of signet ring cells are generally clearly indented by the vacuoles and display malignant

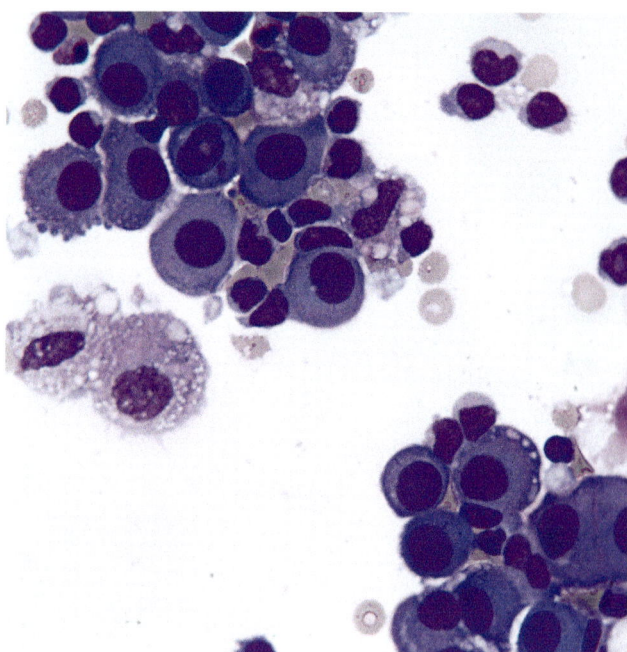

**Fig. 1.11** Cytoplasmic blebs on the surface of the mesothelial cells and glycogen vacuoles at the periphery of the cytoplasm; MGG

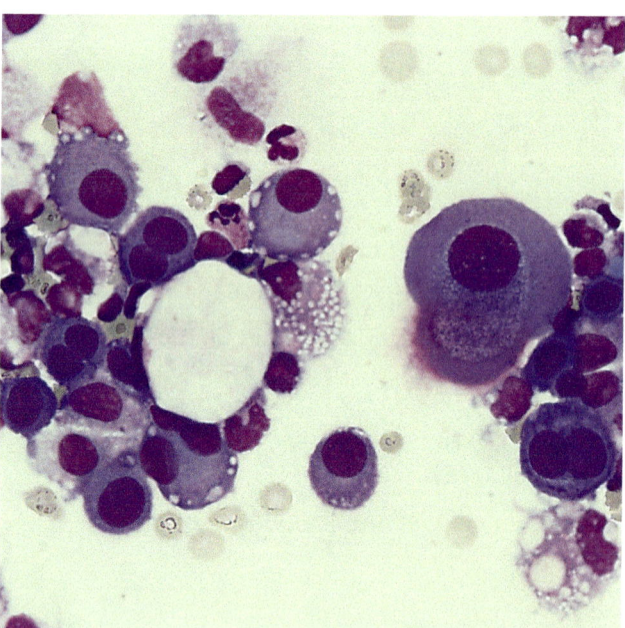

**Fig. 1.12** Mesothelial cells showing multiple small fat vacuoles around the nucleus and glycogen vacuoles at the periphery; MGG

features such as hyperchromasia, coarse chromatin, and irregular contours (Fig. 1.14a, b). They may be pushed aside to the degree that the outer border of the nucleus forms an angle with the outer border of the cytoplasm (Fig. 1.14c). Additionally, degenerative vacuoles are crystal clear, while secretory vacuoles have substance in them which can be highlighted by mucin stains [5, 29] (Fig. 1.14d–f).

Mitotic figures are not rare in mesothelial cells; they should not lead to an incorrect diagnosis of malignancy [8, 27] (Fig. 1.15).

When mesothelial cells come together in groups, slit-like spaces called "windows" are seen between adjacent cells (Fig. 1.16). They are the reflection of the long slender microvilli on their surface [5, 27]. The presence of "windows" in a group of cells is a clue regarding their mesothelial origin (Fig. 1.17). However, it should be noted that "windows" can be seen between adenocarcinoma cells as well (Fig. 1.18). Two different studies showed that "windows" are detected in 13 and 44% of adenocarcinoma cases, and in most of these cases, slit-like spaces between neoplastic cells represented mucin secretion [30, 31].

Molding is a characteristic feature of mesothelial cells. They may form cell-in-cell arrangements (Fig. 1.19) and even Indian files. Cell-in-cell appearance, which is described as one cell embracing the other, is a typical feature of mesothelial cells but more common and more prominent in malignant mesotheliomas than in reactive mesothelial proliferations [28].

Mesothelial groups typically have flower-like, knobby contours (Fig. 1.20). In contrast, adenocarcinoma cells form groups with common borders, such as cell balls and papillae. Knobby-contoured cell clusters are a feature of mesothelial cells both seen in reactive proliferations and in malignant mesotheliomas. However, not infrequently (36.9%), they may also be present in adenocarcinomas [28] (Fig. 1.21). On the other hand, in some cases of mesothelial hyperplasia, papillary structures may develop, creating a pitfall in the differential diagnosis [5] (Fig. 1.22).

Mesothelial cell clusters may contain collagen cores in their center, which are highlighted by Romanowsky stains as a homogeneous metachromatic substance surrounded by cells (Fig. 1.23). These groups may have smooth contours (also called collagen balls) and may be mistaken for metastatic carcinoma. They are more common in peritoneal fluids [29, 32]. Mesothelial cells can also present as large monolayered sheets, especially in washings [27].

When serous membranes are irritated and injured, mesothelial cells proliferate and may show both cellular and structural atypia. Cluster formation, spherical groups with collagen cores, multinucleation, hyperchromasia, high N/C ratio, distinct nucleoli, relatively frequent mitotic figures, and cytoplasmic vacuoles in mesothelial cells may be the cause of overdiagnosis [33] (Figs. 1.24, 1.25 and 1.26). There are several well-known conditions causing atypia in mesothelial cells (Table 1.3), [5, 8, 27, 29] so that clinical information is important. Morphologic features should be interpreted cautiously in order to avoid overdiagnosing or underdiagnosing serous effusions, and when needed, immunocytochemistry is of great help in differentiating reactive atypical mesothelial cells from carcinoma cells (see Appendix). Positive mesothelial markers support the mesothelial origin of the cells in

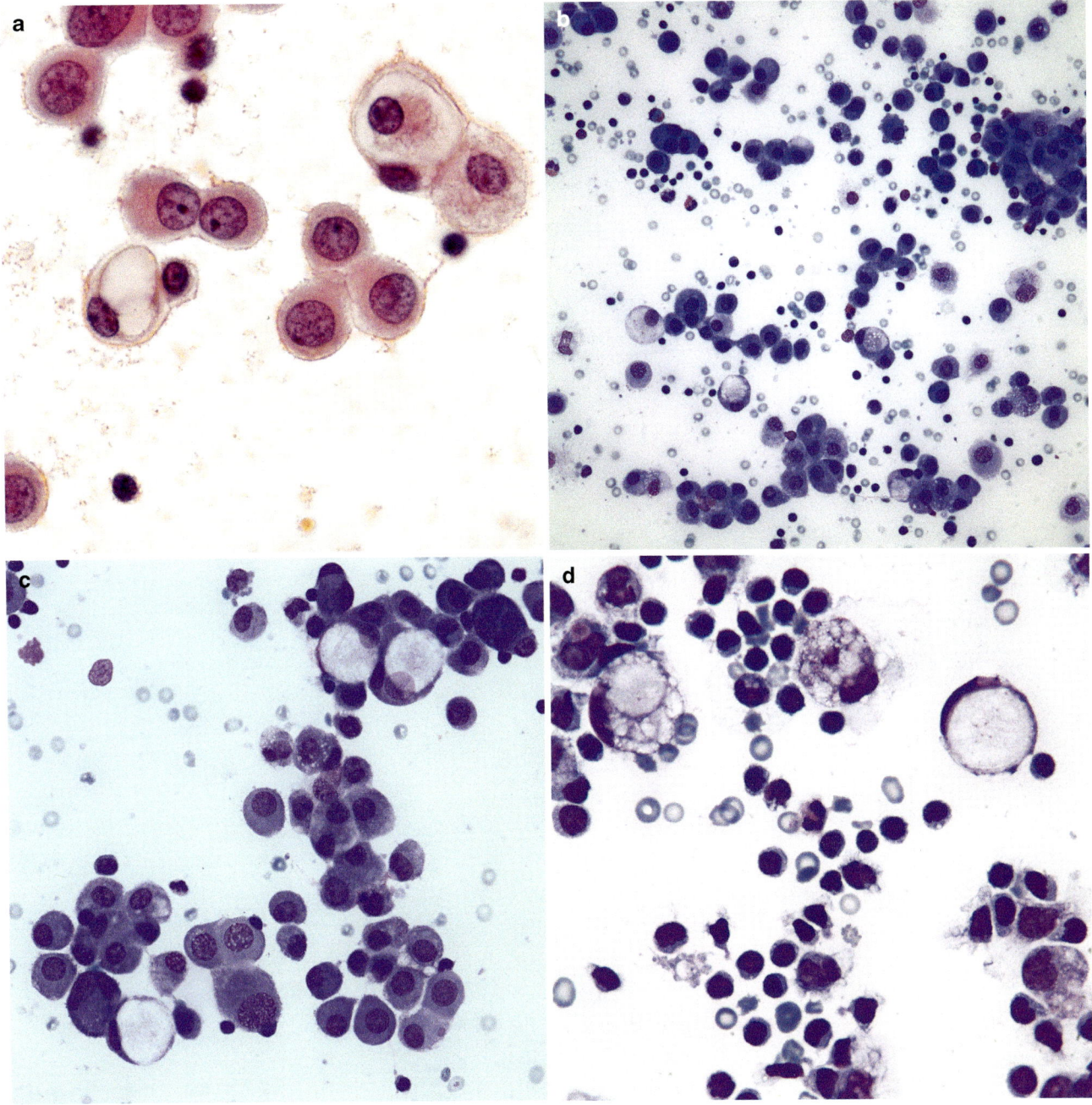

**Fig. 1.13** (**a**, **b**) Degenerative/hydropic vacuoles in mesothelial cells; (**c**) vacuoles overlapping the mesothelial nuclei; (**d**) degenerative vacuoles in macrophages; (**a**) PAP, (**b–d**) MGG

question. However, negative staining for nonmesothelial markers is even more useful, as it confirms that there are no foreign cells in the effusion [32–36].

## Macrophages

Macrophages are present in most effusions. Their size is approximately equal to the size of mesothelial cells but may be variable. They are observed as single cells, sometimes forming loose groups. Their nuclei are usually eccentric and show folding and grooves. The chromatin is fine, and nucleoli are inconspicuous (Fig. 1.27a). Macrophages have a pale, ill-defined, vacuolated cytoplasm, sometimes with large vacuoles causing a signet ring cell-like appearance [1, 8] (Figs. 1.13d and 1.27b). Nuclear features which are not compatible with malignancy and immunocytochemistry help in distinguishing macrophages from carcinoma cells. Immunocytochemically, macrophages do not express epithelial markers and stain positive for CD68 [8].

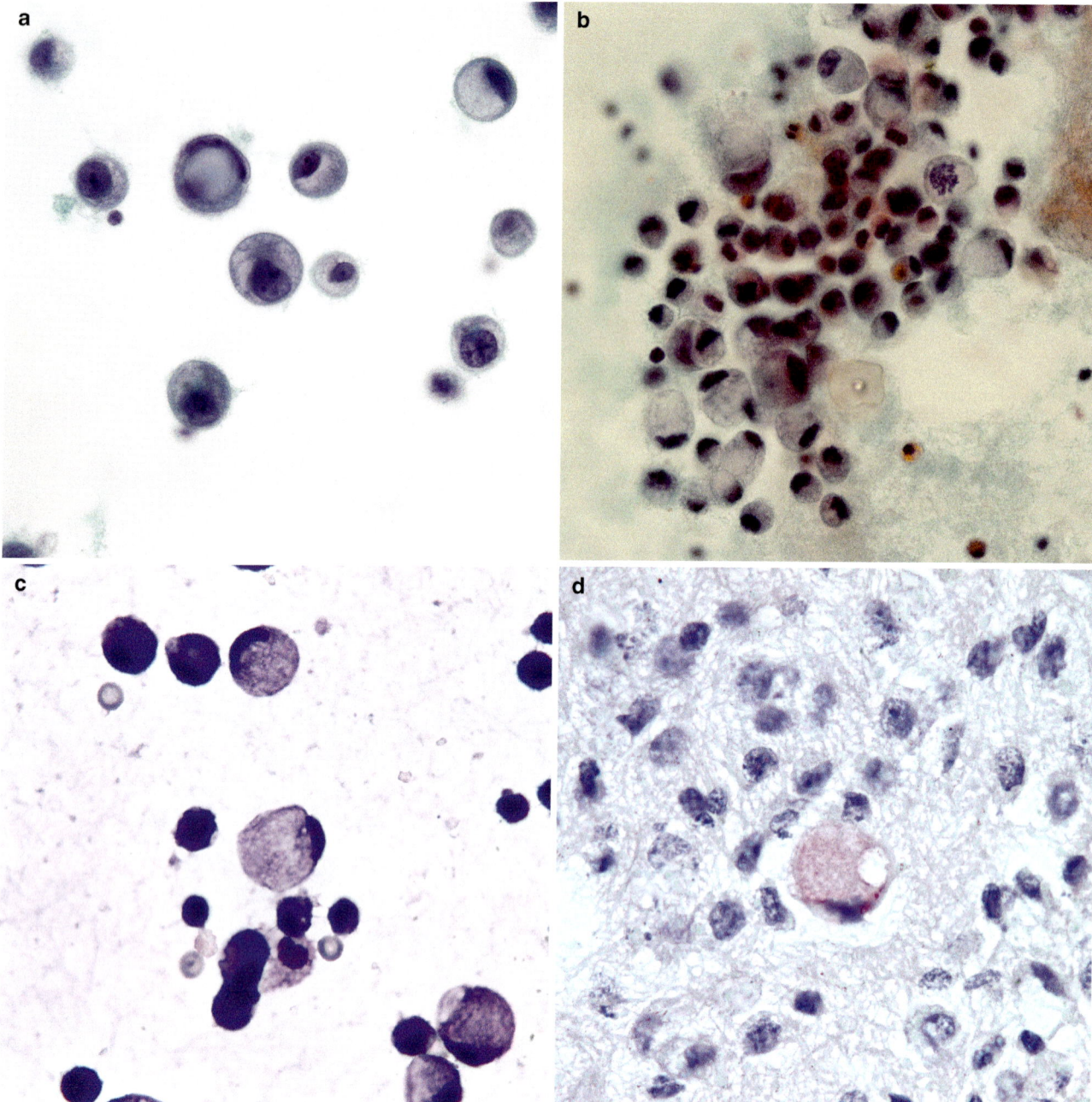

**Fig. 1.14** (**a**) The nuclei of malignant cells are indented by secretory vacuoles; (**b**) signet ring cells displaying hyperchromasia, coarse chromatin, irregular nuclear contours, and mitosis; (**c**) the outer border of the nucleus forming an angle with the outer border of the cytoplasm in a signet ring cell; (**d**) malignant cells showing mucin in their cytoplasm; (**e, f**) signet ring cells containing abundant mucin, their cytoplasm does not appear crystal clear; (**a, b, e**) PAP, (**c, f**) MGG, (**d**) mucicarmine

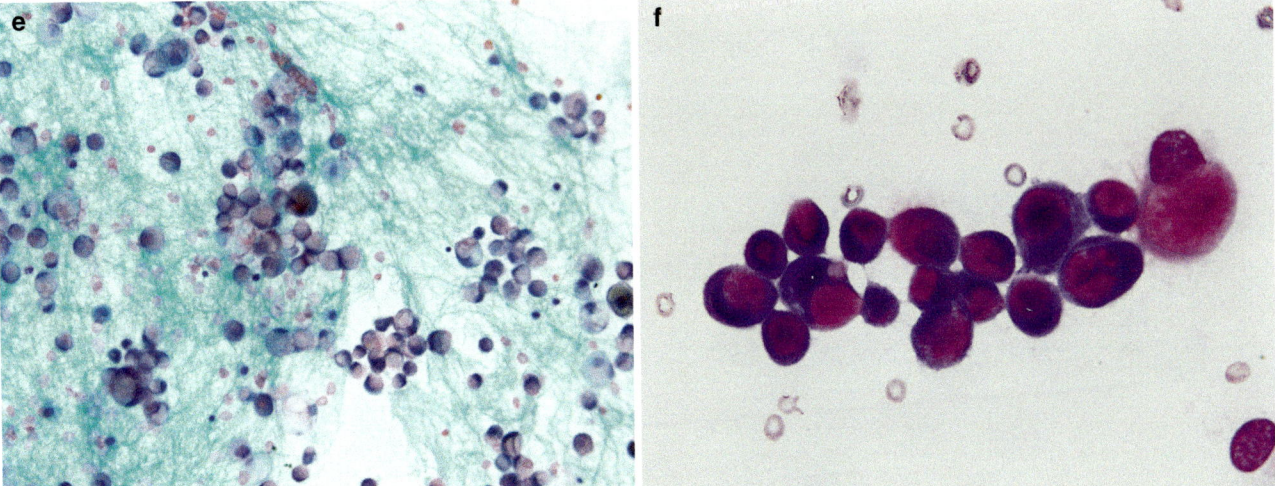

**Fig. 1.14** (continued)

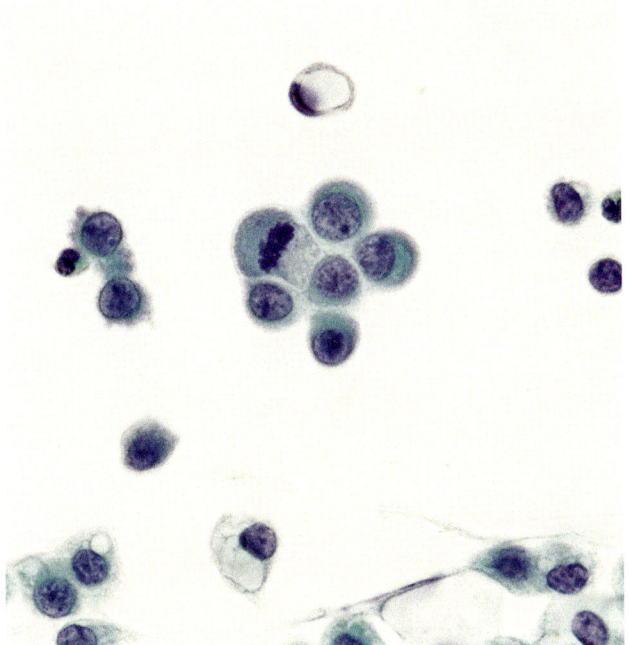

**Fig. 1.15** Mitotic figure in a mesothelial cell; PAP

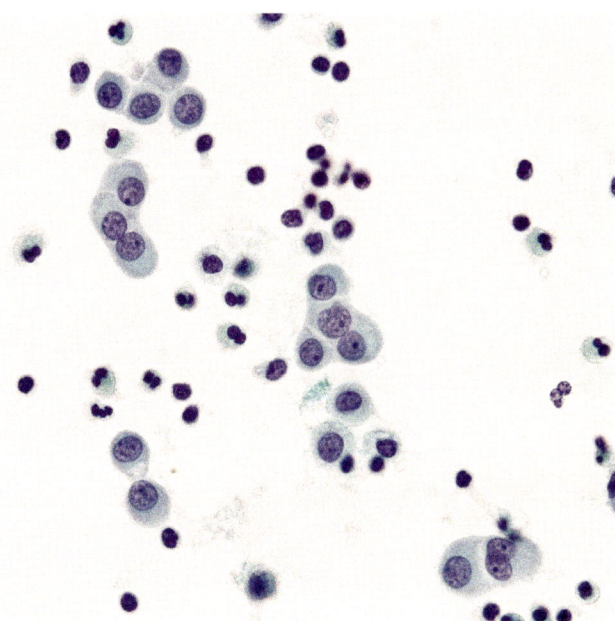

**Fig. 1.16** Slit-like spaces—"windows"—between adjacent mesothelial cells; PAP

It may be difficult to distinguish macrophages from mesothelial cells (Fig. 1.28). However, the former have nuclei that are more oval to elongated, sometimes bean-shaped. Phagocytized debris may be present in their cytoplasm. The cytoplasm does not show an endoplasmic/ectoplasmic demarcation. Macrophages may form groups but without molding, cell-in-cell appearance, windows, or knobby contours. In some effusions they may be numerous, with few accompanying mesothelial cells, and if they show atypical features, immunostains may be necessary to iden-

tify their origin. Adding CD68, calretinin and pan-cytokeratin to the panel will resolve the potential confusion, as macrophages do not stain for mesothelial or epithelial markers [5, 8].

The presence of macrophages with phagocytized erythrocytes and hemosiderin pigment is a sign of recent and old hemorrhage, respectively (Fig. 1.29). Lipid vacuoles may be the indicator of tissue destruction caused by malignancy, pancreatitis, etc. Melanin pigment in macrophages may be seen in patients with malignant melanoma [5].

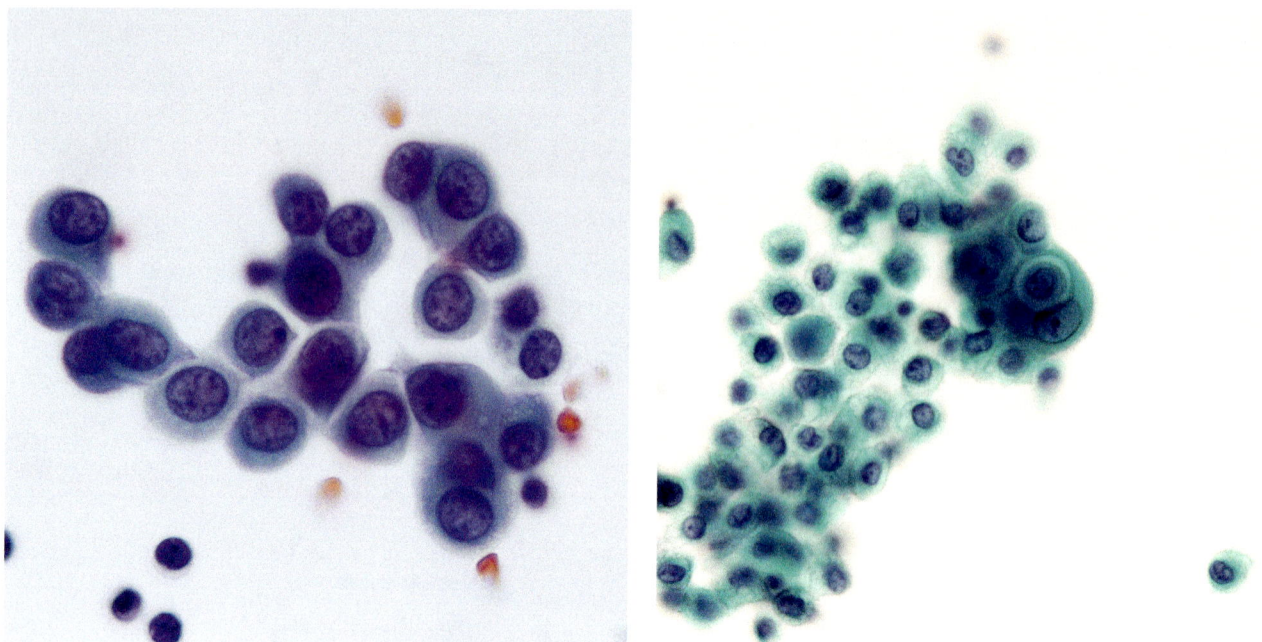

**Fig. 1.17** "Windows" between cells in a mesothelial group; PAP

**Fig. 1.19** Cell-in-cell appearance in a mesothelial group; PAP

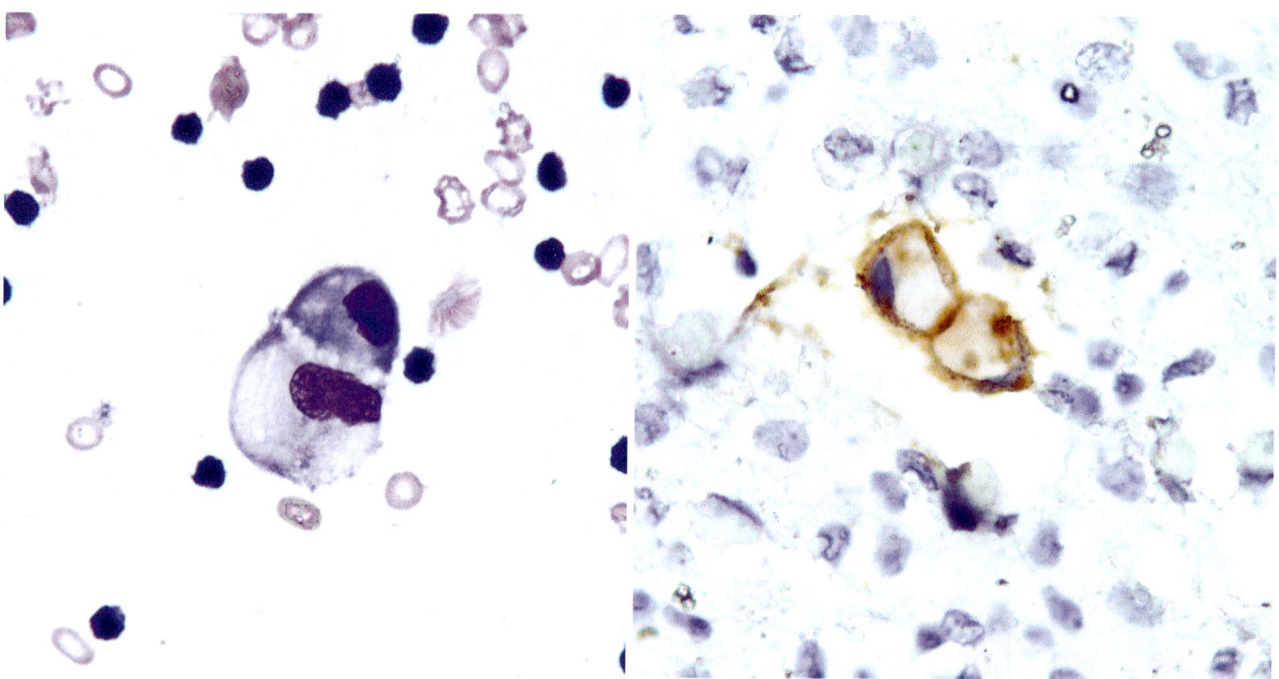

**Fig. 1.18** Slit-like space between two adenocarcinoma cells looking like "windows" of the mesothelial cells, MGG. *Inset*: Ber-EP4 positivity in these carcinoma cells

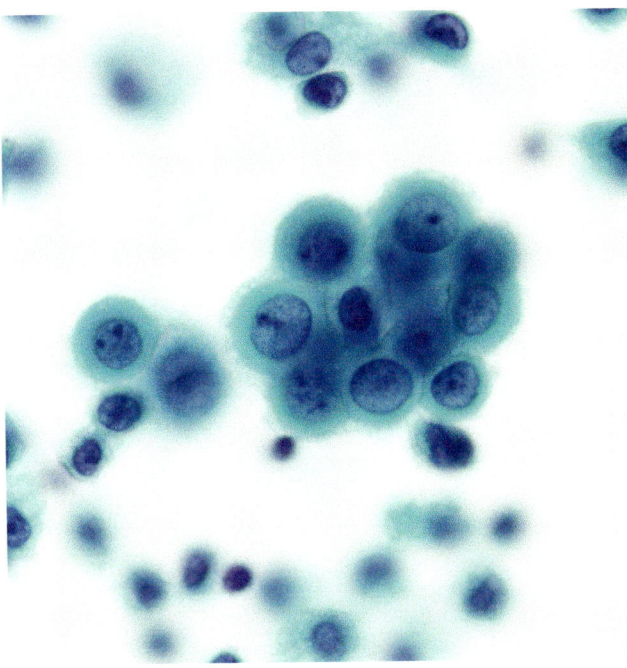

**Fig. 1.20** Knobby contours of mesothelial clusters; PAP

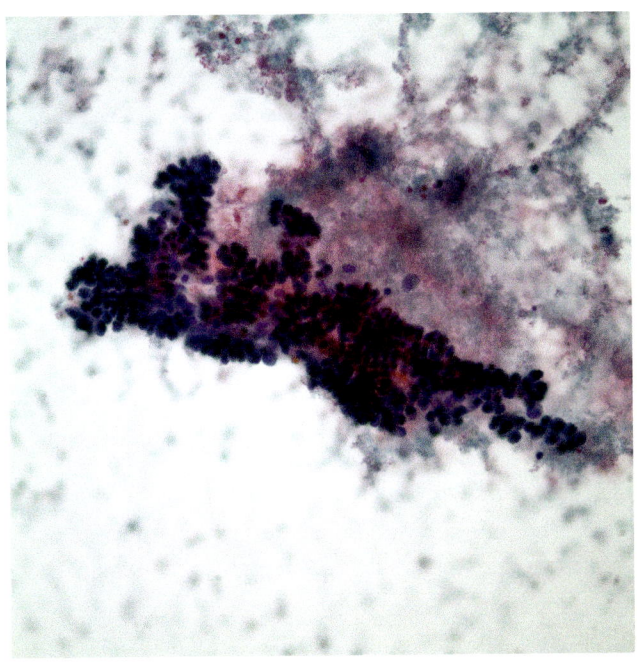

**Fig. 1.22** Reactive mesothelial cells forming papillary structures; PAP

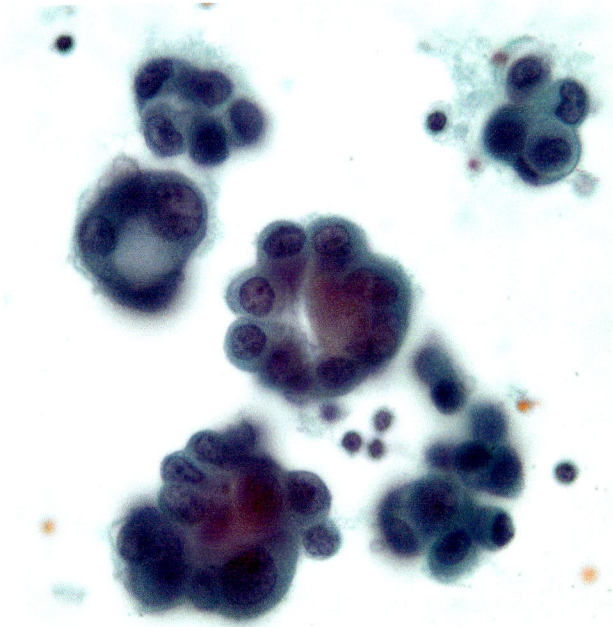

**Fig. 1.21** Adenocarcinoma displaying groups with knobby contours; PAP

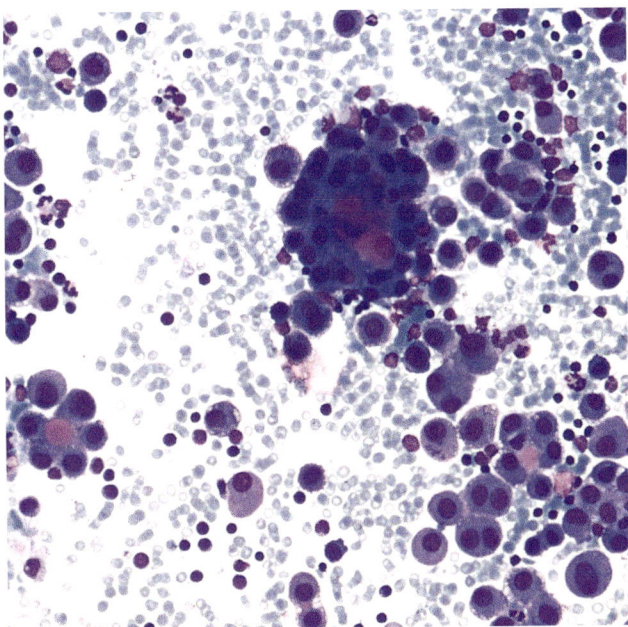

**Fig. 1.23** Collagen cores in mesothelial cell clusters; MGG

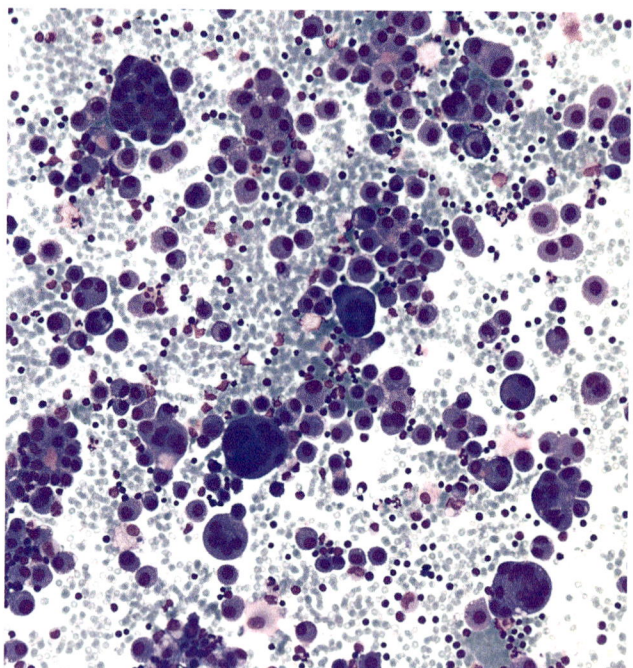

**Fig. 1.24** Multinucleation and cluster formation in a reactive mesothelial proliferation; MGG

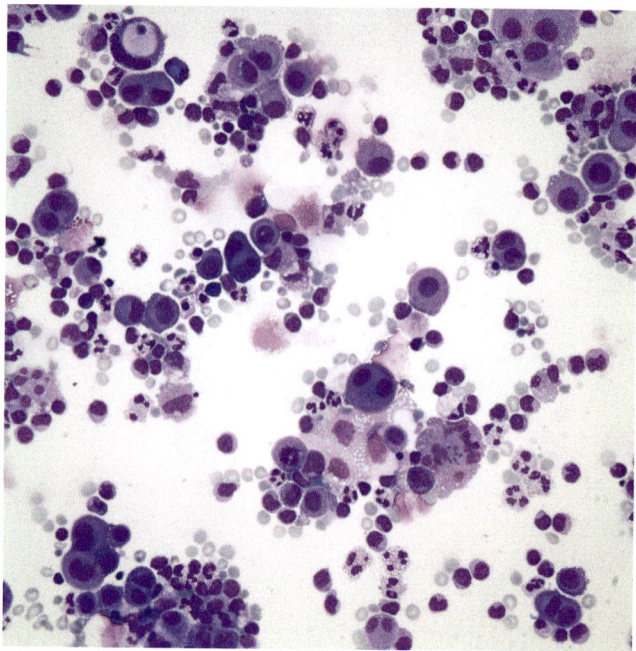

**Fig. 1.26** Mitotic figures, multinucleation, and cytoplasmic vacuoles in reactive mesothelial cells; MGG

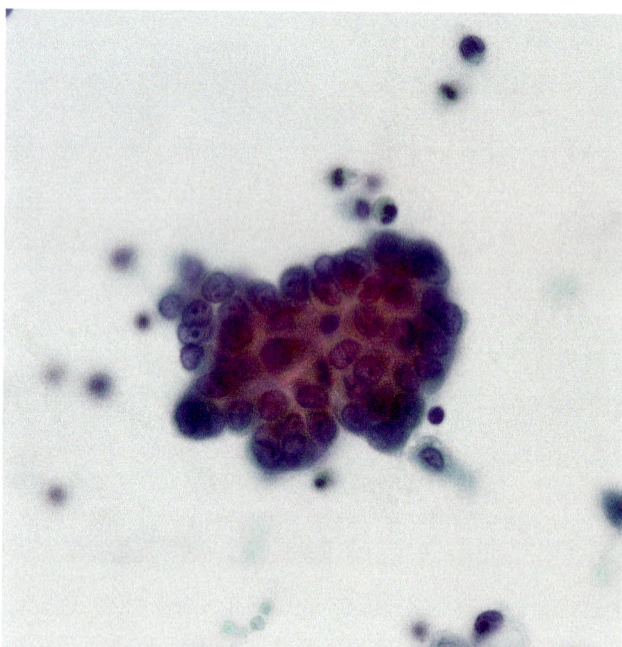

**Fig. 1.25** Cluster formation, high N/C ratio, distinct nucleoli, and some degree of hyperchromasia in a reactive mesothelial proliferation; PAP

**Table 1.3** Disorders that may cause reactive atypia in mesothelial cells

| Causes of atypia in reactive mesothelial proliferations |
| --- |
| Heart failure |
| Liver disease/cirrhosis, hepatitis |
| Renal failure/uremia |
| Pulmonary embolism/infarction |
| Infections |
| Pancreatitis |
| Peritoneal dialysis |
| Collagen vascular diseases |
| Radiation |
| Asbestos |

## Lymphocytes

Lymphocytes are almost always present in effusions. They may be few or many, and their presence is a nonspecific finding. A wide range of etiologies is described for lymphocytosis in effusions [3, 9] (Table 1.4). Any type of reactive, infectious, or neoplastic effusion may contain lymphocytes. In most of these conditions, plasma cells may accompany lymphocytes. In long-standing fluids, such as a persistent

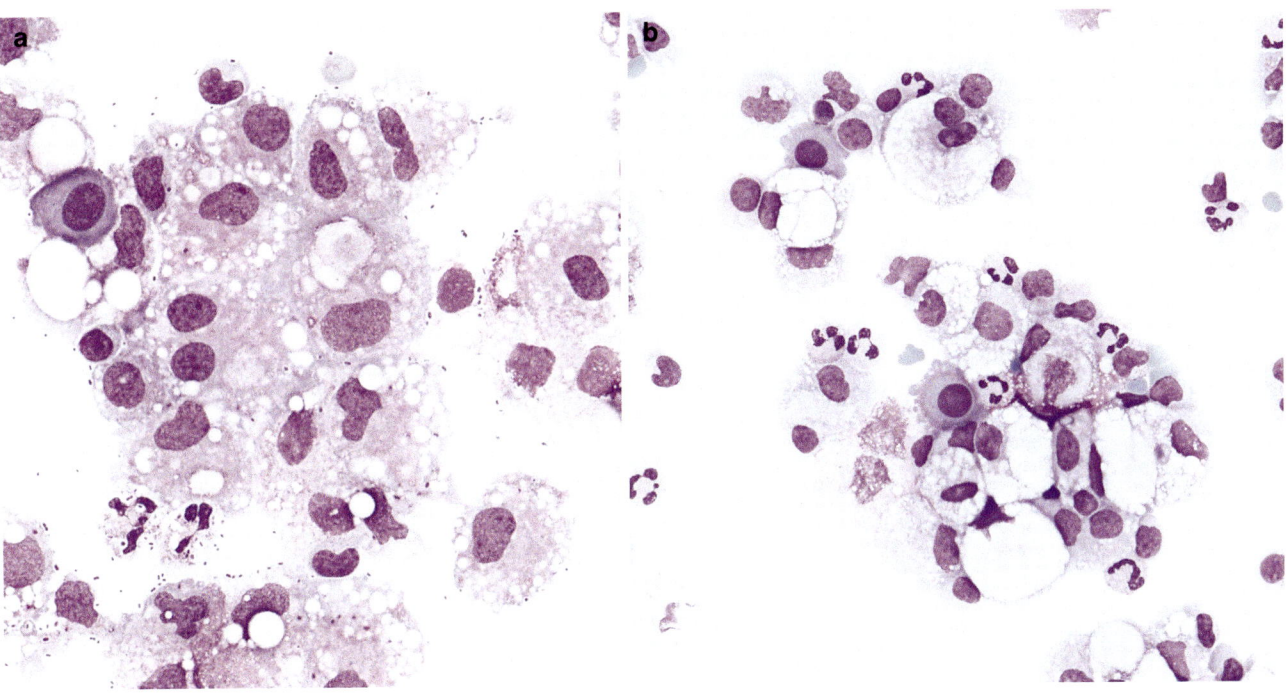

**Fig. 1.27**  (**a, b**) Macrophages with oval- or bean-shaped nuclei, fine chromatin, inconspicuous nucleoli, and vacuolated cytoplasm admixed with mesothelial cells; MGG

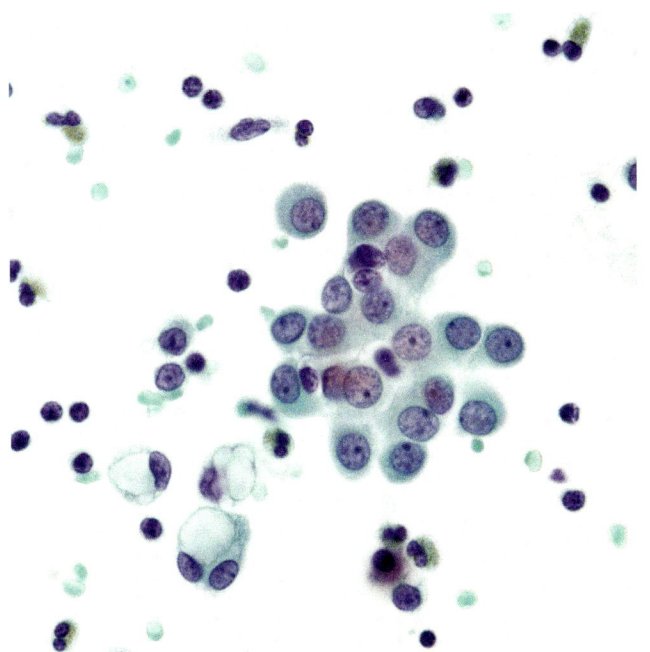

**Fig. 1.28**  Macrophages at the left lower corner and a group of mesothelial cells in the center; PAP

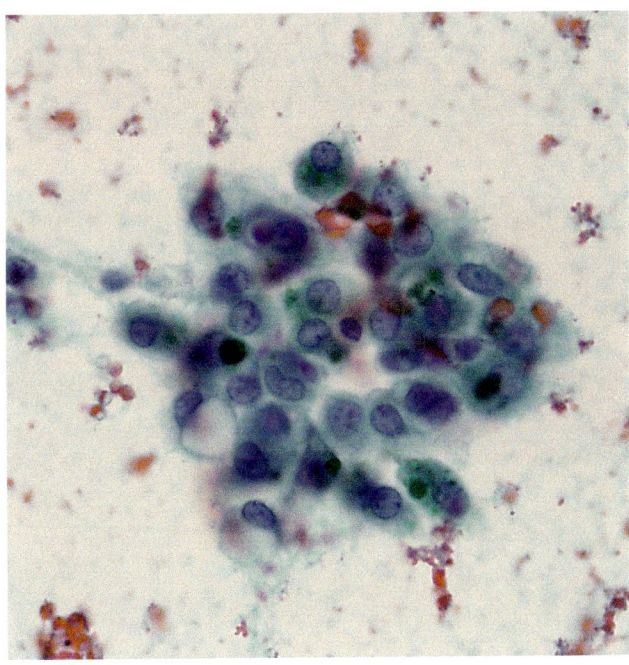

**Fig. 1.29**  Phagocytized hemosiderin pigment in the cytoplasm of macrophages as a sign of old hemorrhage; PAP

**Table 1.4** Common causes of effusions according to the predominant inflammatory cell type

| Predominant cell type | Underlying disease |
|---|---|
| Lymphocytes | Congestive heart failure |
| | Chronic renal failure, uremia |
| | Cirrhosis of the liver |
| | Infections |
| |    Tuberculosis |
| |    Viral |
| | Collagen vascular diseases |
| | Acute lung rejection |
| | Malignancy |
| Neutrophils | Purulent infection, empyema |
| | Embolism and infarction |
| | Gastrointestinal rupture |
| | Collagen vascular diseases |
| Eosinophils | Idiopathic |
| | Air introduction |
| | Infections |
| |    Parasitic |
| |    Fungal |
| | Embolism and infarction |
| | Hypersensitivity (asthma, drug reaction, peritoneal dialysis, etc.) |
| | Asbestosis |
| | Malignancy |

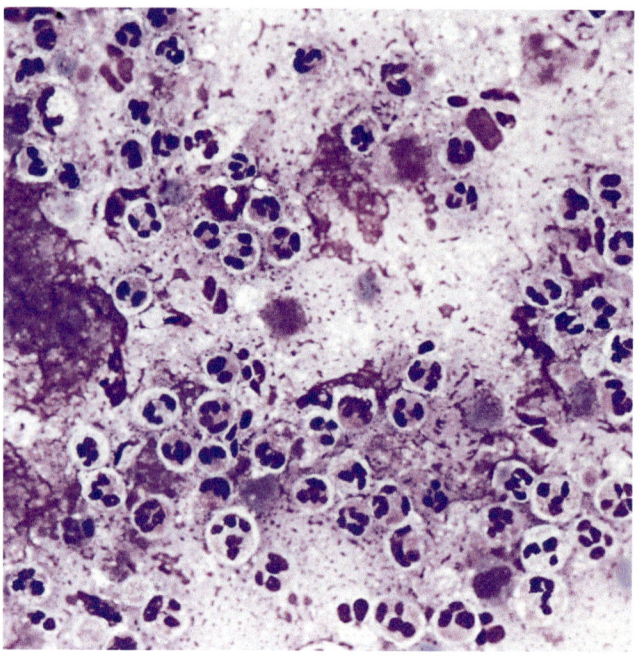

**Fig. 1.31** Neutrophils as the dominating cell type in an effusion; MGG

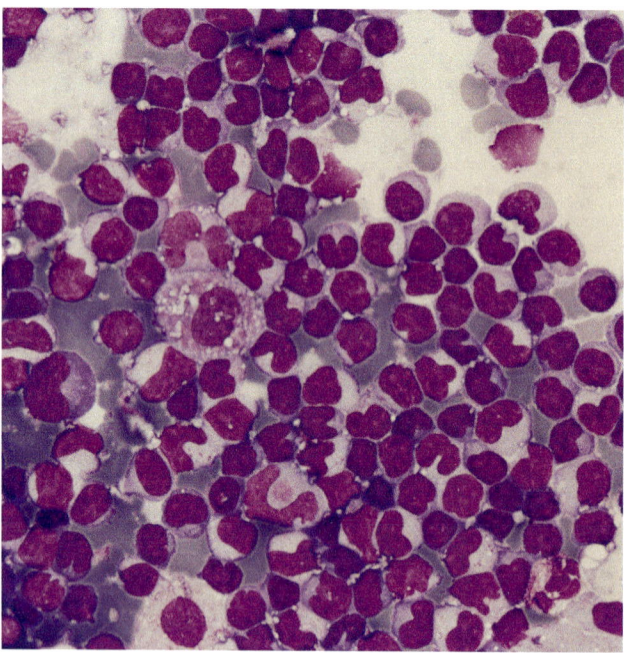

**Fig. 1.30** Benign lymphocytic effusion containing a polymorphic population; MGG

effusion due to heart failure, the number of lymphocytes increases [5].

A polymorphic population showing different levels of maturation is the characteristic of benign lymphocytic effusions (Fig. 1.30). However, one should not rely on this feature in differentiating lymphomas from reactive conditions, since few lymphoma cells admixed with reactive lymphocytes, or the lymphoma itself, if composed of polymorphic cells, may mimic benign lymphocytosis. If the clinical and morphologic findings are suspicious for lymphoma, ancillary tests are needed for correct diagnosis [37].

The diagnosis of tuberculosis should be borne in mind within the category of benign lymphocytic effusions. It is the most common cause of lymphocyte-rich pleural effusions. Mesothelial cells are few in tuberculous effusions, and as many as 90% of the cells are lymphocytes [3, 38].

## Neutrophils

It is possible to find a few neutrophils in any effusion. The presence of neutrophils is considered significant when their count exceeds 25% (Fig. 1.31). Etiologic factors are variable, with parapneumonic effusion, empyema, embolism/infarction, and pancreatitis being the most common causes (Table 1.4). Neutrophils are rarely seen in malignant effusions unless there is a superimposed infection [3, 5, 39].

Indeed, any type of injury causing exudates attracts neutrophils at the acute phase. One example is the early tuberculous effusion. The mononuclear cells—macrophages and lymphocytes—reach the serous cavity within 72 h, and as the effusion becomes older, the number of lymphocytes increases. Transudates practically never contain neutrophils [3, 6].

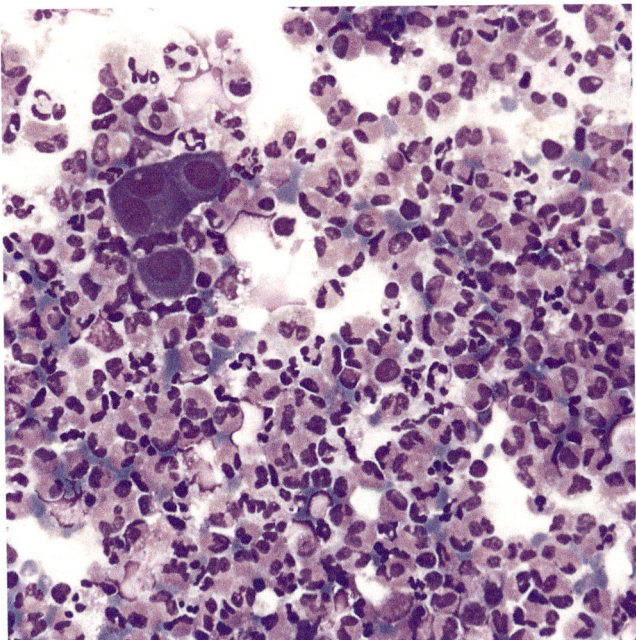

**Fig. 1.32** A small group of mesothelial cells with many eosinophils in the background; MGG

## Eosinophils

Eosinophilia in an effusion is defined by an eosinophil count of more than 10% (Fig. 1.32). Eosinophilic effusions are most common in the pleural cavity. Even though variable etiologies attract eosinophils to the serous cavities, the most common causes are pneumothorax, infections, asbestosis, and hypersensitivity states such as asthma and drug reactions [3, 9, 40]. One-third of the cases are idiopathic (Table 1.4).

Air introduction into the pleural cavity causes eosinophilia, probably as an allergic reaction to particles in the air (5). It has been suggested that as thoracocentesis introduces air into the pleural cavity, the number of eosinophils in an effusion increases with repeated procedures. However, there are reports in the literature which disagree with this statement, arguing that no significant change occurs in the number of eosinophils after thoracocentesis and that there is no relationship between eosinophilia and the number of procedures [41, 42].

About 20% of eosinophilic effusions are due to a malignant neoplasm. The previous belief that eosinophilia significantly reduces the risk of malignancy has been disproved by some studies [42]. However, the higher the percentage of eosinophils in an effusion (>40%), the lower the likelihood of malignancy. The presence of eosinophilia makes tuberculosis very unlikely as an etiologic factor [43]. Most of the cases with very high eosinophil numbers are idiopathic [41].

Charcot-Leyden crystals may develop in eosinophilic effusions. They are more common if the preparation is delayed and specimens are stored in the refrigerator [44].

## Benign Cells and Noncellular Material Rarely Found in Effusions/Pitfalls in Cytological Diagnosis

### Megakaryocytes/Bone Marrow Cells

The presence of megakaryocytes in serous effusions is a very rare condition. In a series of 4844 pleural and 3279 peritoneal effusions, only five specimens were found to contain megakaryocytes, all from patients with myeloproliferative disease or diffuse neoplastic involvement of the bone marrow [45] (Fig. 1.33a, b). The presence of megakaryocytes is best explained by extramedullary hematopoiesis on the serous membranes. Myeloproliferative diseases, hemolytic anemias, hereditary spherocytosis, and Gaucher disease have been reported to cause pulmonary/pleural extramedullary hematopoiesis [46]. Patients with space-occupying lesions in the bone marrow, such as extensive metastatic involvement, may develop leukoerythroblastosis, a condition described as the presence of immature cells of the erythrocytic and granulocytic series in the circulation. In the presence of peripheral blood in serous fluids, these specimens may also contain immature hematopoietic cells.

Megakaryocytes should be differentiated from malignant cells. They are huge cells with large multilobed nuclei, indistinct nucleoli, and abundant cytoplasm. Sometimes smaller forms are observed with high N/C ratios and unilobed nuclei which may mimic carcinoma cells more closely (Fig. 1.33c, d). They may present as anucleated cytoplasmic masses as well. Immune markers such as factor VIII, CD61, and CD41 are useful in their identification. Familiarity with the morphology of bone marrow elements and recognizing immature hematopoietic cells in the background are important [29, 45, 47]. The presence of megakaryocytes should be reported, as it is almost always an indirect sign of a malignant tumor, either hematopoietic or carcinomatous, with bone marrow involvement [45].

### Benign ciliated Epithelial Cells/Ciliary Tufts

Ciliated columnar cells or their detached ciliated apical portion (ciliary tufts) may be desquamated into peritoneal fluids (Fig. 1.34a, b). The origin of ciliated cells is the fallopian tube, usually in the second half of the cycle (cyclic shedding). They may otherwise originate from endosalpingiosis or benign ovarian serous tumors [32, 48]. They are more common in peritoneal washings than in effusions. Detached

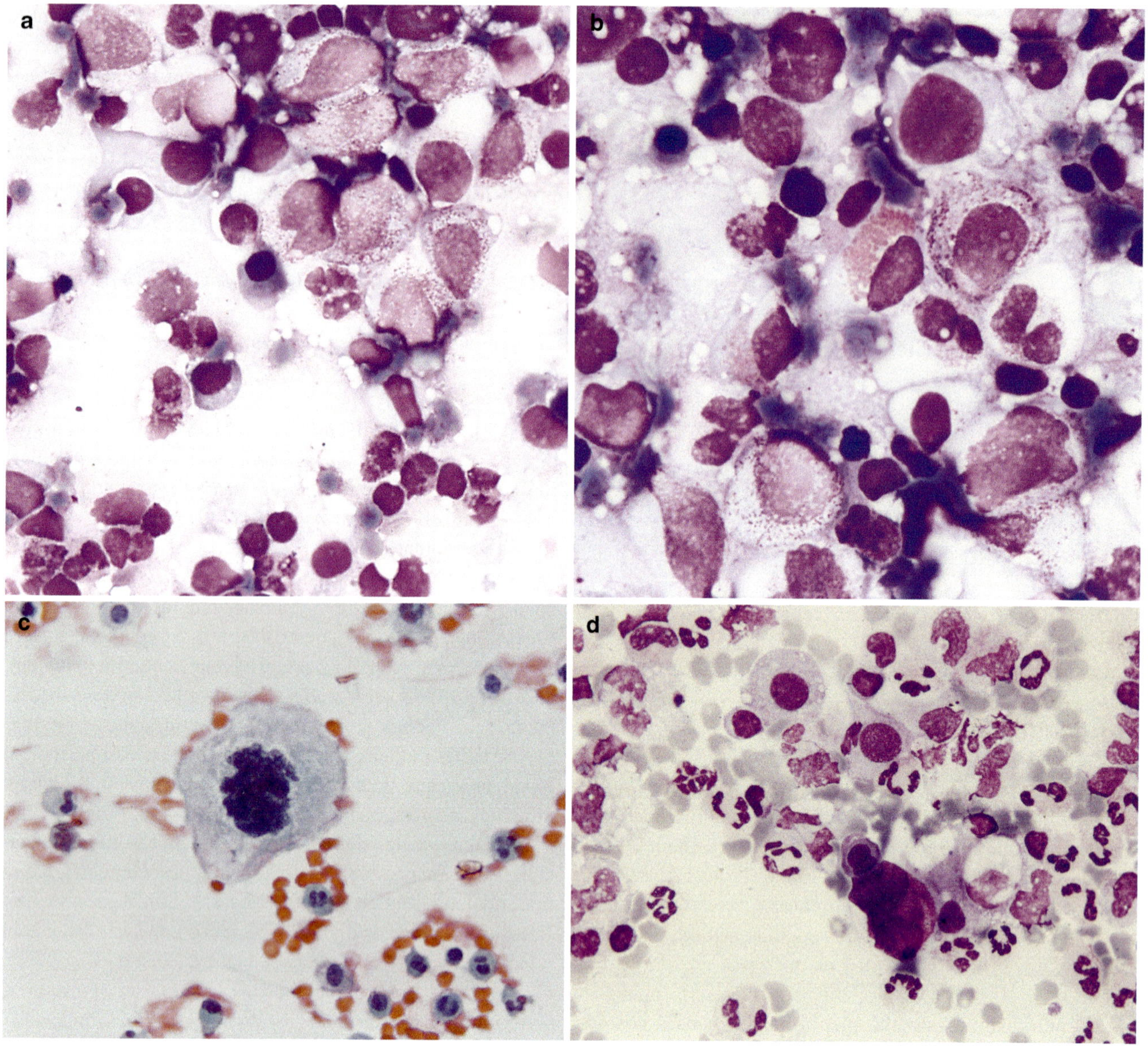

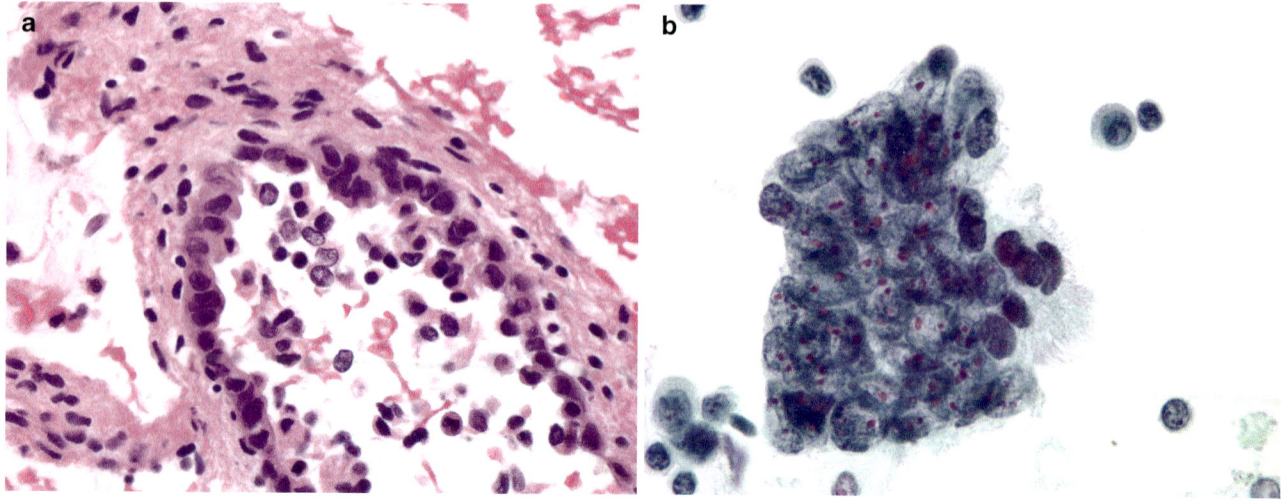

**Fig. 1.33** (**a**, **b**) Bone marrow elements—erythroid and myeloid precursors—in an effusion from a patient with widespread metastases, (**c**, **d**) megakaryocytes in the ascitic fluid of a patient with primary myelofibrosis; (**a**, **b**, **d**) MGG, (**c**) PAP

**Fig. 1.34** (**a**, **b**) Benign ciliated cells originating from the fallopian tube desquamating into the peritoneal fluid; (**a**) H&E, (**b**) PAP

ciliary tufts may be mistaken to be parasites when examined in wet preparations because of their appearance and motility, but they are generally correctly identified in fixed specimens prepared for cytological examination [49, 50]. Benign- ciliated cells have bland oval nuclei with finely dispersed chromatin and a uniform nuclear membrane [32, 48, 50]. These cells stain for epithelial immune markers such as Ber-EP4 and should not be misdiagnosed as carcinoma cells as a result of this fact [51].

Not only endosalpingiosis but also endometriosis may mimic metastatic tumors such as low-grade serous carcinoma. The presence of cilia and lack of single atypical cells or marked nuclear atypia are features favoring a benign process [52]. However, cilia or cilia-like structures are rarely identified on cells from ovarian borderline serous tumors and even more rarely on mesothelial cells [53].

## Psammoma Bodies

Psammoma bodies are occasionally encountered in serous effusions. They are commonly associated with malignant tumors, especially ovarian carcinoma (Fig. 1.35), but their presence is not diagnostic of malignancy. Psammoma bodies were present in 3.7% of cases in a series of 3335 effusions [54]. In this series, most of the effusions with psammoma bodies (91%) were peritoneal, 8.1% were pleural, and only one case was pericardial. All pleural and pericardial effusions were malignant, consisting of carcinomas of the thyroid, lung, and ovary. However, 36.6% of peritoneal effusions

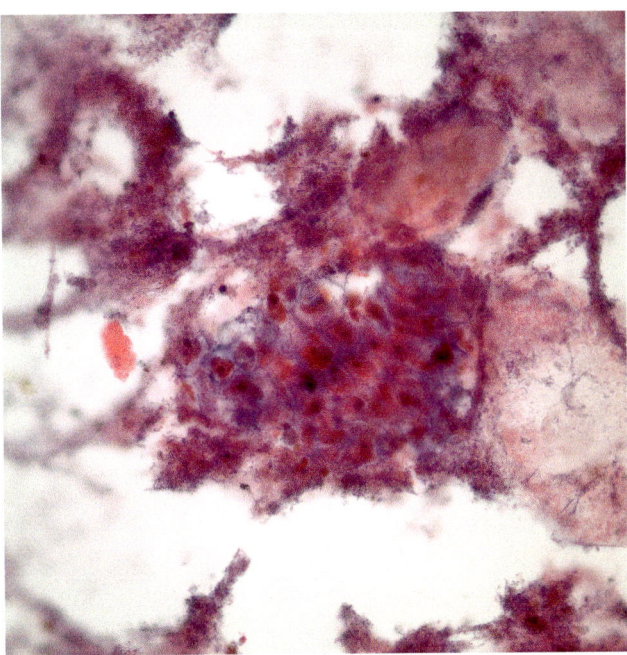

**Fig. 1.36** Fecal matter as a contaminant in a peritoneal effusion; PAP

containing psammoma bodies were associated with benign disorders, such as papillary mesothelial hyperplasia, endosalpingiosis, endometriosis, and ovarian cystadenoma/ cystadenofibroma. Detecting psammoma bodies in serous cavities other than the peritoneum is a strong indicator of malignancy, but in peritoneal effusions the associated cellular features should be carefully examined before malignancy is suspected [5, 54].

## Contaminants

Skin and appendages, fibroadipose tissue, muscle, cartilage, hepatocytes, lung and gut tissue, and fecal matter (Fig. 1.36) may be seen in serous effusions, generally as pickups of the needle. Rarely, they represent fistulas [5, 29].

## Cytologic Features of Benign Conditions in Effusions

### Heart Failure

Patients with heart failure often develop pleural effusions. Pericardial effusion and peritoneal effusion may also occur in heart failure. Pleural effusions are usually bilateral. When unilateral, they are commonly right-sided for unknown reasons. Effusions caused by heart failure are typically transudates and contain mesothelial cells, lymphocytes, and sometimes macrophages. In long-standing effusions,

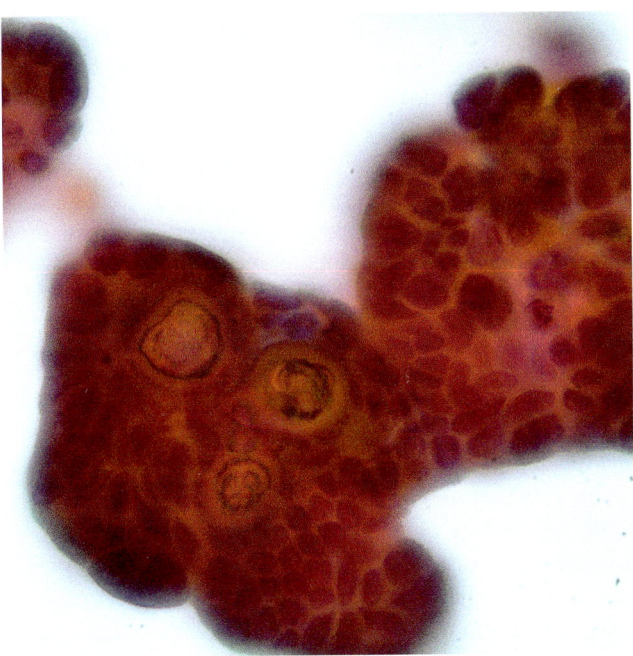

**Fig. 1.35** Psammoma bodies in serous carcinoma of the ovary; PAP

hemosiderin-laden macrophages may appear. Effusions due to heart failure rarely cause a diagnostic dilemma on cytological examination [55, 56].

## Cirrhosis

Effusions are usually the result of hypoalbuminemia in cirrhosis and are transudates. Reactive changes, sometimes with nuclear atypia, may be seen [5]. Many macrophages are usually encountered. Lymphocytes are present in the background. Bacterial peritonitis may develop in long-standing ascites, resulting in effusions rich in neutrophils [2, 8].

## Renal Failure/Uremia

Uremic effusions are usually hemorrhagic and are exudates rich in lymphocytes. Pericardial effusions are the most common, but pleural and peritoneal effusions may also develop. Reactive mesothelial atypia is frequent in uremic effusions. Erythrophagocytosis and hemosiderin may be seen in macrophages [57].

Dialysis may result in the formation of peritoneal, pleural, and pericardial effusions. Lymphocytes, occasionally eosinophils, predominate. Reactive atypia may be seen in mesothelial cells. Peritonitis may complicate dialysis [58–60].

## Pancreatitis

Peritoneal and pleural effusions are well-recognized complications of pancreatitis. Amylase level is high in these effusions. In most cases, effusions are the result of chronic pancreatitis. Acute pancreatitis causes pleural effusion, and the presence of pleural effusion is a poor prognostic sign for patients suffering from this disease [61, 62]. Cytological examination reveals reactive mesothelial cells and inflammatory cells, the latter consisting mainly of neutrophils and macrophages with lipid and/or bile phagocytosis, as well as proteinaceous debris in the background. Mesothelial cells may show atypical features.

## Embolism/Infarction

Pulmonary embolism is one of the most common causes of pleural effusion. It is estimated that each year 300,000–500,000 patients develop pleural effusions secondary to pulmonary embolism in the USA [63]. The effusion is almost always exudative and bloody. Clinically, the D-dimer test supports the diagnosis, and computed tomographic angiogram is used to show the emboli in the pulmonary arteries. The two complications of pleural effusion in patients with

pulmonary embolism are hemothorax and pleural infection [53]. In the early phases of the effusion, neutrophils predominate but are not many in number unless the fluid is infected. Subsequently, lymphocytes, macrophages, and eosinophils replace the neutrophils, and hemosiderin-laden macrophages appear [2]. The mesothelial cells in the effusion may show atypical features mimicking metastatic carcinoma. Caution is warranted in diagnosing malignancy when there is clinical evidence of pulmonary embolism. Ancillary tests are needed in equivocal cases.

## Tuberculosis

Tuberculous pleuritis should be considered in any patient with an exudative pleural effusion rich in lymphocytes. The incidence of pulmonary tuberculosis in the USA has been shown to decrease steadily through a 10-year period (1993–2003), while the ratio of pleural to pulmonary tuberculosis has remained stable [64]. Tuberculosis may not be a frequently encountered cause of pleural effusions in western countries. However, in developing countries where the disease is endemic, it is the most common cause of exudative pleural effusions. The incidence of tuberculous pleuritis among tuberculosis patients varies geographically and ranges from 4% in the USA to 10% in Spain and up to 20–30% in developing countries [65, 66].

In a series of 132 patients with pleural tuberculosis, adenosine deaminase (ADA) activity was the most sensitive test, and detecting antibodies against mycobacterium antigens was the most specific test for the diagnosis. The sensitivity of culture was 42% [67]. Smears for bacteria are virtually always negative in tuberculous effusions [15]. In a recent review, it has been shown that the ability of ADA to rule-in or rule-out tuberculosis is affected by the prevalence of the disease in that setting. The complementary use of interferon-γ or interleukin-27 increases the efficacy of ADA to rule-in or rule-out tuberculosis, respectively [66]. Due to limitations of conventional tests and the delayed culture results, new tests such as inflammatory and immune response markers, nucleic acid amplification tests, and scoring systems based on a combination of clinical and biological markers are being evaluated. Valdes et al. found in their study that younger age, high levels of TNF-α, LDH, ADA, C-reactive protein, and low levels of CEA were significant predictors in distinguishing tuberculous from malignant pleural effusions [68].

Tuberculosis is characterized by hypercellular lymphocytic effusions which are poor in mesothelial cells. Lymphocytes are of T-cell origin and mainly CD4+ helper cells. In effusions, lymphocytosis was found to be the best predictive factor for the presence of tuberculous infection, whereas the presence of mesothelial cells and eosinophils was shown to be a negative predictor. However, the absence of mesothelial cells is not a constant finding, as occasional

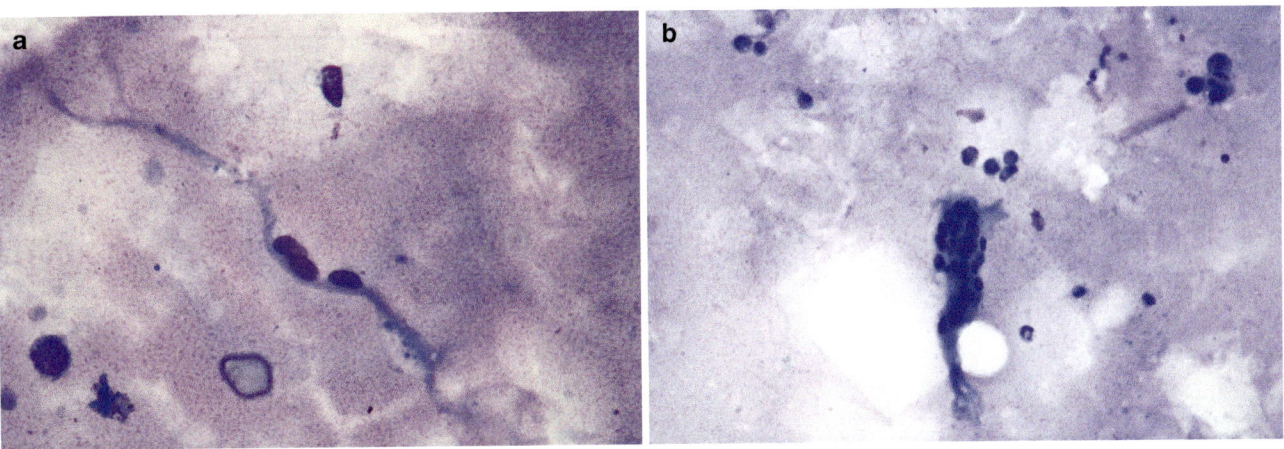

**Fig. 1.37** Slender, elongated cell (**a**) and multinucleated histiocytic giant cell (**b**) in the pleural effusion of a patient with rheumatoid arthritis; (**a, b**) MGG. (Courtesy of Koray Ceyhan, Professor of Pathology, Ankara University Faculty of Medicine, Ankara, Turkey)

cases present with many mesothelial cells, the majority of which are from HIV+ patients [69, 70]. A hypercellular specimen containing many lymphocytes (>50%) and few mesothelial cells (<10%) is a characteristic of tuberculosis. If more than 10% of the cells are mesothelial in an effusion from an HIV patient, tuberculosis is virtually excluded [69].

The differential diagnosis includes lymphoma, especially small lymphocytic lymphoma (SLL)/chronic lymphocytic leukemia (CLL). The cells of SLL/CLL are positive for B-cell markers, in contrast to the T-cell predominance of lymphocytes in tuberculous effusions [65].

## Rheumatoid Arthritis

Pleural effusion is an uncommon but well-known manifestation of rheumatoid arthritis. It develops in 2–4% of the patients, more frequently in males, usually in the setting of a previously diagnosed rheumatoid arthritis. Patients are typically older than 35 years with high titers of rheumatoid factor (RF). However, pleural effusion may precede the development of joint manifestations and consequently remains undiagnosed for months [71, 72]. The effusion is an exudate with low glucose level and reduced pH. Among exudative pleural effusions, rheumatoid arthritis-associated effusions constitute 0.6% [72]. In some patients pericardial involvement may additionally occur.

Effusions caused by rheumatoid arthritis have characteristic morphological features, reflecting the histopathological findings in the pleura. The mesothelial lining is replaced by pseudostratified palisading epithelioid histiocytes, multinucleated giant cells, and necrosis which appear like "an opened out rheumatoid nodule exposing its necrotic/fibrinoid content to the pleural cavity." [73] This histiocytic layer may easily detach, and all its three components are seen in the effusion fluid: slender, elongated histiocytes/macrophages, multinucleated giant cells, and an amorphous

granular material in the background [71–73] (Figs. 1.37a, b and 1.38a, b). The fluids are usually devoid of mesothelial cells. The elongated histiocytes with oval nuclei and long and tadpole-like cytoplasmic tails are the typical cells of rheumatoid effusions and are sometimes called "comet cells" [74]. Various transitional forms occur between the elongated histiocytes and the multinucleated giant cells. Both cell types have similar nuclear and cytoplasmic features with regular chromatin, inconspicuous nucleoli, finely granular cytoplasm, and distinct cell borders. Giant cells may contain more than 20 nuclei and are indistinguishable from the giant cells of any other granulomatous inflammation elsewhere in the body. The granular necrotic material may be abundant in the background, dominating the cytological picture. It has a "fluffy" appearance and usually forms aggregates (Fig. 1.38). Neutrophils, lymphocytes, and small mononuclear macrophages may also be present in the effusion [71–73].

## Systemic Lupus Erythematosus (SLE)

Patients with SLE commonly develop pleural and pericardial effusions, affecting nearly one-third of patients. Peritoneal effusions are rare [75]. Effusions are usually exudates and show a normal glucose level, in contrast to rheumatoid effusions. The predominant cell type is either neutrophils or lymphocytes. Nuclear fragmentation and apoptosis are frequent in the background. The characteristic finding is the presence of LE cells, but they are rarely observed and cannot be depended on to make the diagnosis in most cases (Fig. 1.39a).

The LE cell is a neutrophil or a macrophage phagocytizing a round homogeneous basophilic material called hematoxylin body (Fig. 1.39b). Hematoxylin bodies are apoptotic blebs representing the cell death caused by the penetration of anti-DNA antibodies into the cells [76]. Some authors describe LE cells as only neutrophils, not macrophages,

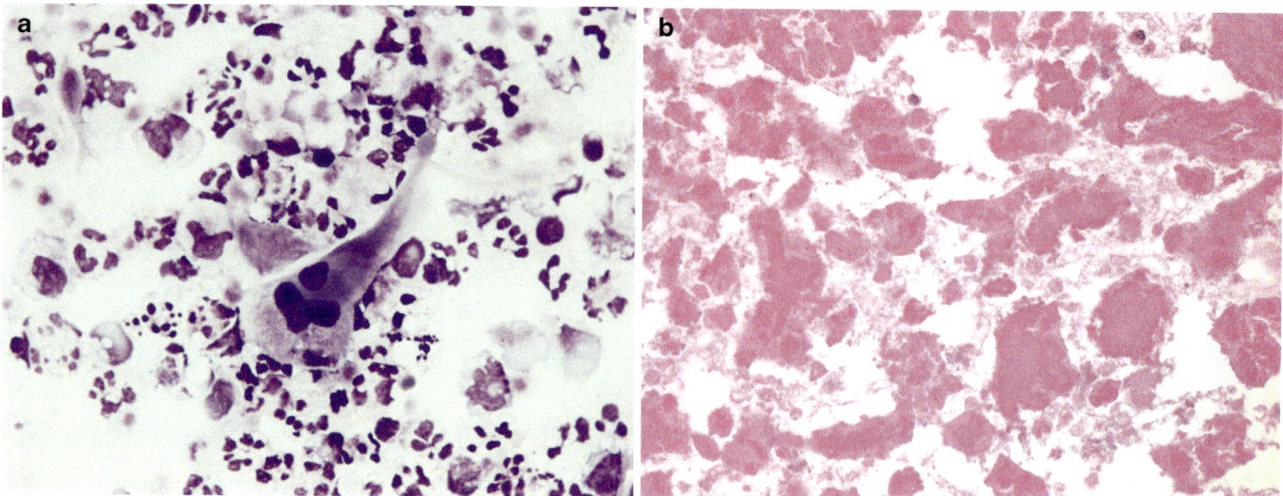

**Fig. 1.38** (**a**) Elongated histiocytic giant cell with a long cytoplasmic tail, and mixed inflammatory cells in the pleural fluid of a patient with rheumatoid arthritis; (**b**) Amorphous "fluffy" material in the background of a rheumatoid effusion; (**a**) MGG, (**b**) H&E

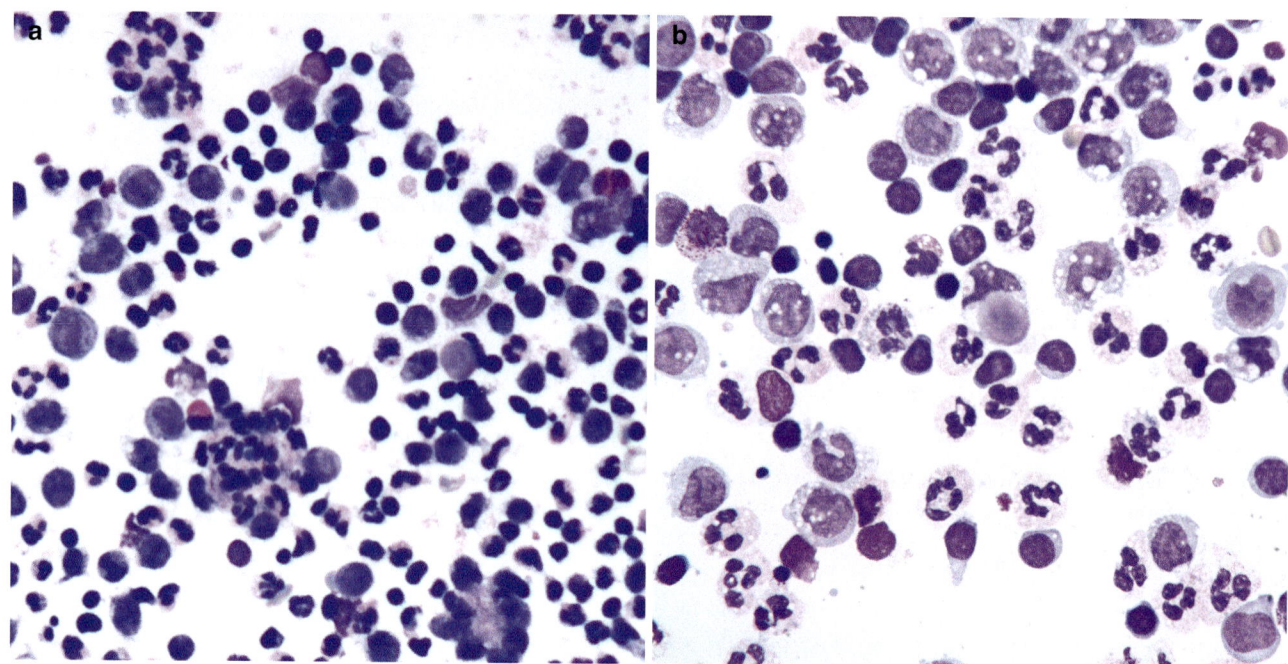

**Fig. 1.39** (**a**) Two LE cells are seen within a mixed population of inflammatory cells; (**b**) LE cell, a macrophage phagocytizing a round homogeneous basophilic material; MGG

which phagocytose the basophilic homogeneous material, and name macrophages with the same phagocytosis as "tart" cells. Described this way, LE cells are said to be highly specific for SLE [77]. Though characteristic, LE cells maybe observed in drug-induced SLE-like syndromes as well. LE cells are more common in fluids that are kept at room temperature and processed with some delay [5, 78].

Pleural effusion may be the first manifestation of SLE. In unexplained effusions from women of childbearing age, or in persistent effusions rich in neutrophils without any response to antibiotics, the presence of LE cells should be carefully searched for [79, 80].

## Radiation and Chemotherapy Effects

The cytopathological diagnosis of effusions obtained from patients with malignant tumors treated by radiation and/or chemotherapy has significant therapeutic and prognostic implications. The atypical changes in mesothelial cells caused by radiation may lead to an erroneous diagnosis. Several nuclear and cytoplasmic changes related to radiation have been reported in the literature: cytomegaly, multinucleation, variation in nuclear size, hyperchromasia, cytoplasmic vacuolization, and the presence of bizarre cells [81–83] (Fig. 1.40a, b). Caution is warranted in the interpretation of

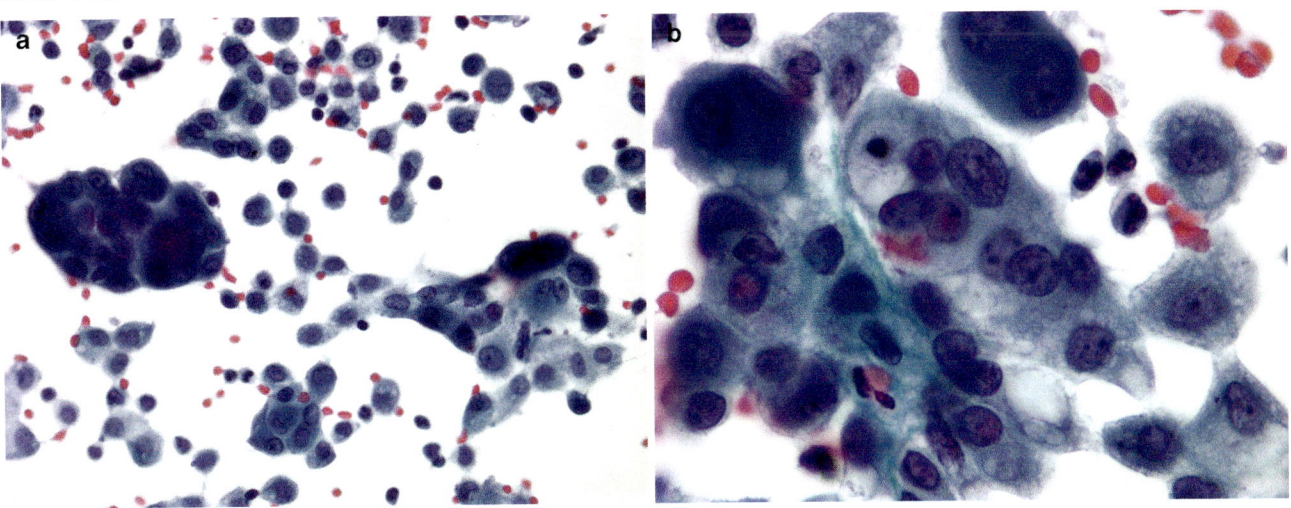

**Fig. 1.40** (**a**, **b**) Cytomegaly, multinucleation, variation in nuclear size, hyperchromasia, and cytoplasmic vacuolization in reactive mesothelial cells, caused by radiation; PAP

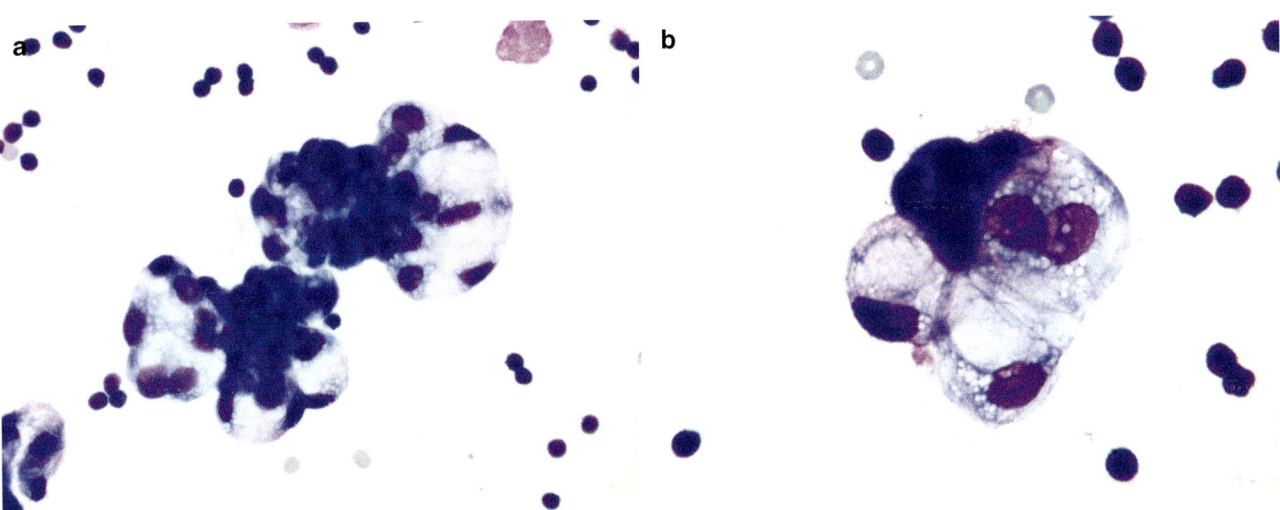

**Fig. 1.41** (**a**, **b**) Tight clustering, vacuolization, and variation in nuclear size and shape mimicking malignancy in reactive mesothelial cells due to chemotherapy; MGG

morphological alterations in mesothelial cells (Fig. 1.41a, b). On the other hand, abnormal features should not be overlooked and directly attributed to the radiation and/or chemotherapy history. In a series comparing the cytological features of pleural effusions from patients treated with and without radiation, only the presence of bizarre cells in specimens from patients who received radiation was found to be significantly different [83]. Immunocytochemistry would be an invaluable tool to resolve the problematic cases.

### Differential Diagnosis

Overcalling and undercalling effusion samples are well-known problems. The reason why mimicry is so common in effusion cytology may be the physical environment. The

mesothelial cells and "foreign" cells exfoliated into the fluid may resemble one another. Nevertheless, despite their superficial resemblance, persisting morphological differences should allow us to separate entities and make a correct interpretation [29]. In doubtful cases, ancillary tests are needed.

### Reactive Mesothelial Hyperplasia vs. Metastatic Carcinoma

Differentiating reactive mesothelial proliferations from metastatic carcinomas can be difficult in some cases due to either the atypical features of reactive mesothelial cells or the bland appearance of some carcinomas, resembling mesothelial proliferations [29]. The pattern and the cellular features should be evaluated together. Cells in reactive mesothelial

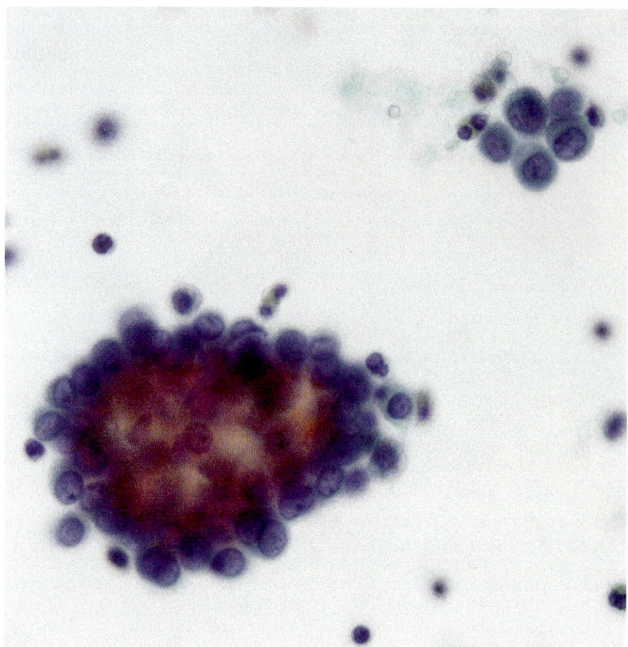

**Fig. 1.42** Reactive mesothelial proliferation; the cells forming the cluster and the cells in the background resemble each other; PAP

proliferations resemble one another (Fig. 1.42), and even the most atypical reactive mesothelial cells retain their characteristics. The presence of a discrete cell population is the major finding of metastatic carcinoma in serous effusions (Fig. 1.43). Unless all cells are neoplastic, carcinoma cells contrast with the mesothelial cells [33].

Mesothelial cell nuclei are centrally or paracentrally located, with fine chromatin and smooth contours. Nucleoli may be conspicuous but are regular (Figs. 1.2, 1.3, 1.4 and 1.5). Adenocarcinomas have eccentric nuclei with features of malignancy (Fig. 1.44), while their cytoplasm is delicate. The dark nuclei of adenocarcinomas are highlighted within this delicate cytoplasm. On the other hand, the cytoplasm of mesothelial cells is dense with a lacy skirt. Their nuclei may sometimes look hyperchromatic but do not form a real contrast with the cytoplasm (Fig. 1.4). If a clear-cut benign mesothelial cell is attached to a cell in doubt, it is accepted that both are mesothelial in origin [5] (Fig. 1.45).

Secretory vacuoles are seen in adenocarcinomas, displacing and indenting the nuclei (Figs. 1.14 and 1.44). Hydropic vacuoles occupying most of the cytoplasm may be observed in mesothelial cells, but these vacuoles do not contain mucin,

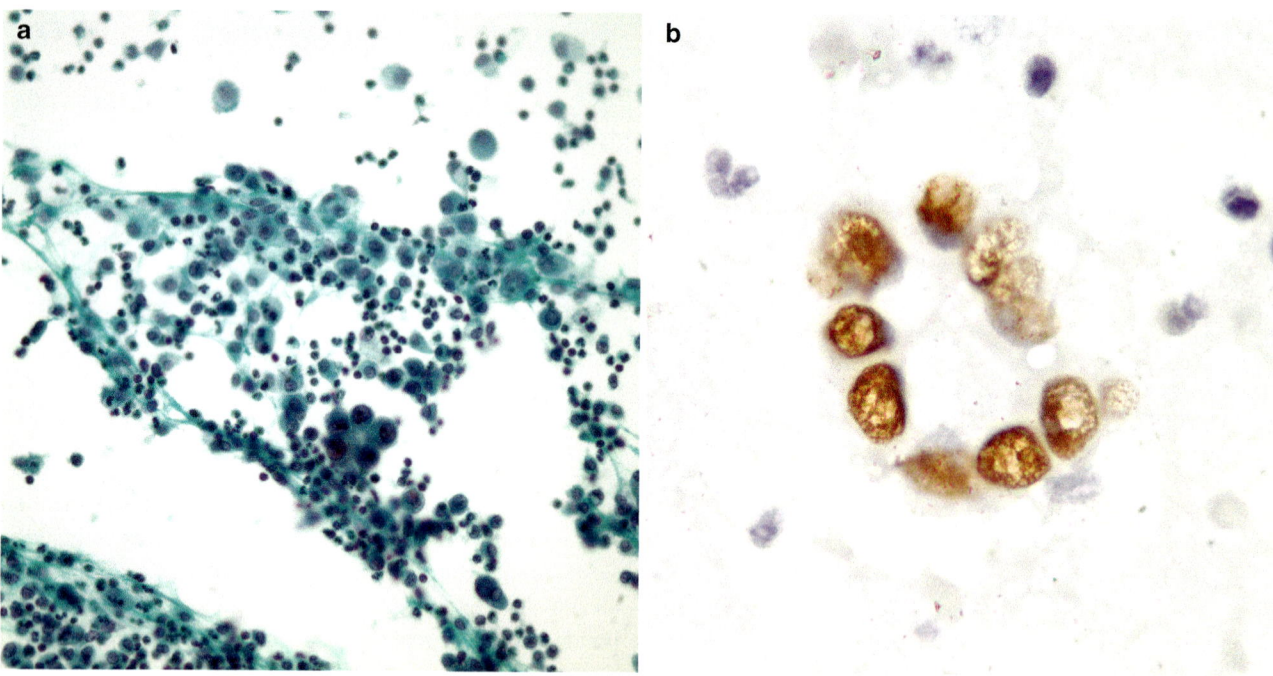

**Fig. 1.43** Lung adenocarcinoma; a small but discrete group of carcinoma cells looking different than other cells in the background; (**a**) PAP, (**b**) TTF-1 positivity in carcinoma cells

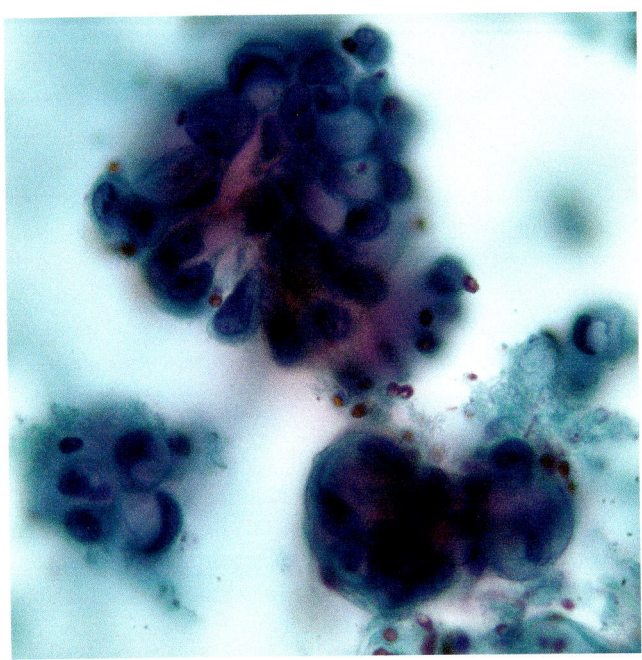

**Fig. 1.44** Adenocarcinoma with hyperchromatic eccentric nuclei indented by vacuoles; PAP

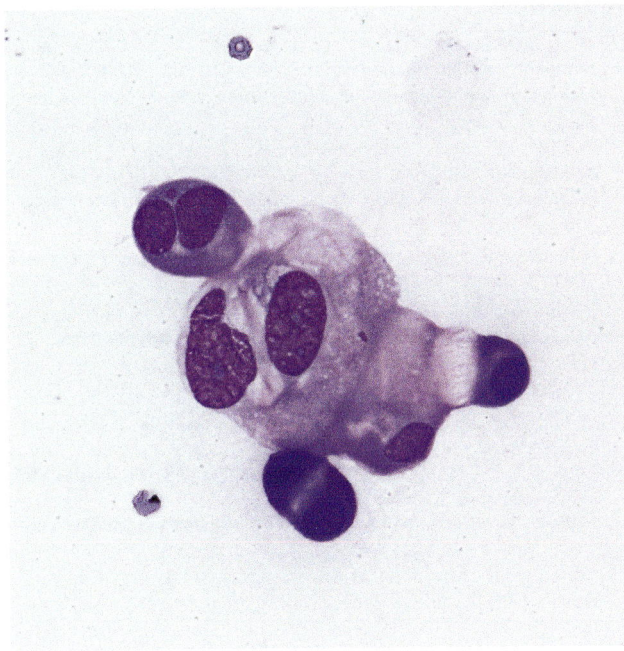

**Fig. 1.45** Atypia in reactive mesothelial cells; MGG

adenocarcinomas form tight clusters with common borders like cell balls and papillae [5, 27]. Any three-dimensional tight group detected in a serous effusion should be alerting for metastatic carcinoma.

The sensitivity of morphologic examination in diagnosing metastatic carcinoma in effusions varies from 40% to 80%, mainly depending on the experience of the cytopathologist and the quality of the preparations. It was shown that if cyto-morphology is combined with immunocytochemistry, the sensitivity increases from 84 to 94%, and the specificity increases from 92 to 100% [35].

Ber-EP4, MOC-31, claudin-4, CEA, and B72.3 are immunocytochemical markers that are used to highlight the presence of carcinoma cells within a reactive proliferation of mesothelial cells [33, 34]. Ber-EP4 and MOC-31 target the same antigen on the cell surface and are highly sensitive and specific markers for carcinoma, especially for adenocarcinoma. Claudin-4, a relatively recent marker, also shows high sensitivity and specificity for the differential between mesothelial proliferations and metastatic carcinomas [84]. On the other hand, mesothelial markers such as calretinin and D2–40 which would show that the cells in question are actually mesothelial are also useful in identifying the origin of atypical cells [34]. The expression of immunocytochemical markers varies in different carcinomas, and the antibodies that will be included in the panel should be selected according to the differential diagnosis. Antibodies that are rather organ-specific, such as TTF-1, estrogen receptor, PSA, etc., which may both be diagnostic for metastatic carcinoma and aid in locating the primary site, can also be used in correlation with the clinical features [85–88]. Recommended antibody panels for the most common differential diagnostic settings in effusion cytology are detailed in the Appendix.

## Reactive Mesothelial Hyperplasia vs. Malignant Mesothelioma

In mesotheliomas, the malignant cells look like native mesothelial cells. If the cells are sufficiently well differentiated to be recognized as mesothelial, it becomes difficult to call them malignant based on morphology [33, 89]. On the other hand, atypia in reactive proliferations may alert the pathologist to the diagnosis of malignant mesothelioma in an appropriate clinical setting. An important clue to the diagnosis of malignant mesothelioma is the presence of "more and bigger cells in more and bigger clusters." [5] High cellularity with many large aggregates suggests malignancy, especially in pleural effusions [89]. Benign effusions show fewer mesothelial cells and smaller, less complex groups. Cell-in-cell arrangements are more common in malignant proliferations [5, 28]. Macronucleoli favor malignancy. In general, clear-cut malignant nuclear features are not seen in malignant mesotheliomas but may be observed in some

and the nuclei are not indented, look benign, and do not differ from the nuclei of the other cells in the background [5, 27, 33] (Fig. 1.13).

Mesothelial cells form loose groups which are generally composed of few cells. Intercellular windows, cell-in-cell arrangement, and knobby contours are typical features of mesothelial groups (Figs. 1.17, 1.19, and 1.20). In contrast,

cases, in which the diagnosis of malignancy is easy to reach [89]. Pattern analysis is more important than individual cell features in differentiating reactive mesothelial proliferations from malignant mesotheliomas (Figs. 1.46 and 1.47).

The immunocytochemistry panel available for the differential diagnosis between benign and malignant mesothelial proliferations is limited but is nevertheless of some value. p53, EMA (thick membranous staining), E-cadherin, and Glut-1 have been reported to be positive in mesotheliomas and negative in reactive proliferations and have been considered to be useful markers in this setting. Desmin, another useful marker, has been shown to be positive in benign but negative in malignant mesothelial proliferations [90–93]. Loss of BAP1 expression is a recently introduced feature of malignant mesotheliomas which is reliably used in distinguishing benign from malignant mesothelial proliferations [94]. As detailed in Chap. 5 and the Appendix, the authors of this book find EMA, desmin, and BAP1 to be especially useful in this setting. Other ancillary techniques in this differential, as well as in the differential diagnosis between malignant mesothelioma and adenocarcinoma, are detailed in Chap. 11.

Differentiating malignant mesothelioma from benign mesothelial proliferations is a problematic area. The question of how far we can go in effusion cytology is still a controversial issue, and the diagnostic accuracy depends on the experience of the cytopathologist and the ancillary techniques available.

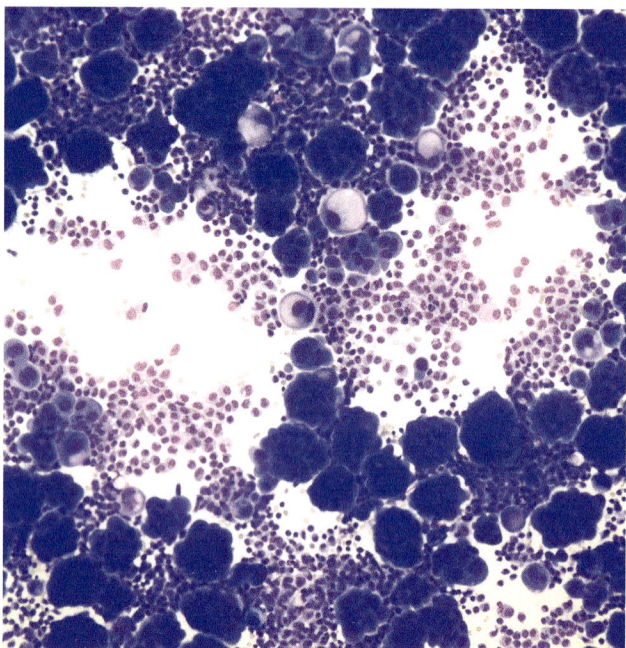

**Fig. 1.46** Malignant mesothelioma showing hypercellularity with many three-dimensional groups; MGG

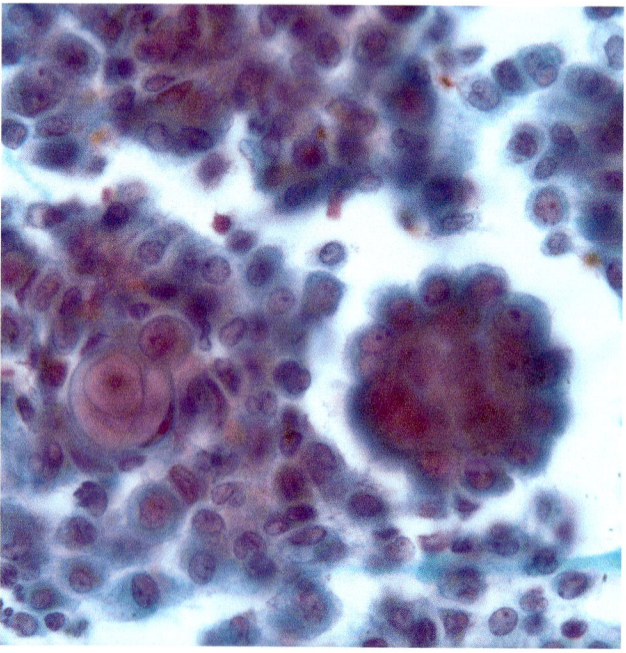

**Fig. 1.47** Malignant mesothelioma with knobby-contoured clusters and cell-in-cell arrangement; PAP

## References

1. Shidham VB. Introduction. In: Shidham VB, Atkinson BF, editors. Cytopathologic diagnosis of serous fluids. Chap. 1. Philadelphia: Saunders Elsevier; 2007. p. 1–17.
2. Tao LC. Etiology of effusions. In: Tao LC, editor. Cytopathology of malignant effusions. Johnston WW series ed. ASCP theory and practice of cytopathology. vol 6. Chap. 1. Chicago: ASCP Press; 1996. p. 1–55.
3. Sahn SA. The value of pleural fluid analysis. Am J Med Sci. 2008;335:7–15.
4. Wong JW, Pitlik D, Abdul-Karim FW. Cytology of pleural, peritoneal and pericardial fluids in children. A 40-year summary. Acta Cytol. 1997;41:467–73.
5. DeMay RM. Fluids. In: DeMay RM, editor. The art and science of cytopathology. vol 1. Chap. 8. Chicago: ASCP Press; 1996. p. 257–325.
6. Porcel JM. Pearls and myths in pleural fluid analysis. Respirology. 2011;16:44–52.
7. Heffner JE. Discriminating between transudates and exudates. Clin Chest Med. 2006;27:241–52.
8. Yousef MM, Michael CW. Body cavity fluids. In: Gattuso P, Reddy VB, Masood S, editor. Differential diagnosis in cytopathology. Chap. 3. New York: Cambridge University Press; 2010. p. 99–150.
9. Sahn SA. Getting the most from pleural fluid analysis. Respirology. 2012;17:270–7.
10. Wilcox ME, Chong CAKY, Stanbrook MB, Tricco AC, Wong C, Straus SE. Does this patient have an exudative pleural effusion? The rational clinical examination systematic review. JAMA. 2014;311:2422–31.
11. Light RW, Macgregor MI, Luchsinger PC, Ball WC Jr. Pleural effusion: the diagnostic separation of transudates and exudates. Ann Intern Med. 1972;77:507–13.
12. Romero-Candeira S, Hernandez L. The separation of transudates and exudates with particular reference to the protein gradient. Curr Opin Pulm Med. 2004;10:294–8.

13. Porcel JM, Azzopardi M, Koegelenberg CF, Maldonado F, Rahman NM, Lee YCG. The diagnosis of pleural effusions. Expert Rev Respir Med. 2015;9:801–15.

14. Huggins JT. Chylothorax and cholesterol pleural effusion. Semin Respir Crit Care Med. 2010;31:743–50.

15. Light RW. Update on tuberculous pleural effusion. Respirology. 2010;15:451–8.

16. Porcel JM, Esquerda A, Bielsa S. Diagnostic performance of adenosine deaminase activity in pleural fluid: a single center experience with over 2100 consecutive patients. Eur J Intern Med. 2010;21:419–23.

17. Antony VB, Godbey SW, Kunkel SL, et al. Recruitment of inflammatory cells to the pleural space. Chemotactic cytokines, IL-8, and monocyte chemotactic peptide-1 in human pleural fluids. J Immunol. 1993;151:7216–23.

18. Sherr HP, Light RW, Merson MH, Wolf RO, Taylor LL, Hendrix TR. Origin of pleural fluid amylase in esophageal rupture. Ann Intern Med. 1972;76:985–6.

19. Kramer MR, Saldana MJ, Cepero RJ, Pitchenik AE. High amylase levels in neoplasm-related pleural effusion. Ann Intern Med. 1989;110:567–9.

20. Villena V, López-Encuentra A, García-Luján R, Echave-Sustaeta J, Martínez CJ. Clinical implications of appearance of pleural fluid at thoracentesis. Chest. 2004;125:156–9.

21. Light RW. Clinical practice. Pleural effusion. N Engl J Med. 2002;346:1971–7.

22. Maldonado F, Hawkins FJ, Daniels CE, Doerr CH, Decker PA, Ryu JH. Pleural fluid characteristics of chylothorax. Mayo Clin Proc. 2009;84:129–33.

23. Creaney J, Dicka IM, Robinson BW. Comparison of mesothelin and fibulin-3 in pleural fluid and serum as markers in malignant mesothelioma. Curr Opin Pulm Med. 2015;21:352–6.

24. Psallidas I, Kalomenidis I, Porcel JM, Robinson BW, Stathopoulos GT. Malignant pleural effusion: from bench to bedside. Eur Respir Rev. 2016;25:189–98.

25. Rooper LM, Ali SZ, Olson MT. A minimum fluid volume of 75 mL is needed to ensure adequacy in a pleural effusion: a retrospective analysis of 2540 cases. Cancer (Cancer Cytopathol). 2014;122:657–65.

26. Porcel JM, Esquerda A, Vives M, Bielsa S. Etiology of pleural effusions: analysis of more than 3,000 consecutive thoracenteses. Arch Bronconeumol. 2014;50:161–5.

27. Pereira TC, Saad RS, Liu Y, Silverman JF. The diagnosis of malignancy in effusion cytology: a pattern recognition approach. Adv Anat Pathol. 2006;13:174–84.

28. Stevens MW, Leong ASY, Fazzalari NL, Dowling KD, Henderson DW. Cytopathology of malignant mesothelioma: a stepwise logistic regression analysis. Diagn Cytopathol. 1992;8:333–41.

29. Boerner SL. Mimicry and pitfalls in effusion cytology. Pathol Case Rev. 2006;11:85–91.

30. Gordon HY, Sack MJ, Baloch ZW, DeFrias DVS, Gupta PK. Occurrence of intercellular spaces (windows) in metastatic adenocarcinoma in serous fluids: a cytomorphologic, histochemical and ultrastructural study. Diagn Cytopathol. 1999;20:115–9.

31. Murugan P, Siddaraju N, Habeebullah S, Basu D. Significance of intercellular spaces (windows) in effusion fluid cytology: a study of 46 samples. Diagn Cytopathol. 2008;36:628–32.

32. Selvaggi SM. Diagnostic pitfalls of peritoneal washing cytology and the role of cell blocks in their diagnosis. Diagn Cytopathol. 2003;28:335–41.

33. Bedrossian CWM. Diagnostic problems in serous effusions. Diagn Cytopathol. 1998;19:131–7.

34. Ordonez NG. What are the current best immunohistochemical markers for the diagnosis of epithelioid mesothelioma? A review and update. Hum Pathol. 2007;38:1–16.

35. Metzgeroth G, Kuhn C, Schultheis B, Hehlmann R, Hastka J. Diagnostic accuracy of cytology and immunocytology in carcinomatous effusions. Cytopathology. 2008;19:205–11.

36. Grefte JM, de Wilde PC, de Salet-van Pol MR, Tomassen M, Raaymakers-van Geloof WL, Bulten J. Improved identification of malignant cells in serous effusions using a small, robust panel of antibodies on paraffin-embedded cell suspensions. Acta Cytol. 2008;52:35–44.

37. Das DK. Serous effusions in malignant lymphomas: a review. Diagn Cytopathol. 2006;34:335–47.

38. Valdes L, Alvarez D, Valle JM, Pose A, Jose ES. The etiology of pleural effusions in an area with high incidence of tuberculosis. Chest. 1996;109:158–62.

39. Hampson C, Lemos JA, Klein JS. Diagnosis and management of parapneumonic effusions. Semin Respir Crit Care Med. 2008;29:414–26.

40. Cugell DW, Kamp DW. Asbestos and the pleura. Chest. 2004;125:1103–17.

41. Krenke R, Nasilowski J, Korczynski P, et al. Incidence and aetiology of eosinophilic pleural effusion. Eur Respir J. 2009;34:1111–7.

42. Rubins JB, Rubins HB. Etiology and prognostic significance of eosinophilic pleural effusions. A prospective study. Chest. 1996;110:1271–4.

43. Adelman M, Albelda SM, Gottlieb J, Haponik EF. Diagnostic utility of pleural fluid eosinophilia. Am J Med. 1984;77:915–20.

44. Krishnan S, Statsinger AL, Kleinman M, Bertoni MA, Sharma P. Eosinophilic pleural effusion with Charcot-Leyden crystals. Acta Cytol. 1983;27:529–32.

45. Kumar NB, Naylor B. Megakaryocytes in pleural and peritoneal fluids: prevalence, significance, morphology and cytohistological correlation. J Clin Pathol. 1980;33:1153–9.

46. Bowling MR, Cauthen CG, Perry CD, et al. Pulmonary extramedullary hematopoiesis. J Thorac Imaging. 2008;23:138–41.

47. Koch M, Kurian EM. Pleural fluid extramedullary hematopoiesis case report with review of the literature. Diagn Cytopathol. 2016;44:41–4.

48. Kobayashi TK, Moritani S, Urabe M, et al. Cytologic diagnosis of endosalpingiosis with pregnant women presenting in peritoneal fluid: a case report. Diagn Cytopathol. 2004;30:422–5.

49. Kuritzkes DR, Rein M, Horowitz S, et al. Detached ciliary tufts mistaken for peritoneal parasites: a warning. Rev Infect Dis. 1988;10:1044–7.

50. Sidawy MK, Chandra P, Oertel YC. Detached ciliary tufts in female peritoneal washings. A common finding. Acta Cytol. 1987;31:841–4.

51. Risberg B, Davidson B, Dong HP, Nesland JM, Berner A. Flow cytometric immunophenotyping of serous effusions and peritoneal washings: comparison with immunocytochemistry and morphological findings. J Clin Pathol. 2000;53:513–7.

52. Shield P. Peritoneal washing cytology. Cytopathology. 2004;15:131–41.

53. Bharani V, Singh P, Gupta N, Srinivasan R. Significance of flower pot cells in effusion cytology. Diagn Cytopathol. 2017;45:925–7.

54. Parwani AV, Chan TY, Ali SZ. Significance of psammoma bodies in serous cavity fluid: a cytopathologic analysis. Cancer. 2004;102:87–91.

55. Natanzon A, Kronzon I. Pericardial and pleural effusions in congestive heart failure-anatomical, pathophysiologic, and clinical considerations. Am J Med Sci. 2009;338:211–6.

56. Porcel JM. Pleural effusions from congestive heart failure. Semin Respir Crit Care Med. 2010;31:689–97.

57. Berger HW, Rammohan G, Neff MS, Buhain WJ. Uremic pleural effusion. Ann Intern Med. 1975;82:362–4.

58. Piraino B, Sheth H. Peritonitis—does peritoneal dialysis modality make a difference? Blood Purif. 2010;29:145–9.

59. Ejaz AA, Fitzpatrick PM, Durkin AJ, et al. Pathophysiology of peritoneal fluid eosinophilia in peritoneal dialysis patients. Nephron. 1999;81:125–30.

60. Han SH, Reynolds TB, Fong TL. Nephrogenic ascites. Analysis of 16 cases and review of the literature. Medicine (Baltimore). 1998;77:233–45.

61. Browne GW, Pitchumoni CS. Pathophysiology of pulmonary complications of acute pancreatis. World J Gastroenterol. 2006;12:7087–96.

62. Pai CG, Suvarna D, Bhat G. Endoscopic treatment as first-line therapy for pancreatic ascites and pleural effusion. J Gastroenterol Hepatol. 2009;24:1198–202.

63. Light RW. Pleural effusion in pulmonary embolism. Semin Respir Crit Care Med. 2010;31:716–22.

64. Baumann MH, Nolan R, Petrini M, Lee YC, Light RW, Schneider E. Pleural tuberculosis in the United States: incidence and drug resistance. Chest. 2007;131:1125–32.

65. Udwadia ZF, Sen T. Pleural tuberculosis: an update. Curr Opin Pulm Med. 2010;16:399–406.

66. Skouras VS, Kalomenidis I. Pleural fluid tests to diagnose tuberculous pleuritic. Curr Opin Pulm Med. 2016;22:367–77.

67. Trajman A, Kaisermann C, Luiz RR, et al. Pleural fluid ADA, IgA-ELISA and PCR sensitivities for the diagnosis of pleural tuberculosis. Scand J Clin Lab Invest. 2007;67:877–84.

68. Valdes L, San-Jose E, Ferreiro L, Golpe A, Gonzales-Barcala FJ, Toubes ME, et al. Predicting malignant and tuberculous pleural effusions through demographics and pleural fluid analysis of patients. Clin Respir J. 2015;9:203–13.

69. Ellison E, Lapuerta P, Martin SE. Cytologic features of mycobacterial pleuritis: logistic regression and statistical analysis of a blinded, case-controlled study. Diagn Cytopathol. 1998;19:173–6.

70. Lau KY. Numerous mesothelial cells in tuberculous pleural effusions. Chest. 1989;96:438–9.

71. Chou CW, Chang SC. Pleuritis as a presenting manifestation of rheumatoid arthritis: diagnostic clues in pleural fluid cytology. Am J Med Sci. 2002;323:158–61.

72. Avnon LS, Abu-Shakra M, Flusser D, Heimer D, Sion-Vardy N. Pleural effusion associated with rheumatoid arthritis: what cell predominance to anticipate? Rheumatol Int. 2007;27:919–25.

73. Naylor B. The pathognomonic cytologic picture of rheumatoid pleuritis. Acta Cytol. 1990;34:465–73.

74. Brucato A, Tombini V, Guffanti C. Clinical image: comet cells in rheumatoid arthritis. Arthritis Rheum. 2006;54:243.

75. Ishiguro N, Tomino Y, Fujito K, Nakayama S, Koide H. A case of massive ascites due to lupus peritonitis with a dramatic response to steroid pulse therapy. Jpn J Med. 1989;28:608–11.

76. Ruiz-Argüelles A, Alarcón-Segovia D. Novel facts about an old marker: the LE cell. Scand J Clin Lab Invest Suppl. 2001;235:31–7.

77. Gulhane S, Gangane N. Detection of lupus erythematosus cells in pleural effusion: an unusual presentation of systemic lupus erythematosus. J Cytol. 2012;29:77–9.

78. Reda MG, Baigelman W. Pleural effusion in systemic lupus erythematosus. Acta Cytol. 1980;24:553–7.

79. Wang DY, Chang DB, Kuo SH, et al. Systemic lupus erythematosus presenting as pleural effusion: report of a case. J Formos Med Assoc. 1995;94:746–9.

80. Park JY, Malik A, Dumoff KL, Gupta PK. Case report and review of lupus erythematosus cells in cytology fluids. Diagn Cytopathol. 2007;35:806–9.

81. de Torres EF, Guevara EC. Pleuritis by radiation: report of two cases. Acta Cytol. 1981;25:427–9.

82. von Haam E. The effect of chemotherapy and radiotherapy upon the cells of transudates and exudates. Monogr Clin Cytol. 1977;5:93–123.

83. Wojno KJ, Olson JL, Sherman ME. Cytopathology of pleural effusions after radiotherapy. Acta Cytol. 1994;38:1–8.

84. Kim NI, Kim GE, Lee JS. Diagnostic usefulness of Claudin-3 and Claudin-4 for immunocytochemical differentiation between metastatic adenocarcinoma cells and reactive mesothelial cells in effusion cell blocks. Acta Cytol. 2016;60(3):232–9.

85. Zhu W, Michael CW. WT1, monoclonal CEA, TTF1, and CA125 antibodies in the differential diagnosis of lung, breast, and ovarian adenocarcinomas in serous effusions. Diagn Cytopathol. 2007;35:370–5.

86. Pomjanski N, Grote HJ, Doganay P, Schmiemann V, Buckstegge B, Böcking A. Immunocytochemical identification of carcinomas of unknown primary in serous effusions. Diagn Cytopathol. 2005;33:309–15.

87. Pu RT, Pang Y, Michael CW. Utility of WT-1, p63, MOC31, mesothelin, and cytokeratin (K903 and CK5/6) immunostains in differentiating adenocarcinoma, squamous cell carcinoma, and malignant mesothelioma in effusions. Diagn Cytopathol. 2008;36:20–5.

88. Westfall DE, Fan X, Marchevsky AM. Evidence-based guidelines to optimize the selection of antibody panels in cytopathology: pleural effusions with malignant epithelioid cells. Diagn Cytopathol. 2010;38:9–14.

89. Whitaker D. Cytopathology of malignant mesothelioma. Cytopathology. 2000;11:139–51.

90. Davidson B, Nielsen S, Christensen J, et al. The role of desmin and N-cadherin in effusion cytology: a comparative study using established markers of mesothelial and epithelial cells. Am J Surg Pathol. 2001;25:1405–12.

91. Saad RS, Cho P, Liu YL, Silverman JF. The value of epithelial membrane antigen expression in separating benign mesothelial proliferation from malignant mesothelioma. Diagn Cytopathol. 2005;32:156–9.

92. Kitazume H, Kitamura K, Mukai K, et al. Cytologic differential diagnosis among reactive mesothelial cells, malignant mesothelioma, and adenocarcinoma: utility of combined E-cadherin and calretinin immunostaining. Cancer. 2000;90:55–60.

93. Hasteh F, Grace YL, Weidner N, Michael CW. The use of immunohistochemistry to distinguish reactive mesothelial cells from malignant mesothelioma in cytologic effusions. Cancer Cytopathol. 2010;118:90–6.

94. Andrici J, Sheen A, Sioson L, Wardell K, Clarkson A, Watson N, et al. Loss of expression of BAP1 is a useful adjunct, which strongly supports the diagnosis of mesothelioma in effusion cytology. Mod Pathol. 2015;28(10):1360–8.

# Lung Carcinoma

2

Claire W. Michael

## Introduction

### Epidemiology

Lung cancer is considered the most common source of new cancer worldwide and contributes the highest number of deaths from cancer, with an estimated 1.8 million new cases diagnosed in 2012 (12.9% of all cancer deaths) [1]. In the United States, more than 222,500 new cases and approximately 155,870 deaths are expected in 2017 [2]. The Surveillance, Epidemiology, and End Results (SEER) group, who studied the incidence of lung cancer in 17 geographic areas, reported that the highest incidence occurred in Europe and North America and the lowest incidence in Africa, Latin America, and the Caribbean [1, 2].

Among males, squamous cell carcinoma predominates, except for selected countries (North America, China, and Japan), in which adenocarcinoma predominates. Among females, adenocarcinoma is the dominant histological type worldwide, except in England and Poland, where squamous cell carcinoma predominates, and Scotland, where small cell carcinoma is the most common subtype [3, 4].

Smoking increases the risk for lung carcinoma, as does occupational exposure to asbestos and silica [4].

Lung carcinoma continues to be the most common cause of malignant effusion, accounting for 37% of 840 malignant effusions evaluated in a recent study [5]. About 40% of patients with lung carcinoma present with pleural effusions at some time during the course of their disease. In half of these patients, the effusions progress enough to require thoracocentesis, with less than 20% of them attributed to a benign etiology [6].

In a study evaluating 584 malignant pleural effusions, lung carcinoma was the etiology for 167 effusions, representing 49.1% of cases among male patients and 15% among female patients. Histologically, 41.3% of these specimens were adenocarcinomas, 24.6% small cell carcinoma, 20.3% squamous cell carcinoma, 9.6% large cell undifferentiated carcinoma, 3.6% adenosquamous carcinoma, and 0.6% carcinoid [7]. A similar study of positive pleural effusions evaluated 143 patients who died of malignancy and underwent autopsy. Lung carcinoma was the source of effusion in 28.7% of males and 20.6% of females [8].

## Clinical Presentation

Pleural effusion develops in a considerable percentage of patients with lung carcinoma. The effusion results from one of two mechanisms: (1) reduced drainage as a result of obstruction of the pleural lymphatics through various routes, invasion, direct seeding, or from obstruction of the hilar lymph nodes [9] and (2) overproduction and capillary leak resulting frequently in the very rapid accumulation of malignant effusions [10]. Pleural effusion may initially present as a transudate but quickly develops into an exudate. The presence of a confirmed malignant effusion would upgrade the staging of a lung tumor of any size to stage T-IXA according to the TNM classification of the lung. Meanwhile, it is important to recognize that in rare cases where the effusion remains a transudate and consistently negative by cytological examination, the presence of effusion should not be considered in the staging [11, 12].

The most common symptom is dyspnea, resulting from the reduced compliance of the chest wall, diaphragm, and lung volume. The trachea may be shifted to the contralateral side. Physical examination will reveal reduced breath sounds and dullness to percussion.

## Diagnosis

Standard chest X-ray is the first radiological test performed, and it can detect as little as 50 mL of pleural fluid on a lateral

2

C. W. Michael
Department of Pathology, University Hospitals Cleveland Medical Center, Case Western Reserve University, Cleveland, OH, USA
e-mail: claire.michael@case.edu

© Springer International Publishing AG, part of Springer Nature 2018
B. Davidson et al. (eds.), *Serous Effusions*, https://doi.org/10.1007/978-3-319-76478-8_2

view and 200 mL on the posterior–anterior view [13]. Computerized tomography (CT) can play a great role in distinguishing malignant from benign pleural disease with a sensitivity of 72% and specificity of 83%. It was noted that nodular and parietal pleural thickening of more than 1 cm and mediastinal pleural involvement are highly suggestive of malignancy. In addition, malignant effusions tend to involve the entire pleural surface, while pleural calcifications suggest reactive pleurisy [14]. Magnetic resonance imaging (MRI) is useful in demonstrating tumor invasion into the chest wall and diaphragm. Positron emission tomography (PET) has been very helpful in identifying malignant effusions, with 95% sensitivity and 80% specificity. A negative PET can be very useful to rule out a malignant effusion. However, it is important to recognize that some benign pleural diseases can be PET-avid [15].

Thoracocentesis and cytological examination of the pleural fluid are necessary to establish the diagnosis and remain the standard initial evaluation [16]. The effusion can also be subjected to other analyses, such as cell count and chemical analysis, particularly pH and glucose. It is critical to understand that these tests can only be performed on the initial thoracentesis fluid and might not be valid on subsequent thoracentesis [16]. Most malignant effusions have a high lymphocyte count, and a considerable number have a high eosinophil count. A pH < 7.30 or glucose <60 mg/dL suggest malignancy. The presence or absence of blood in pleural effusions was not found to be useful in predicting cancer. In fact, in a study evaluating 390 patients who were diagnosed with cancer and underwent thoracentesis, 82.5% of the cytologically positive fluids were not bloody [17].

Cytological evaluation has a wide range of reported diagnostic yield ranging from 62 to 90%, particularly when mesothelioma is included in the differential. Immunocytochemical staining is frequently necessary in order to confirm the diagnosis.

When cytology fails to establish a diagnosis, in approximately 47% of patients, several diagnostic procedures can be approached, such as repeated thoracentesis, closed pleural biopsy, or thoracoscopy. The method of choice varies by geographic location, performer experience, and available resources. Closed pleural biopsy is not generally performed, as the additional diagnostic yield is only 7% above a negative cytology. Thoracoscopic pleural biopsy is performed via video assistance (VATS) as the method of choice by many experts to obtain a biopsy. Thoracoscopy offers many advantages:

1. Can expedite the diagnosis as it obviates the need for repeated thoracentesis and/or pleural biopsy.
2. Offers direct visualization of virtually the entire pleural surface, and thus the clinician can localize and perform

direct biopsy of the nodule even when they occur as isolated scattered islands of tumor.
3. Tissue can be retrieved for intraoperative frozen section and immediate assessment.
4. If required, pleurodesis can be performed in the same setting.

Thoracoscopy is generally considered safe and has high sensitivity and specificity for the diagnosis of cancer in malignant effusions [15, 16].

## Treatment

Management of a malignant pleural effusion is performed for palliative reasons only, as it does not change the prognosis or survival. In the absence of respiratory symptoms, therapeutic intervention is not indicated. Thoracentesis is the first management of choice since it will also improve the breathlessness and indicate the rate of reaccumulation. Repeated thoracocentesis is not advised, as it may lead to complications such as adhesions and infections and is only performed in patients with expected very short life expectancy [16].

For recurrent effusions, chemical pleurodesis is the method of choice, as it induces inflammation and fibrin deposition, consequently resulting in adhesions between the layers of pleura. As a result pain and fever are common side effects. While talc is the most common chemical used for pleurodesis, other agents, including bleomycin, tetracycline, cisplatin, etc., have been used with comparable success. Respiratory failure and acute respiratory distress syndrome (ARDS) have been reported in patients who underwent talc pleurodesis, and this complication has been attributed to systemic absorption of small-sized talc particles. However, this was not reported when preparations with strictly large particles are used [15]. Pleurodesis is usually limited to patients with recurrent effusions resulting in respiratory distress, malignant effusions that are not responsive to chemotherapy, and lung expansion to the chest wall after thoracentesis and patients with life expectancy longer than 2–3 months [18].

Long-term indwelling pleural catheter is used when pleurodesis is not recommended. It provides immediate relief of dyspnea in over 90% of patients while allowing them to function independently at home. Complications include catheter dislodgment, infection, and loculation. An alternative, especially in patients with inadequate lung expansion, is pleuroperitoneal shunting. This method can achieve effective palliation in 95% of patients. However, complications such as shunt occlusion and infection were reported in 14.8% of patients [13].

Surgical resection is contraindicated in patients with malignant pleural effusion. However, a recent study evaluated the effect of intraoperative intrathoracic hyperthermotherapy (IIH) and hyperthermochemotherapy (IIHC) in patients who were discovered to have malignant effusion or dissemination at the time of surgery. The study found that the use of IIH and IIHC may be beneficial in the prevention of future pleural effusion rather than in improving prognosis [19].

## Morphology

Histologically, the major types of carcinoma of the lung are, in the order of frequency, squamous cell carcinoma, small cell carcinoma, adenocarcinoma, and large cell anaplastic carcinoma. However, in effusions, the incidence of these tumors is different, mainly due to their access and propensity to invade the pleura. While squamous and small cell carcinoma are very common, they are traditionally centrally located and thus do not manifest as effusion unless they erode into the pleural surface. In contrast, adenocarcinoma tends to arise peripherally and has tendency to invade the pleura and directly seed the pleural lymphatics. Consequently, adenocarcinoma is the most common type encountered in effusions [20–23].

## Adenocarcinoma (ADC) [21, 23]

## Morphology

The most common presentation is in the form of numerous variably sized clusters in a background of single malignant cells (Figs. 2.1 and 2.2). The presence of the native reactive mesothelial cells can be helpful in identifying their alien nature. However, cancer cells frequently predominate the

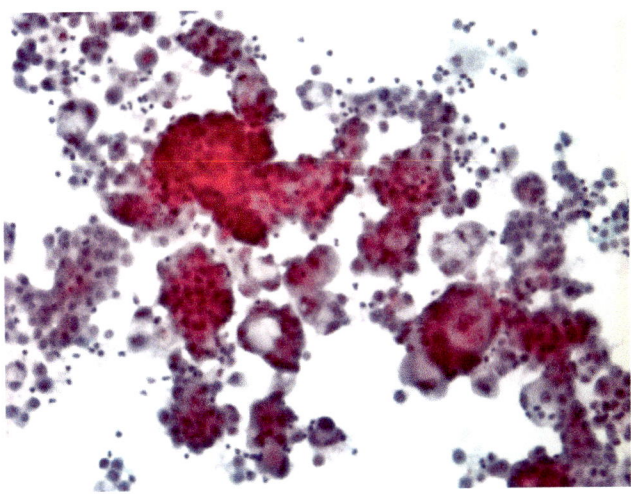

**Fig. 2.1** Lung ADC presenting as variably sized clusters and single malignant cells in a background of benign mesothelial cells; PAP

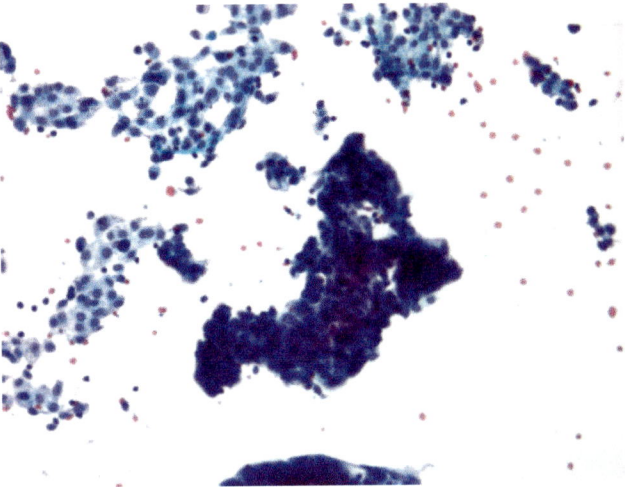

**Fig. 2.2** Lung ADC presenting as large geographic sheets of malignant cells in a background of benign mesothelial cells; PAP

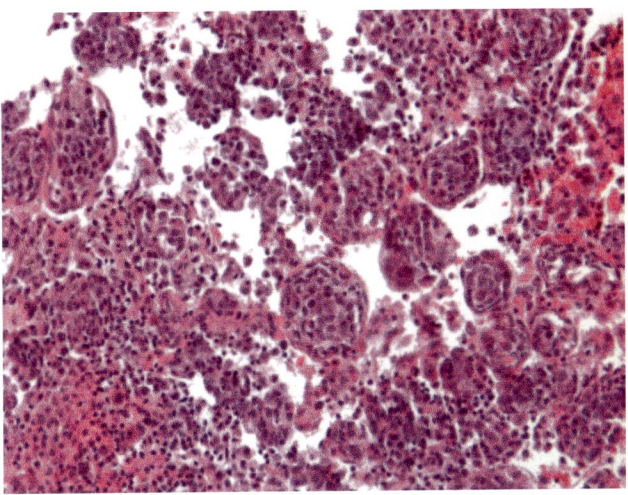

**Fig. 2.3** Cell block of a lung ADC presenting predominantly as cohesive spheres mimicking mesothelioma; H&E

fluid (Fig. 2.3). The clusters are comprised of medium-sized tightly cohesive cells with finely vacuolated cytoplasm, enlarged nuclei, and increased nuclear-to-cytoplasmic (N/C) ratio. The cellular clusters vary from small groups to large cell balls similar to the spheres seen in mesothelioma (Fig. 2.4). They tend to exhibit a common cell border at least partially, although they may also exhibit scalloping of their borders. The nuclei may be moderately to significantly enlarged, with coarse irregularly distributed chromatin and prominent nucleoli. Mitotic figures may be detected. It is not unusual to see large disfiguring cytoplasmic vacuoles (Fig. 2.5). These vacuoles, particularly when small, may mimic intercellular windows of mesothelium (Fig. 2.6). In very well-differentiated ADC, particularly those that have a lepidic growth pattern, the clusters may be loose, with prominent scalloped borders, and the cells arranged like petals

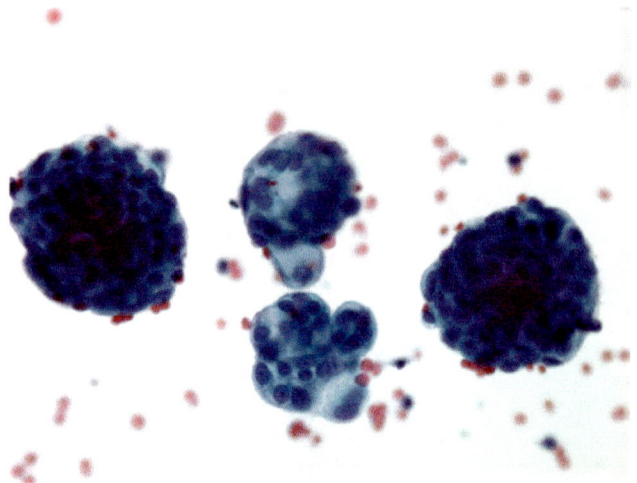

**Fig. 2.4** Correlating smear showing medium-sized cellular spheres, some with common cell border and others with scalloped surface mimicking mesothelioma; PAP

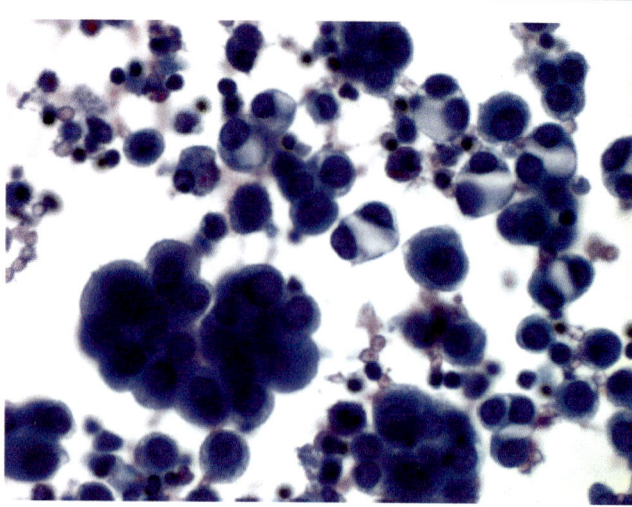

**Fig. 2.6** Lung ADC presenting as clusters with scalloped borders in a background of opposing cells with degenerative cytoplasmic vacuoles mimicking windows. This pattern should not be mistaken for mesothelioma; PAP

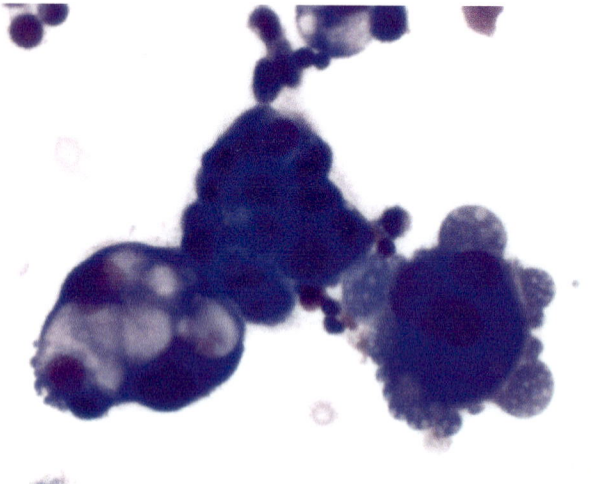

**Fig. 2.5** Malignant cells frequently exhibit large and disfiguring cytoplasmic degenerative vacuoles; Diff-Quik

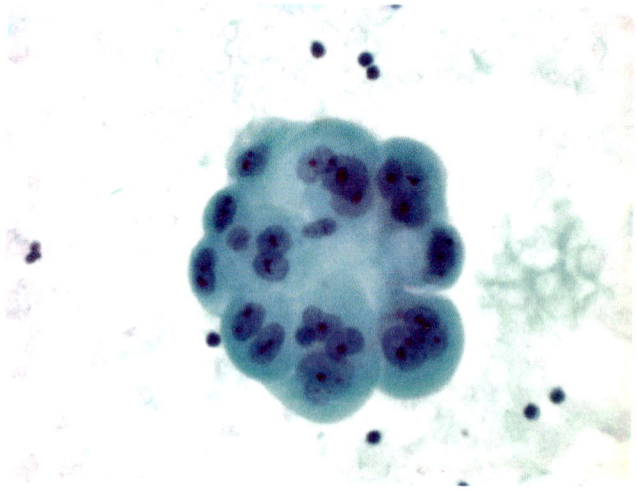

**Fig. 2.7** Malignant effusion from a patient with previous history of ADC with lepidic growth pattern. The malignant cells are arranged in a flat flowerlike pattern. The hobnailing cells are arranged like petals around a central core; PAP

around a central core (Fig. 2.7). Intranuclear pseudoinclusions and psammoma bodies may also be detected. The background malignant cells are usually larger, with more prominent atypia, and in many cases multinucleated cells are also seen (Fig. 2.8).

Poorly differentiated ADC may present mainly as single discohesive cells with very rare groups (Fig. 2.9). The nuclei are eccentric in location, enlarged, and obviously abnormal, with coarse chromatin, irregular nuclear membranes, and prominent nucleoli. The N/C ratio is high, and bizarre-appearing cells are not unusual (Fig. 2.10). Occasional cases may not manifest a high degree of atypia and therefore would be difficult to separate from reactive mesothelium. ADC cells of lung primary may rarely contain cytoplasmic glyco-

gen. However, contrary to mesothelioma, in the rare cells containing glycogen, it tends to fill the cytoplasm, rather than form submembranous elongated vacuoles as in the case of mesothelium (Fig. 2.11).

## Differential Diagnosis

1. *Reactive mesothelium*: This differential is mainly significant in samples presenting as single cells with subtle cytological atypia (Fig. 2.12). The malignant cells may also have vacuoles that mimic intercellular windows,

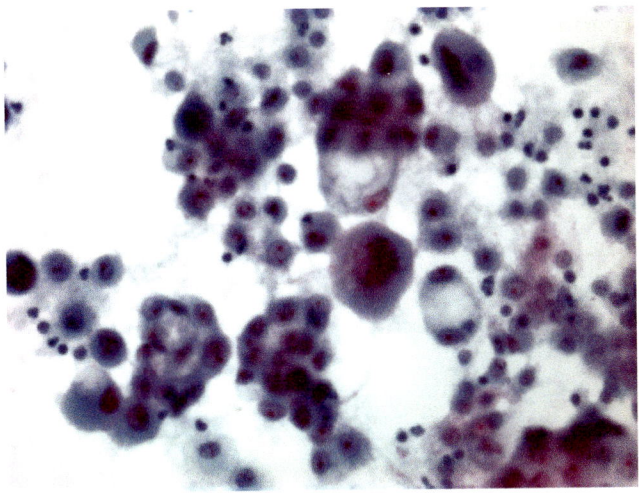

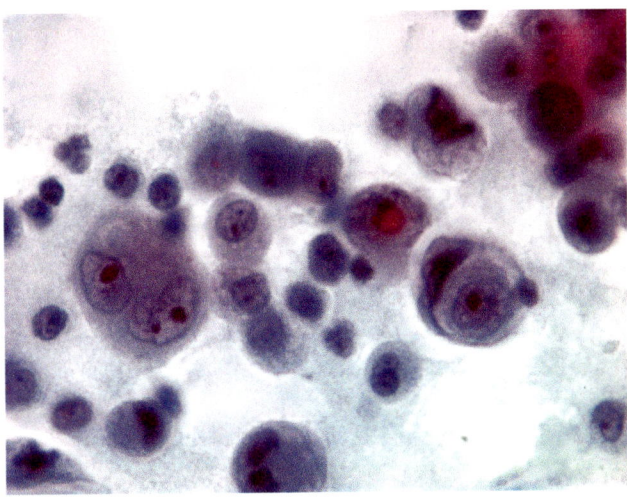

**Fig. 2.8** Background single cells in lung ADC usually appear larger than those within the clusters and exhibit obvious atypical features. The cells are frequently multinucleated, and degenerative cytoplasmic vacuoles are common; PAP

**Fig. 2.10** Discohesive ADC cells may contain bizarre cells and show cell-within-cell pattern; PAP

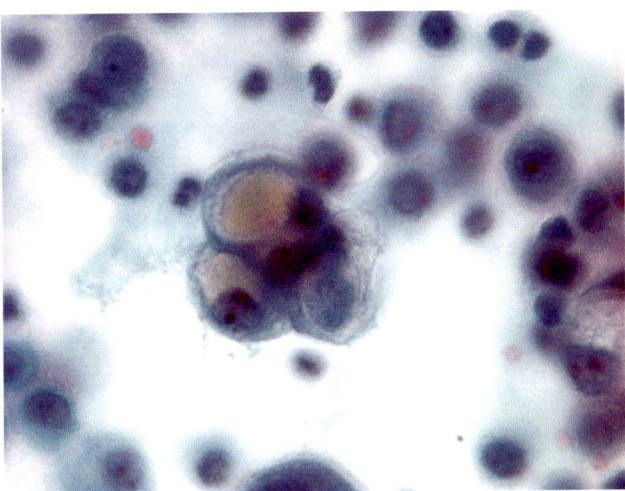

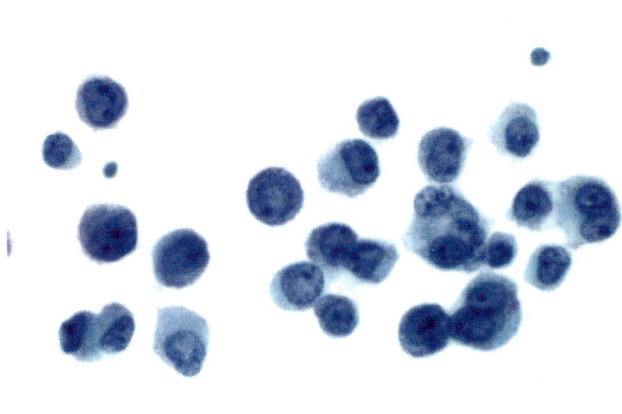

**Fig. 2.11** Lung ADC may rarely contain intracytoplasmic glycogen. However, contrary to mesothelioma, the glycogen occupies a diffuse area of the cytoplasm and may displace the nucleus rather than being in submembranous elongated vacuoles; PAP

**Fig. 2.9** Poorly differentiated lung ADC presenting as single malignant cells. The nuclei are eccentric in location and show hyperchromasia, irregular nuclear contours, and prominent nucleoli; PAP

although careful evaluation will reveal the presence of disfiguring large vacuoles elsewhere in the smear. ADC cells lack the characteristic two-tone cytoplasm and the submembranous glycogen vacuoles of mesothelial cells. Their nuclei tend to be eccentric rather than central and are more atypical than those of mesothelium.

2. *Malignant mesothelioma*: This differential presents itself whether the tumor manifests as single cells or as tight clusters in the background of large multinucleated cells (Fig. 2.13). Moreover, it is well-known that lung adenocarcinoma can grow along the pleural surface and present on radiographic evaluation primarily as pleural thickening rather than a parenchymal nodule [24]. However, the cells lack the features of mesothelial origin, and they present with significant cytological atypia rarely encountered in mesothelioma (Figs. 2.14 and 2.15). While the

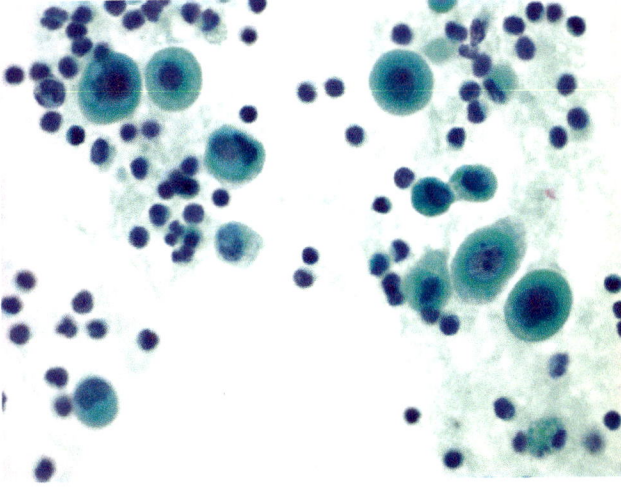

**Fig. 2.12** Lung ADC presenting as few discohesive single cells with mild cytological atypia that could be mistaken for reactive mesothelial cells; PAP

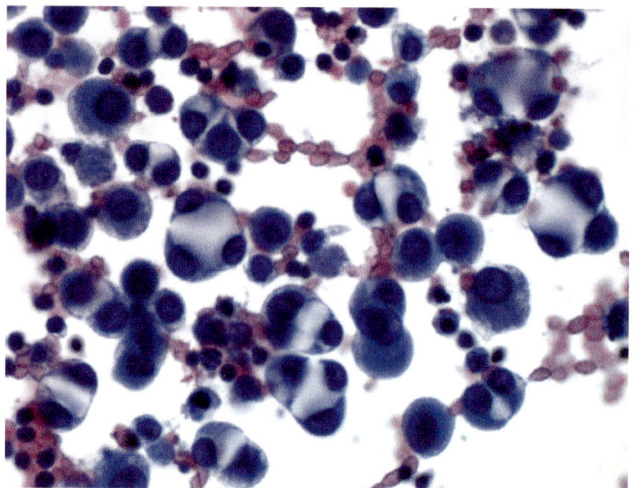

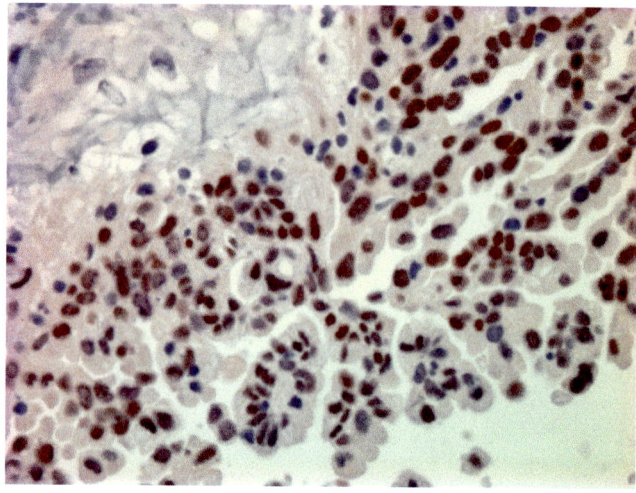

**Fig. 2.13** Cellular effusion from a patient who radiologically had a thickened pleural rind. The cells are arranged as short rows and small clusters with intercellular spaces mimicking windows, a pattern that can be easily mistaken for mesothelioma. However, notice that the spaces are actually intracytoplasmic vacuoles. The cells are obviously atypical and do not have the otherwise characteristic features of mesothelial origin; PAP

**Fig. 2.15** Correlating pleura-based ADC showing positive nuclear reaction with TTF-1 confirming the pulmonary ADC origin

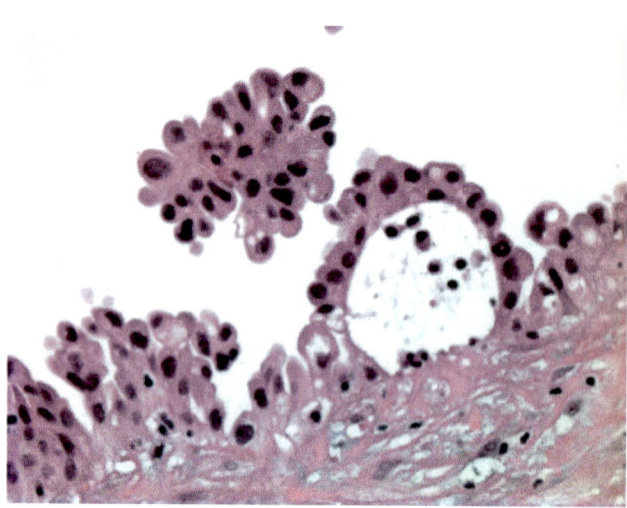

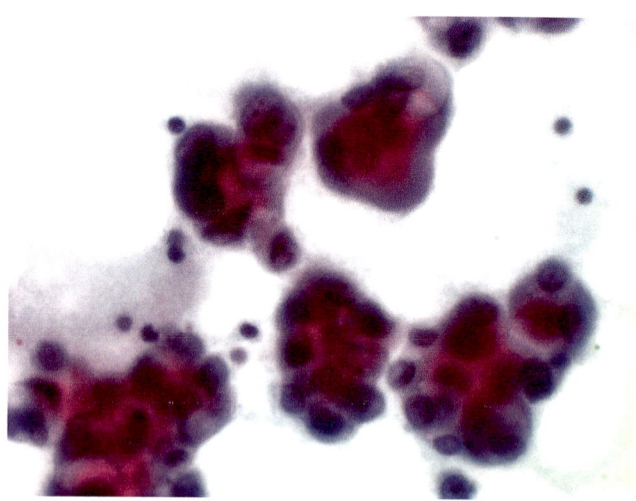

**Fig. 2.16** ADC of the breast presenting as medium-sized clusters in a pleural effusion. Clinical history and immunostains are essential to resolve the differential with lung ADC; PAP

**Fig. 2.14** Correlating pleural biopsy reveals a cellular pleura-based proliferation. The cells were negative for calretinin and D2-40 and positive for traditional ADC markers; H&E

presence of large multinucleated cells is a common feature, adenocarcinoma lacks the monotonous cytology and the wide range of cell size characteristically seen in mesothelioma.

3. *Other adenocarcinomas*: When presenting as tightly cohesive clusters, lung ADC may be difficult to distinguish from breast carcinoma (Fig. 2.16), carcinoma of Müllerian origin (particularly ovarian serous carcinoma), and in rare occasions carcinoma of the gastrointestinal tract (GIT) (Fig. 2.17). When presenting as single cells, the differential should include GIT, especially gastric carcinoma and breast carcinoma (Fig. 2.18). Ancillary tests are usually required to establish the primary origin.

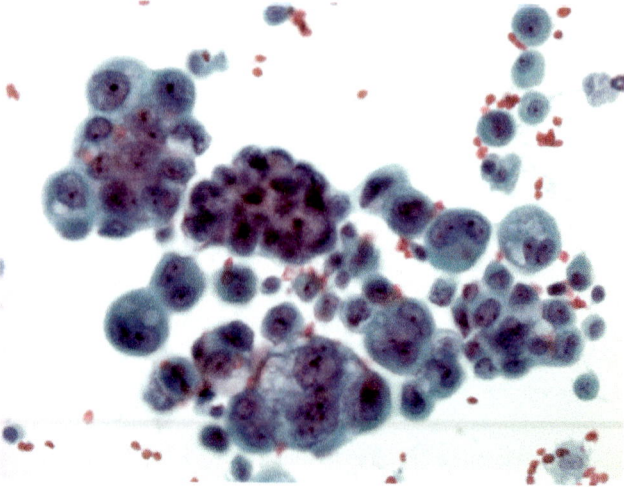

**Fig. 2.17** ADC of the pancreas presenting as clusters very similar to those of pulmonary ADC; PAP

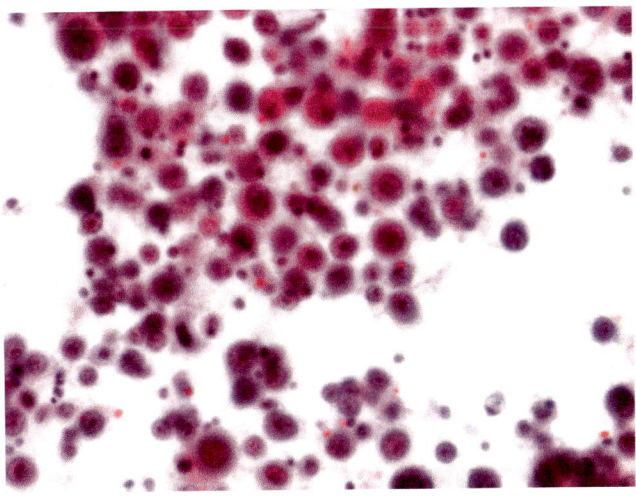

**Fig. 2.18** Gastroesophageal ADC presenting as single abnormal cells very similar to the poorly differentiated lung ADC; PAP

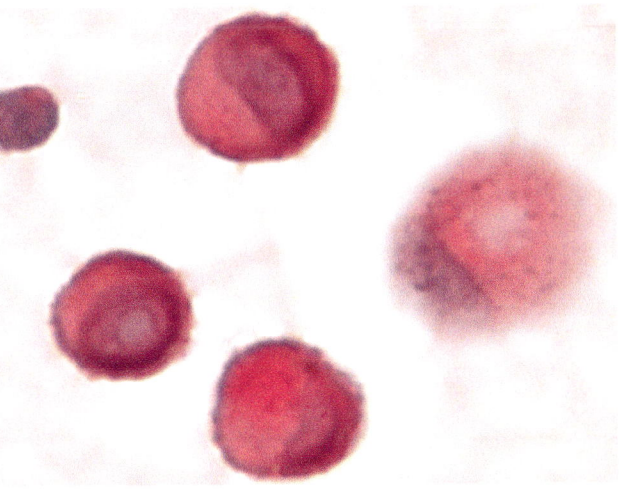

**Fig. 2.19** Intracytoplasmic mucin can be detected in about 50% of lung ADC; mucicarmine stain

## Ancillary Tests

In selecting the panel of immunostains, one should consider which differential is in question. Some immunostains will serve to differentiate ADC from mesothelioma or reactive mesothelium, and these should include stains that confirm the epithelial identity of the tumor and those that exclude the diagnosis or, in other words, confirm a mesothelial origin. Other stains are used to confirm pulmonary origin and should be selected as a complement to the panel once ADC is confirmed. Kaur et al. confirmed the value of morphologic assessment combined with immunostains in evaluating pleural fluids from patients suspected of lung carcinoma and found that it had comparable results with biopsy samples for the diagnosis and subclassification of lung carcinoma even in cases where radiology failed to identify the definitive lung lesion [25].

## Tests Useful in Confirming the Diagnosis of ADC

### Mucin-Directed Stains

Both mucicarmine and PAS-D can be used to detect neutral mucin. Lung adenocarcinoma was reported to have intracytoplasmic mucin in about 50% of cases, while mesothelioma is negative for mucin [26, 27]. Mucicarmine was reported to be less sensitive than PAS-D (Fig. 2.19).

### ADC Markers [27–32]

*Epithelial membrane antigen (EMA)*: It is directed against polymorphic epithelial mucins and is generally positive in carcinoma and mesothelioma. However, in carcinoma, it tends to exhibit diffuse strong cytoplasmic staining, while in

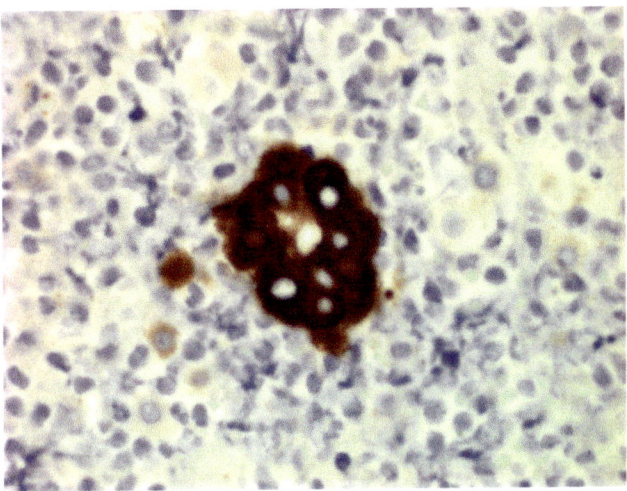

**Fig. 2.20** Lung ADC showing diffuse cytoplasmic staining with EMA

mesothelioma, it shows a distinctive margination at the brush border (Figs. 2.20 and 2.21).

*Carcinoembryonic antigen (CEA)*: It is among the most extensively studied antigens and reported to react with the majority of lung ADC (Fig. 2.22). Its reactivity varies widely depending on the clone used, and positive staining was reported in up to 30% of mesotheliomas in the old literature. However, this does not hold true with the use of newer clones, and it is believed to be negative in the majority of mesotheliomas, according to the more recent literature.

*B72.3*: It recognizes a tumor-associated glycoprotein (TAG-72) and is present in a wide range of ADC. It was reported to stain between 44 and 85% of lung ADC and may exhibit weak reaction in up to 20% of mesotheliomas (Fig. 2.23).

*Ber-EP4*: It is directed against 34 and 39 kDa glycoproteins present on the cell membrane of most epithelial cells. It

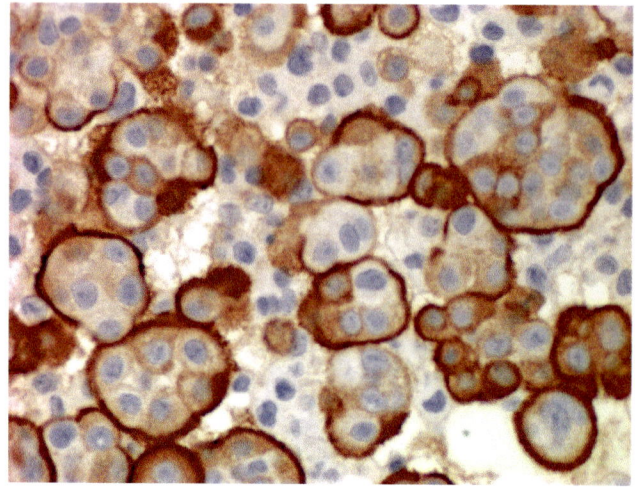

**Fig. 2.21** Mesotheliomas positively react with EMA. However, contrary to ADC, the staining has distinctive margination at the brush border

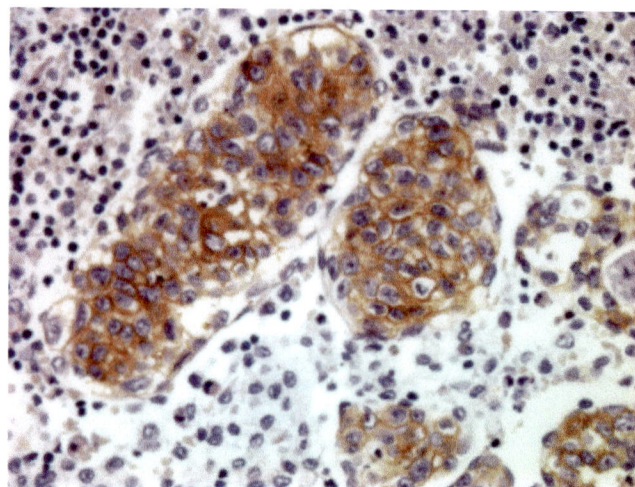

**Fig. 2.24** Lung ADC showing membranous staining for Ber-EP4

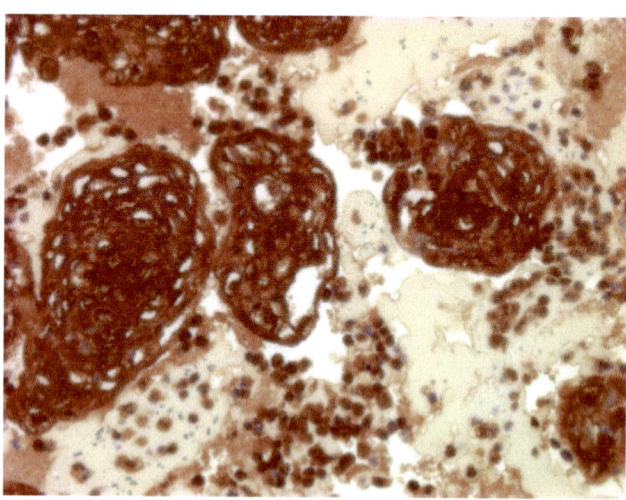

**Fig. 2.22** Lung ADC showing diffuse cytoplasmic staining for CEA

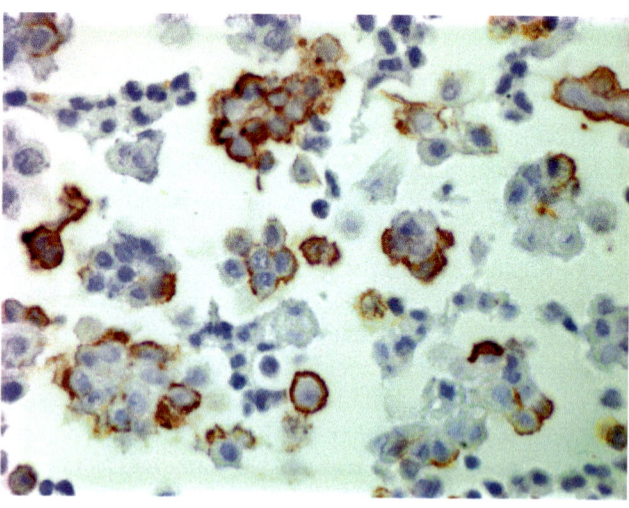

**Fig. 2.25** Lung ADC showing membranous staining with the MOC-31 antibody

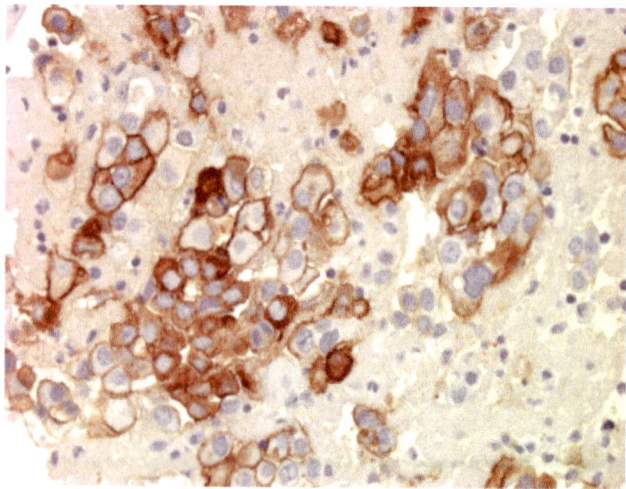

**Fig. 2.23** Lung ADC showing positive membranous reaction with the B72.3 antibody

was reported to stain between 60% and 100% of lung ADC (Fig. 2.24). It may stain up to 27% of mesotheliomas. However, the staining tends to have a focal pattern.

*MOC-31*: It reacts with a 38 kDa glycoprotein present on the cell membrane of epithelial cells and was reported to stain 67% of lung ADC (Fig. 2.25). Similar to Ber-EP4, it may stain focally in up to 10% of mesotheliomas. Lv et al. evaluated the potential use of combined MOC-31 and calretinin in the work-up of patients suspected of lung carcinoma. MOC-31 was expressed in 90.2% of pleural fluids with lung cancer and 2.9% from patients with benign lung disease, while calretinin was expressed in 87% of benign lung effusions and 6.5% in effusions with lung cancer with a combined sensitivity of 100% and specificity of 98.6% [33].

*CD15 (Leu-M1)*: It belongs to the cluster designation 15 and was found to recognize many ADC. It is reported to recognize the majority of lung adenocarcinomas, although it is believed to be less sensitive in effusions than in histological sections [28, 34]. It rarely reacts with mesothelioma.

*Blood group-related antigens*: These antigens were found in cells other than erythrocytes. Earlier studies showed that mesotheliomas do not express these antigens, while many ADC do. The BG-8 antibody, directed against Lewis$^y$ blood group antigen, was extensively studied and reported to react with 90–100% of pulmonary ADC and with less than 9% of mesotheliomas [35, 36]. On the other hand, CA19-9, a sialylated Lewis antigen, is commonly expressed in pancreatic, gastrointestinal, and ovarian ADC but is less sensitive for pulmonary ADC, reacting with only 35–57% of tumors [37].

*E-cadherin and N-cadherin*: These are transmembrane glycoproteins that mediate calcium-dependent intercellular adhesion. It is believed that E-cadherin detects a large number of pulmonary ADC but is negative in mesothelioma, while N-cadherin has the opposite profile. Studies of effusions have nevertheless shown less consistent results [38–40].

*CD138*: Syndecan-1 is a transmembrane heparan sulfate proteoglycan that is detected on the surface of plasma cells and epithelial cells. Saqi et al. evaluated its utility in the work-up of malignant effusions. CD138 was found to be expressed in a distinct membranous pattern without background staining (Fig. 2.26). Used in the separation of ADC from mesothelioma, CD138 was expressed in 55% of ADC and 8% of mesotheliomas, with 94% positive predictive value, 97% specificity, and 55% sensitivity. It stained 69% of the lung ADC. Other studies showed comparable results, with a range of 41–100% staining of pulmonary ADC [41–43].

*MUC4*: It belongs to the membrane-bound mucin family with MUC1 and MUC3. MUC4 is expressed early in the primitive gut and is commonly expressed in normal bronchial mucosa. Llinares et al. explored its utility in distinguishing pulmonary ADC from mesothelioma and reported

it to be 100% specific and 91.4% sensitive for lung carcinoma. However, it is important to remember that it may also be detected in extrapulmonary ADC [44].

## Markers Related to Pulmonary Origin

*Peripheral airway cell markers*: It has been noted that surfactant protein (SP-A) is detected in alveolar type II pneumocytes and Clara cells, while SP-C is only detected in type II pneumocytes, and CC10 is specific for Clara cell 10 kDa protein. Based on this, Takezawa and colleagues explored the utility of these markers in identifying pulmonary ADC in effusions and separating it from other neoplasms [45]. Among the 52 samples studied, 20 were lung ADC, 6 small cell carcinoma, 11 extrapulmonary carcinomas, and 15 benign effusions. SP-A positively reacted with 10/20 lung ADC, while 6/20 reacted with proSP-C. All 20 cases were negative to CC10. These markers were nonreactive with the remaining effusions.

*TTF-1*: Thyroid transcription factor 1 is a nuclear transcription factor expressed in the normal lung and thyroid and their malignant counterparts. It is highly expressed in both ADC and small cell carcinoma of the lung (Fig. 2.27). Studies of effusions have shown TTF-1 to have up to 92% sensitivity for separating lung ADC from mesothelioma, staining 61/66 cases, [46] and up to 100% specificity [47, 48]. Recently, TTF-1 has been reported to react focally with some extrapulmonary metastatic carcinomas, such as those of colon, gastric, and endometrial origin [49–51].

*Napsin A*: This is an aspartic protease involved in the N- and C-terminal processing of proSP-B expressed in type II pneumocytes. It was reported to be diagnostically superior to SP-A and was detected in up to 87.5% of lung ADC [52]. In a study by Dejmek et al., the authors compared Napsin A and TTF-1 in 50 pleural effusions, of which 12 cases were pulmonary ADC. Napsin A detected more cases than TTF-1 (10/12 vs. 8/12) and was noted to stain more cells per case

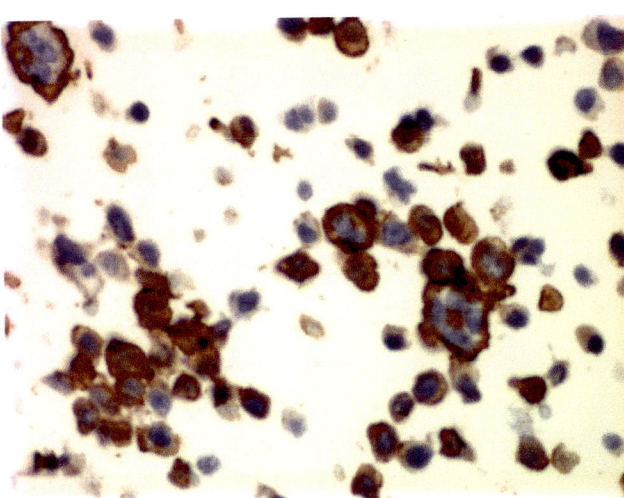

**Fig. 2.26** Lung ADC showing distinct membranous staining for CD138

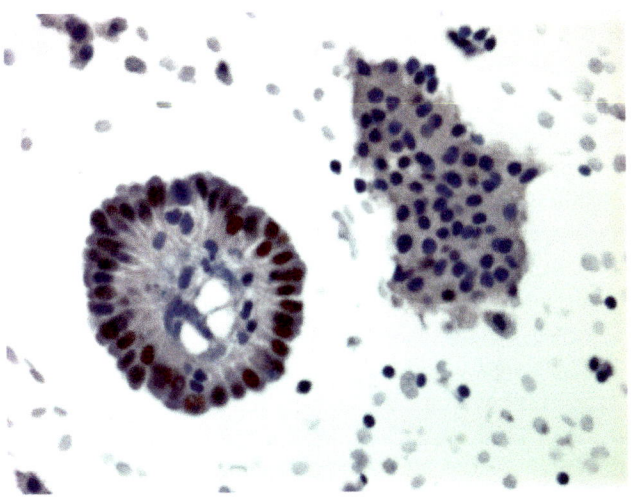

**Fig. 2.27** Lung ADC showing characteristic TTF-1 nuclear staining

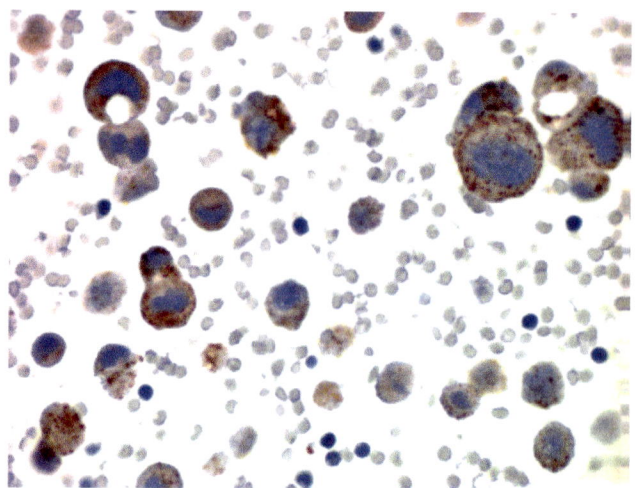

**Fig. 2.28** Lung ADC showing characteristic Napsin A granular cytoplasmic staining

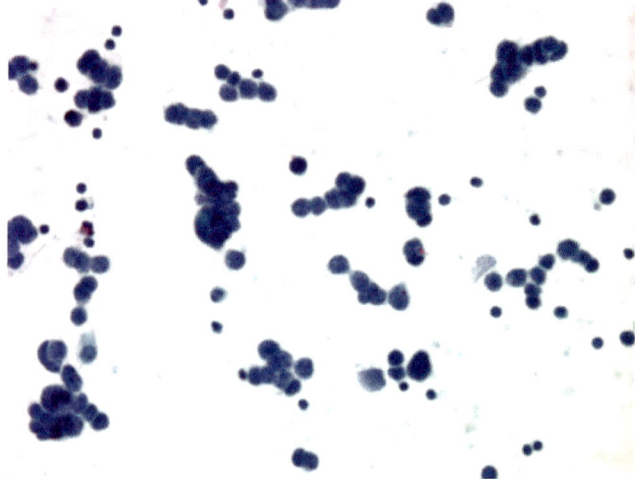

**Fig. 2.29** Smcc in a typical moderately cellular effusion. Notice the presence of short rows of cells and rare clusters. Within these rows, the cells have tight molding, throwing them at times into crescent shapes; PAP

(Fig. 2.28). The authors suggested that Napsin A could be particularly useful in cases with low cellularity [53]. El Hag et al. evaluated TTF-1 and Napsin A in the work-up of malignant effusions. They concluded that both Napsin A and TTF-1 performed well in distinguishing lung ADC from extrapulmonary metastatic ADC (EP-ADC). TTF-1 reacted with 65% of lung ADC and 1.8% of EP-ADC, while Napsin A reacted with 54% of lung ADC and was nonreactive with all EP-ADC. Interestingly, Napsin A reacted with 78% (7/9 cases) of the poorly differentiated cases, while only 45% (4/9 cases) were identified by TTF-1 [54].

*Cytokeratins 7 and 20*: These markers are not specific to pulmonary origin but play an important role in the differential with other primaries. Lung ADC is generally CK7-positive and CK20-negative [55]. It is important to recognize that mucinous ADC has the opposite profile [56].

## Small Cell Carcinoma (Smcc)

## Morphology

Smcc is rarely encountered in fluids, and studies have been published mainly in the form of case reports. The fluids are low to moderate in cellularity at best. The cells exfoliate mainly as single cells or small groups and tend to rapidly degenerate and therefore may be difficult to detect.

In well-preserved samples, the neoplastic cells are seen as small cords, long-arching cords, and small clusters and in rare cases as large clusters (Figs. 2.29 and 2.30).

The cells are relatively small, not exceeding the size of three resting lymphocytes, and have a high N/C ratio. Because fluids are a hospitable medium, more cytoplasm than traditionally seen for Smcc can be seen. The nuclei are

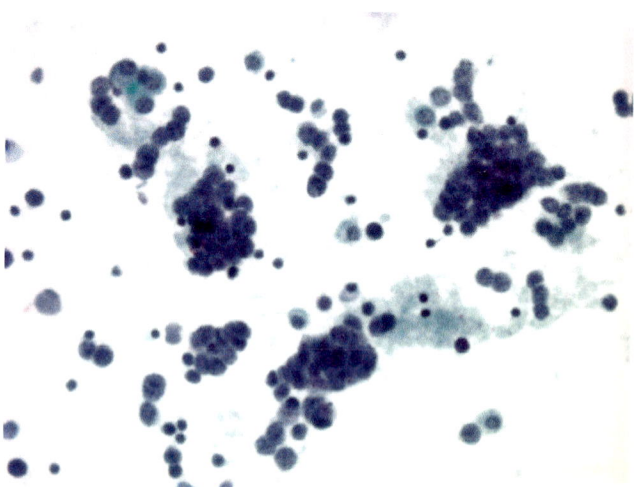

**Fig. 2.30** Rarely, Smcc effusions are cellular and present with cell clusters in addition to the cell cords. Notice the tight molding of cells within the clusters and almost lack of visible cytoplasm when compared to ADC; PAP

hyperchromatic, and the chromatin has a coarse granular quality, obscuring the nucleoli. Nuclear molding is very pronounced, and consequently the cellular cords appear stacked like the "vertebrae in the vertebral column" or "rouleau arrangement" (Fig. 2.31). Cellular clusters frequently show an "onion-ring arrangement" as the semilunar cells mold around a central round nucleus (Fig. 2.32). The nuclear shapes are widely variable with irregular, angulated, semilunar, biconcave, or rounded form. This variability is a result of the cells attempting to accommodate each other and each fitting snugly within the adjacent cell [57–62].

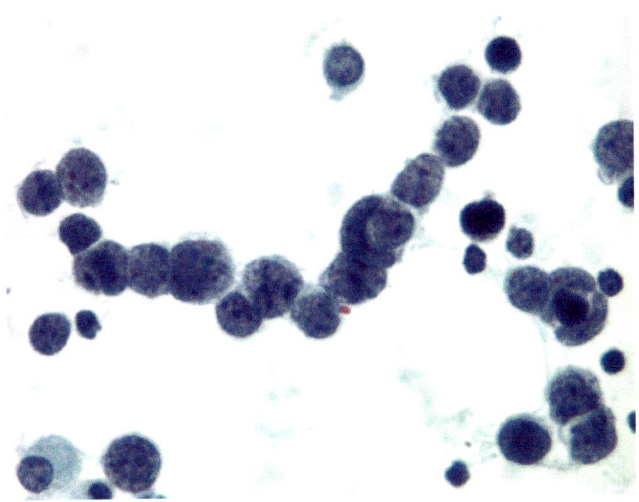

**Fig. 2.31** Smcc cells presenting as long-arching cords with a rouleau-like arrangement. Within the cord, the cells form a crescent shape as a result of the tight molding; PAP

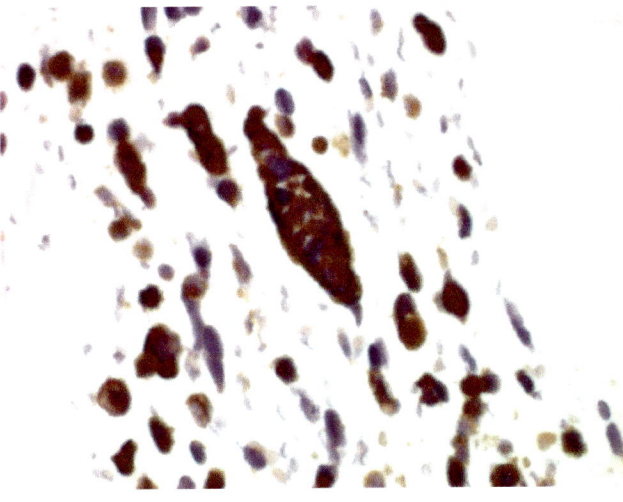

**Fig. 2.33** Smcc showing strong positive cytoplasmic reaction with pancytokeratin stain

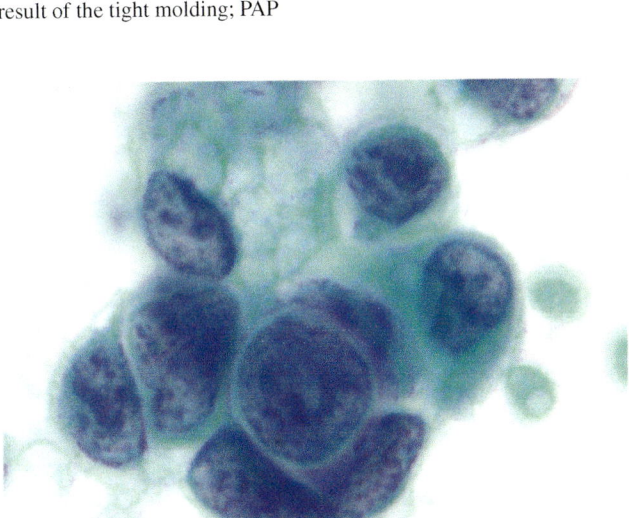

**Fig. 2.32** A small cluster of Smcc in which the tight molding results in crescent-like cells around a central rounded nucleus, forming an onion ring-like pattern; PAP

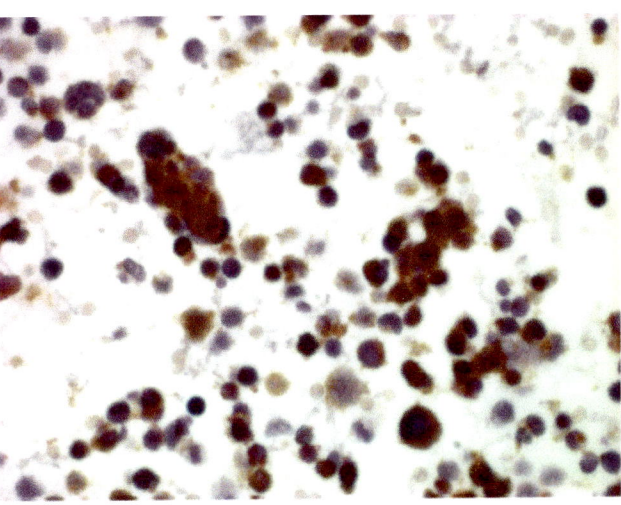

**Fig. 2.34** Smcc showing strong positive cytoplasmic reaction with cytokeratin 7 stain

## Ancillary Tests [63–65]

Despite the potential of Smcc to rapidly degenerate in fluids, it tends to retain its reactivity to immunomarkers.

*Cytokeratins*: Smcc is typically positive for the broad-spectrum antibody cytokeratin CAM5.2, as well as for CK8, CK18, CK5/6, CK7, and CK19. Staining is typically in a dot-like pattern. CK20, while commonly expressed in neuro-endocrine tumors of the skin, is expressed in less than 10% of Smcc of lung origin (Figs. 2.33 and 2.34).

*Neuroendocrine markers:* The combination of chromogranin, synaptophysin, and CD56 represents the best balance between sensitivity and specificity.

*Chromogranin A*: It is the major constituent of the secretory granules and is highly specific. However, its detection is directly proportional to the number of neurosecretory granules detected by electron microscopy and consequently is not easily detected in Smcc (Fig. 2.35).

*Synaptophysin*: It is a calcium-binding glycoprotein that is an integral membrane constituent of the neuronal synaptic vesicles and therefore, while not specific, is highly sensitive and can detect Smcc with sparse granules (Fig. 2.36).

*Neuron-specific enolase (NSE)*: This is a gamma-dimeric form of an enzyme that is present in the cells of the diffuse neuroendocrine system. While this marker is very sensitive, it lacks specificity due to cross-reactivity between gamma-dimers and heterodimers (Fig. 2.37).

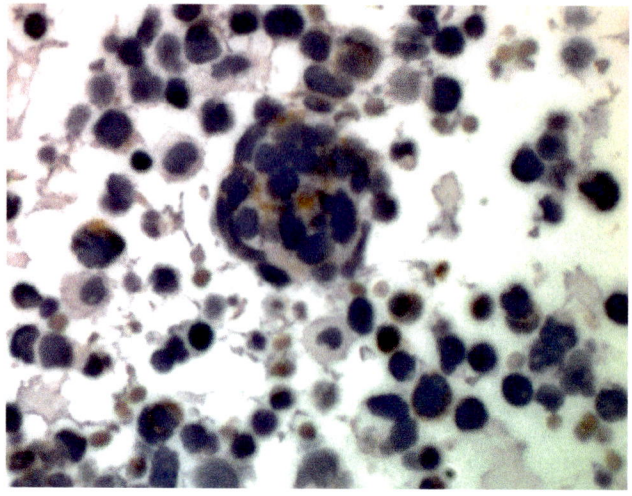

**Fig. 2.35** Smcc showing focal positive reaction with chromogranin A stain

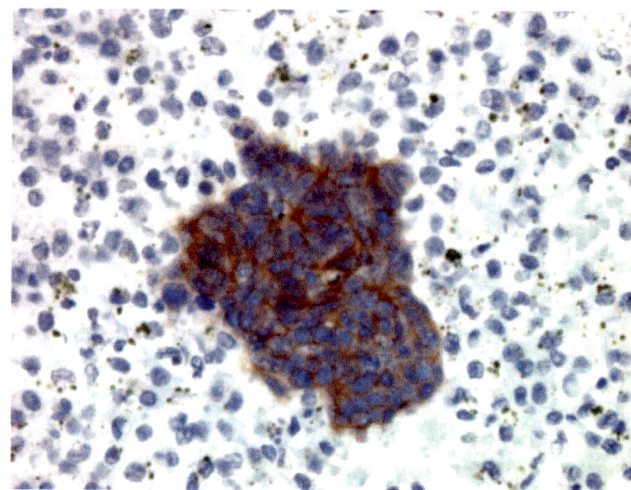

**Fig. 2.38** Smcc showing distinct cytoplasmic staining for CD56

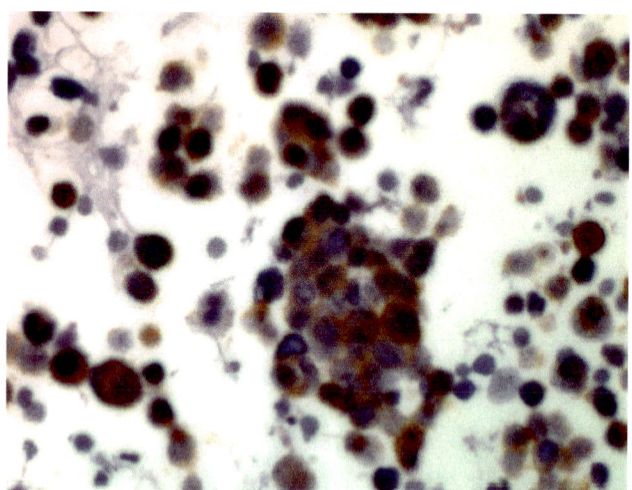

**Fig. 2.36** Smcc showing positive synaptophysin staining

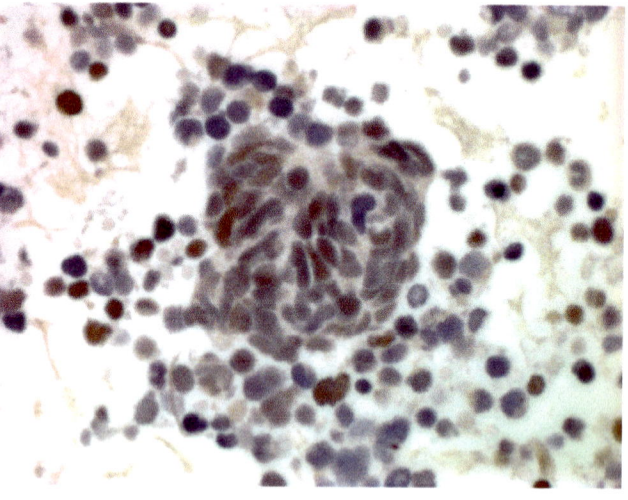

**Fig. 2.39** Smcc showing strong positive nuclear reaction for TTF-1

*CD56*: This is a member of the neural cell adhesion molecule family and, though not specific for neuroendocrine tumors, has been reported to stain 95–100% of pulmonary Smcc (Fig. 2.38). Positive reaction has also been reported in neuroendocrine tumors of extrapulmonary origin, including ovarian, endometrial, and renal tumors.

*Thyroid transcription factor 1 (TTF-1)*: This has been reported to stain up to 94% of pulmonary Smcc (Fig. 2.39). Positive reaction has also been reported infrequently in extrapulmonary Smcc, including tumors of salivary gland, cervical, and urinary bladder origin.

## Differential Diagnosis

The differential would include other small blue cell tumors:

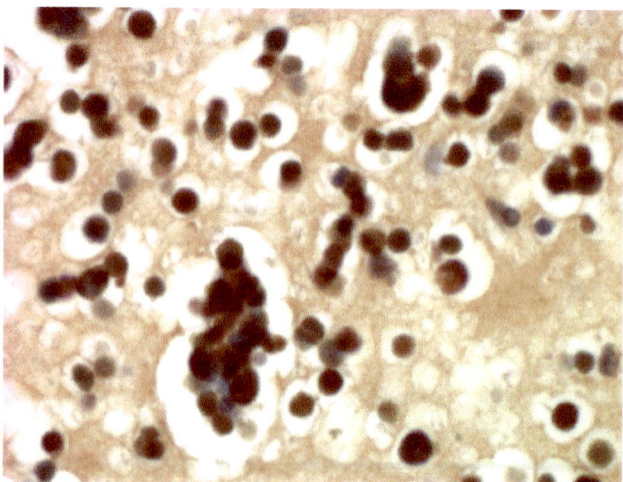

**Fig. 2.37** Smcc showing strong cytoplasmic NSE staining

*Lymphocytosis and lymphoma*: Lymphocytes tend to present as single cells and lack the linear arrangement and tight molding so characteristic of Smcc. The cells are usually monomorphic in appearance and may have a skirt of blue cytoplasm, nuclear grooves, or nucleoli depending on the type of lymphoma. The nuclei are rounded and lack the angulated and semilunar shapes seen in Smcc. Immunostaining and flow cytometry are helpful in confirming the lymphocytic origin and monoclonality.

*Small blue round cell tumors*: These include Ewing's sarcoma/primitive neuroectodermal tumor, rhabdomyosarcoma, Wilms' tumor, and neuroblastoma. These tumors rarely present as effusions without a known primary, and the clinical history is therefore essential in the differential. Morphologically, they all present as single cells or small groups of round to oval cells with scant cytoplasm and high N/C ratio. However, they lack the linear arrangement, onion-ring pattern, and extensive molding of Smcc. With the exception of neuroblastoma, which stains positively with neuroendocrine markers, all these tumors are negative for all the markers described above.

*Extrapulmonary small cell carcinoma*: These may be morphologically indistinguishable from the pulmonary ones. Luckily, they are extremely rare in effusions and usually have a known history of the primary site. Cutaneous tumors, i.e., Merkel cell tumor, stain in a dot-like pattern with CK20, which is traditionally negative in pulmonary Smcc. TTF-1 tends to stain the majority of the pulmonary Smcc and is less frequently expressed by Smcc of extrapulmonary origin.

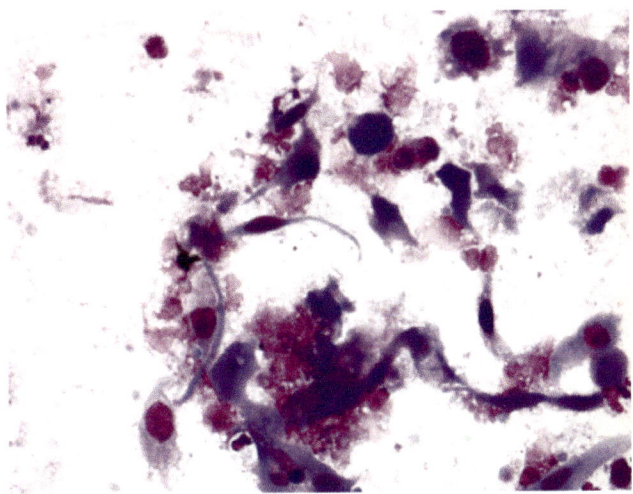

**Fig. 2.40** Well-differentiated keratinizing Sqcc presenting as spindled, tadpole, and polygonal cells. The cytoplasm has the classic robin blue color characteristic of keratinizing cells, and the nuclei are hyperchromatic; Diff-Quik

mainly in the third-type cells. Keratinization may be evident (Figs. 2.40 and 2.41).

With less differentiation, the fluids may become more cellular and consist predominantly of third-type cells. The malignant cells manifest mainly as large flat sheets or cellular spheres and therefore could easily be confused with ADC or mesothelioma (Fig. 2.42). Frequently, these clusters exhibit a swirling pattern reminiscent of squamous eddies and appear two-dimensional. Contrary to ADC, the borders of these cellular groups are rarely smooth, but rather undulating and frequently appear as if they are budding (Fig. 2.43).

The poorly differentiated third-type cells are usually rounded and have dense refractile cyanophilic cytoplasm. The cell border is well defined. Keratinization normally occurs from the periphery of the cytoplasm inward toward the nucleus. However, in these less differentiated cells, keratinization tends to abruptly stop midway (abnormal keratinization) and consequently result in refractile rings as if successive zones of keratinization are occurring which create an endo-ectoplasmic demarcation (Figs. 2.44 and 2.45). The endo-ectoplasmic border can be ruffled or thrown into linear folds and when viewed in stretched cells appear as spirals, also known as "Herxheimer's spirals."

In the background, it is common to see cells within cells, as well as small groups of two or more cells that tightly swirl around each other in an attempt to form squamous pearls (Fig. 2.46). Sometimes, the cells stack in long cords with an appearance similar to the vertebrae in the vertebral column (Fig. 2.47). However, contrary to Smcc, the cells do not mold around each other, instead being flattened where they oppose each other in a manner that mimics cell windows, but without a space. This appearance is most likely the result of opposing cell junctions [67–70].

## Squamous Cell Carcinoma (Sqcc)

### Morphology

Metastatic Sqcc in effusions is exceedingly rare. The largest series published is a bi-institutional study of 46 cases collected from a total of 9297 effusions covering a period of 33 years [66]. Pulmonary Sqcc was the most common origin and contributed 13/34 pleural and 2/4 pericardial fluid samples, but only 1/8 peritoneal samples. Morphologically, there are no specific features that would discriminate pulmonary from extrapulmonary Sqcc [66].

Well-differentiated keratinizing Sqcc are usually low in cellularity but easily recognized. A variety of squamous shapes can be detected, including tadpole cells, which are elongated with a bulbous end containing the nucleus; fiber cells, which are spindled in shape and contain central elongated nuclei; third-type cells, which are rounded with dense refractile cytoplasm that may stain eosinophilic or cyanophilic; and polygonal cells and anucleated squames reminiscent to those seen in cervical smears. The nuclei are hyperchromatic, and prominent nucleoli tend to be visible,

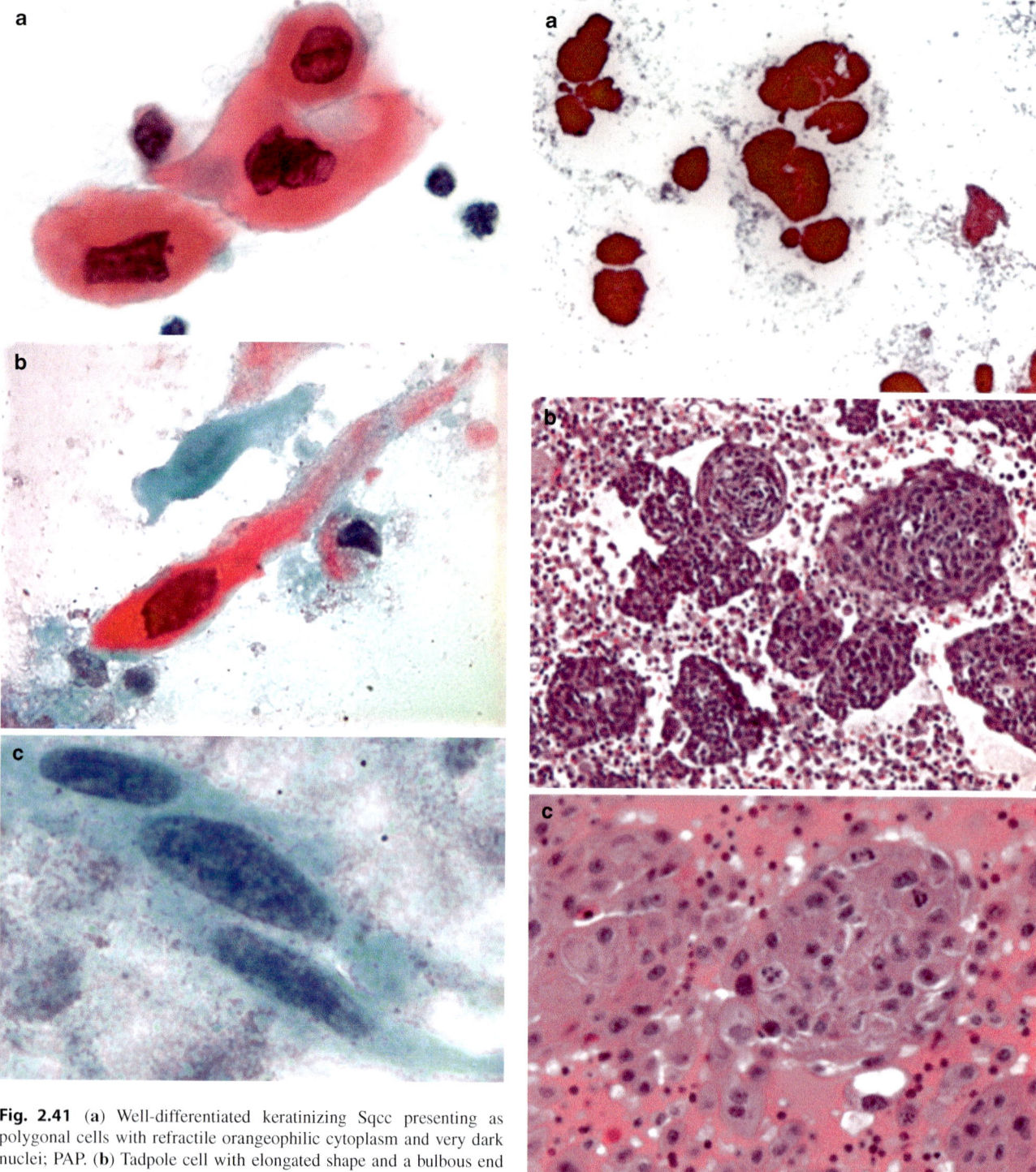

**Fig. 2.41** (**a**) Well-differentiated keratinizing Sqcc presenting as polygonal cells with refractile orangeophilic cytoplasm and very dark nuclei; PAP. (**b**) Tadpole cell with elongated shape and a bulbous end containing the nucleus. Notice the polychromatic staining of the cytoplasm; PAP. (**c**) Fiber cells are spindled in shape and contain central elongated nuclei; PAP

Despite the characteristically dense cytoplasm, it is not unusual to see cytoplasmic vacuoles, mainly in the single cells and small clusters. Although fine vacuoles may be seen, vacuoles tend to be large and disfiguring, as in ADC (Figs. 2.48 and 2.49).

**Fig. 2.42** (**a**) Moderately differentiated Sqcc presenting as large irregular cellular groups. Although at first glance these groups appear very similar to spheres seen in ADC or mesothelioma, in Sqcc they tend to be much larger and to have irregular shapes; PAP. (**b**) Corresponding cell block showing numerous cellular groups/spheres with evidence of swirling reminiscent of squamous eddies. Notice the well-defined cell borders within the cellular groups in contrast to the syncytial appearance traditionally seen in ADC; PAP. (**c**) High magnification of the cell block showing the distinct cell borders and intercellular junctions indicative of the squamous nature of these cells; PAP

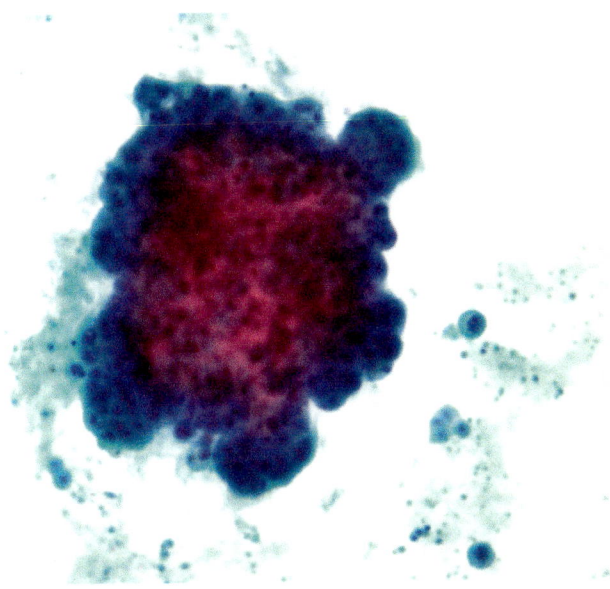

**Fig. 2.43** In contrast to ADC and mesothelioma, this cell group from Sqcc has a very undulating circumference and appears as if there are budding clusters sprouting from the surface; PAP

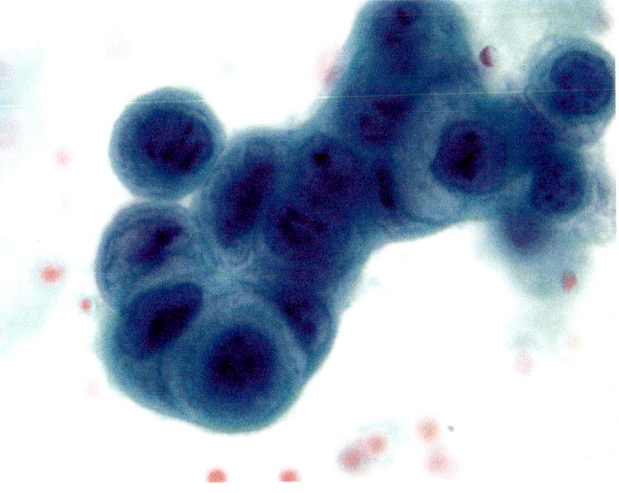

**Fig. 2.45** Cell cluster from a poorly differentiated Sqcc distinctly showing well-defined borders and a central refractile wavy line corresponding to the "Herxheimer's spirals"; PAP

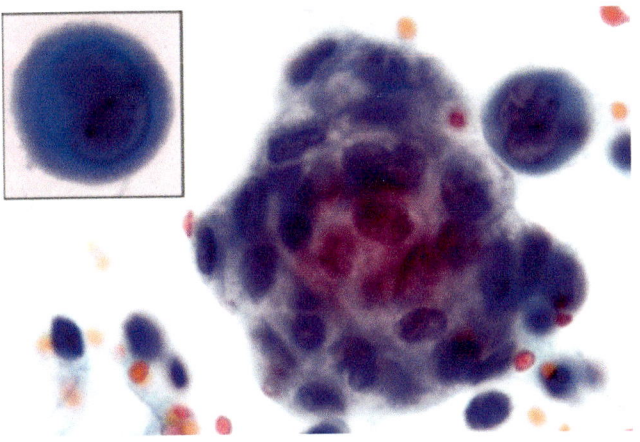

**Fig. 2.44** Third-type cells in clusters and as single cells are rounded cells with basophilic cytoplasm and well-defined cell borders. The two-tone cytoplasm has a well-defined refractile central line corresponding to the immature abnormal keratinization; PAP. *Inset* shows a higher magnification of a single cell; PAP

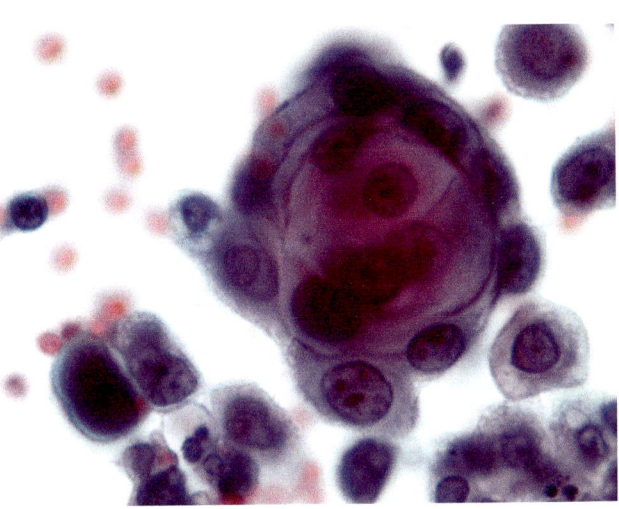

**Fig. 2.46** Small groups of cells tightly wrapped around each other attempting to form squamous pearls; PAP

## Differential Diagnosis

1. *Malignant mesothelioma*: Sqcc can be easily confused with mesothelioma. The cells have an endo-ectoplasmic demarcation, tend to whorl around each other mimicking cellular clasping, and form cell rows with cellular connections that mimic windows. However, closer examination will reveal that the two-tone cytoplasm in squamous cells is the reverse of that seen in mesothelial cells and that cell borders are distinct and dense rather than the fine submembranous vacuoles or brush border of the mesothelium. While mesothelioma rarely exhibits definitive malignant features, Sqcc is usually obviously atypical with abnormal nuclear features and numerous mitotic figures.

2. *ADC*: The large cellular groups and scattered cells with cytoplasmic vacuoles may resemble ADC. However, rather than the syncytial appearance typically seen in ADC, the cell borders within the clusters are typically well defined. Examination at low magnification reveals a swirling appearance within these clusters which is reminiscent of squamous eddies.

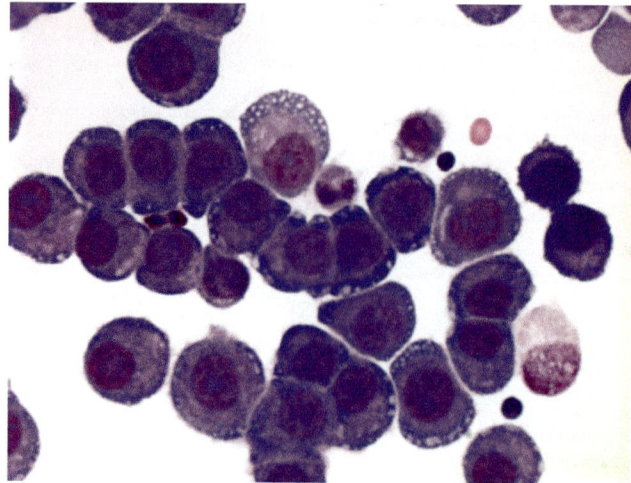

**Fig. 2.47** Sqcc may form long twisted cords which should not be mistaken with those of mesothelioma. In Sqcc, the opposing cell surfaces have flat rather than the biconcave surface seen in mesothelial cell windows, and a real space is seldom seen. The cells have obvious malignant features, in contrast to the usual bland appearance of mesothelioma; Diff-Quik stain

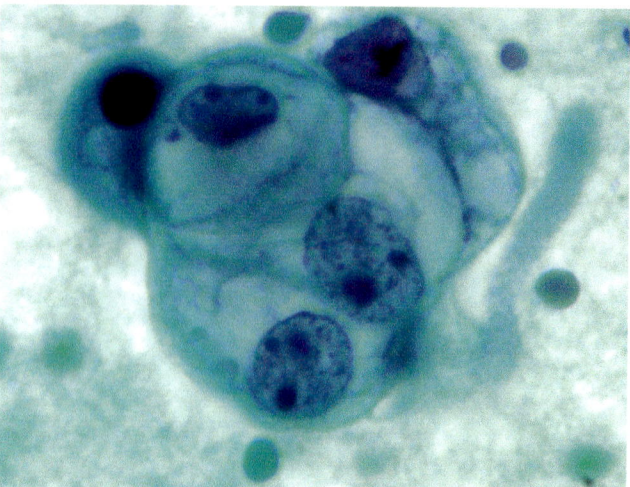

**Fig. 2.49** Small groups of Sqcc with cytoplasmic vacuoles mimicking ADC. These vacuolated cells are usually a minority population; PAP

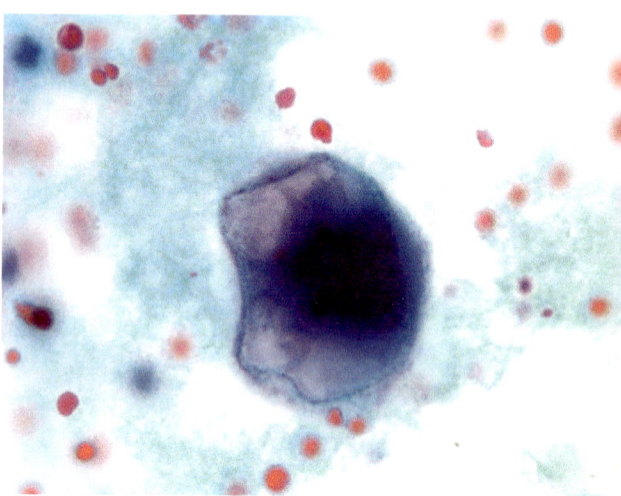

**Fig. 2.48** Large and sometimes disfiguring cytoplasmic vacuoles may be seen in effusions of Sqcc, especially in single cells; PAP

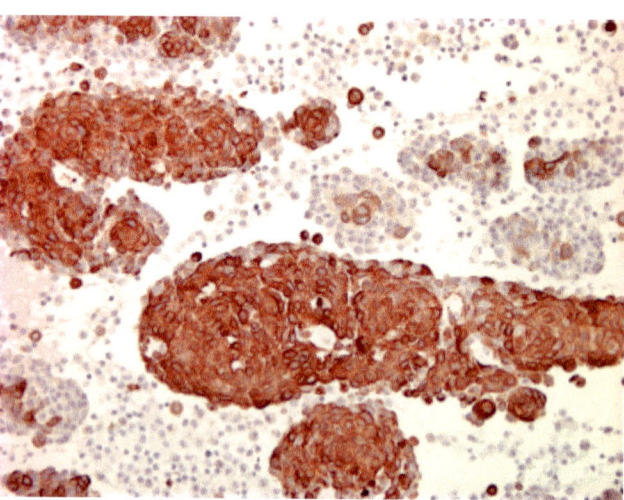

**Fig. 2.50** Sqcc clusters showing diffuse strong cytoplasmic staining for cytokeratin 5/6

## Ancillary Tests [71–76]

Sqcc reacts with many of the markers used to identify ADC and mesothelioma, and therefore, a panel of stains should always be utilized and judiciously interpreted. In pleural fluids, the differential includes mainly lung ADC and mesothelioma, while in peritoneal fluids the differential should include ovarian ADC. ADC of other body sites that traditionally present as cellular clusters, such as breast carcinoma, would enter the differential diagnosis depending on the patient's history.

## Mesothelial Markers

*Podoplanin*: reportedly expressed in up to 50% of Sqcc, between 86 and 100% of mesotheliomas, and up to 15% of serous ovarian carcinomas.

*Calretinin*: one of the best markers for mesothelioma but can be expressed in 6–10% of lung ADC and up to 40% of Sqcc.

*Keratins 5 and 6*: generally expressed as strong and diffuse reaction in Sqcc; also highly expressed in mesothelioma (up to 93%) and in about 10% of lung ADC (Fig. 2.50).

*Cytokeratin 7*: expressed in both mesothelioma and lung ADC, but only in about 20–50% of Sqcc.

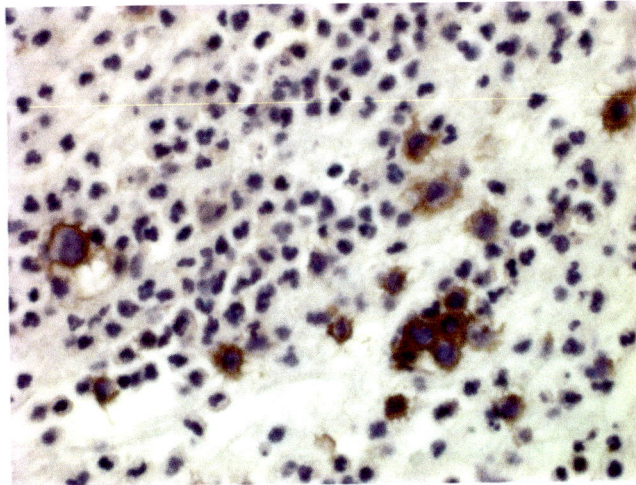

**Fig. 2.51** Sqcc presenting as single cells positively reacting with the thrombomodulin antibody

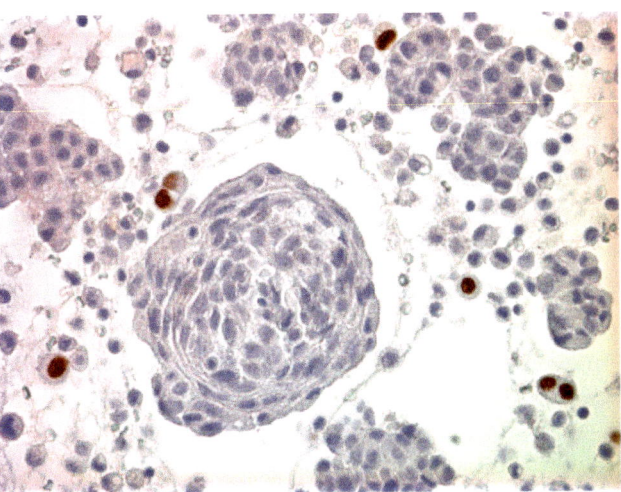

**Fig. 2.53** Sqcc clusters are completely negative for WT1, which is strongly staining the background mesothelial cells

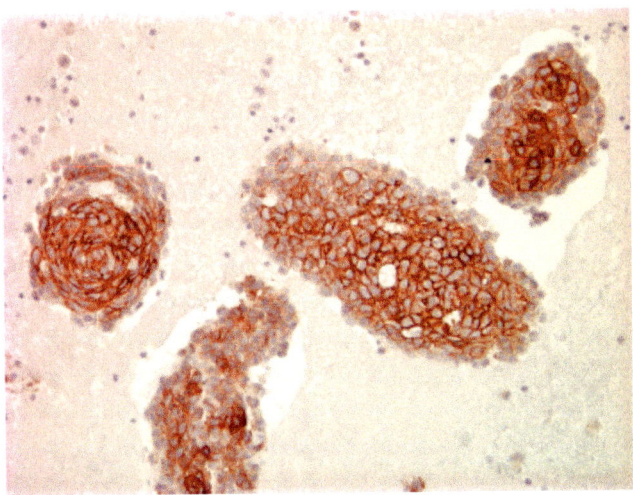

**Fig. 2.52** Sqcc clusters staining positive for mesothelin

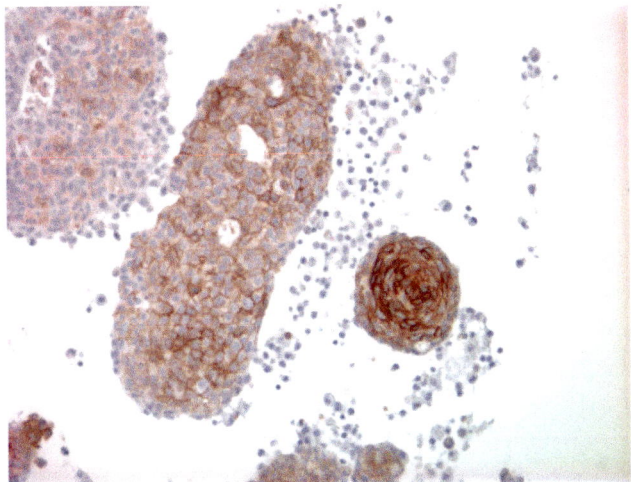

**Fig. 2.54** Sqcc clusters showing distinct membranous staining with the MOC-31 antibody

*Thrombomodulin:* not useful in the differential diagnosis, as it is reportedly expressed in 34–100% of mesotheliomas, the majority of Sqcc, and 5–77% of ADC (Fig. 2.51).

*Mesothelin:* can be expressed in up to 100% of mesotheliomas but was also reported to stain about 40% of lung ADC and 27% of lung Sqcc. However, the staining in the latter two is usually cytoplasmic and focal, while in mesothelioma, the reaction occurs along the cell membrane. Mesothelin has been reported to stain ADC of extrapulmonary sites (Fig. 2.52).

*WT1:* very useful in this differential, since it is consistently negative in Sqcc and lung ADC but reportedly expressed in 43–93% of mesotheliomas. Of note, it is additionally expressed in 83–100% of ovarian serous ADC. It is therefore very useful as a confirmatory negative marker for Sqcc (Fig. 2.53).

## Epithelial Markers

*MOC-31:* It reacts with up to 97% of Sqcc, 90–100% of lung ADC, and 98% of ovarian serous ADC. In contrast, only 2–10% of mesotheliomas express MOC-31 (Fig. 2.54).

*Ber-EP4:* It is expressed in up to 87% of Sqcc, 100% of lung and ovarian ADC, and 13–18% of mesotheliomas.

*Carcinoembryonic antigen (CEA):* It is reportedly expressed in up to 77% of Sqcc, although in the author's experience, Sqcc is not that frequently positive. It is expressed in 50–100% of lung ADC, but mesothelioma and ovarian ADC are virtually negative (Fig. 2.55).

*B72.3:* The reported reactivity for Sqcc ranged between 45 and 84%. It is also highly expressed in 75–85% of lung

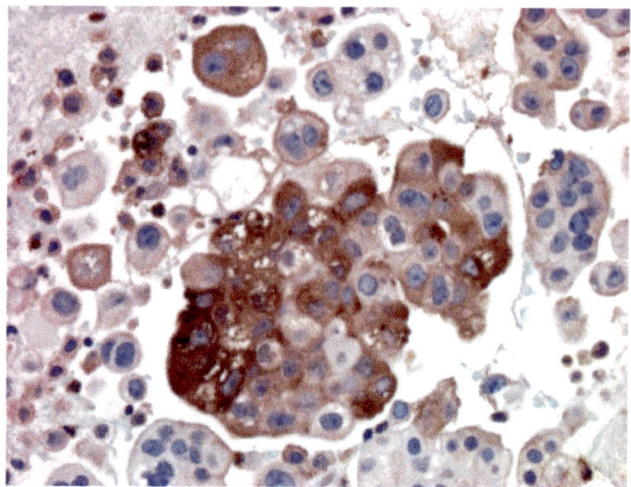

**Fig. 2.55** Sqcc clusters showing cytoplasmic positive reaction for CEA

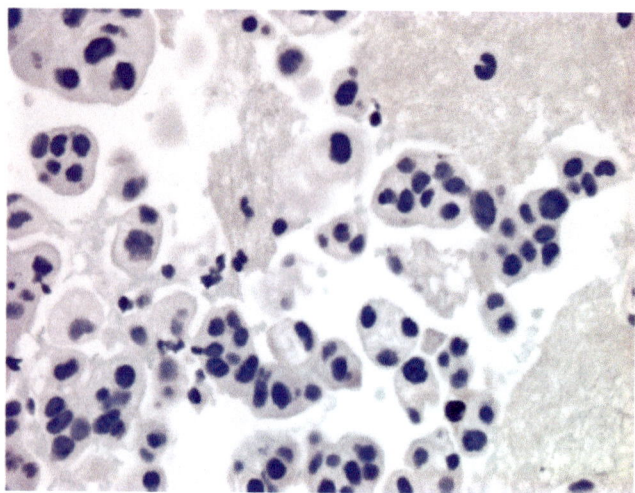

**Fig. 2.57** Sqcc clusters are nonreactive with TTF-1

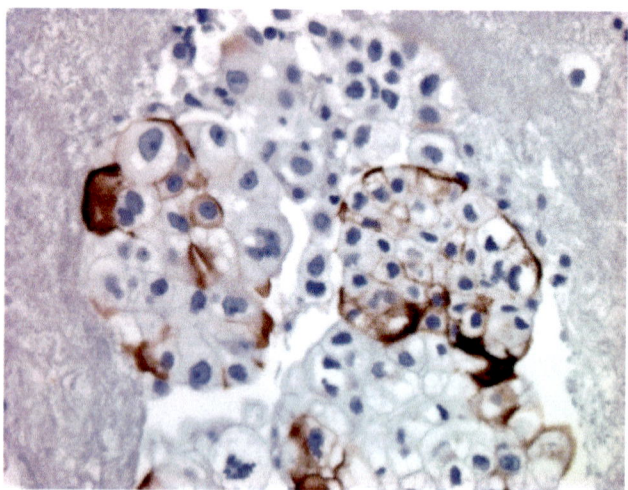

**Fig. 2.56** Sqcc clusters showing focal cytoplasmic and membranous staining for B72.3

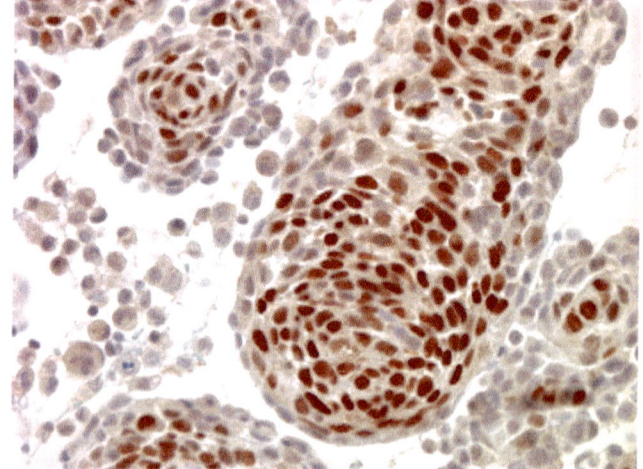

**Fig. 2.58** Sqcc clusters showing distinct nuclear reaction for p63

and up to 75% of ovarian ADC. It is usually negative in mesothelioma (Fig. 2.56).

*BG-8*: Up to 83% of Sqcc are positive, as well as 89–100% of lung ADC and 73% of ovarian ADC, compared to only 3–7% of mesotheliomas.

*Leu-M1 (CD15)*: It has no value in the differential diagnosis between Sqcc and ADC since it is expressed in about 30% of Sqcc compared to 50–70% of lung ADC and 30–60% of ovarian ADC. It is rarely expressed in mesothelioma.

## Other Markers

*TTF-1*: expressed in up to 75% of lung ADC but invariably negative in mesothelioma and Sqcc (Fig. 2.57).

*p63 and p40*: expressed as strong nuclear staining in 80–100% of Sqcc but rarely expressed in mesothelioma or

lung ADC. It is therefore very useful as a confirmatory positive marker for Sqcc (Fig. 2.58). Bishop et al. reported that p40 is superior to p63 in a tissue-based study, staining no more than 5% of cells in rare ADC, while p63 stained up to 26% of ADC [76]. A recent cytology study disputed these results in effusions and reported that in 20 effusions with lung ADC, p40 positively reacted with 40% of cases, while p63 reacted with only 15% [77].

## References

1. Ferlay J, Soerjonataram I, Ervik M, Dikshit R, Eser S, Mathers C, Rebelo M, Parkin DM, Forman D, Bray F. GLOBOCAN 2012 v1.1 cancer incidence and mortality worldwide: IARC CancerBase No. 11 [Internet]. Lyon: International Agency for Research on Cancer; 2014. http://globocan.iarc.fr. Accessed 16 Jan 2015.
2. Howlader N, Noone AM, Krapcho M, Miller D, Bishop K, Kosary CL, Yu M, Ruhl J, Tatalovich Z, Mariotto A, Lewis DR, Chen HS, Fewer EJ, Cronin KA, editors. SEER cancer statistics review,

1975–2014, Bethasda, MD: National Cancer Institute. https://seer.cancer.gov/csr/1975_2014/, bases on November 2016 SEER data submission, posted to the SEER web site, April 2017.

3. Parkin DM, Muir CS. Cancer incidence in five continents. Comparability and quality of data. IARC Sci Publ. 1992;120:45–173.

4. Travis WD, Brambilla E, Burke A, Marx A, Nicholson AG. WHO classification of tumours of the lung, pleura, thymus and heart. In: Travis WD, Brambilla E, Burke AP, Marx A, Nicholson AG, editors. Pathology and genetics of tumours of the lung, pleura, thymus and heart. 4th ed. Lyon: IARC Press; 2015.

5. Porcel JM, Esquerda A, Vives M, Bilsa S. Etiology of pleural effusion: analysis of more than 3,000 consecutive thoracenteses. Arch Bronconeumol. 2014;50:161–5.

6. Porcel JM, Gasol A, Bielsa S, Civit C, Light RW, Salud A. Clinical features and survival of lung cancer patients with pleural effusions. Respirology. 2015;20:654–9.

7. Johnston WW. The malignant pleural effusion. A review of cytopathologic diagnoses of 584 specimens from 472 consecutive patients. Cancer. 1985;56:905–9.

8. DiBonito L, Falconieri G, Colautti I, Bonifacio D, Dudine S. The positive pleural effusion. A retrospective study of cytopathologic diagnoses with autopsy confirmation. Acta Cytol. 1992;36:329–32.

9. Renshaw AA, Madge R, Sugarbaker DJ, Swanson S. Malignant pleural effusions after resection of pulmonary adenocarcinoma. Acta Cytol. 1998;42:1111–5.

10. Light RW, Hamm H. Malignant pleural effusion: would the real cause please stand up? Eur Respir J. 1997;112:242S–8S.

11. Eberhardt WE, Mitchell A, Crowley L, et al. The IASLC lung cancer staging project: proposals for the revisions of the M descriptors in the forthcoming eighth edition of the TNM classification of lung cancer. J Thorac Oncol. 2015;10(110):1515–22.

12. Rami-Porta R, Asamura H, Travis WD, Rusch VW. Lung. In: Amin MB, editor. AJCC cancer staging manual. 8th ed. Cham: Springer; 2017.

13. Lombardi G, Zustovich F, Nicoletto MO, Donach M, Artioli G, Pastorelli D. Diagnosis and treatment of malignant pleural effusion: a systematic literature review and new approaches. Am J Clin Oncol. 2010;33:420–3.

14. Leung AN, Muller NL, Miller RR. CT in differential diagnosis of diffuse pleural disease. AJR Am J Roentgenol. 1990;154:487–92.

15. Azzopardi M, Porcel JM, Koegelenberg CF, Lee YCG, Fysh ETH. Current controversies in the management of malignant pleural effusions. Semin Respir Crit Care Med. 2014;35:723–31.

16. Yoneda KY, Mathur PN, Gasparini S. The evolving role of interventional pulmonary in the interdisciplinary approach to the staging and management of lung cancer: Part III: diagnosis and management of malignant pleural effusions. Clin Lung Cancer. 2007;8(9):535–47.

17. Ozcakar B, Martinez CH, Morice RC, et al. Does pleural fluid appearance really matter? The relationship between fluid appearance and cytology, cell counts, and chemical laboratory measurements in pleural effusions of patients with cancer. J Cardiothorac Surg. 2010;5:63.

18. Heffner JE, Klein JS. Recent advances in the diagnosis and management of malignant pleural effusions. Mayo Clin Proc. 2008;83:235–50.

19. Kimura M, Tojo T, Naito H, Nagata Y, Kawai N, Taniguchi S. Effects of a simple intraoperative intrathoracic hyperthermotherapy for lung cancer with malignant pleural effusion or dissemination. Interact Cardiovasc Thorac Surg. 2010;10:568–71.

20. Sahn SA. Pleural effusion in lung cancer. Clin Chest Med. 1982;3:443–52.

21. Bedrossian CWM, editor. Malignant effusions: a multimodal approach to cytologic diagnosis. New York: Igaku-Shoin; 1994.

22. Tao LC, editor. Cytopathology of malignant effusions. Chicago: ASCP Press; 1996.

23. Michael CW, Bedrossian CWM, Chhieng D. Effusion cytology. In: Michael CW, editor. Papanicolaou society of cytopathology monograph series. New York, NY: Cambridge University Press; 2015.

24. Tang P, Vatsia SK, Teichberg S, Kahn E. Pulmonary adenocarcinoma simulating malignant mesothelioma. Arch Pathol Lab Med. 2001;125:1598–600.

25. Kaur G, Nijhawan R, Gupta N, Singh N, Rajwanshi A. Pleural fluid cytology samples in cases of suspected lung cancer: an experience from tertiary care center. Diagn Cytopathol. 2017;45:195–201.

26. Cibas ES, Corson JM, Pinkus GS. The distinction of adenocarcinoma from malignant mesothelioma in cell blocks of effusions: the role of routine mucin histochemistry and immunohistochemical assessment of carcinoembryonic antigen, keratin proteins, epithelial membrane antigen, and milk fat globule-derived antigen. Hum Pathol. 1987;18:67–74.

27. Shield PW, Callan JJ, Devine PL. Markers for metastatic adenocarcinoma in serous effusion specimens. Diagn Cytopathol. 1994;11:237–45.

28. Fetsch PA, Abati A. Immunocytochemistry in effusion cytology: a contemporary review. Cancer. 2001;93:293–308.

29. Westfall DE, Fan X, Marchevsky AM. Evidence-based guidelines to optimize the selection of antibody panels in cytopathology: pleural effusions with malignant epithelioid cells. Diagn Cytopathol. 2010;38:9–14.

30. Lozano MD, Panizo A, Toledo GR, Sola JJ, Pardo-Mindan J. Immunocytochemistry in the differential diagnosis of serous effusions: a comparative evaluation of eight monoclonal antibodies in Papanicolaou stained smears. Cancer. 2001;93:68–72.

31. Ordonez NG. Role of immunohistochemistry in differentiating epithelial mesothelioma from adenocarcinoma. Review and update. Am J Clin Pathol. 1999;112:75–89.

32. Maguire B, Whitaker D, Carrello S, Spagnolo D. Monoclonal antibody Ber-EP4: its use in the differential diagnosis of malignant mesothelioma and carcinoma in cell blocks of malignant effusions and FNA specimens. Diagn Cytopathol. 1994;10:130–4.

33. Lv M, Leng J-H, Hao Y-Y, Sun Y, Cha N, Wu G-P. Expression and significance of MOC-31 and calretinin in pleural fluid of patients with lung cancer. Diagn Cytopathol. 2015;43:527–31.

34. Comin CE, Novelli L, Boddi V, Paglierani M, Dini S. Calretinin, thrombomodulin, CEA, and CD15: a useful combination of immunohistochemical markers for differentiating pleural epithelial mesothelioma from peripheral pulmonary adenocarcinoma. Hum Pathol. 2001;32:529–36.

35. Riera JR, Astengo-Osuna C, Longmate JA, Battifora H. The immunohistochemical diagnostic panel for epithelial mesothelioma: a reevaluation after heat-induced epitope retrieval. Am J Surg Pathol. 1997;21:1409–19.

36. Noguchi M, Nakajima T, Hirohashi S, Akiba T, Shimosato Y. Immunohistochemical distinction of malignant mesothelioma from pulmonary adenocarcinoma with anti-surfactant apoprotein, anti-Lewisa, and anti-Tn antibodies. Hum Pathol. 1989;20:53–7.

37. Fetsch PA, Abati A, Hijazi YM. Utility of the antibodies CA 19–9, HBME-1, and thrombomodulin in the diagnosis of malignant mesothelioma and adenocarcinoma in cytology. Cancer. 1998;84:101–8.

38. Simsir A, Fetsch P, Mehta D, Zakowski M, Abati A. E-cadherin, N-cadherin, and calretinin in pleural effusions: the good, the bad, the worthless. Diagn Cytopathol. 1999;20:125–30.

39. Han AC, Filstein MR, Hunt JV, Soler AP, Knudsen KA, Salazar H. N-cadherin distinguishes pleural mesotheliomas from lung adeno-carcinomas: a ThinPrep immunocytochemical study. Cancer. 1999;87:83–6.

40. Schofield K, D'Aquila T, Rimm DL. The cell adhesion molecule, E-cadherin, distinguishes mesothelial cells from carcinoma cells in fluids. Cancer. 1997;81:293–8.

41. Saqi A, Yun SS, Yu GH, et al. Utility of CD138 (syndecan-1) in distinguishing carcinomas from mesotheliomas. Diagn Cytopathol. 2005;33:65–70.

42. Chu PG, Arber DA, Weiss LM. Expression of T/NK-cell and plasma cell antigens in nonhematopoietic epithelioid neoplasms. An immunohistochemical study of 447 cases. Am J Clin Pathol. 2003;120:64–70.

43. O'Connell FP, Pinkus JL, Pinkus GS. CD138 (syndecan-1), a plasma cell marker immunohistochemical profile in hematopoietic and nonhematopoietic neoplasms. Am J Clin Pathol. 2004;121:254–63.

44. Llinares K, Escande F, Aubert S, et al. Diagnostic value of MUC4 immunostaining in distinguishing epithelial mesothelioma and lung adenocarcinoma. Mod Pathol. 2004;17:150–7.

45. Takezawa C, Takahashi H, Fujishima T, et al. Assessment of differentiation in adenocarcinoma cells from pleural effusion by peripheral airway cell markers and their diagnostic values. Lung Cancer. 2002;38:273–81.

46. Mimura T, Ito A, Sakuma T, et al. Novel marker D2-40, combined with calretinin, CEA, and TTF-1: an optimal set of immunodiagnostic markers for pleural mesothelioma. Cancer. 2007;109:933–8.

47. Gomez-Fernandez C, Jorda M, Delgado PI, Ganjei-Azar P. Thyroid transcription factor 1: a marker for lung adenocarcinoma in body cavity fluids. Cancer. 2002;96:289–93.

48. Zhu W, Michael CW. WT1, monoclonal CEA, TTF1, and CA125 antibodies in the differential diagnosis of lung, breast, and ovarian adenocarcinomas in serous effusions. Diagn Cytopathol. 2007;35:370–5.

49. Tan D, Zander DS. Immunohistochemistry for assessment of pulmonary and pleural neoplasms: a review and update. Int J Clin Exp Pathol. 2008;1:19–31.

50. Agoff SN, Lamps LW, Philip AT, et al. Thyroid transcription factor-1 is expressed in extrapulmonary small cell carcinomas but not in other extrapulmonary neuroendocrine tumors. Mod Pathol. 2000;13:238–42.

51. Pomplun S, Wotherspoon AC, Shah G, Goldstraw P, Ladas G, Nicholson AG. Immunohistochemical markers in the differentiation of thymic and pulmonary neoplasms. Histopathology. 2002;40:152–8.

52. Suzuki A, Shijubo N, Yamada G, et al. Napsin A is useful to distinguish primary lung adenocarcinoma from adenocarcinomas of other organs. Pathol Res Pract. 2005;201:579–86.

53. Dejmek A, Naucler P, Smedjeback A, et al. Napsin A (TA02) is a useful alternative to thyroid transcription factor-1 (TTF-1) for the identification of pulmonary adenocarcinoma cells in pleural effusions. Diagn Cytopathol. 2007;35:493–7.

54. El-Hag M, Schmidt L, Roh M, Michael CW. Utility of TTF-1 and Napsin-A in the work up of malignant effusions. Diagn Cytopathol. 2016;44:299–304.

55. Chu P, Wu E, Weiss LM. Cytokeratin 7 and cytokeratin 20 expression in epithelial neoplasms: a survey of 435 cases. Mod Pathol. 2000;13:962–72.

56. Li HC, Schmidt L, Greenson JK, Chang AC, Myers JL. Primary pulmonary adenocarcinoma with intestinal differentiation mimicking metastatic colorectal carcinoma: case report and review of literature. Am J Clin Pathol. 2009;131:129–33.

57. Spriggs AI, Boddington MM. Oat-cell bronchial carcinoma. Identification of cells in pleural fluid. Acta Cytol. 1976;20:525–9.

58. Spieler P, Gloor F. Identification of types and primary sites of malignant tumors by examination of exfoliated tumor cells in serous fluids. Comparison with the diagnostic accuracy on small histologic biopsies. Acta Cytol. 1985;29:753–67.

59. Smith R, Nguyen GK. Unusual cytologic manifestation of small-cell lung cancer in associated pleural effusion. Diagn Cytopathol. 2004;30:266–7.

60. Salhadin A, Nasiell M, Nasiell K, et al. The unique cytologic picture of oat cell carcinoma in effusions. Acta Cytol. 1976;20:298–302.

61. Khunamornpong S, Siriaunkgul S, Suprasert P. Cytology of small-cell carcinoma of the uterine cervix in serous effusion: a report on two cases. Diagn Cytopathol. 2001;24:253–5.

62. Pereira TC, Saad RS, Liu Y, Silverman JF. The diagnosis of malignancy in effusion cytology: a pattern recognition approach. Adv Anat Pathol. 2006;13:174–84.

63. DeLellis RA. The neuroendocrine system and its tumors: an overview. Am J Clin Pathol. 2001;115(Suppl):S5–S16.

64. Chhieng DC, Ko EC, Yee HT, Shultz JJ, Dorvault CC, Eltoum IA. Malignant pleural effusions due to small-cell lung carcinoma: a cytologic and immunocytochemical study. Diagn Cytopathol. 2001;25:356–60.

65. Cerilli LA, Ritter JH, Mills SE, Wick MR. Neuroendocrine neoplasms of the lung. Am J Clin Pathol. 2001;116(Suppl):S65–96.

66. Smith-Purslow MJ, Kini SR, Naylor B. Cells of squamous cell carcinoma in pleural, peritoneal and pericardial fluids. Origin and morphology. Acta Cytol. 1989;33:245–53.

67. Huang CC, Michael CW. Cytomorphological features of metastatic squamous cell carcinoma in serous effusions. Cytopathology. 2014;25:112–9.

68. Nieto-Llanos S, Vera-Roman JM. Squamous cell carcinoma of the bladder with metastasis diagnosed cytologically in a pleural effusion. Acta Cytol. 1999;43:1191–2.

69. Hoda SA, Rosen PP. Cytologic diagnosis of metastatic penile carcinoma in pleural effusion. Arch Pathol Lab Med. 1992;116:198–9.

70. Gamez RG, Jessurun J, Berger MJ, Pambuccian SE. Cytology of metastatic cervical squamous cell carcinoma in pleural fluid: report of a case confirmed by human papillomavirus typing. Diagn Cytopathol. 2009;37:381–7.

71. Pu RT, Pang Y, Michael CW. Utility of WT-1, p63, MOC31, mesothelin, and cytokeratin (K903 and CK5/6) immunostains in differentiating adenocarcinoma, squamous cell carcinoma, and malignant mesothelioma in effusions. Diagn Cytopathol. 2008;36:20–5.

72. Ordonez NG. What are the current best immunohistochemical markers for the diagnosis of epithelioid mesothelioma? A review and update. Hum Pathol. 2007;38:1–16.

73. Ordonez NG. The diagnostic utility of immunohistochemistry in distinguishing between epithelioid mesotheliomas and squamous carcinomas of the lung: a comparative study. Mod Pathol. 2006;19:417–28.

74. Li Q, Bavikatty N, Michael CW. The role of immunohistochemistry in distinguishing squamous cell carcinoma from mesothelioma and adenocarcinoma in pleural effusion. Semin Diagn Pathol. 2006;23:15–9.

75. Bassarova AV, Nesland JM, Davidson B. D2-40 is not a specific marker for cells of mesothelial origin in serous effusions. Am J Surg Pathol. 2006;30:878–82.

76. Bishop JA, Teruya-Feldstein J, Westra WH, Pelosi G, Travis WD, Rekhtman N. p40 (ΔN063) is superior to p63 for the diagnosis of pulmonary squamous cell carcinoma. Mod Pathol. 2012;25:405–15.

77. Alexander M, Chiaffarano J, Zhou F, Cangiarella J, Yee-Chang M, Simsir A. Can p40 (polyclonal) replace p63 (Clone 4A4) in the cytologic diagnosis of pulmonary non-small cell carcinoma? Am J Clin Pathol. 2017;147:580–8.

# Ovarian Cancer

Ben Davidson

## Introduction

### Epidemiology

Ovarian cancer is the seventh most common cancer among women worldwide and ranks eighth in lethality, accounting globally for an estimated 238,700 newly diagnosed cases and 151,900 fatalities in 2012. The disease has variable incidence in different geographic regions and among different ethnic groups, with a high incidence in developed countries, where it ranks fifth in incidence and sixth in mortality [1]. Ovarian cancer is rarely diagnosed in women under the age of 30 years, and disease incidence increases with age, with a median age of diagnosis at 63 years [2].

The majority of cases are sporadic, but 15–20% of the affected women have genetic predisposition for breast or ovarian cancer, most commonly related to germline mutations in the *BRCA1* or *BRCA2* genes. Mutations in other genes whose protein products are involved in DNA repair and/or are tumor suppressors, including *RAD51C*, *RAD51D*, *BRIP1*, *BARD1*, *PALB2*, *CHEK2*, *MRE11A*, *RAD50*, *ATM*, and *TP53*, are additionally implicated, as are mutations in the DNA mismatch repair genes *MLH1*, *PMS2*, *MSH2*, or *MSH6* associated with the hereditary nonpolyposis colorectal cancer (HNPCC) or Lynch syndrome. Among environmental factors, use of oral contraceptives reduces the risk of developing ovarian cancer, whereas hormone replacement therapy in postmenopausal women increases it. Parity, prior tubal ligation, salpingectomy, and unilateral or bilateral oophorectomy are additional factors conferring reduced risk of ovarian cancer [2].

## Clinical Presentation, Diagnosis, and Treatment

Ovarian cancer is diagnosed at advanced stage in the majority of cases due to insidious onset, characterized by non-specific symptoms such as abdominal discomfort and pain, dyspepsia, vomiting, alteration of bowel habit, urinary frequency, menstrual irregularities, fatigue, weight loss, anorexia, and depression. Pelvic or abdominal mass may be palpable, and abdominal distention due to peritoneal effusion (ascites) may be present. Extra-abdominal disease may present as respiratory difficulty due to pleural effusion or enlarged inguinal or supraclavicular lymph nodes. Less frequently, parenchymal metastases to distant organs are found. The diagnosis is based on clinical findings, ultrasonography and/or abdominal-pelvic CT, and serum measurement of CA 125 levels [3, 4].

Ovarian cancer staging is based on the 2013 FIGO system by the International Federation of Gynecology and Obstetrics [5]. Patients with localized ovarian cancer or ovarian cancer with regional spread have 5-year survival at 92% and 73%, respectively, whereas this figure is 29% for those with distant metastasis [6]. This makes early detection of ovarian cancer crucial for improving disease outcome. However, screening for ovarian cancer has not altered the course of this disease to date [2]. In view of the suboptimal performance of CA 125 alone in this setting, use of a larger panel of serum biomarkers, e.g., CA 125 combined with human epididymis antigen 4 (HE4), CA 72.4, and anti-TP53 autoantibodies, has been advocated. Other approaches include analysis of circulating microRNA (miRNA), cell-free DNA (cfDNA), circulating tumor cells (CTC), and exosomes, as well as advanced imaging [7]. Prophylactic surgery, i.e., bilateral salpingo-oophorectomy, is advocated for women at high-risk of developing the disease [2].

Established clinicopathologic prognostic factors in addition to FIGO stage include histological type, tumor grade, and residual tumor volume [3].

B. Davidson, M.D., Ph.D.
Department of Pathology, The Norwegian Radium Hospital, Oslo University Hospital, Oslo, Norway

Faculty of Medicine, Institute of Clinical Medicine, University of Oslo, Oslo, Norway
e-mail: bend@medisin.uio.no; bdd@ous-hf.no

© Springer International Publishing AG, part of Springer Nature 2018
B. Davidson et al. (eds.), *Serous Effusions*, https://doi.org/10.1007/978-3-319-76478-8_3

The majority of ovarian cancer patients undergo standard therapy consisting of surgery followed by adjuvant chemotherapy. The former includes total abdominal hysterectomy, bilateral salpingo-oophorectomy, omentectomy, lymphadenectomy, and maximal debulking of tumor nodules on all peritoneal surfaces, in addition to tapping of ascites or peritoneal washing. When complete resection is not possible, cytoreductive surgery is performed, as it increases the effectiveness of subsequent chemotherapy. Standard first-line chemotherapy consists of combination paclitaxel in combination with a platinum-based compound (cisplatin or carboplatin) or platinum-based therapy alone. Neoadjuvant chemotherapy, i.e., administration of platinum-based chemotherapy prior to cytoreductive surgery, is an alternative treatment approach in patients with stage III/IV ovarian cancer [2, 3]. Intraperitoneal (IP) administration of platinum compounds and taxanes has been investigated for a possible role as standard care for advanced ovarian cancer but has not become standard therapy in the majority of institutions, partly due to concerns regarding the toxicity and complications associated with IP drug administration [8]. While more radical surgery and optimization of chemotherapy protocols have increased the 5-year survival rate to 45%, the percentage of patients cured of ovarian cancer has remained at about 30% [7].

Targeted therapy is discussed in Chap. 9.

## Histological Classification

Ovarian carcinoma (OC) accounts for about 90% of all malignant diseases of the ovary and is the main topic of this chapter, as the overwhelming majority of malignant effusions of ovarian origin are from carcinomas or carcinosarcomas (CS). Recent years have brought major changes to our understanding of ovarian carcinogenesis, with obvious effect on the classification of these tumors.

OC has been previously divided into type I and type II disease based on clinical, pathological, and molecular genetic studies. Type I tumors, consisting of low-grade serous carcinoma (LGSC), mucinous carcinoma (MC), endometrioid carcinoma (EC), and clear cell carcinoma (CCC), arise from borderline tumors and grow slowly. They are characterized by *KRAS* and *BRAF* mutations. Type II tumors, including high-grade serous carcinoma (HGSC), CS, and undifferentiated carcinomas, are highly aggressive and grow rapidly. Type II tumors are characterized by *TP53* and *BRCA* mutations and frequent gross genomic instability [9]. While this division is informative in many ways, it is now evident that OC consists of five distinct diseases—HSGC, LGSC, CCC, MC, and EC—in terms of origin, morphology, immunohistochemistry (IHC) profile, genetic characteristics, and clinical course. It is further accepted that many, though probably not all HGSC have their origin in the fimbriae of the fallopian tube rather than the ovary or perito-

neum [10, 11]. The latter observation impacts on both the assigning of primary site and staging of many HGSC and on the adoption of prophylactic approaches.

## Effusions in OC

Malignant effusions are a frequent clinical finding in advanced carcinomas of different origin, particularly primary tumors of the lung and breast. However, none of these malignancies has the practically universal predilection that OC, particularly of the serous type, has for the serosal cavities. This undoubtedly reflects the presence of widespread intra-abdominal disease in advanced-stage OC, although tumor cell homing to this anatomic site is of major significance as well. The accumulation of effusion fluid within the serosal cavities is believed to be the result of lymphatic obstruction by metastatic cancer cells, increased production of fluid by cells lining these cavities, and increased vascular permeability, as well as new vessel formation (angiogenesis), fibrin accumulation, and changes in the peritoneal stroma [12–16]. Ascites is found in 75% of patients with advanced-stage disease at diagnosis [17] and predicts the presence of malignant disease in the differential diagnosis from borderline tumors or benign ones, especially at advanced stage [18].

The clinical significance of ascites has been investigated in several studies. Although some authors have reported that positive ascites is not an independent prognostic marker in OC [17, 19, 20], the majority of large studies support the opposite view [21–25]. Involvement of the pleural space occurs in 33–55% of patients with stage IV disease and is the most common site for distant metastasis in the majority of series [26–31]. Pleural effusion defines stage IV, designated FIGO IVA disease, even in the absence of solid metastases [5]. Despite the fact that pleural effusion constitutes distant metastasis and is generally associated with poor survival, patients diagnosed at this stage have been shown to benefit from maximal surgical debulking in several studies [26–28, 31, 32], although the choice upfront therapy may be dependent on resectability of the abdominal disease and the extent of pleural disease [33]. Survival did not depend on the site of stage IV disease (pleural effusion, parenchymal metastasis, or extra-abdominal lymph node) but rather resectability of the abdominal disease, in the recent study by Jamieson et al. [32]. Pericardial involvement is infrequent in OC, reported in 6/97 patients with stage IV disease in the series of Dauplat et al. [30].

## Morphology

### HGSC and LGSC

HGSC of extrauterine origin, including tumors originating from the fallopian tube, the ovary, and the peritoneum, is the most frequent histologic type of OC. In a population-based study from Canada, HGSC comprised 68.1% of all OC, whereas LGSC comprised only 3.4% of cases. HGSC and LGSC were further overrepresented in the group of patients with advanced-stage disease, in which these entities made up 87.7% and 5.3% of tumors, respectively [34]. Based on the author's experience, these entities constitute the overwhelming majority of OC effusions, with the remaining cases being CCC and CS. The presence of EC and MC in effusions is rare.

Serous carcinomas have highly variable morphology, although definite classification as LGSC vs. HGSC based on effusion morphology may be difficult in many cases.

LGSC are composed of cells in well-defined papillary structures, often with calcifications in the form of psammoma bodies in their core. The latter may mask the presence of tumor cells in the so-called psammocarcinoma (Fig. 3.1a), although the majority of LGSC contain fewer (if any) psammoma bodies and present in the form of papillary groups with a varying degree of atypia (Fig. 3.1b). In LGSC, atypia is often minimal; nuclei are round, fairly uniform and cen-

trally located; and nucleoli are small and round (Fig. 3.1c). Vacuolization is often seen (Fig. 3.2a, b) and may occasionally create confusion with mucinous carcinoma. LGSC specimens obtained post-chemotherapy may lack papillary architecture and form less well-defined groups that are nonspecific for this entity or for serous carcinoma in general (Fig. 3.3a, b). Cells in such tumors have higher grade of nuclear atypia with coarse chromatin and large nucleoli. Nuclei are often eccentrically located.

HGSC consist characteristically of cohesive cell groups, some with papillary architecture, with overt high-grade atypia (Fig. 3.4a–c). Rarely, tumors consist mainly of large cell balls which may be reminiscent of breast carcinoma (Fig. 3.4d, e). Poorly differentiated tumors may present as single cells of moderate to large size and variable nuclear-to-cytoplasmic (n/c) ratio, including multinucleated tumor cells (Fig. 3.5a–c). Cells with intracytoplasmic and intranuclear vacuoles resembling those in breast carcinoma may be observed (Fig. 3.5a). Multiple mitotic figures, including atypical ones, are usually found (Fig. 3.5b). Phagocytosis of other cells may rarely be seen (Fig. 3.6a, b).

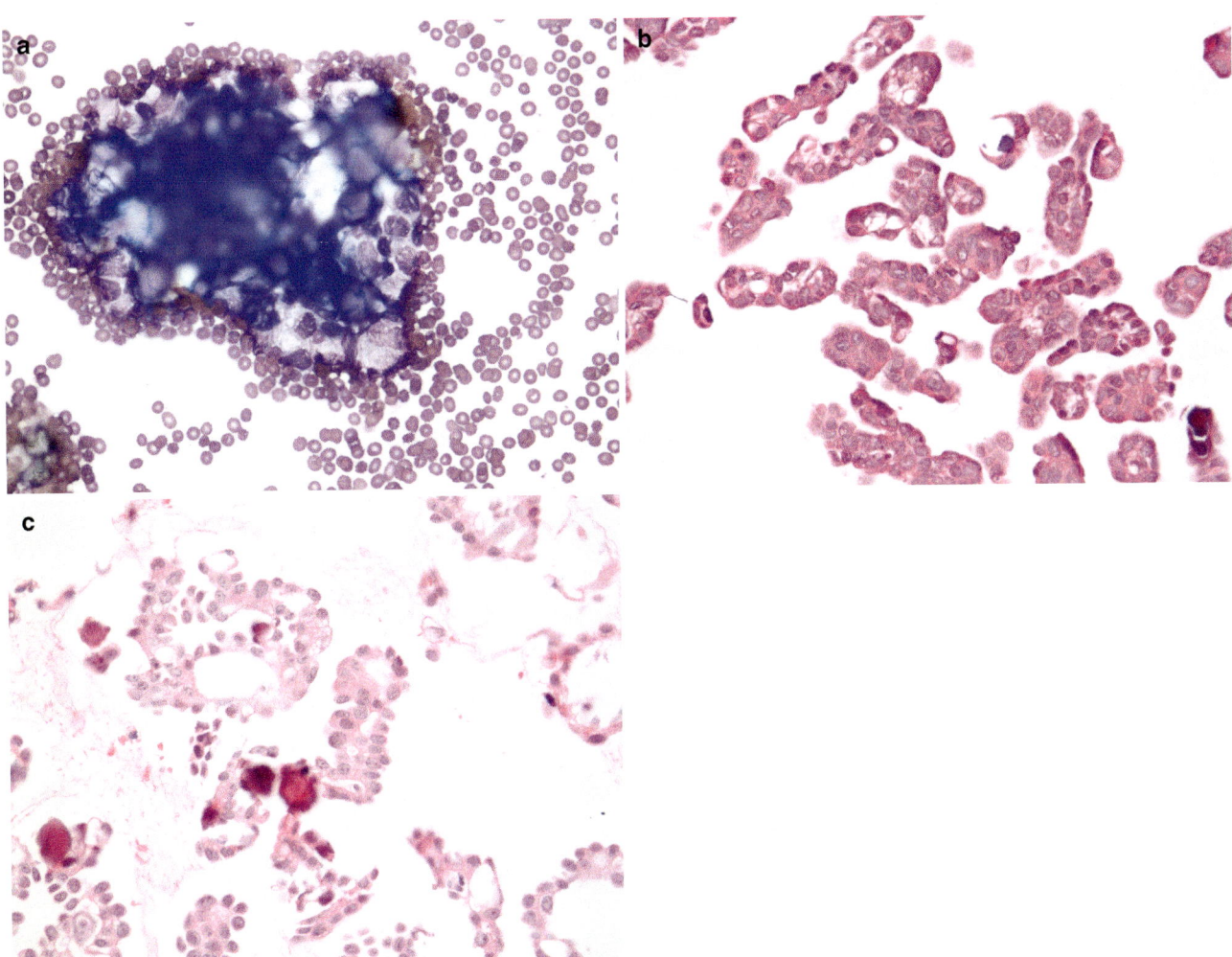

**Fig. 3.1** (**a–c**) Low-grade serous adenocarcinoma (LGSC; a: so-called psammocarcinoma); (**a**) Diff-Quik, (**b, c**) H&E

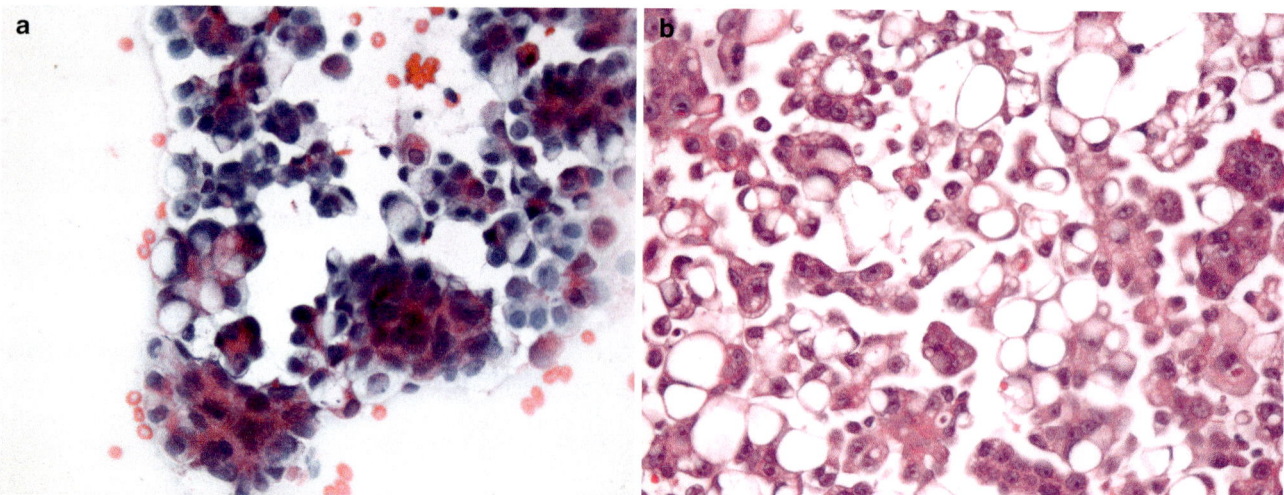

Fig. 3.2 (a, b) Vacuolization in LGSC cells; (a) PAP, (b) H&E

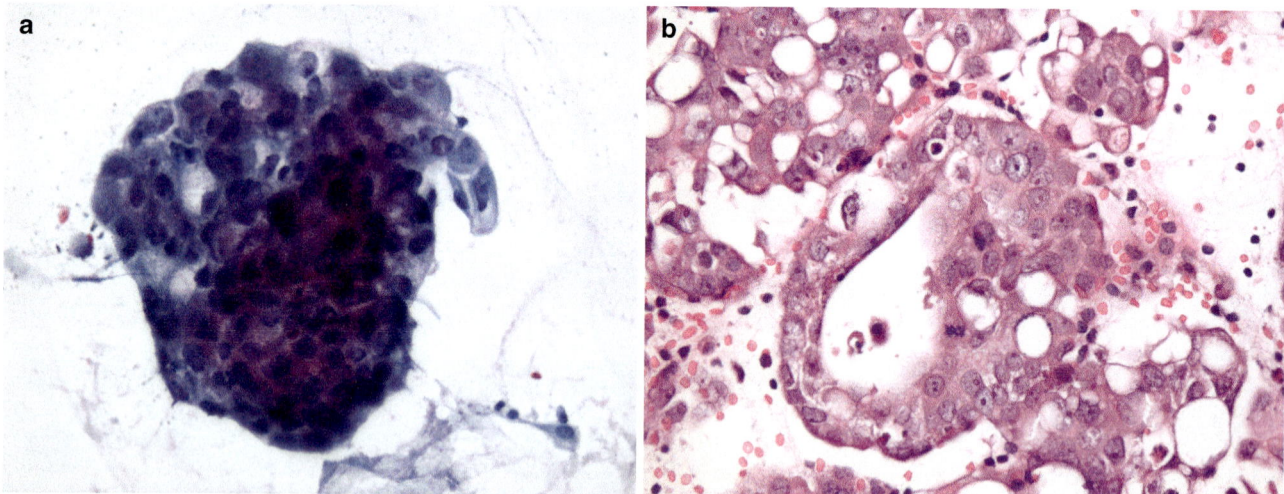

Fig. 3.3 (a, b) LGSC post-chemotherapy showing moderate atypia; (a) PAP, (b) H&E

HGSC effusions are often tapped after neo-adjuvant chemotherapy has been administered or at disease recurrence. Cells exposed to chemotherapy have bizarre morphology, with giant, often multinucleated cells that lie singly or in small groups consisting of few cells (Fig. 3.7a, b). Even in tumors with lesser atypia prior to chemotherapy, pleomorphic cells may be found intermingled with less atypical cells in papillary structures (Fig. 3.7c, d).

## Differential Diagnosis

As is true for all effusions with metastatic cancer, an important clue to the diagnosis of malignancy is the presence of two cell populations, i.e., tumor cells and reactive cells. The latter vary considerably and may consist predominantly of reactive mesothelial cells, be dominated by leukocytes or contain large populations of both cell classes (Fig. 3.8). The leukocytic infiltrates are usually composed predominantly of macrophages and lymphocytes, but neutrophils may predominate in a minority of cases, occasionally in very large numbers.

Pattern recognition is essential in reaching a correct differential diagnosis, as comprehensively reviewed by Pereira et al. [35].

The differential diagnosis of LGSC constitutes the following:

1. Fallopian tube epithelium (mainly in peritoneal washings) or endosalpingiosis.
2. Benign ovarian tumors located at the ovarian surface (predominantly serous cystadenofibroma).

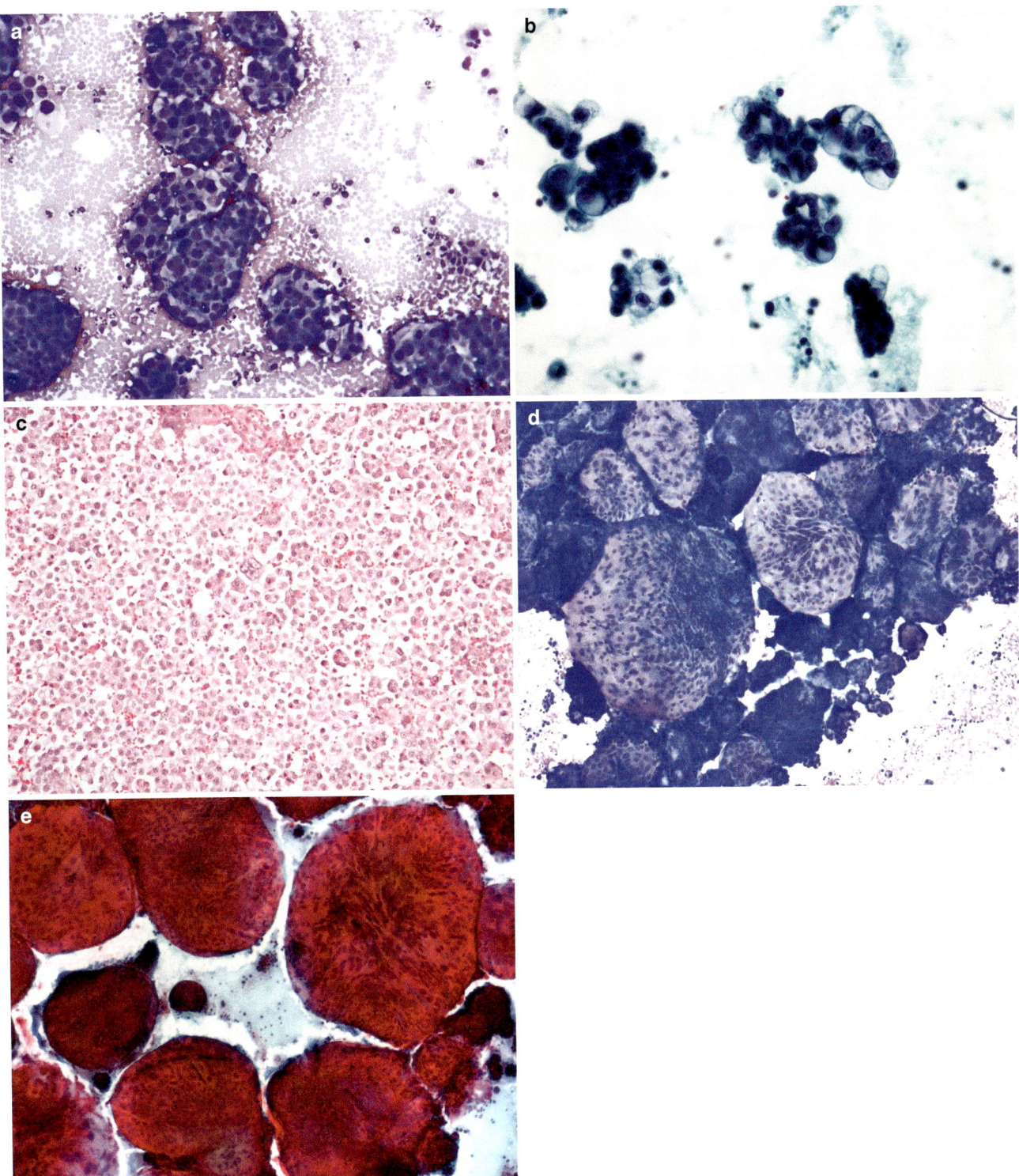

**Fig. 3.4** High-grade serous adenocarcinoma (HGSC): (**a–c**) papillary group with overt atypia; (**d, e**) cell balls in HGSC; (**a, d**) Diff-Quik, (**b, e**) PAP, (**c**) H&E

3. Serous borderline tumors, particularly when the ovarian capsule is breached or when the tumor originates from the ovarian surface.
4. Reactive mesothelial cells (RMC) and macrophages.
5. Malignant mesothelioma (MM).

6. Metastatic serous carcinoma of the uterine corpus.
7. Metastatic nongenital papillary carcinoma. These may essentially originate from any organ, but morphological resemblance is most problematic with renal and pancreatobiliary adenocarcinomas.

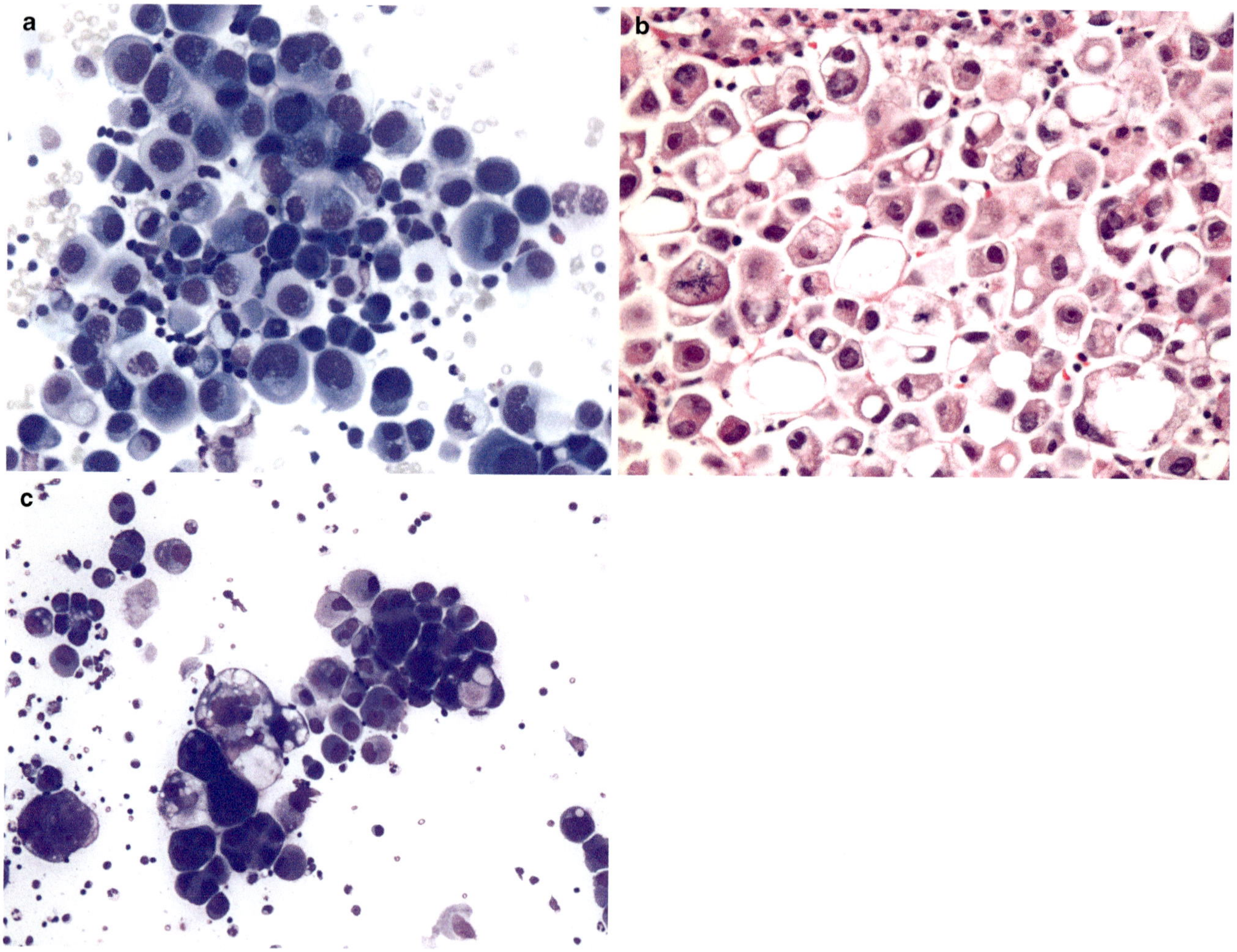

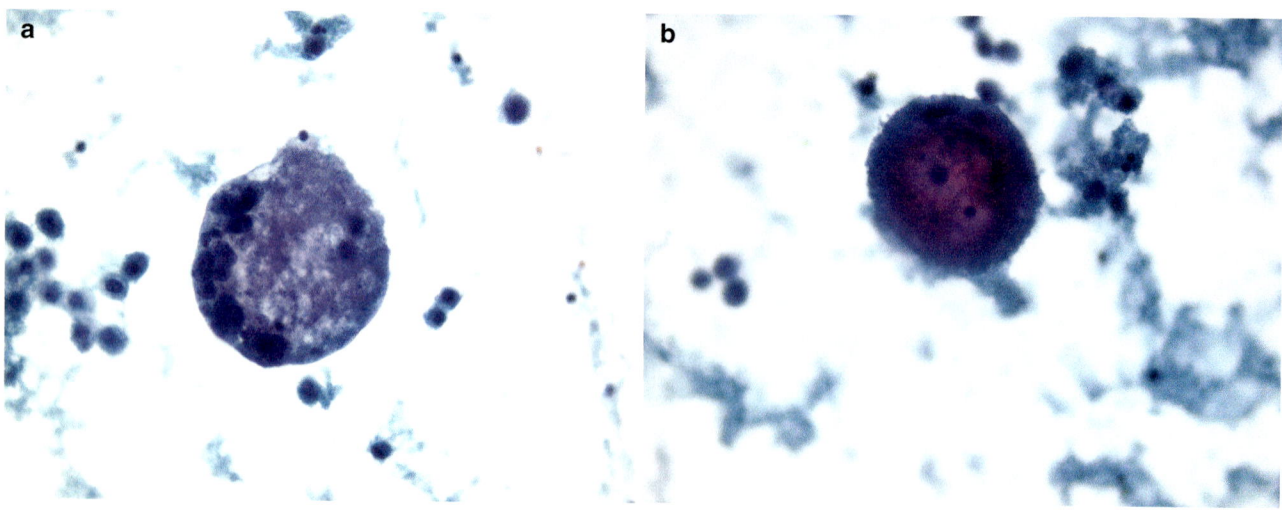

**Fig. 3.5** (**a–c**) Dissociated HGSC cells; (**a, c**) Diff-Quik, (**b**) H&E

**Fig. 3.6** (**a, b**) Cancer cell phagocytosis. Leukocytes in giant, partially degenerated adenocarcinoma cells; (**a, b**) PAP

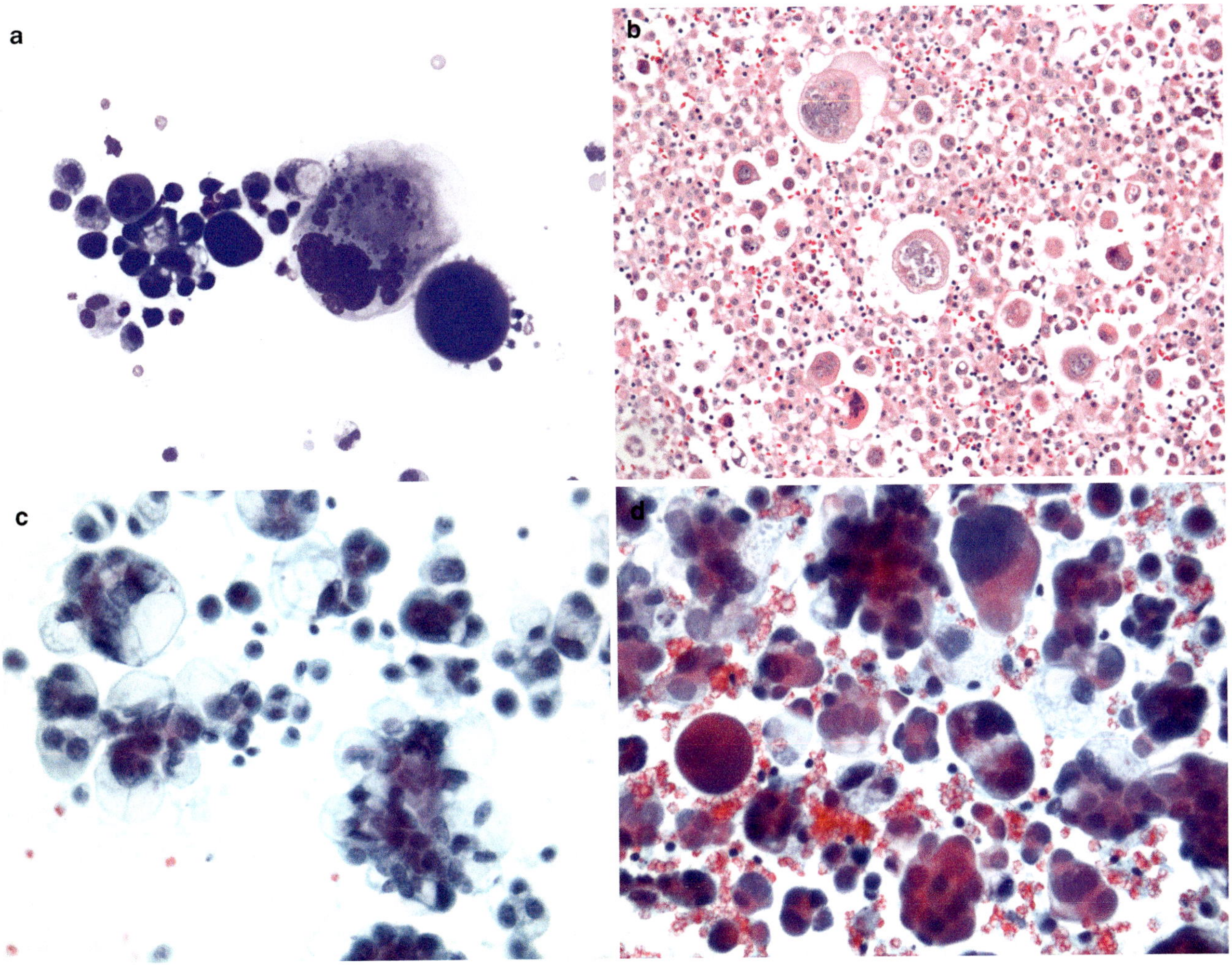

**Fig. 3.7** (**a**–**d**) Chemotherapy-induced alterations in HGSC cells; (**a**) Diff-Quik, (**b**) H&E, (**c**, **d**) PAP

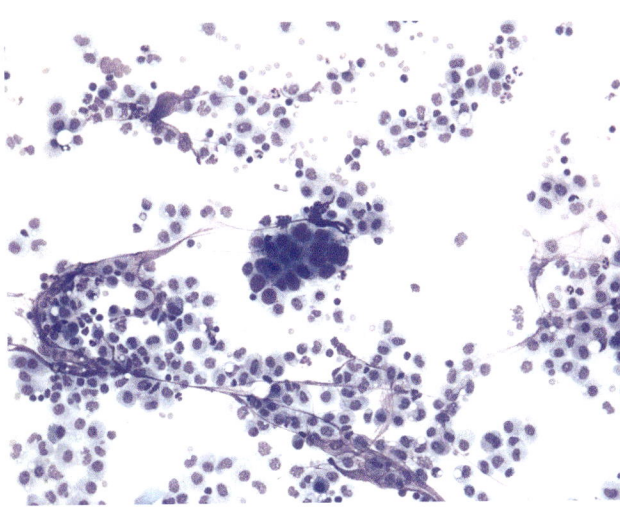

**Fig. 3.8** HGSC cell group surrounded by many reactive cells; Diff-Quik

HGSC need to be differentiated from metastases from other organs, primarily from lung and breast carcinoma within the pleural cavity and breast, genital tract, and gastrointestinal (GI) carcinoma in peritoneal effusions. Poorly differentiated tumors, especially with single-lying tumor cells, must be differentiated from any malignant tumor, including carcinoma, hematological malignancies, germ cell or stromal/sex cord tumors of the ovary, sarcoma, and melanoma.

Benign epithelium, benign serous tumors, and borderline tumors are unlikely diagnoses in the face of pronounced atypia but may be extremely difficult to differentiate from carcinomas with minimal atypia. Effusions originating from serous borderline tumors may have mild–moderate degree of atypia, making their differentiation from serous carcinoma essentially impossible without evaluation of the surgical specimen (Fig. 3.9a), although occasional tumors may have benign appearance (Fig. 3.9b, c).

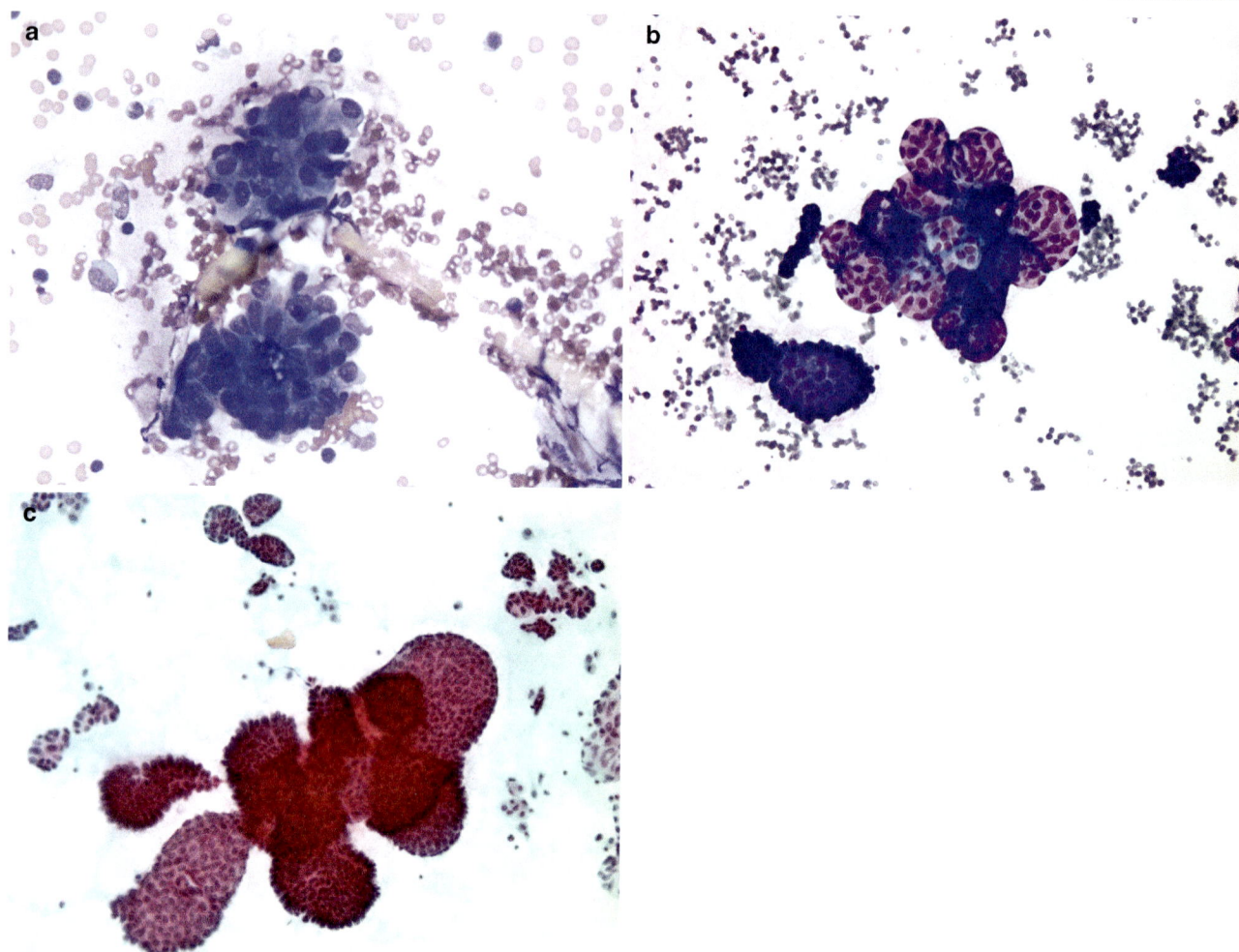

**Fig. 3.9** (**a–c**) Serous borderline tumor in peritoneal effusions. (**a**) tumor cells with atypia; (**b**, **c**) tumor cells with minimal atypia; (**a**, **b**) Diff-Quik, (**c**) PAP

Reactive mesothelium may similarly be difficult to separate from serous carcinoma, and a set of morphological characteristics rather than a single one needs to be applied (see Chap. 1), as even so-called specific features, such as the presence of intercellular windows, have been shown to be non-specific [36].

The diagnosis of serous carcinoma based on IHC is discussed below.

## CCC

CCC constitute about 5% of ovarian carcinomas in the Western world and are more common in Asian countries. In the author's effusion series, approximately 3% of cases are of this histotype. In surgical specimens, this tumor assumes a variety of growth patterns, including papillary, tubulocystic, solid, and hobnail patterns [37].

The morphology of ovarian CCC in effusions is as heterogeneous as it is in surgical specimens. Hobnailing is often present but may be less distinct than in surgical specimens in some

cases. Cell groups may have papillary or tubulocystic arrangement (Fig. 3.10a) and may appear as non-specific clusters common to all adenocarcinomas (Fig. 3.10b) or as open acinar structures with one cell layer (Fig. 3.10c). The acinar structures may surround an empty lumen or, more frequently, have a metachromatic core in Diff-Quik-stained sections (Fig. 3.10d), which stains eosinophilic in H&E sections. The latter structure is the only diagnostic feature of this tumor in effusions, as the remaining ones are non-specific. It was termed "raspberry body" by Ito et al. and shown to stain positive for PAS, Alcian Blue, colloidal iron, and PAS-methenamine silver. These stain positive for laminin and collagen type IV and were shown to represent excessive synthesis of basal lamina by electron microscopy [38]. This characteristic eosinophilic material may occasionally take the form of a ring (Fig. 3.10e) or diffusely cover the tumor cell cluster. The presence of this extracellular material has been highlighted as a central feature of CCC in a recent series of five specimens [39].

CCC cells in effusions have variable size, some attaining huge proportions (Fig. 3.10f). Vacuolization may be fine, may be in the form of large intracytoplasmic vacuoles fill-

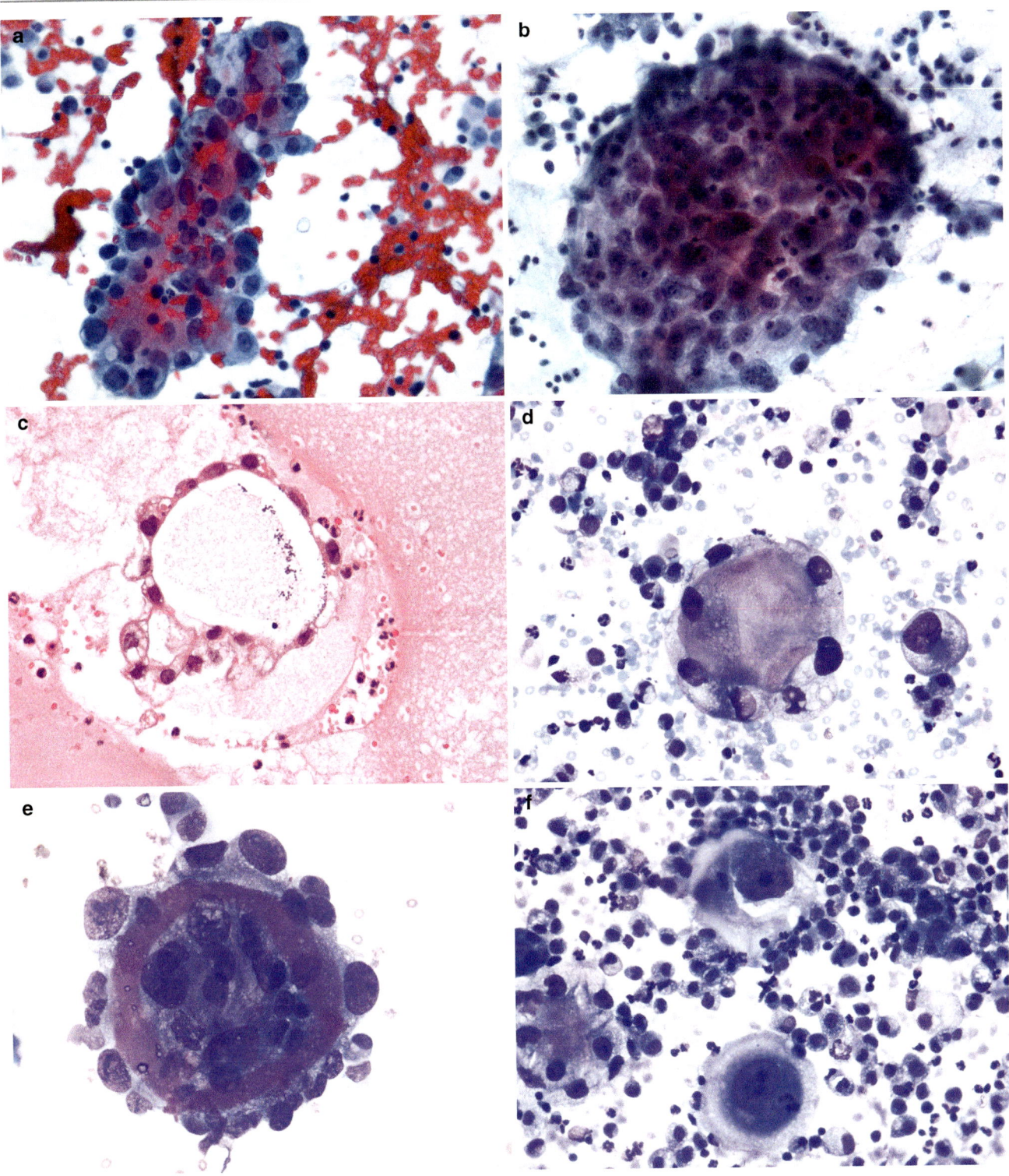

**Fig. 3.10** (**a–i**) The many faces of clear cell carcinoma (CCC). (**a**) papillary group; (**b**) non-specific; (**c**) open acinar; (**d**) metachromatic material in the tumor group core; (**e**) metachromatic material as a ring in the basal aspect of the tumor group; (**f**) giant tumor cells; (**g**, **h**) vacu- olization of carcinoma cells; (**i**) granular cytoplasm; (**j**) malignant mesothelioma groups with cores containing metachromatic material; (**a**, **b**, **g**, **i**) PAP, (**d–f**), (**j**) Diff-Quik, (**c**, **h**) H&E

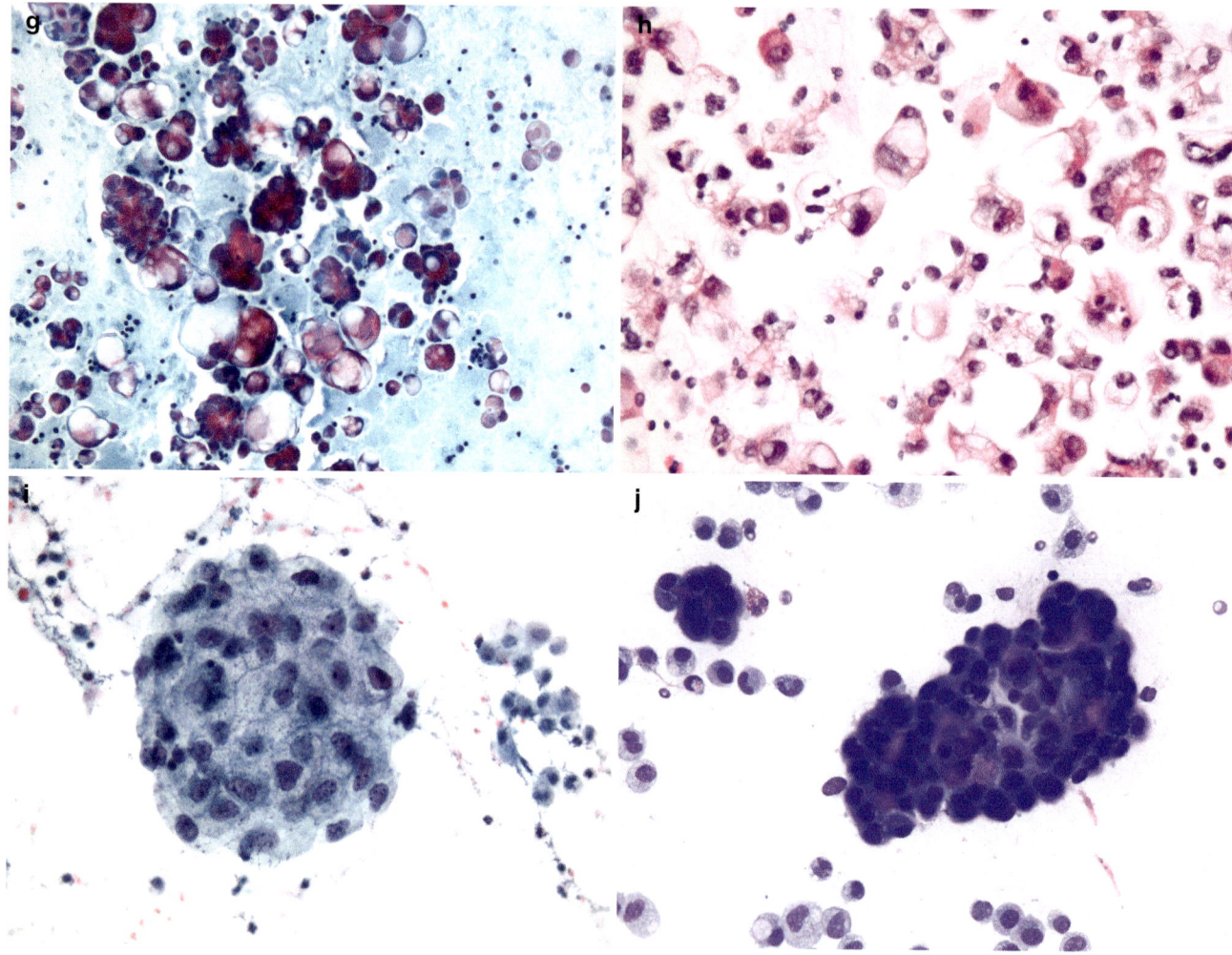

**Fig. 3.10** (continued)

ing the entire cytoplasm or is altogether absent (Fig. 3.10g, h). In other cases, the cytoplasm is lacy or finely granular (Fig. 3.10i). Cells may have coarse chromatin, but this is more often rather fine in texture. Nucleoli are large and eosinophilic. Mitotic figures may be found but are only rarely abundant. In the abovementioned series of Damiani et al., the cytoplasm was granular or clear, nuclei were large or pleomorphic, and hobnailing was observed in all cases [39].

## Differential Diagnosis

CCC of the ovary cannot be differentiated from its counterpart in the uterine corpus or from the rare primary tumor of the fallopian tube based on morphology. The differential diagnosis otherwise includes the following entities:

1. Serous carcinoma (genital or other) or serous borderline tumor with vacuolization.
2. EC, especially with secretory features.
3. Clear cell borderline tumor.
4. Metastatic renal cell carcinoma.

5. Clear cell or deciduoid variant of malignant mesothelioma.
6. MC (ovarian or other).
7. Germ cell tumors (especially yolk sac tumor).
8. Stromal/sex cord tumors.
9. Other tumors with clear cell features (e.g., sarcomas).
10. Macrophages or reactive mesothelial cells.

The morphological differentiation of carcinomas from macrophages or benign mesothelial cells is discussed in Chap. 1. Non-epithelial tumors are a less likely diagnosis when acinar or tubular structures are found, and the finding of true signet-ring cells suggests that one is dealing with a MC rather than CCC. As discussed above, the finding of extracellular metachromatic material is highly suggestive of CCC, although this finding should not be confused with the extracellular material found in MM (Fig. 3.10j) or the rare granulosa cell tumor (see below).

Despite the morphological clues, the use of IHC is mandated in some cases, especially when the primary tumor site is unknown. With the exception of clear cell borderline tumor and the abovementioned genital counterparts of ovarian CCC, all tumors listed above can be differentiated from CCC based on IHC (see below).

## MC

MC of the ovary infrequently metastasizes to the serosal cavities. In our database, these cases constitute <1% of malignant effusions with an ovarian primary. Tumor cells may have nonspecific features, such as papillary groups, or form true glandular/acinar structures (Fig. 3.11a, b). Cell balls may be additionally seen (Fig. 3.11c). Dissociated cells are often found, and signet-ring morphology is evident in poorly differentiated tumors (Fig. 3.11d). Mucinous carcinoma cells often have thick cell membrane. The cytoplasm is vacuolated, either finely or with large mucin vacuoles (Fig. 3.11b–f), although this may be difficult to appreciate in some cells. The n/c ratio is usually low to moderate, and nuclei do not exceed moderate size in most cases. Nucleolar size is variable, as is the mitotic activity. Larger cells, occasionally with binucleation or multinucleation, may be infrequently found (Fig. 3.11e).

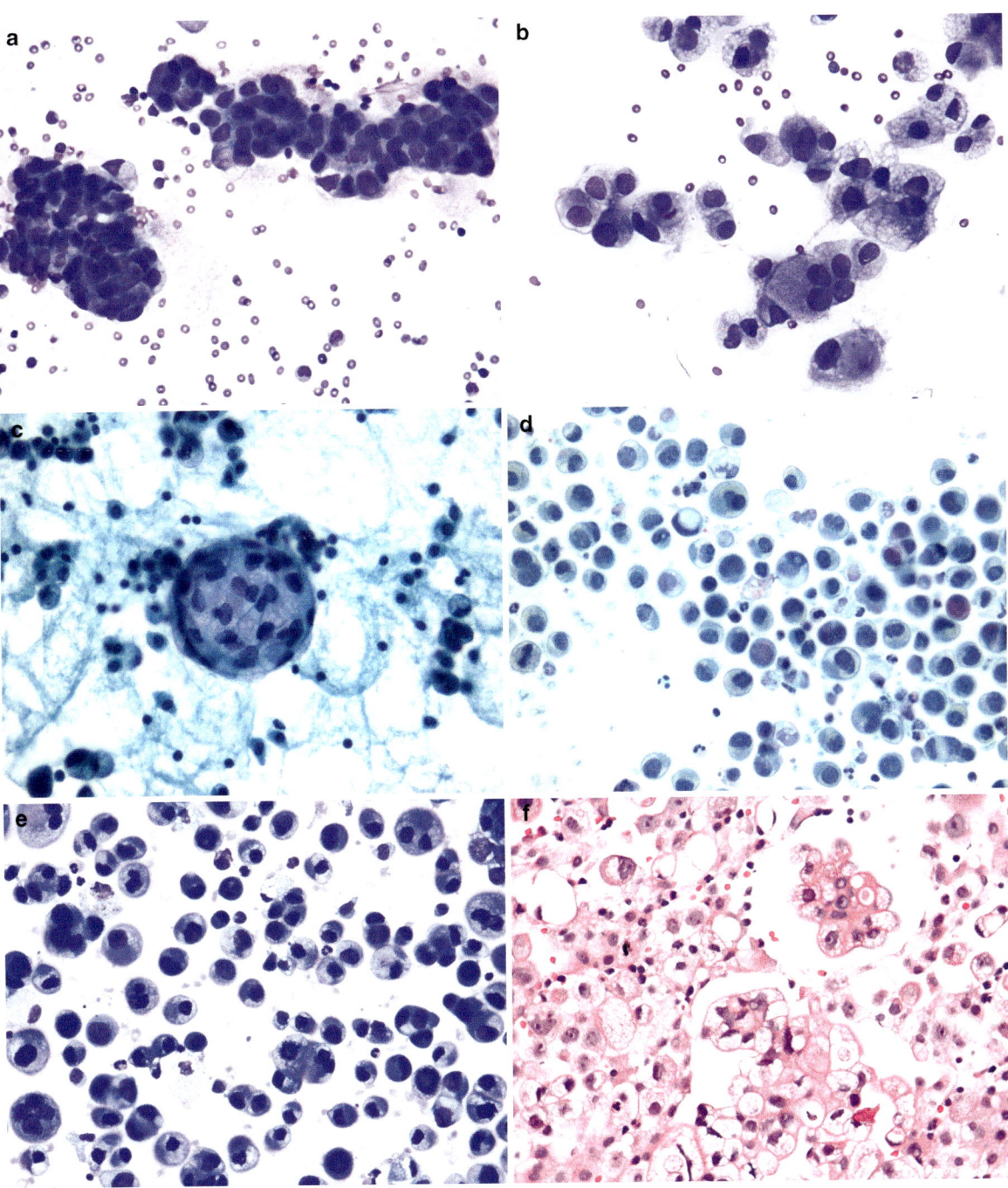

**Fig. 3.11** (**a–f**) The many faces of mucinous carcinoma (MC). (**a**) papillary; (**b**) acinar; (**c**) cell ball; (**d, e**) dissociated cells, some with signet-ring cell morphology; (**f**) small cytoplasmic vacuoles; (**a, b, e**) Diff-Quik, (**c, d**) PAP, (**f**) H&E

## Differential Diagnosis

The differential diagnosis of mucinous ovarian carcinoma overlaps considerably with that of CCC and includes the following entities:

1. MC of GI origin, including cases diagnosed clinically as pseudomyxoma peritonei.
2. EC of Müllerian origin.
3. CCC (ovarian, uterine, renal, other).
4. Clear cell or deciduoid variant of malignant mesothelioma.
5. Germ cell tumors.
6. Macrophages or reactive mesothelial cells.

MC of the ovary cannot be morphologically differentiated from tumors originating in the GI tract or other primaries, such as breast and lung. IHC is unfortunately of very limited value in making the important distinction between MC of the ovary and metastasis from a primary in the upper GI tract,

although it may be useful in separating mucinous OC from colon carcinoma (see below). In unresolved cases, clinical and radiological evaluation of the possible site of origin is critical. IHC is of more help in differentiating MC from the remaining entities in the above list (see below).

## EC

As its mucinous counterpart, EC of the ovary metastasizes infrequently to the serosal cavities, constituting approximately 1% of malignant effusions with an ovarian primary in our database. Metastases from tumors of mixed histology do metastasize to the serosal cavities, but the metastases usually have non-EC morphology.

Well-differentiated EC forms glandular structures that are reminiscent of those seen in surgical specimens from the ovary or the uterine corpus and even more so of endometrial cytology (Fig. 3.12a–c). The glands may be dilated, with an

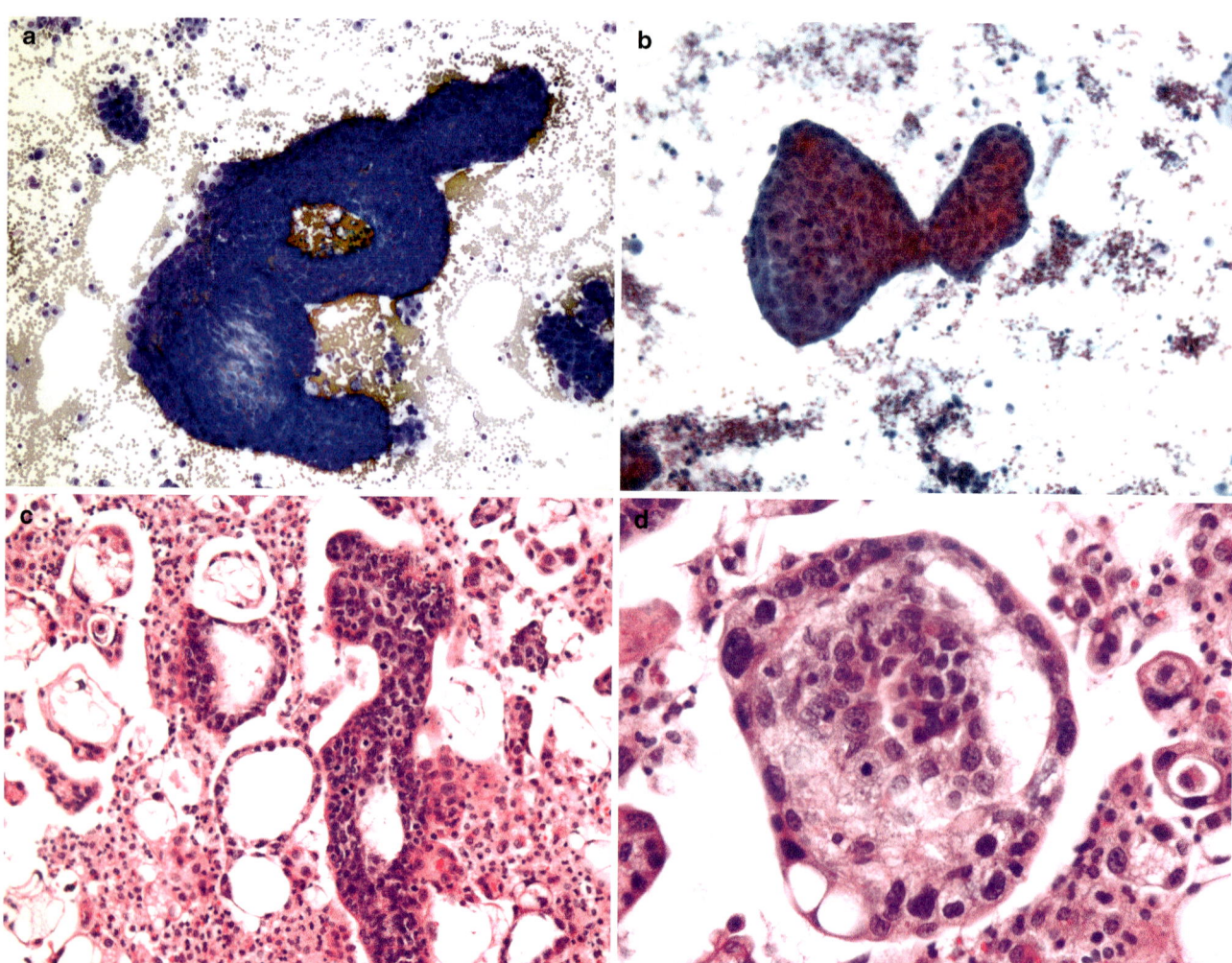

**Fig. 3.12** (**a–f**) The morphologic spectrum in endometrioid carcinoma (EC). (**a, b**) gland structures with typical endometrial architecture; (**c**) endometrial type glands and open glands; (**d**) near-total absence of lumen; (**e, f**) variable atypia (papillary group in **e**); (**g**) cytoplasmic vacuolization; (**h**) dissociated cells with marked atypia; (**a, f, h**) Diff-Quik, (**b, e**) PAP, (**c, d, g**) H&E

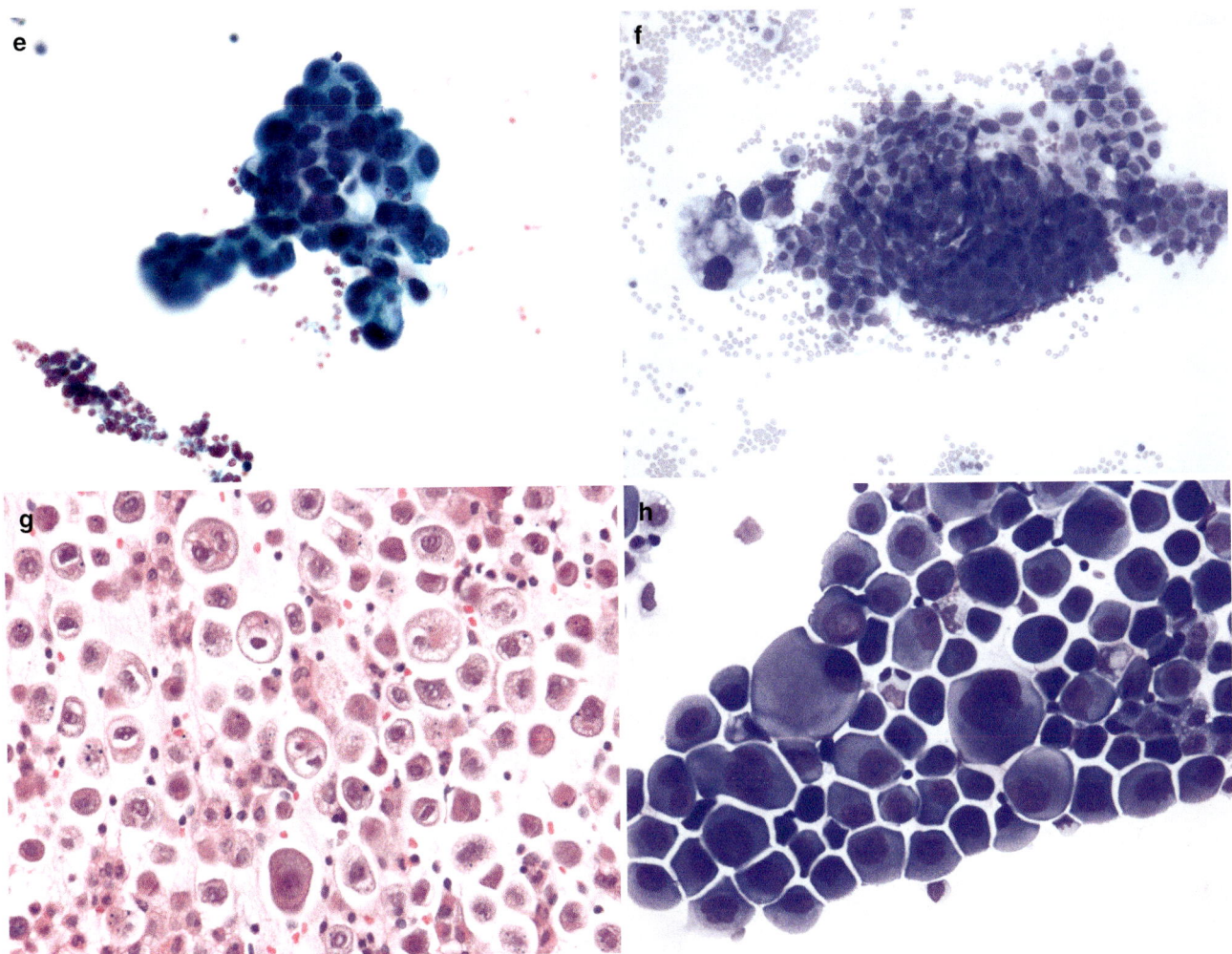

**Fig. 3.12** (continued)

empty lumen in H&E sections, or have partially or totally obliterated lumen (Fig. 3.12c, d). Nuclei are elongated or oval. Nuclear atypia is variable but may be pronounced (Fig. 3.12e, f). Mitotic activity may be pronounced (Fig. 3.12c). Less differentiated tumors consist of dissociated cells, some with vacuolated cytoplasm that is indistinguishable from MC (Fig. 3.12g). Previous exposure to chemotherapy results, as in serous carcinoma, in the appearance of bizarre-looking cells of variable size, some reaching very large proportions (Fig. 3.12h).

**Differential Diagnosis**

The differential diagnosis of ovarian EC depends on the degree of differentiation. In well-differentiated cases, it includes the following:

1. Endometriosis.
2. Metastatic adenocarcinoma of GI or non-GI (breast, lung, other) origin, especially of the colon.
3. MC of Müllerian origin.
4. Germ cell tumors (mainly yolk sac tumor).

In poorly differentiated tumors, especially those with dissociated cells, the differential diagnosis needs to include other tumor types, including mesothelioma, sarcoma, melanoma, and hematological cancers.

EC of the ovary or fallopian tube cannot be morphologically differentiated from tumors of the same type originating in the uterine corpus. However, EC of the uterine corpus rarely metastasizes to effusions, unless the tumor has invaded the entire wall and reached the serosal surface. In such cases, clinical data are essential to establishing the correct diagnosis. IHC cannot distinguish between EC of the ovary and uterine corpus. It is nevertheless useful in differentiating this tumor from the remaining entities in the above list (see below).

**Other Carcinomas**

Rare cases of malignant Brenner tumor metastasis in ascites have been reported, in which the cells displayed squamous features [40, 41]. Mixed carcinomas, as abovementioned, may be encountered. Undifferentiated OC commonly metastasizes to effusions, and their morphology at this site is as non-specific as it is in the primary organ. CS metastases are from the epithelial component in the vast majority of cases, most frequently as HGSC (Fig. 3.13a–c), although the presence of sarcomatous elements has been recorded in rare cases [42] (see Chap. 7).

The author diagnosed a case of a primary peritoneal small cell carcinoma that has metastasized to the pleural cavity in a young woman (Fig. 3.14a–c). No hypercalcemia was present. The tumor was positive for hormone receptors, vimentin and pan-cytokeratin AE1/AE3, and was negative for all IHC and molecular markers of hematological cancers and specific sarcoma entities. It proved rapidly fatal.

## Other Ovarian Tumors

Sex cord-stromal tumors of the ovary may very rarely give rise to a malignant effusion. Several reports of granulosa cell tumor of adult type in effusions have been published [43–48]. In a recent report of two cases in ascites and pleural effusion, the presence of Call-Exner bodies and nuclei with longitudinal grooves (coffee-bean nuclei) was regarded as morphological evidence supporting this diagnosis [48]. A granulosa cell tumor of adult type in a peritoneal effusion, with Call-Exner bodies and coffee-bean nuclei, was seen by the author (Fig. 3.15a–c). A case of granulosa cell tumor of juvenile type in ascites was described [49], and one case of Sertoli-Leydig tumor at this anatomic site has been pub-

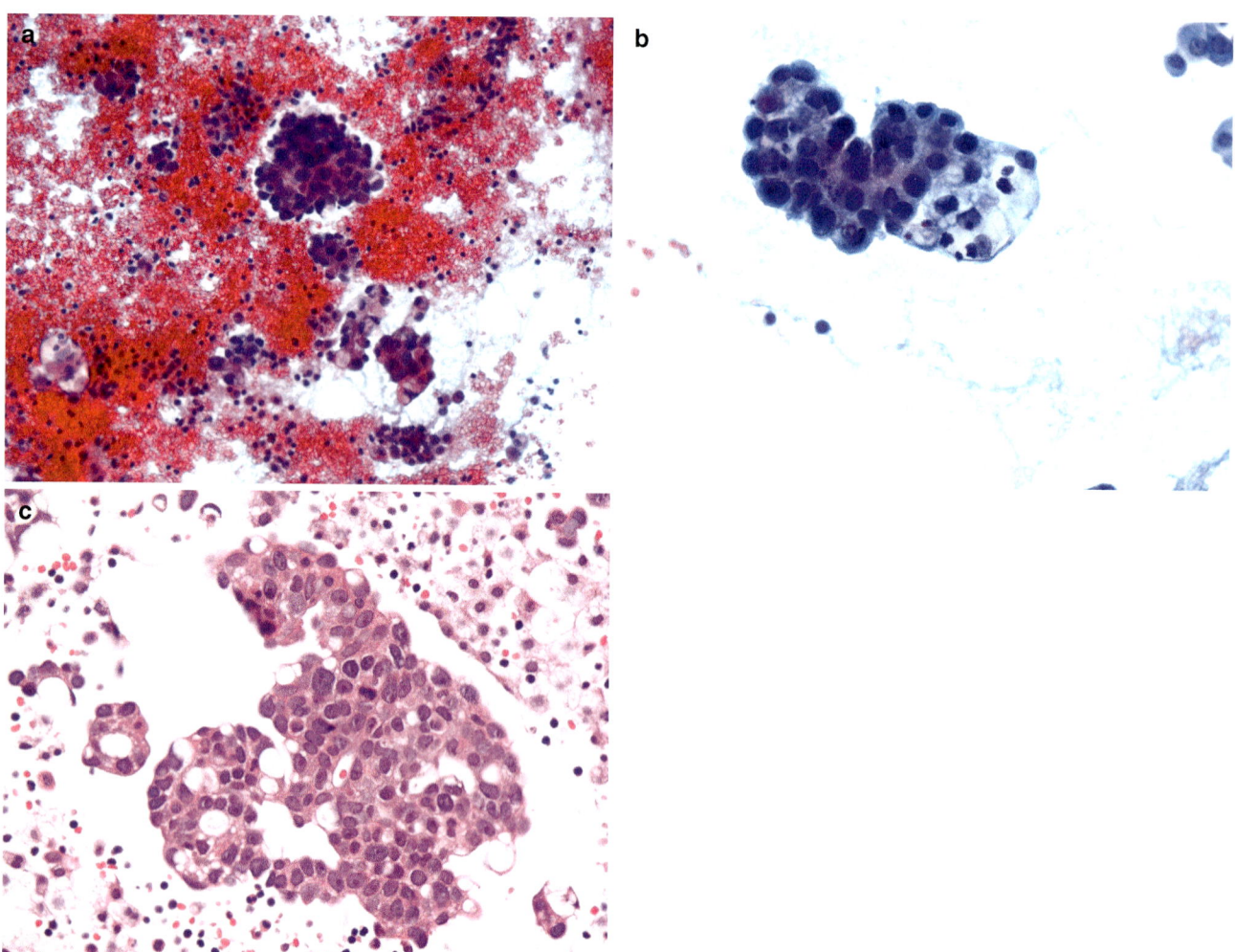

**Fig. 3.13** (**a–c**) Carcinosarcoma in a peritoneal effusion. Metastasis is in the form of malignant epithelial elements (**a, b**) PAP, (**c**) H&E

lished [50]. Immunostaining for inhibin may aid in confirming the diagnosis in such cases.

Several reports of ovarian germ cell tumors spreading to effusions have been published [51–57]. This group of tumors is discussed in Chap. 7, as they may have origin in organs other than the ovary.

Sarcomas of the ovary are rare tumors, and their metastasis to effusions is still less frequently observed, with publications limited to case reports, including the author's report of ovarian angiosarcoma metastasis in ascites [58] (see Chap. 7) and a single report of ovarian adenosarcoma in ascites [59].

## Ancillary Techniques

The differentiation of OC from other malignancies, and occasionally from the abovementioned benign proliferations, requires ancillary methods. OC cells carry a large number of genetic aberrations at both the chromosome and gene level (see Chap. 9). However, none of these has been universally accepted to be useful in diagnosing this tumor. Consequently, molecular tests may aid only in excluding other diagnoses. For all practical purposes, IHC is the method of choice in this diagnostic setting.

Evaluating published data regarding the IHC profile of OC in effusions is made difficult by the fact that many studies have analyzed adenocarcinomas of various origin, often with only few OC specimens included. Another limitation is the fact that the histological type of the OC cases studied is rarely detailed in older studies. One may assume that the majority of cases analyzed in this setting are serous carcinomas, making the literature regarding CCC and EC in effusions very scarce. Nevertheless, the more robust positive and negative diagnostic markers are generally similarly expressed in surgical specimens and in effusions, allowing one to rely on studies of the former specimens as well. The following

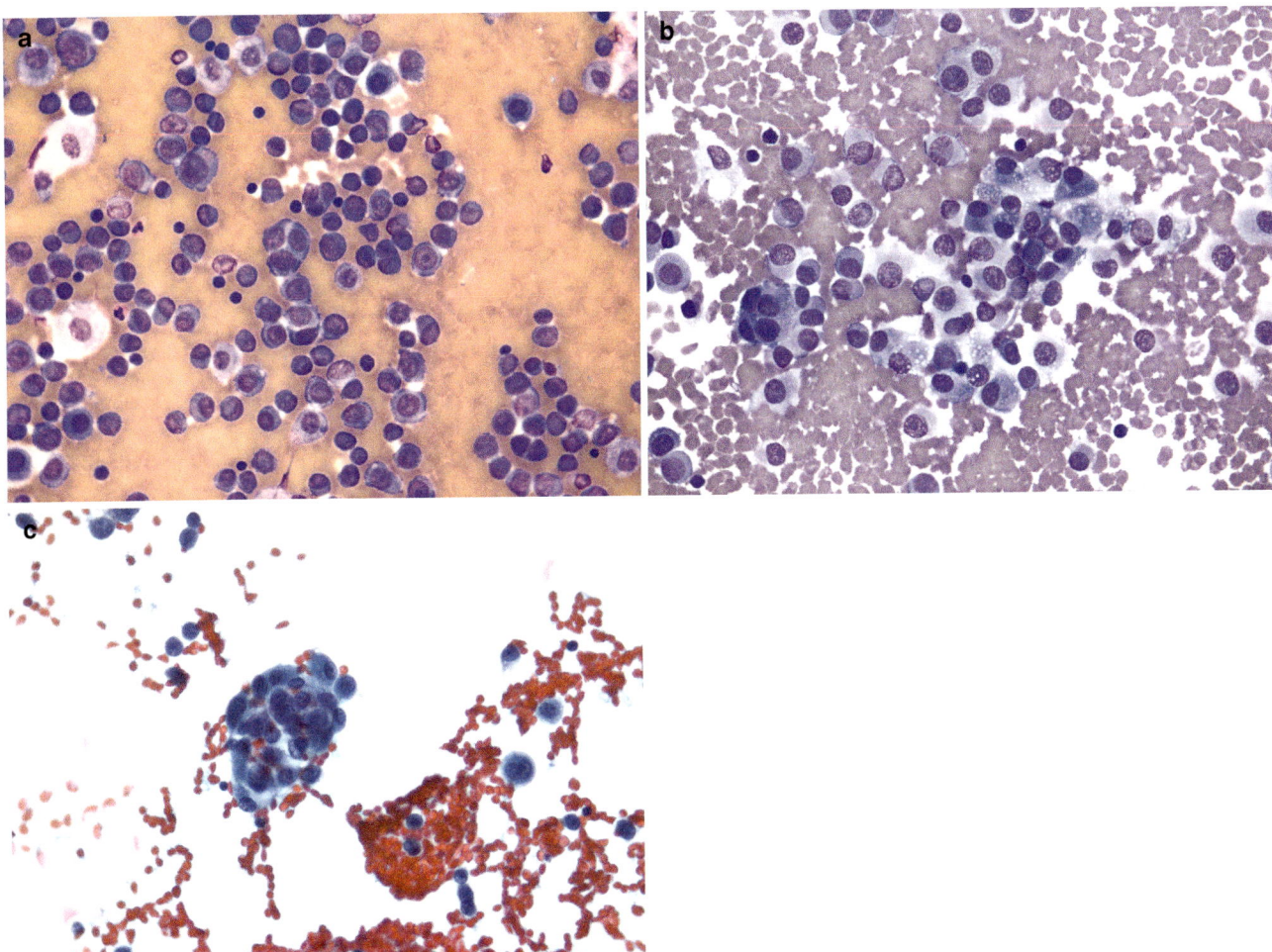

**Fig. 3.14** (a–c) Primary peritoneal small cell carcinoma, metastasis in a pleural effusion. Small cells with high n/c ratio, predominantly dissociated, few in small clusters. (a, b) Diff-Quik, (c) PAP

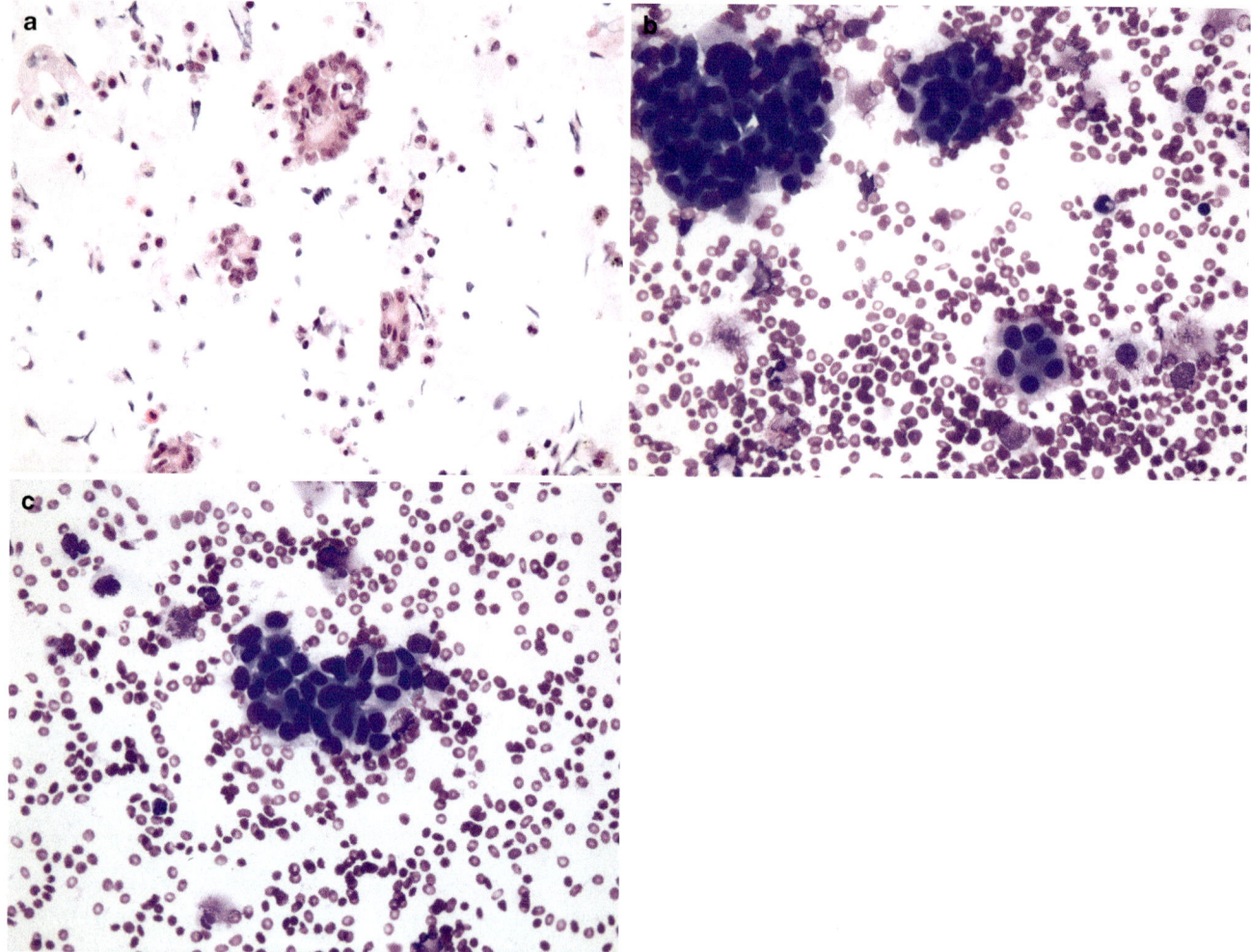

**Fig. 3.15** (a–c) Granulosa cell tumor, adult type, in a peritoneal effusion. Nondescript tumor groups are seen (**b**, upper part), but typical acinar structures with metachromatic/eosinophilic core are easily discerned (**a**): H&E, (**b**, **c**): Diff-Quik

discussion attempts to summarize the current status in this area, focusing on studies in which at least ten tumors of each diagnostic category were included.

## Serous OC Vs. MM and RMC

The most useful positive markers of OC in this differential diagnosis include Ber-EP4, B72.3, and BG8 as general adenocarcinoma markers [60–63] (Fig. 3.16a–c) and PAX8 as marker of Müllerian origin (Fig. 3.16d) [64–67]. MOC-31 and EpCAM antibodies recognize the epithelial surface molecule EpCAM (Fig. 3.16e), as does Ber-EP4, and are favored by some authors. These markers are highly sensitive and specific in differentiating OC from RMC. However, it is noteworthy that epithelioid MM not infrequently expresses Ber-EP4 and MOC-31, at least focally. Two additional OC-specific markers in this setting are estrogen receptor

(ER) (Fig. 3.16f) and Leu-M1, although the sensitivity of the latter is lower than that of the abovementioned markers [60–62]. Additional markers reported to be overexpressed in OC compared to MM and/or RMC in effusions include PAX2, CA 19-9, MUC4, claudin-3, claudin-4, cyclin E, non-integrin 67 kDa laminin receptor, MMP7, and CD24 [67–76] (Fig. 3.17a–d; see also Chap. 9).

The most useful mesothelial marker is calretinin, which stains the overwhelming majority of MM and RMC. It is infrequently expressed in serous carcinoma and then only focally [77–79]. Desmin is expressed in RMC and is absent from OC, making it very useful for this differential diagnosis. However, it is negative or only focally expressed in MM [77].

The author's group reported on the potential role of tenascin-X in differentiating MM from OC in effusions and solid specimens, as it is overexpressed in the former tumor (Fig. 3.18a, b) [78], and the same was reported for hyaluronic

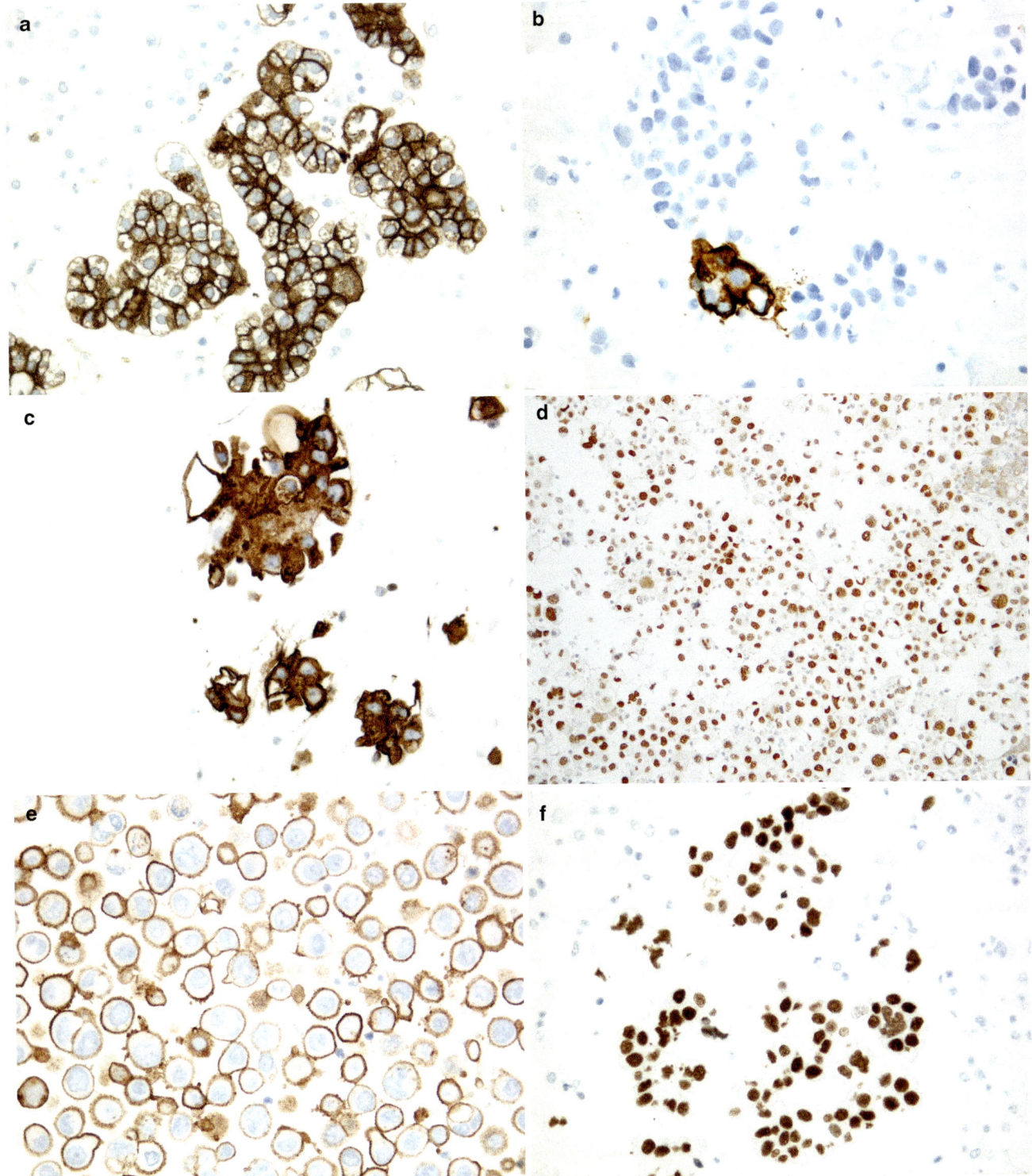

**Fig. 3.16** (**a–f**) Immunohistochemistry, carcinoma markers. (**a**) Ber-EP4, (**b**) B72.3, (**c**) BG8, (**d**) PAX8, (**e**) MOC-31, (**f**) ER

acid [80]. Epithelial membrane antigen (EMA) is expressed in MM in a characteristic thick brush-like membrane pattern, whereas it usually stains OC in a combined membrane and cytoplasmic pattern (Fig. 3.18c). However, exceptions do occur (Fig. 3.18d) [78], making this marker unreliable as a

single one. RMC are as a rule EMA-negative or express it weakly in their cytoplasm.

Loss of BAP1 (BRCA1-associated protein 1) expression has been reported to be specific for MM in the differential diagnosis from both RMC and metastatic carcinoma [81–83].

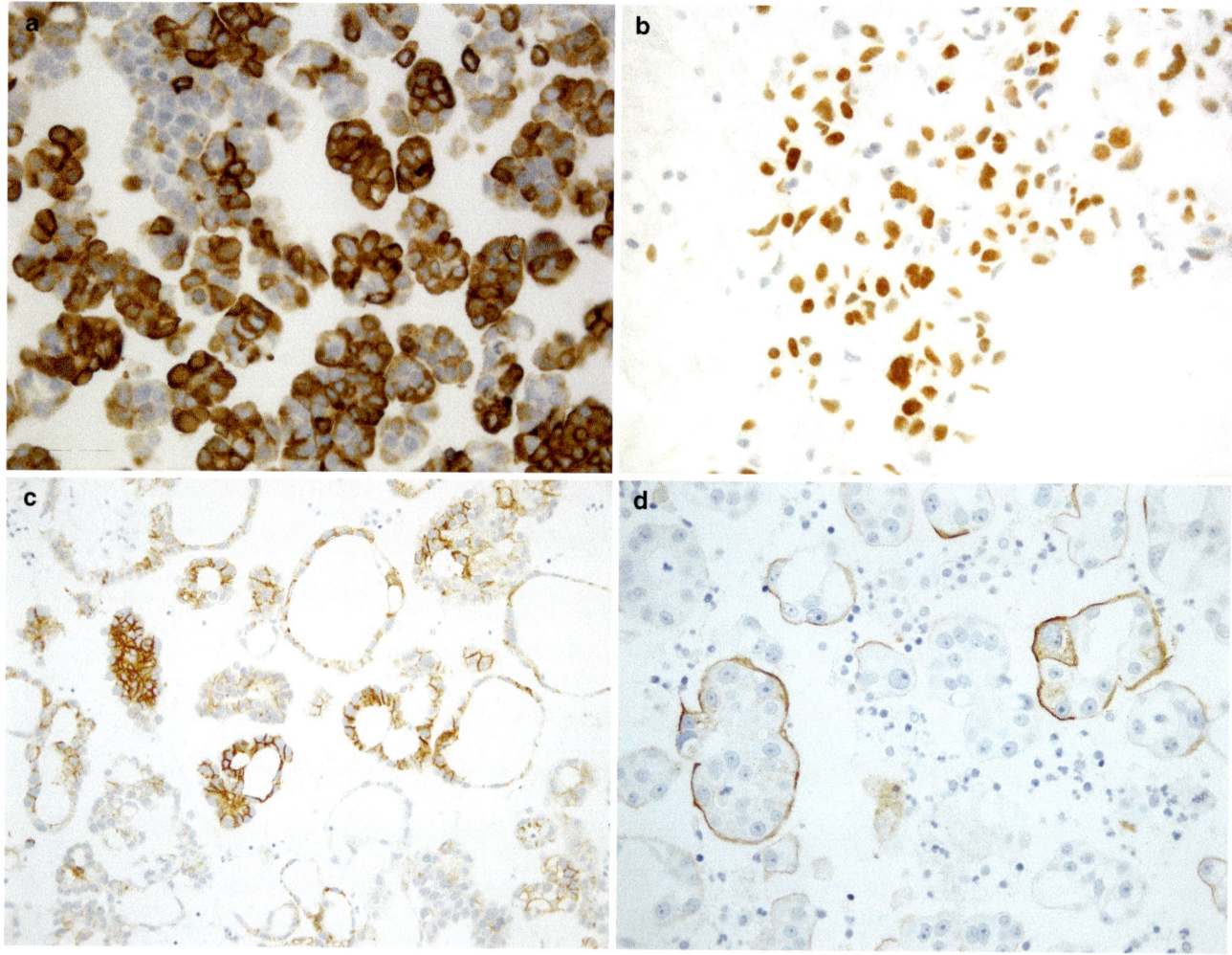

**Fig. 3.17** (**a, b**) New potential markers for ovarian/peritoneal carcinoma. (**a**) MUC4 (membrane and cytoplasm), (**b**) cyclin E (nuclei), (**c**) claudin-4 (membrane), (**d**) CD24 (membrane)

Of the markers that are of no diagnostic use in this setting, CEA is the best example of one that is negative in all three entities [84], whereas CA 125, Wilms' tumor antigen 1 (WT1), pan-cytokeratin, CK5/6, CK7, and vimentin are expressed in all three (Fig. 3.19a–d) [77, 84, 85]. HBME-1 is expressed in both OC and MM [86].

One unresolved issue is related to antibodies against the lymphatic marker podoplanin. In analysis of 290 effusions, the author showed that D2–40 performed poorly in the differential diagnosis between OC and MM (Fig. 3.20a, b) [87]. Hanna et al. used another antibody against podoplanin and reported expression in 94% MM vs. 7% OC in a smaller series [88]. Whether this antibody is more specific than the one used in our series remains to be tested in larger series, although these two antibodies were reported to perform similarly in surgical specimens [89].

## Serous OC Vs. Fallopian Tube Epithelium, Endosalpingiosis, Benign Serous Ovarian Tumors, and Serous Borderline Tumors

These benign entities and serous borderline tumors have similar expression pattern of many of the abovementioned markers (Fig. 3.21a). This makes it necessary to obtain detailed clinical and radiological data of cases in which the degree of atypia of papillary groups in effusion is minimal or mild and occasionally to wait for evaluation of the surgical specimen prior to reporting the effusion, especially when the material for evaluation is a peritoneal washing. Based on the experience of the author, B72.3 is the best marker for distinguishing OC and borderline tumors from benign entities but does not differentiate between the former two (Fig. 3.21b). Aberrant p53 expression (strong nuclear staining in >75% of

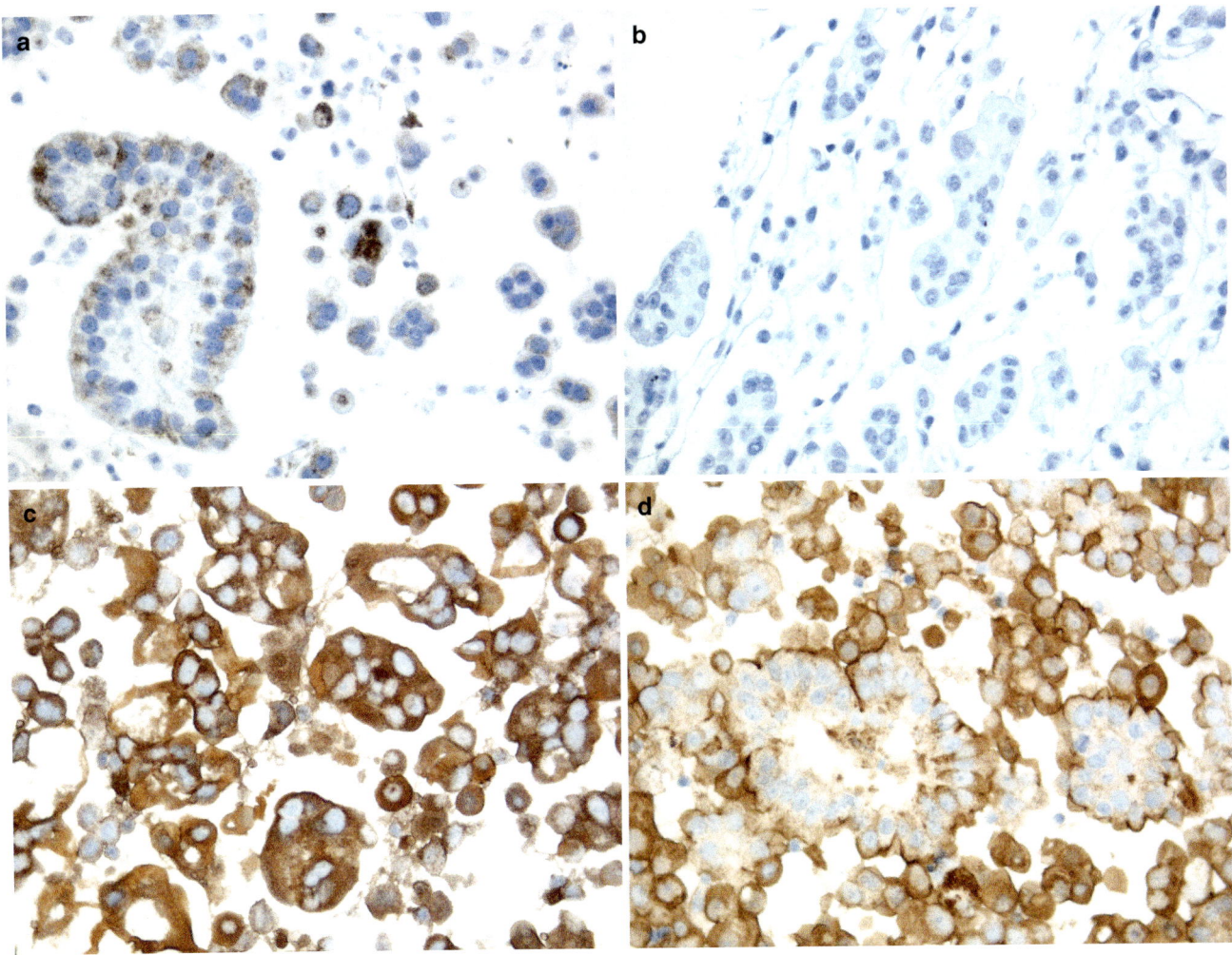

**Fig. 3.18** (**a**, **b**) Tenascin-X in the differential diagnosis between mesothelioma and serous ovarian carcinoma. (**a**) Tenascin-X-positive epithelioid mesothelioma, (**b**) negative staining in serous carcinoma (**c**, **d**) EMA in HGSC. (**c**) combined cytoplasmic and membrane staining, typical for adenocarcinoma; (**d**) accentuated membrane staining which mimics the pattern seen in malignant mesothelioma.

cells or entirely negative staining) favors HGSC over LGSC, borderline tumors, and benign proliferations, but its diagnostic role is primarily in differentiating HGSC from LGSC (Fig. 3.21c, d). It remains to be seen whether some of the new markers listed above will prove to be a useful addition to B72.3.

## Serous OC/PPC Vs. Other Metastatic Carcinomas

There is little data with respect to expression differences between serous OC and serous carcinoma of the uterine corpus in effusions. However, WT1 has been shown to differentiate between these lesions in surgical specimens, as it is often only focally expressed in uterine serous carcinoma [90, 91]. The combination of WT1 and MUC5AC was reported to differentiate between pancreatic serous carcinoma (WT1-negative, MUC5AC-positive) and OC (WT1-positive, MUC5AC-negative) in 100% of studied specimens [92]. A pilot study by the author supports this observation (Fig. 3.22a, b). WT1 is generally negative in non-serous adenocarcinomas of female genital origin, as well as in the majority of carcinomas of other origin (see also Appendix in this book).

In addition to its role in differentiating OC from RMC and MM, PAX8 differentiates OC and uterine carcinomas from metastatic carcinomas of other origin, including breast, lung, and GI primaries [65–67]. In the series of Wiseman et al., cell block sections from 54 Müllerian and 98 non-Müllerian carcinoma effusions were stained for PAX2 and PAX8, and expression of these proteins was found in 24 and 96% of the former, compared to 0 and 4% of the latter, suggesting that both markers may be useful in this diagnostic setting [67].

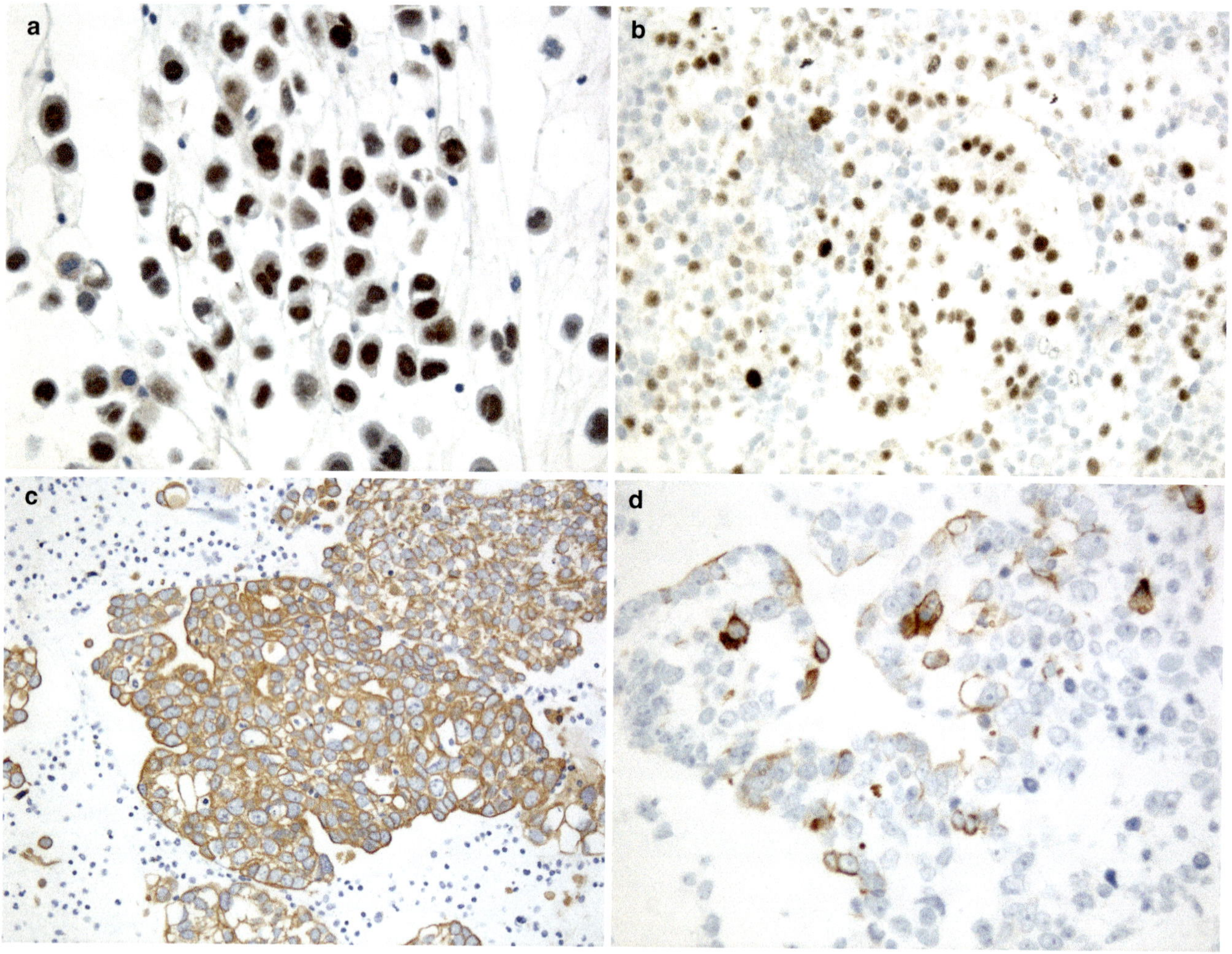

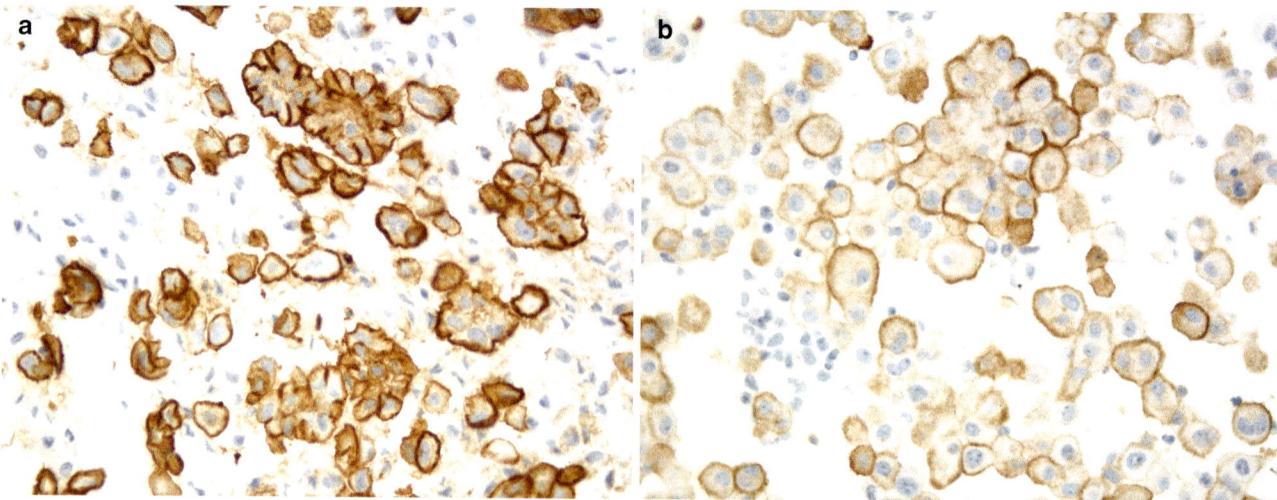

**Fig. 3.19** (**a–d**) Non-specific markers. (**a**, **b**) WT-1. WT-1 immunostaining in HGSC (**a**) and malignant mesothelioma (**b**); (**c**, **d**) cytokeratins. CK7 (**c**) and CK5/6 (**d**) in ovarian carcinoma

**Fig. 3.20** D2–40. Staining in seen in serous ovarian carcinoma (**a**) and in malignant mesothelioma (**b**)

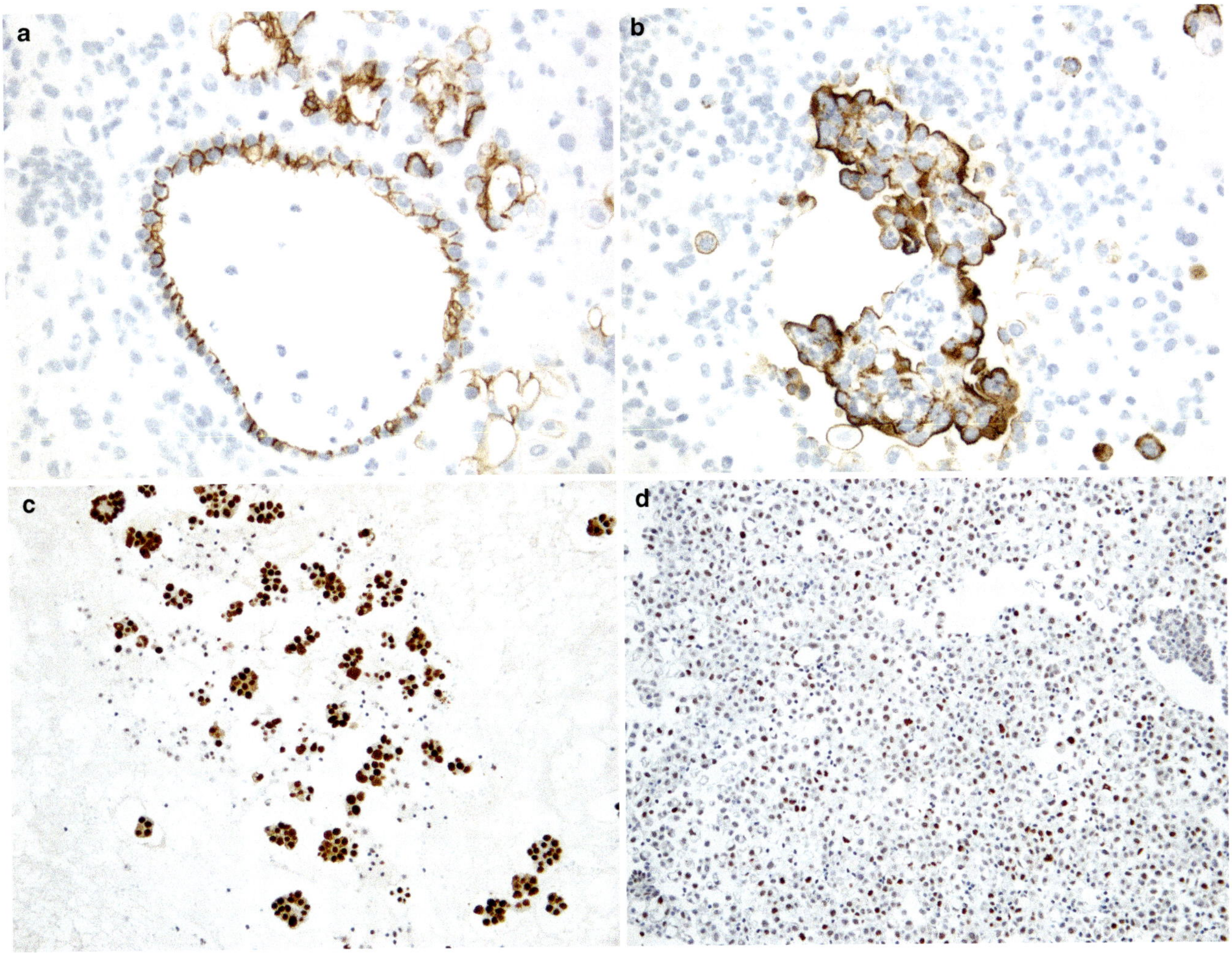

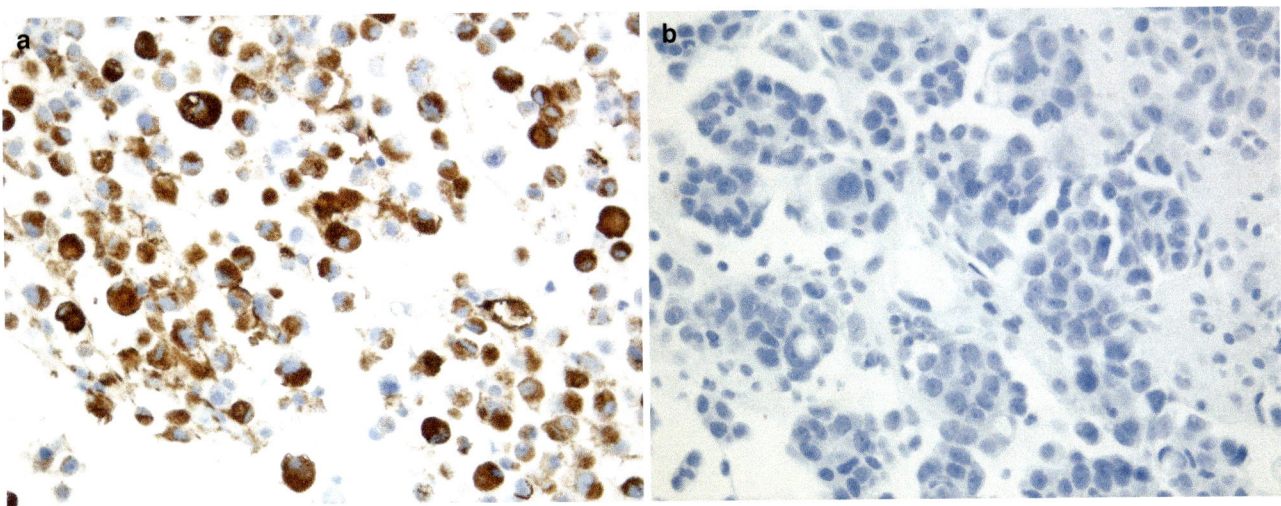

**Fig. 3.21** Immunohistochemistry as differentiator between serous borderline tumor, LGSC and HGSC. (**a**) Ber-EP4; (**b**) B72.3 in serous border-line tumor; (**c**) aberrant p53 in HGSC; (**d**) wild-type p53 in LGSC

**Fig. 3.22** MUC5AC. (**a**) Expression is seen in metastatic pancreatic carcinoma; (**b**) negative staining in HGSC

Data regarding the differential diagnosis between renal and ovarian carcinomas is predominantly from studies of CCC (see below).

## CCC

Large series focusing on the immunophenotype of CCC in effusions are rare, as this tumor is only infrequently found at this anatomic site. Based on studies of tissue sections, CCC are usually WT1-negative and ER-negative, a characteristic that aids in their differentiation from serous carcinoma (both markers) and endometrioid carcinoma (ER) [93].

Hepatocyte nuclear factor-1β (HNF-1β) was shown to be a CCC-specific marker that does not stain serous, endometrioid, or mucinous OC in a series of 21 effusions [94]. The author's experience only partly concurs with this observation. HNF-1β does stain the majority of CCC and is negative in the majority of serous carcinomas (Fig. 3.23a, b). However, EC of both ovarian and uterine origin are often stained, as are carcinomas of other origin [95]. Napsin A is another useful marker supporting the diagnosis of CCC, as is loss of ARID1A (Fig. 3.23c, d), though the latter is also seen in EC.

Differentiation of CCC from clear cell borderline tumor may be impossible, as is the case with serous tumors. However, this is an exceedingly rare problem in effusion cytology. Markers that have been shown to be useful in separating renal from ovarian CCC in tissue sections are renal cell carcinoma antigen (RCC) and CD10 as markers of the former and CK7 (and ER and PR, when expressed) as marker of the latter [96, 97]. Mesothelin is another marker that may be useful in this context, as it is expressed in OC but not in RCC [96]. PAX2 and carbonic anhydrase IX were shown to stain CCC of both origins and is therefore of little use in this context [98–100].

Differentiation of CCC from carcinomas of other origin, benign or malignant mesothelial cells, non-epithelial cancers, and macrophages is fairly easily achieved applying the panels discussed elsewhere in this book.

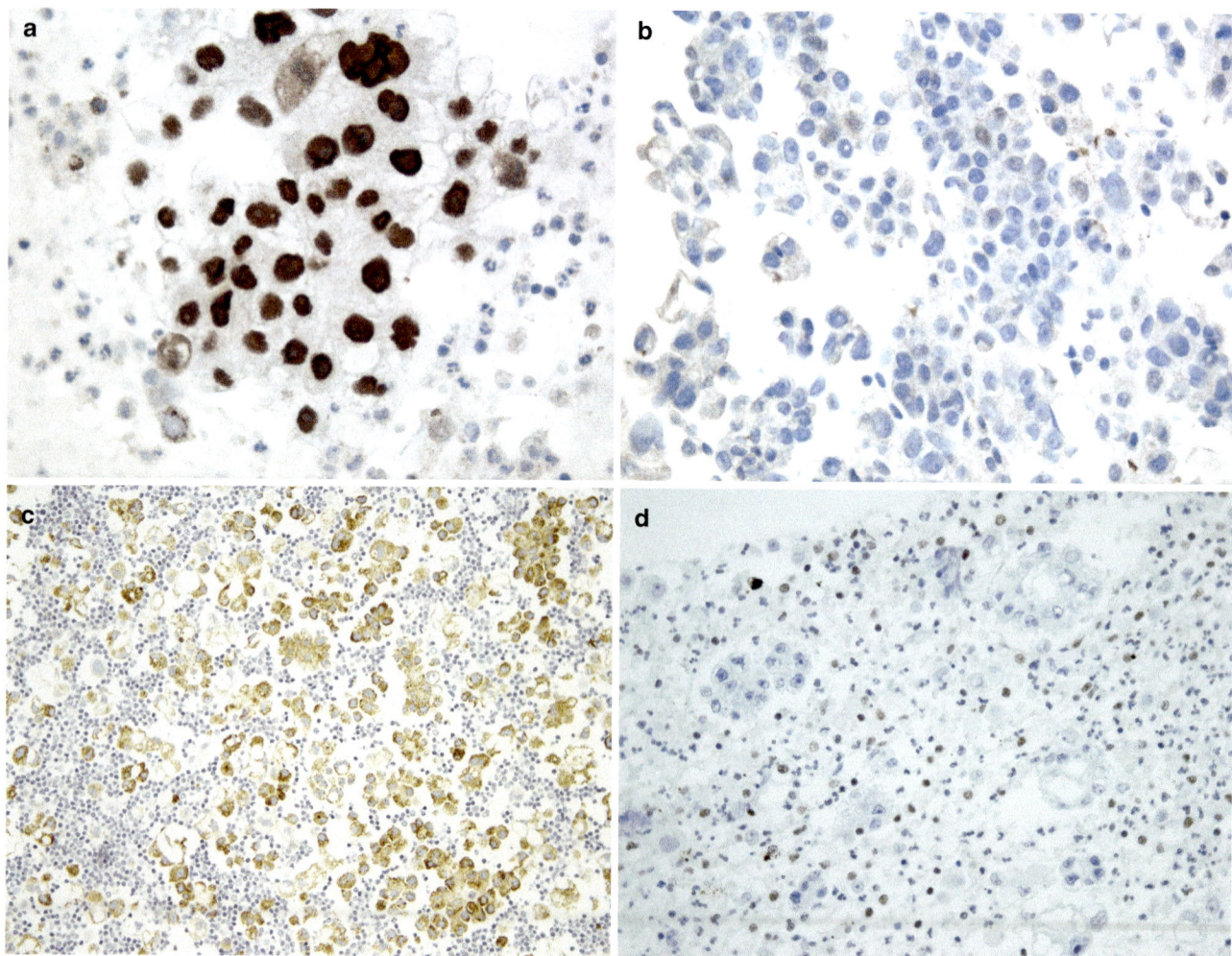

**Fig. 3.23** (**a**, **b**) HNF-1β in ovarian carcinoma. CCC cells are strongly stained at the nucleus, whereas a serous carcinoma stains focally at the cytoplasm, with very weak nuclear staining in isolated cells. (**c**) Napsin A expression in CCC. (**d**) Loss of ARID1A in CCC

## MC

As stated above, differentiation of mucinous OC from other mucinous carcinomas based on IHC may be difficult. Differentiation of this tumor from colorectal carcinoma is often possible based on CK7/CK20 expression, as mucinous OC are CK7+/CK20- or CK7+/CK20±, whereas colorectal carcinomas are CK7−/CK20+. Exceptions do occur, however. Upper GI carcinomas may have the same CK7/CK20 expression pattern as mucinous OC does. CEA, CDX2, and villin are expressed both ovarian and non-ovarian MC based on the author's experience, although CDX2 expression is generally more widespread in the latter. SATB2 may be helpful in this differential diagnosis as a colorectal carcinoma marker, but no studies of effusion specimens investigating this marker have been published to date.

As is true for the other types of OC, differentiation from mucinous borderline tumor may be impossible but is fortunately rarely needed.

Differentiation of mucinous from other types of OC is easier using markers specific for the former, including CEA (may be focally expressed in ovarian EC but not diffusely as in mucinous OC) and CDX2, as well as negative markers such as WT1 and ER. HNF-4α was reported to be mucinous OC-specific in this differential diagnosis [101].

As is the case for CCC, differentiation of MC from benign or malignant mesothelial cells, non-epithelial cancers, and macrophages is generally easy using sufficiently broad panels, as discussed elsewhere in this book.

## EC

As is true for all non-serous carcinomas, guidelines for choosing the relevant IHC panel are largely based on studies of surgical specimens. EC express ER and PR and are WT1-negative [93], whereas CEA expression is focal or absent, features that help in the differential diagnosis from other OC histotypes, as well as from metastatic tumors. For the latter, addition of CDX2, SATB2, CK7, and CK20 to the panel may be useful.

## References

1. Torre LA, Bray F, Siegel RL, Ferlay J, Lortet-Tieulent J, Jemal A. Global cancer statistics, 2012. CA Cancer J Clin. 2015;65:87–108.
2. Matulonis UA, Sood AK, Fallowfield L, Howitt BE, Sehouli J, Karlan BY. Ovarian cancer. Nat Rev Dis Primers. 2016;2:16061.
3. Berek JS, Bast RC Jr. Ovarian cancer. In: Kufe DW, Bast Jr RC, Hait WM, Hong WK, Pollock RE, Weichselbaum RR, Holland JF, Frei III E, editors. Cancer medicine. 7th ed. Hamilton: BC Decker Inc.; 2006. p. 1543–68. Chapter 104.
4. Jacob IJ, Shepherd JH, Oran DH, Blackett AD, Luesley DM, Berchuck A, Hudson CN, editors. Ovarian cancer. Oxford: Oxford University Press; 2002.
5. Prat J. Ovarian, fallopian tube and peritoneal cancer staging: rationale and explanation of new FIGO staging 2013. Best Pract Res Clin Obstet Gynaecol. 2015;29:858–69.
6. Siegel RL, Miller KD, Jemal A. Cancer statistics, 2017. CA Cancer J Clin. 2017;67:7–30.
7. Yang WL, Lu Z, Bast RC Jr. The role of biomarkers in the management of epithelial ovarian cancer. Expert Rev Mol Diagn. 2017;17:577–91.
8. Karam A, Ledermann JA, Kim JW, Sehouli J, Lu K, Gourley C, Katsumata N, Burger RA, Nam BH, Bacon M, Ng C, Pfisterer J, Bekkers RLM, Casado Herráez A, Redondo A, Fujiwara H, Gleeson N, Rosengarten O, Scambia G, Zhu J, Okamoto A, Stuart G, Ochiai K. Participants of the 5th ovarian cancer consensus conference fifth ovarian cancer consensus conference of the Gynecologic Cancer InterGroup: first-line interventions. Ann Oncol. 2017;28:711–7.
9. Kurman RJ, Visvanathan K, Roden R, Wu TC, Shih IM. Early detection and treatment of ovarian cancer: shifting from early stage to minimal volume of disease based on a new model of carcinogenesis. Am J Obstet Gynecol. 2008;198:351–6.
10. Prat J. Ovarian carcinomas: five distinct diseases with different origins, genetic alterations, and clinicopathological features. Virchows Arch. 2012;460:237–49.
11. Singh N, McCluggage WG, Gilks CB. High-grade serous carcinoma of tubo-ovarian origin: recent developments. Histopathology. 2017;71:339–56.
12. Hirabayashi K, Graham J. The genesis of ascites in ovarian cancer. Am J Obstet Gynecol. 1970;106:492–7.
13. Feldman GB, Knapp RC, Order SE, Hellman S. The role of lymphatic obstruction in the formation of ascites in a murine ovarian carcinoma. Cancer Res. 1972;32:1663–6.
14. Nagy JA, Masse EM, Herzberg KT, Meyers MS, Yeo KT, Yeo TK, Sioussat TM, Dvorak HF. Pathogenesis of ascites tumor growth: vascular permeability factor, vascular hyperpermeability, and ascites tumor accumulation. Cancer Res. 1995;55:360–8.
15. Nagy JA, Meyers MS, Masse EM, Herzberg KT, Dvorak HF. Pathogenesis of ascites tumor growth: fibrinogen influx and fibrin accumulation in tissues lining the peritoneal cavity. Cancer Res. 1995;55:369–75.
16. Nagy JA, Morgan ES, Herzberg KT, Manseau EJ, Dvorak AM, Dvorak HF. Pathogenesis of ascites tumor growth: angiogenesis, vascular remodeling, and stroma formation in the peritoneal lining. Cancer Res. 1995;55:376–85.
17. Sorbe B, Frankendal B. Prognostic importance of ascites in ovarian carcinoma. Acta Obstet Gynecol Scand. 1983;62:415–8.
18. Shen-Gunther J, Mannel RS. Ascites as a predictor of ovarian malignancy. Gynecol Oncol. 2002;87:77–83.
19. Rice LW, Mark SD, Berkowitz RS, Goff BA, Lage JM. Clinicopathologic variables, operative characteristics, and DNA ploidy in predicting outcome in ovarian epithelial carcinoma. Obstet Gynecol. 1995;86:379–85.
20. Ayhan A, Gultekin M, Taskiran C, Dursun P, Firat P, Bozdag G, Celik NY, Yuce K. Ascites and epithelial ovarian cancers: a reappraisal with respect to different aspects. Int J Gynecol Cancer. 2007;17:68–75.
21. Chi DS, Liao JB, Leon LF, Venkatraman ES, Hensley ML, Bhaskaran D, Hoskins WJ. Identification of prognostic factors in advanced epithelial ovarian carcinoma. Gynecol Oncol. 2001;82:532–7.
22. Clark TG, Stewart ME, Altman DG, Gabra H, Smyth JF. A prognostic model for ovarian cancer. Br J Cancer. 2001;85:944–52.
23. Puls LE, Duniho T, Hunter JE, Kryscio R, Blackhurst D, Gallion H. The prognostic implication of ascites in advanced-stage ovarian cancer. Gynecol Oncol. 1996;61:109–12.
24. Makar AP, Baekelandt M, Tropé CG, Kristensen GB. The prognostic significance of residual disease, FIGO substage, tumor histology, and grade in patients with FIGO stage III ovarian cancer. Gynecol Oncol. 1995;56:175–80.

25. Omura GA, Brady MF, Homesley HD, Yordan E, Major FJ, Buchsbaum HJ, Park RC. Long-term follow-up and prognostic factor analysis in advanced ovarian carcinoma: the gynecologic oncology group experience. J Clin Oncol. 1991;9:1138–50.

26. Curtin JP, Malik R, Venkatraman ES, Barakat RR, Hoskins WJ, Stage IV. Ovarian cancer: impact of surgical debulking. Gynecol Oncol. 1997;64:9–12.

27. Bristow RE, Montz FJ, Lagasse LD, Leuchter RS, Karlan BY. Survival impact of surgical cytoreduction in stage IV epithelial ovarian cancer. Gynecol Oncol. 1999;72:278–87.

28. Akahira JI, Yoshikawa H, Shimizu Y, Tsunematsu R, Hirakawa T, Kuramoto H, Shiromizu K, Kuzuya K, Kamura T, Kikuchi Y, Kodama S, Yamamoto K, Sato S. Prognostic factors of stage IV epithelial ovarian cancer: a multicenter retrospective study. Gynecol Oncol. 2001;81:398–403.

29. Bonnefoi H, A'Hern RP, Fisher C, Macfarlane V, Barton D, Blake P, Shepherd JH, Gore ME. Natural history of stage IV epithelial ovarian cancer. J Clin Oncol. 1999;17:767–75.

30. Dauplat J, Hacker NF, Nieberg RK, Berek JS, Rose TP, Sagae S. Distant metastases in epithelial ovarian carcinoma. Cancer. 1987;60:1561–6.

31. Liu PC, Benjamin I, Morgan MA, King SA, Mikuta JJ, Rubin SC. Effect of surgical debulking on survival in stage IV ovarian cancer. Gynecol Oncol. 1997;64:4–8.

32. Jamieson A, Sykes P, Eva L, Bergzoll C, Simcock B. Subtypes of stage IV ovarian cancer; response to treatment and patterns of disease recurrence. Gynecol Oncol. 2017;146:273–8.

33. Escayola C, Ferron G, Romeo M, Torrent JJ, Querleu D. The impact of pleural disease on the management of advanced ovarian cancer. Gynecol Oncol. 2015;138:216–20.

34. Köbel M, Kalloger SE, Huntsman DG, Santos JL, Swenerton KD, Seidman JD, Gilks CB, Cheryl Brown ovarian cancer outcomes unit of the British Columbia Cancer Agency, Vancouver BC. Differences in tumor type in low-stage versus high-stage ovarian carcinomas. Int J Gynecol Pathol. 2010;29:203–11.

35. Pereira TC, Saad RS, Liu Y, Silverman JF. The diagnosis of malignancy in effusion cytology: a pattern recognition approach. Adv Anat Pathol. 2006;13:174–84.

36. Yu GH, Sack MJ, Baloch ZW, DeFrias DV, Gupta PK. Occurrence of intercellular spaces (windows) in metastatic adenocarcinoma in serous fluids: a cytomorphologic, histochemical, and ultrastructural study. Diagn Cytopathol. 1999;20:115–9.

37. Kurman RJ, Carcangiu ML, Herrington CS, Young RH, editors. WHO classification of tumours of female reproductive organs. Lyon: IARC; 2014.

38. Ito H, Hirasawa T, Yasuda M, Osamura RY, Tsutsumi Y. Excessive formation of basement membrane substance in clear-cell carcinoma of the ovary: diagnostic value of the "raspberry body" in ascites cytology. Diagn Cytopathol. 1997;16:500–4.

39. Damiani D, Suciu V, Genestie C, Vielh P. Cytomorphology of ovarian clear cell carcinomas in peritoneal effusions. Cytopathology. 2016;27:427–32.

40. Ahr A, Arnold G, Göhring UJ, Costa S, Scharl A, Gauwerky JF. Cytology of ascitic fluid in a patient with metastasizing malignant Brenner tumor of the ovary: a case report. Acta Cytol. 1997;41(4 Suppl):1299–304.

41. Driss M, Mrad K, Dhouib R, Doghri R, Abbes I, Ben Romdhane K. Ascitic fluid cytology in malignant Brenner tumor: a case report. Acta Cytol. 2010;54:598–600.

42. Motoyama T, Watanabe H. Ascitic fluid cytologic features of a malignant mixed mesodermal tumor of the ovary. Acta Cytol. 1987;31:63–7.

43. Ehya H, Lang WR. Cytology of granulosa cell tumor of the ovary. Am J Clin Pathol. 1986;85:402–5.

44. Lal A, Bourtsos EP, Nayar R, DeFrias DV. Cytologic features of granulosa cell tumors in fluids and fine needle aspiration specimens. Acta Cytol. 2004;48:315–20.

45. Kavuri S, Kulkarni R, Reid-Nicholson M. Granulosa cell tumor of the ovary: cytologic findings. Acta Cytol. 2010;54:551–9.

46. Gupta N, Rajwanshi A, Dey P, Suri V. Adult granulosa cell tumor presenting as metastases to the pleural and peritoneal cavity. Diagn Cytopathol. 2012;40:912–5.

47. Atilgan AO, Tepeoglu M, Ozen O, Bilezikçi B. Peritoneal washing cytology in an adult granulosa cell tumor: a case report and review of literature. J Cytol. 2013;30:74–7.

48. Omori M, Kondo T, Yuminamochi T, Nakazawa K, Ishii Y, Fukasawa H, Hashi A, Hirata S. Cytologic features of ovarian granulosa cell tumors in pleural and ascitic fluids. Diagn Cytopathol. 2015;43:581–4.

49. Murugan P, Siddaraju N, Sridhar E, Soundararaghavan J, Habeebullah S. Unusual ovarian malignancies in ascitic fluid: a report of 2 cases. Acta Cytol. 2010;54:611–7.

50. Valente PT, Schantz HD, Edmonds PR, Hanjani P. Peritoneal cytology of uncommon ovarian tumors. Diagn Cytopathol. 1992;8:98–106.

51. Ikeda K, Tate G, Suzuki T, Mitsuya T. Cytomorphologic features of immature ovarian teratoma in peritoneal effusion: a case report. Diagn Cytopathol. 2005;33:39–42.

52. Geisinger KR, Hajdu SI, Helson L. Exfoliative cytology of nonlymphoreticular neoplasms in children. Acta Cytol. 1984;28:16–28.

53. Selvaggi SM, Guidos BJ. Immature teratoma of the ovary on fluid cytology. Diagn Cytopathol. 2001;25:411–4.

54. Selvaggi SM. Cytologic features of malignant ovarian monodermal teratoma with an ependymal component in peritoneal washings. Int J Gynecol Pathol. 1992;11:299–303.

55. Kashimura M, Tsukamoto N, Matsuyama T, Kashimura Y, Sugimori H, Taki I. Cytologic findings of ascites from patients with ovarian dysgerminoma. Acta Cytol. 1983;27:59–62.

56. Hajdu SI, Nolan MA. Exfoliative cytology of malignant germ cell tumors. Acta Cytol. 1975;19:255–60.

57. Roncalli M, Gribaudi G, Simoncelli D, Servida E. Cytology of yolk-sac tumor of the ovary in ascitic fluid. Report of a case. Acta Cytol. 1988;32:113–6.

58. Davidson B, Abeler VM. Primary ovarian angiosarcoma presenting as malignant cells in ascites: case report and review of the literature. Diagn Cytopathol. 2005;32:307–9.

59. Hirakawa E, Kobayashi S, Miki H, Haba R, Saoo K, Yamakawa K, Ohkura I, Kira Y. Ascitic fluid cytology of adenosarcoma of the ovary: a case report. Diagn Cytopathol. 2001;24:343–6.

60. Delahaye M, van der Ham F, van der Kwast TH. Complementary value of five carcinoma markers for the diagnosis of malignant mesothelioma, adenocarcinoma metastasis, and reactive mesothelium in serous effusions. Diagn Cytopathol. 1997;17:115–20.

61. Motherby H, Kube M, Friedrichs N Nadjari B, Knops K, Donner A, Baschiera B, Dalquen P, Böcking A. Immunocytochemistry and DNA-image cytometry in diagnostic effusion cytology I. Prevalence of markers in tumour cell positive and negative smears. Anal Cell Pathol. 1999;19:7–20.

62. Maguire B, Whitaker D, Carrello S, Spagnolo D. Monoclonal antibody Ber-EP4: its use in the differential diagnosis of malignant mesothelioma and carcinoma in cell blocks of malignant effusions and FNA specimens. Diagn Cytopathol. 1994;10:130–4.

63. Davidson B, Risberg B, Kristensen G, Kvalheim G, Emilsen E, Bjåmer A, Berner A. Detection of cancer cells in effusions from patients diagnosed with gynaecological malignancies. Evaluation of five epithelial markers. Virchows Arch. 1999;435:43–9.

64. McKnight R, Cohen C, Siddiqui MT. Utility of paired box gene 8 (PAX8) expression in fluid and fine-needle aspiration cytology: an immunohistochemical study of metastatic ovarian serous carcinoma. Cancer Cytopathol. 2010;118:298–302.

65. Tong GX, Devaraj K, Hamele-Bena D, Yu WM, Turk A, Chen X, Wright JD, Greenebaum E. Pax8: a marker for carcinoma of Müllerian origin in serous effusions. Diagn Cytopathol. 2011;39:567–74.

66. Zhao L, Guo M, Sneige N, Gong Y. Value of PAX8 and WT1 immunostaining in confirming the ovarian origin of metastatic carcinoma in serous effusion specimens. Am J Clin Pathol. 2012;137:304–9.

67. Wiseman W, Michael CW, Roh MH. Diagnostic utility of PAX8 and PAX2. immunohistochemistry in the identification of metastatic Mullerian carcinoma in effusions. Diagn Cytopathol. 2011;39:651–6.

68. Fetsch PA, Abati A, Hijazi YM. Utility of the antibodies CA 19-9, HBME-1, and thrombomodulin in the diagnosis of malignant mesothelioma and adenocarcinoma in cytology. Cancer. 1998;84:101–8.

69. Davidson B, Baekelandt M, Shih IM. MUC4 is upregulated in ovarian carcinoma effusions and differentiates carcinoma cells from mesothelial cells. Diagn Cytopathol. 2007;35:756–60.

70. Kleinberg L, Holth A, Fridman E, Schwartz I, Shih IM, Davidson B. The diagnostic role of claudins in serous effusions. Am J Clin Pathol. 2007;127:928–37.

71. Lonardi S, Manera C, Marucci R, Santoro A, Lorenzi L, Facchetti F. Usefulness of Claudin 4 in the cytological diagnosis of serosal effusions. Diagn Cytopathol. 2011;39:313–7.

72. Jo VY, Cibas ES, Pinkus GS. Claudin-4 immunohistochemistry is highly effective in distinguishing adenocarcinoma from malignant mesothelioma in effusion cytology. Cancer Cytopathol. 2014;122:299–306.

73. Davidson B, Skrede M, Silins I, Shih IM, Trope' CG, Flørenes VA. Low molecular weight cyclin E forms differentiate ovarian carcinoma from cells of mesothelial origin and are associated with poor survival in ovarian carcinoma. Cancer. 2007;110:1264–71.

74. Reich R, Vintman L, Nielsen S, Kærn J, Bedrossian C, Berner A, Davidson B. Differential expression of the 67 kilodalton laminin receptor in malignant mesothelioma and carcinomas that spread to serosal cavities. Diagn Cytopathol. 2005;33:332–7.

75. Davidson B, Stavnes HT, Hellesylt E, et al. MMP-7 is a highly specific negative marker for benign and malignant mesothelial cells in serous effusions. Hum Pathol. 2016;47:104–8.

76. Davidson B. CD24 is highly useful in differentiating high-grade serous carcinoma from benign and malignant mesothelial cells. Hum Pathol. 2016;58:123–7.

77. Davidson B, Nielsen S, Christensen J, Asschenfeldt P, Berner A, Risberg B, Johansen P. The role of Desmin and N-cadherin in effusion cytology: a comparative study using established markers of mesothelial and epithelial cells. Am J Surg Pathol. 2001;25:1405–12.

78. Yuan Y, Nymoen DA, Tuft Stavnes H, Rossnes AK, Bjørang O, Wu C, Nesland JM, Davidson B. Tenascin-X is a novel diagnostic marker of malignant mesothelioma. Am J Surg Pathol. 2009;33:1673–82.

79. Wieczorek TJ, Krane JF. Diagnostic utility of calretinin immunohistochemistry in cytologic cell block preparations. Cancer. 2000;90:312–9.

80. Afify AM, Stern R, Michael CW. Differentiation of mesothelioma from adenocarcinoma in serous effusions: the role of hyaluronic acid and CD44 localization. Diagn Cytopathol. 2005;32:145–50.

81. Hwang HC, Sheffield BS, Rodriguez S, Thompson K, Tse CH, Gown AM, Churg A. Utility of BAP1 immunohistochemistry and p16 (CDKN2A) FISH in the diagnosis of. malignant mesothelioma in effusion cytology specimens. Am J Surg Pathol. 2016;40:120–6.

82. Cigognetti M, Lonardi S, Fisogni S, Balzarini P, Pellegrini V, Tironi A, Bercich L, Bugatti M, Rossi G, Murer B, Barbareschi M, Giuliani S, Cavazza A, Marchetti G, Vermi W, Facchetti F. BAP1 (BRCA1-associated protein 1) is a highly specific marker for differentiating mesothelioma from reactive mesothelial proliferations. Mod Pathol. 2015;28:1043–57.

83. Andrici J, Sheen A, Sioson L, Wardell K, Clarkson A, Watson N, Ahadi MS, Farzin M, Toon CW, Gill AJ. Loss of expression of BAP1 is a useful adjunct, which strongly supports the diagnosis of mesothelioma in effusion cytology. Mod Pathol. 2015;28:1360–8.

84. Zhu W, Michael CW. WT1, monoclonal CEA, TTF1, and CA125 antibodies in the differential diagnosis of lung, breast, and ovarian adenocarcinomas in serous effusions. Diagn Cytopathol. 2007;35:370–5.

85. Hecht JL, Lee BH, Pinkus JL, Pinkus GS. The value of Wilms tumor susceptibility gene 1 in cytologic preparations as a marker for malignant mesothelioma. Cancer. 2002;96:105–9.

86. Ascoli V, Carnovale-Scalzo C, Taccogna S, Nardi F. Utility of HBME-1 immunostaining in serous effusions. Cytopathology. 1997;8:328–35.

87. Bassarova AV, Nesland JM, Davidson B. D2-40 is not a specific marker for cells of mesothelial origin in serous effusions. Am J Surg Pathol. 2006;30:878–82.

88. Hanna A, Pang Y, Bedrossian CW, Dejmek A, Michael CW. Podoplanin is a useful marker for identifying mesothelioma in malignant effusions. Diagn Cytopathol. 2010;38:264–9.

89. Ordóñez NG. Value of immunohistochemistry in distinguishing peritoneal mesothelioma from serous carcinoma of the ovary and peritoneum: a review and update. Adv Anat Pathol. 2006;13:16–25.

90. Al-Hussaini M, Stockman A, Foster H, McCluggage WG. WT-1 assists in distinguishing ovarian from uterine serous carcinoma and in distinguishing between serous and endometrioid ovarian carcinoma. Histopathology. 2004;44:109–15.

91. Hashi A, Yuminamochi T, Murata S, Iwamoto H, Honda T, Hoshi K. Wilms tumor gene immunoreactivity in primary serous carcinomas of the fallopian tube, ovary, endometrium, and peritoneum. Int J Gynecol Pathol. 2003;22:374–7.

92. Han L, Pansare V, Al-Abbadi M, Husain M, Feng J. Combination of MUC5ac and WT-1 immunohistochemistry is useful in distinguishing pancreatic ductal carcinoma from ovarian serous carcinoma in effusion cytology. Diagn Cytopathol. 2010;38:333–6.

93. Soslow RA. Histologic subtypes of ovarian carcinoma: an overview. Int J Gynecol Pathol. 2008;27:161–74.

94. Kato N, Toukairin M, Asanuma I, Motoyama T. Immunocytochemistry for hepatocyte nuclear factor-1beta (HNF-1beta): a marker for ovarian clear cell carcinoma. Diagn Cytopathol. 2007;35:193–7.

95. Davidson B. Hepatocyte nuclear factor-1β is not a specific marker of clear cell carcinoma in serous effusions. Cancer Cytopathol. 2014;122:153–8.

96. McCluggage WG, Wilkinson N. Metastatic neoplasms involving the ovary: a review with an emphasis on morphological and immunohistochemical features. Histopathology. 2005;47:231–47.

97. Leroy X, Farine MO, Buob D, Wacrenier A, Copin MC. Diagnostic value of cytokeratin 7, CD10 and mesothelin in distinguishing ovarian clear cell carcinoma from metastasis of renal clear cell carcinoma. Histopathology. 2007;51:874–6.

98. Gokden N, Gokden M, Phan DC, McKenney JK. The utility of PAX-2 in distinguishing metastatic clear cell renal cell carcinoma from its morphologic mimics: an immunohistochemical study with comparison to renal cell carcinoma marker. Am J Surg Pathol. 2008;32:1462–7.

99. Al-Ahmadie HA, Alden D, Qin LX, Olgac S, Fine SW, Gopalan A, Russo P, Motzer RJ, Reuter VE, Tickoo SK. Carbonic anhydrase IX expression in clear cell renal cell carcinoma: an immunohistochemical study comparing 2 antibodies. Am J Surg Pathol. 2008;32:377–82.

100. Hynninen P, Vaskivuo L, Saarnio J, Haapasalo H, Kivelä J, Pastoreková S, Pastorek J, Waheed A, Sly WS, Puistola U, Parkkila S. Expression of transmembrane carbonic anhydrases IX and XII in ovarian tumours. Histopathology. 2006;49:594–602.

101. Sugai M, Umezu H, Yamamoto T, Jiang S, Iwanari H, Tanaka T, Hamakubo T, Kodama T, Naito M. Expression of hepatocyte nuclear factor 4 alpha in primary ovarian mucinous tumors. Pathol Int. 2008;58:681–6.

# Breast Carcinoma

Fernando Schmitt and Ben Davidson

## Introduction

Breast cancer is the most commonly diagnosed malignancy in women in the majority of countries, with an estimated 1.7 million new cases and 521,900 deaths in 2012. Disease incidence is highest in North America, Western and Northern Europe, Australia, and New Zealand [1]. In the USA, 61% of new breast cancer cases are diagnosed while localized, 31% are diagnosed in a regional stage, and 6% have already metastasized to distant sites at diagnosis (stage unknown in the remaining 2%) [2]. Breast cancer metastasizes most often to axillary lymph nodes but may involve any organ. Tumor spread to the serosal surfaces is common in patients with metastatic disease, involving primarily the pleural cavity [3, 4] and occasionally the pericardial and peritoneal cavities [5–7]. Breast carcinoma was reported to be the most common tumor diagnosed in pleural effusion in women in a large study of 584 effusions, constituting 37.4% of cases [8]. The risk for metastasis to the pleural or pericardial cavity has been reported to be fourfold for patients with invasive carcinoma of no special type (NST) located in the inner breast quadrants compared to the outer ones [9]. Pleural effusions may occur at any point during the clinical course and may be the presenting sign of malignancy and/or the sole manifestation of metastatic disease [3, 4, 10, 11].

The large majority of effusions in breast cancer patients are the result of involvement of the pleural surfaces by solid metastases. However, the presence of a pleural effusion in a patient with breast cancer does not necessarily imply pleural metastasis. Clinically, effusions that are hemorrhagic and recurrent and that re-accumulate rapidly after drainage are highly suspicious to be secondary to cancer. Although the presence of tumor cells within the pleural space and surface may cause an increase in the amount of pleural fluid secondary to increased oncotic pressure and inflammation-related effects that cause increased capillary permeability, the latter also secondary to production of vascular endothelial growth factor (VEGF), most large effusions are due to obstruction of the pleural lymphatics, preventing the reabsorption of pleural fluid.

## Diagnosis

About 75% of malignant effusions in breast cancer patients are symptomatic. More than 50% of patients complain of dyspnea of varying degree, depending on the size of the effusion. Any new unilateral pleural effusion in a patient with a history of breast cancer and without known metastatic disease justifies diagnostic needle thoracentesis. Similarly, bilateral effusions in a patient with no history of congestive heart failure or other medical causes of bilateral effusions should be aspirated. The vast majority of malignant effusions are exudative, and the fluid should always be sent for cytological examination. Cytologic evaluation of pleural fluid has a higher sensitivity than needle biopsy for the diagnosis of malignant effusions [12]. In patients who are ultimately diagnosed with a malignant effusion, the cytologic detection of cancer cells in effusions can generally be made with the submission of two samples. If the initial specimen is suspicious but not conclusive for malignancy, it is easy to obtain a repeat sample because the malignant fluid rapidly re-accumulates.

F. Schmitt, M.D., Ph.D., F.I.A.C. (✉)
Department of Pathology and Oncology, Medical Faculty of Porto University, Porto, Portugal

Molecular Pathology Unit, Institute of Pathology and Molecular Immunology of Porto University, IPATIMUP, Porto, Portugal

International Academy of Cytology, Freiburg, Germany
e-mail: fschmitt@ipatimup.pt; fernando.schmitt@ipatimup.pt

B. Davidson, M.D., Ph.D.
Department of Pathology, The Norwegian Radium Hospital, Oslo University Hospital, Oslo, Norway

Faculty of Medicine, Institute of Clinical Medicine, University of Oslo, Oslo, Norway
e-mail: bend@medisin.uio.no; bdd@ous-hf.no

© Springer International Publishing AG, part of Springer Nature 2018
B. Davidson et al. (eds.), *Serous Effusions*, https://doi.org/10.1007/978-3-319-76478-8_4

## Morphology

The cytology of a malignant effusion may be highly variable. In some cases, there is an obvious abnormal population of cells distinct from mesothelial cells, macrophages, and other inflammatory cells. Evaluation of the slides at low amplification allows for easy distinction of these cells from the nonneoplastic reactive constituents of an effusion. This is the most common presentation of breast carcinoma cells in effusions (Fig. 4.1a, b). In other specimens, a population of abnormal cells is present that is difficult to distinguish from mesothelial cells. The cells may be in aggregates or single and sometimes the atypia is not so severe. This feature may be misinterpreted as benign, resulting in false-negative diagnosis. This is mainly, but not exclusively, seen with metastases from breast carci-

noma of the lobular subtype (Fig. 4.2a, b). A third pattern is characterized by a background population of inflammatory and mesothelial cells that are so predominant that rare neoplastic cells may be missed. Alternatively, specimens may be sparsely cellular with respect to both malignant and reactive cells (Fig. 4.3a, b). These three patterns have been observed in cytology of breast cancer in effusions by several authors [12–16].

The main challenge to reaching a correct diagnosis is due to the degree of cytological overlap between benign/reactive processes and between malignancies of diverse origins. This is usually not a problem in patients with a previous history of breast cancer in which the effusions appear during disease progression. However, the cytological categorization of an effusion can be of the utmost importance in patients in which an effusion is the presenting symptom of an unknown under-

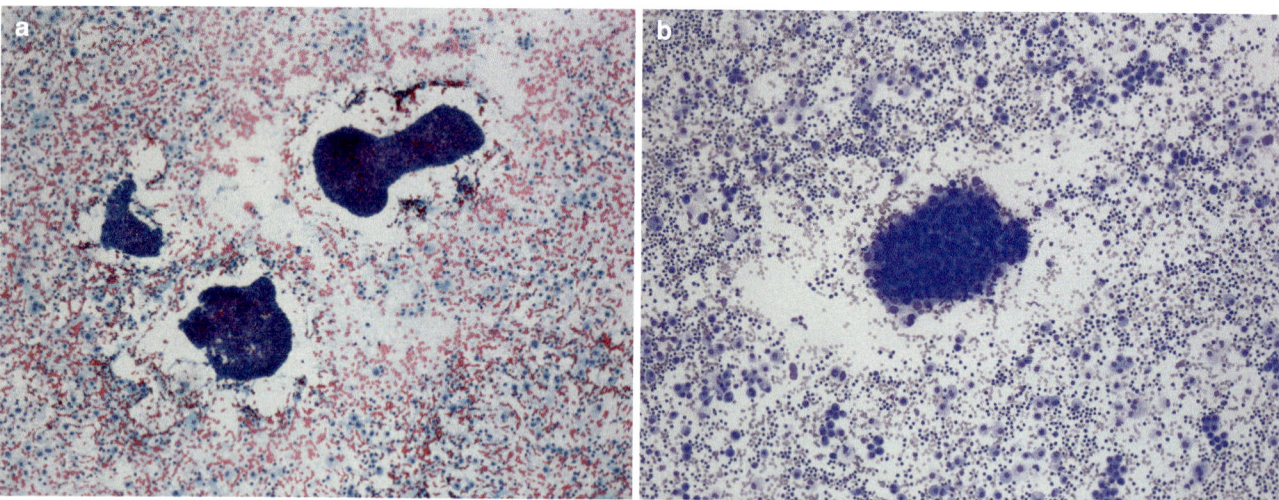

**Fig. 4.1** (a, b) Groups of breast carcinoma cells in a reactive background, predominantly with lymphocytes and mesothelial cells; a: PAP, b: Diff-Quik

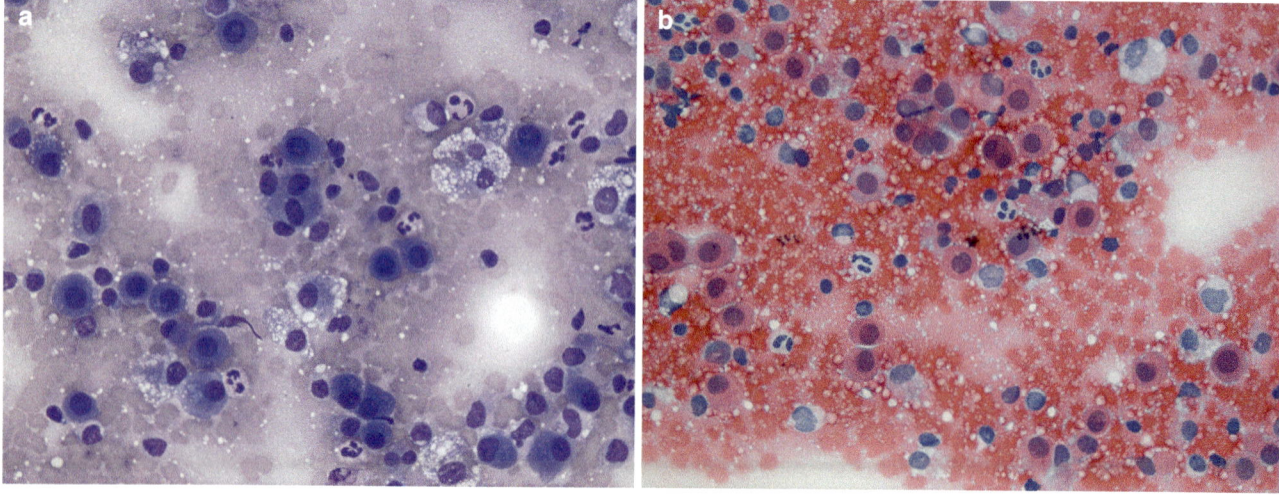

**Fig. 4.2** (a, b) Dissociated medium-sized tumor cells with little atypia, which may mimic reactive mesothelial cells; a: Diff-Quik, b: PAP

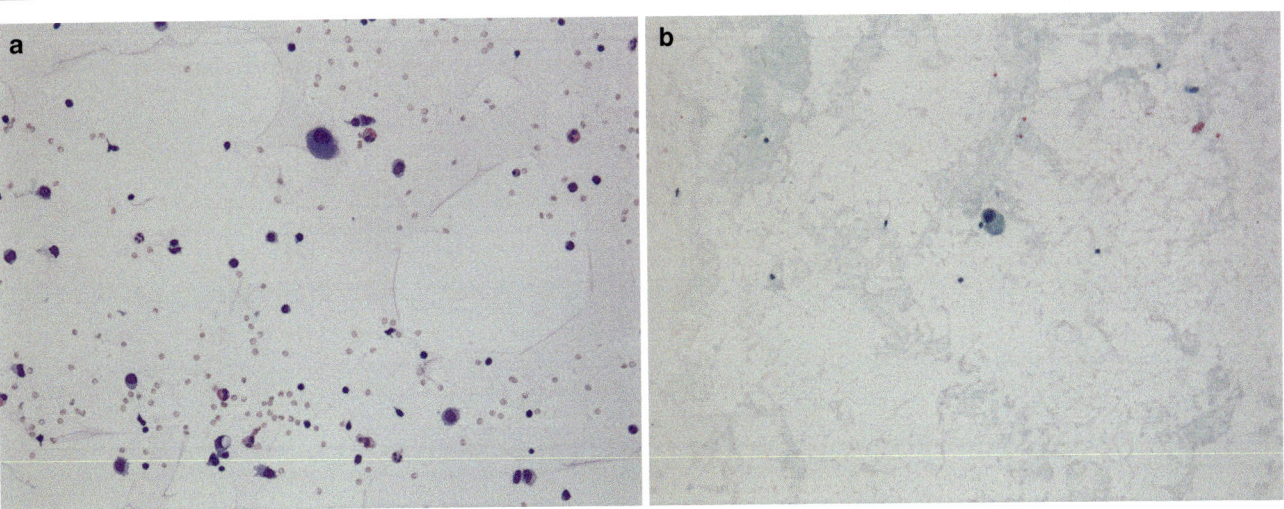

**Fig. 4.3** (**a**, **b**) Sparsely cellular specimen with isolated carcinoma cells, which was originally reported as benign; **a**: Diff-Quik, **b**: PAP

**Table 4.1** Cytomorphological features suggestive of breast primary site in metastatic effusions

| Architecture-based feature | Individual cell features |
|---|---|
| 1. Tridimensional round cell groups—proliferation spheres with sharp edges | 1. Targetoid intracytoplasmic vacuole containing secretion |
| 2. Acini/glands | 2. Signet-ring cells |
| 3. Carcinoma cells in chains and rows | 3. Single and small cells (lobular) |

lying malignancy as first manifestation of the disease. In this case, it is worthwhile to remember that breast and lung carcinomas are the most common causes of pleural effusions, although gastric and ovarian carcinomas are the most common causes of ascites [12–16].

General aspects related to the morphology of breast cancer cells in effusions are similar to those pertaining to adenocarcinomas of other origin in effusions, and in most cases we can identify two cell populations—the reactive ones and the malignant ones. However, as highlighted in Table 4.1, several clues may direct us to consider the breast as the organ of origin for carcinoma cells in effusions, including the presence of cell balls, acini, and intracytoplasmic lumina, as well as detection of many single malignant cells and tumor cell chains.

Carcinoma cells may be present singly or in clusters that may deviate in size from few cells to large three-dimensional cell balls or cannonballs (Fig. 4.4a–c). Typically the edges of the cell balls are smooth, although they may appear knobby, similar to those seen in mesothelial cells (Fig. 4.4c). One of the main cytological features of adenocarcinoma cells is increased nuclear-to-cytoplasmic (n/c) ratio. The nuclei in the cell balls show considerable overlapping and crowding (Fig. 4.5). Cell-in-cell cannibalism which is indicative of a malignant population in general, and not specifically of adenocarcinoma, may be seen.

One of the authors diagnosed a rare case in which tumor cells had a ciliated columnar morphology with minimal atypia (Fig. 4.6a, b).

Proliferation spheres, similar to those formed by a stem cell-like population of CD44$^+$CD24$^{-/low}$ breast cancer cells, originally identified in cells from metastatic pleural effusions of breast carcinoma patients, may be present and aid in diagnosing the tumor as breast carcinoma [17]. These round-to-irregular groups of cells without stromal cores are solid or hollow (Fig. 4.7a, b), in comparison to those observed in mesothelioma, which often show cores (Fig. 4.7c, d). Some authors use the term tissue fragments to highlight the fact that they are true fragments formed in vivo rather than physical aggregations secondary to in vitro processing factors [16]. The neoplastic cells of adenocarcinoma in the proliferation spheres may show ill-defined gland formations. The cytomorphological details are best observed in the cells along the periphery of such groups, with additional details from the single neoplastic cells also present in the background.

Most of the morphological descriptions of breast carcinoma cells in effusions are of invasive carcinoma, NST, previously termed invasive ductal carcinomas. These carcinomas tend to produce large cell balls with smooth borders and acini and have typically eccentric nuclei with high n/c ratios. Although the presence of tumor cell chains, intracytoplasmic lumina, and single malignant cells may suggest a lobular subtype, these are not completely reliable indicators. In general, lobular carcinomas present with cells that are quite monotonous, with high n/c ratio and fairly uniform bland nuclei. There are few descriptions in the literature concerning the particular cytological aspects of breast carcinomas of different histological subtype in effusions [18]. There have been, however, rare reports of pseudomyxoma peritonei secondary to mucinous carcinoma of the breast [13, 14, 16].

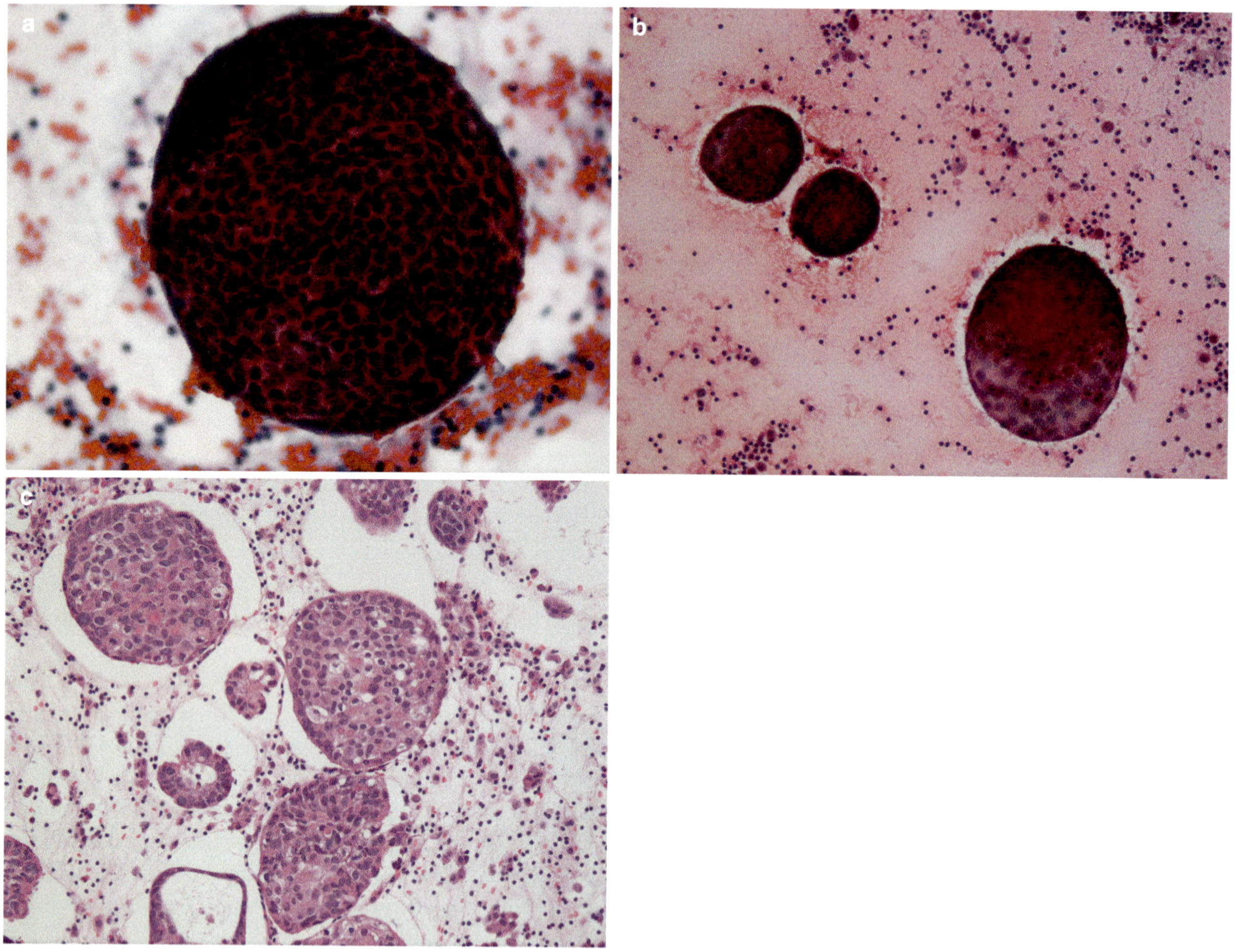

**Fig. 4.4** (**a–c**) Cell balls in breast carcinoma. The outer surface is smooth in **a** and **b**, knobby or irregular in **c**; **a**, **b**: PAP, **c**: H&E

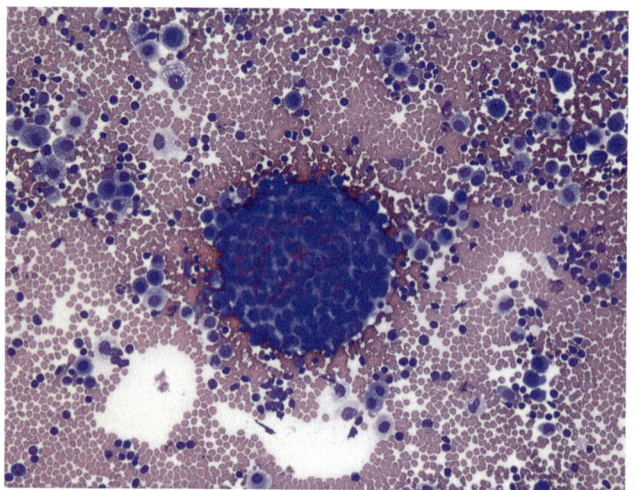

**Fig. 4.5** Breast carcinoma cell ball with overlapping nuclei; Diff-Quik

## Differential Diagnosis

There are three main entities from which breast carcinoma cells on effusions should be distinguished: reactive mesothelial cells, malignant mesothelioma, and other adenocarcinomas.

The distinction of adenocarcinoma from reactive mesothelial cells can be a challenging cytological distinction, particularly in long-standing effusions with reactive mesothelial atypia and in cases of involvement of the pleural cavity by lobular breast carcinoma. In most cases, the individual carcinoma cells show features of malignancy. The cells have high n/c ratio with irregularly shaped nuclear membranes with rounded contours. They may also demonstrate variable degrees of nuclear pleomorphism and multinucleation with atypia. The nuclei are usually eccentric with nucleoli that

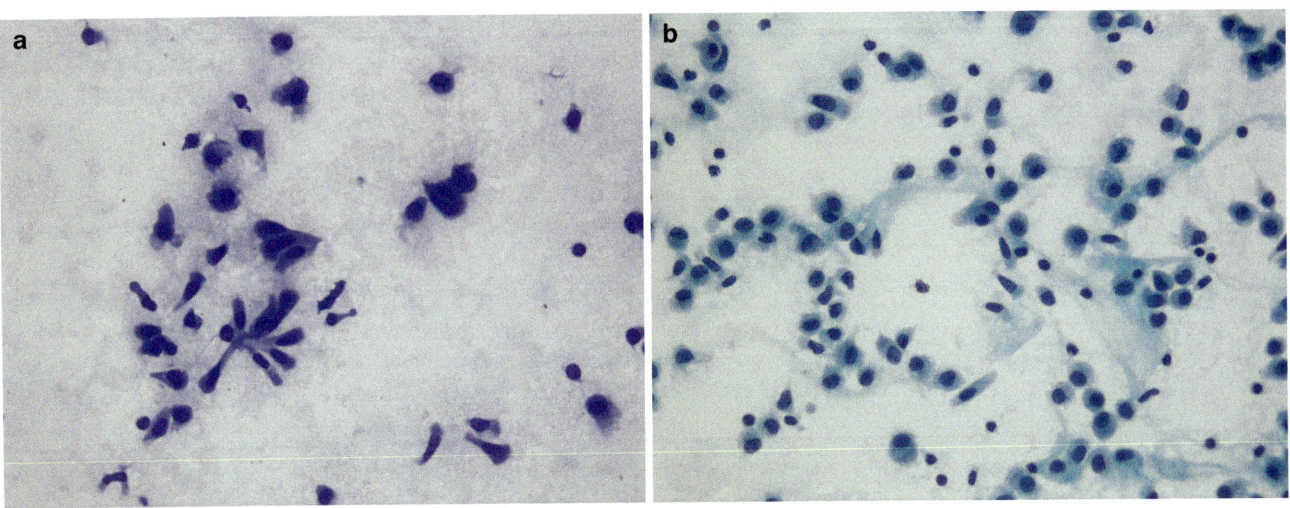

**Fig. 4.6** (**a**, **b**) Ciliated breast carcinoma cells with little atypia in pleural effusion; **a**: Diff-Quik, **b**: PAP

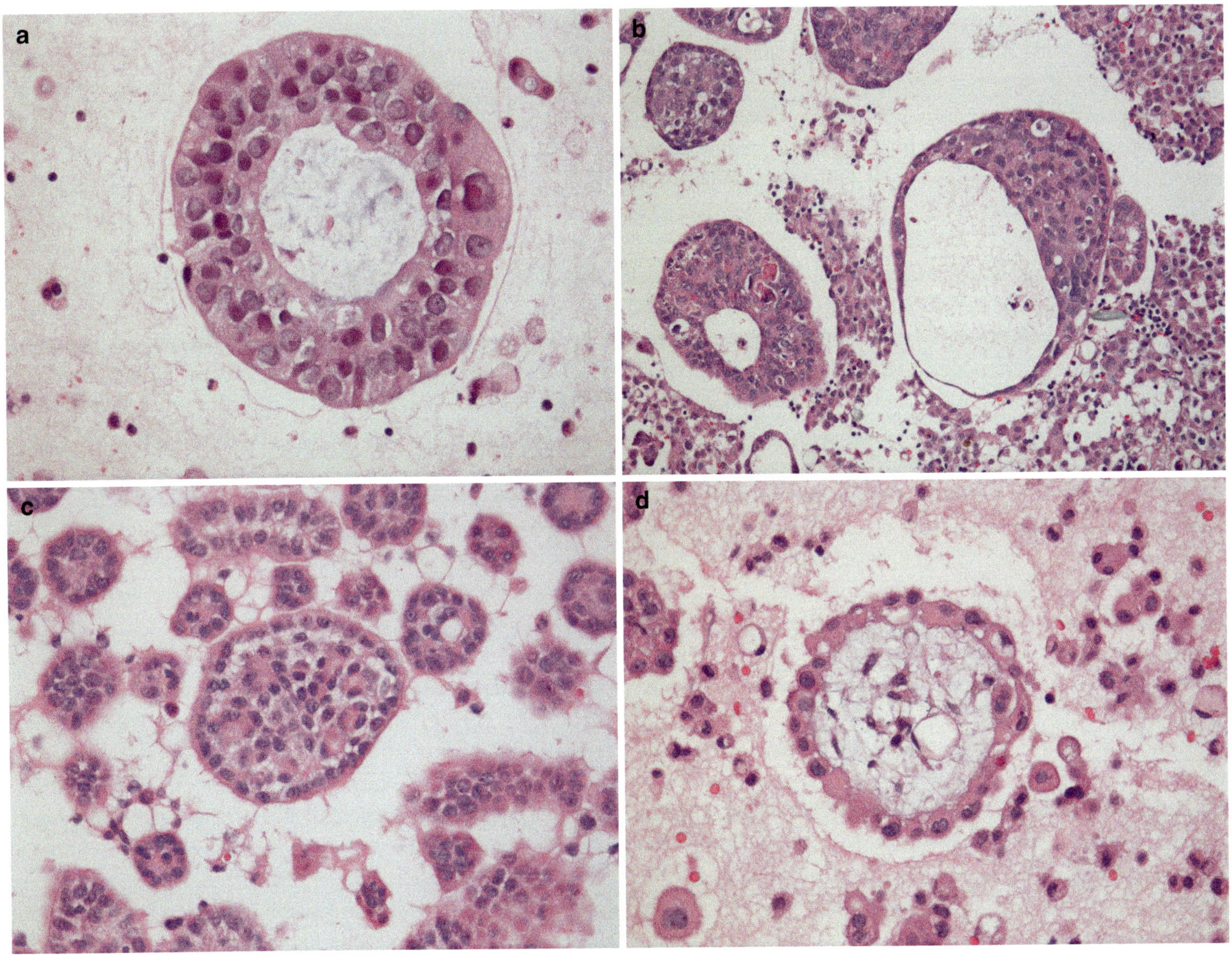

**Fig. 4.7** (**a**–**d**) Proliferation spheres. In breast carcinoma (**a**, **b**), spheres are often hollow, whereas in malignant mesothelioma they have a core with proliferation of smaller lumina (**c**) or accumulation of extracellular material, occasionally with spindle cells; **a**–**d**: H&E

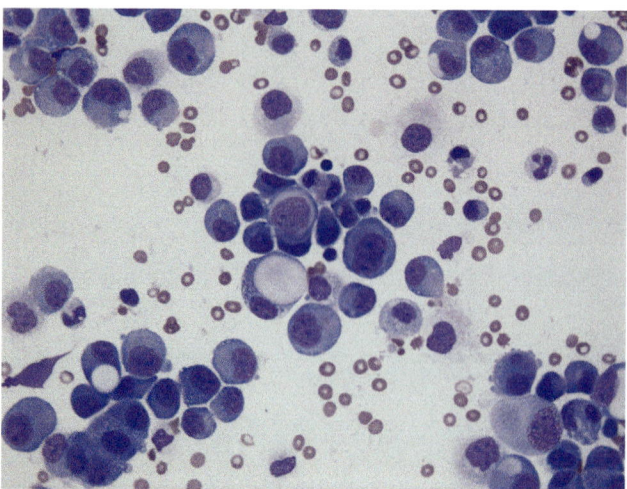

**Fig. 4.8** Lobular carcinoma cells with a single cytoplasmic vacuole pushing the nucleus to the cell periphery; Diff-Quik

may be less prominent compared to other types of adenocarcinoma. The cytoplasmic boundaries may be sharply defined. The presence of true three-dimensional aggregates with rather smooth outlines is strongly suggestive of malignancy in these cases. The true three-dimensional aggregates characteristic of breast carcinoma (cell balls) appear as many overlapping nuclei with an ill-defined cytoplasm. Because carcinoma cells typically have a high n/c ratio, it appears as though there are too many nuclei for the given amount of cytoplasm. In contrast, in the cellular aggregates associated with reactive mesothelial cells, the cytoplasm is more abundant, and the nuclei are not as numerous nor as overlapping. In lobular carcinomas, sometimes the predominance of one type of cells, with less atypia, is a reason for the difficulty in differentiating tumor cells from mesothelial cells. In lobular carcinoma cells, it is not rare to find a single cytoplasmic vacuole pushing the nucleus to the cell periphery (Fig. 4.8). However, degenerative changes in mesothelial cells may result in a single large cytoplasmic vacuole. The lack of nuclear atypia is an important clue. Additionally, the presence of a secretory vacuole with sharp outline with secretions, giving a targetoid appearance, was reported to be highly suggestive of breast carcinoma.

Although clinically, the distinction between mesothelioma and a secondary effusion from metastatic breast carcinoma is an extremely rare condition, the morphological distinction can be posed in some situations, since the incidence rate of mesothelioma in females is not negligible [19]. As is true for other adenocarcinomas, the presence of acinar formations, overt features of malignancy such as high n/c ratios, irregular nuclear borders, atypical mitoses, and cell balls with smooth or less often scalloped edges is more frequently observed in cytology specimens of adenocarcinoma than in mesothelioma. The presence of proliferative spheres without stromal cores also favors breast carcinoma.

Breast carcinoma should be differentiated from other adenocarcinomas, mainly those originating from the ovary, lung, or stomach. Although ovarian carcinomas can show large cell balls with smooth edges like breast carcinoma, ovarian carcinoma cells in general have abundant large vacuoles that push the nuclei to a perimembranous location. Papillary formation, mucin, and psammoma bodies that may be present in ovarian carcinomas are generally absent in breast carcinoma effusions. Effusions associated with lung adenocarcinoma have variable morphology, depending on the appearance of the primary tumor and the degree of differentiation. Papillary clusters, acini, tridimensional aggregates, and single cells may be seen. More pronounced pleomorphism, presence of mucin, and rare formation of cell balls are the main differentiating characteristics from breast carcinoma. Cells of lobular carcinoma have a tendency to form small, caterpillar-like chains similar to those commonly seen in small-cell carcinoma. However, in the latter tumor, cells lack visible cytoplasm, and the nuclei are more hyperchromatic than in lobular carcinoma cells. Finally, gastric carcinoma cells, especially with signet-ring appearance, need to be differentiated from lobular carcinoma cells in effusions. In general, the cells in gastric adenocarcinoma are larger and more pleomorphic than those seen in breast carcinoma.

## Ancillary Techniques

The use of ancillary techniques to distinguish reactive mesothelial cells from mesothelioma and adenocarcinoma in effusions is discussed in different sections of this book. Here we wish to highlight some techniques used to identify breast origin in malignant cells in effusions.

As most adenocarcinomas, breast carcinoma cells in effusions are positive for epithelial markers like cytokeratins (CK), including, among others, pan-CK, CK7, and CK8, as well as MOC-31, Ber-EP4, B72.3, and CEA (Fig. 4.9a–c). It was reported that MOC-31 exhibits superior reactivity compared to Ber-EP4 in detecting invasive breast carcinomas of both lobular type and NST in effusions, whereas these two antibodies perform similarly in detecting other adenocarcinomas [20].

In our hands, CEA, though not very sensitive, is highly specific for malignancy and allows the detection of rare tumor cells intermixed with inflammatory and mesothelial cells (Fig. 4.9d).

A word of caution is mandated regarding CK5, a marker used to characterize mesothelial cells, because a very aggressive subset of breast carcinomas, the so-called basal-like subtype, is also positive for this marker [21] (Fig. 4.9e).

Gross cystic disease fluid protein (GCDFP-15), mammaglobin, and GATA-3 are three markers considered as helpful to confirm a diagnosis of metastatic breast carci-

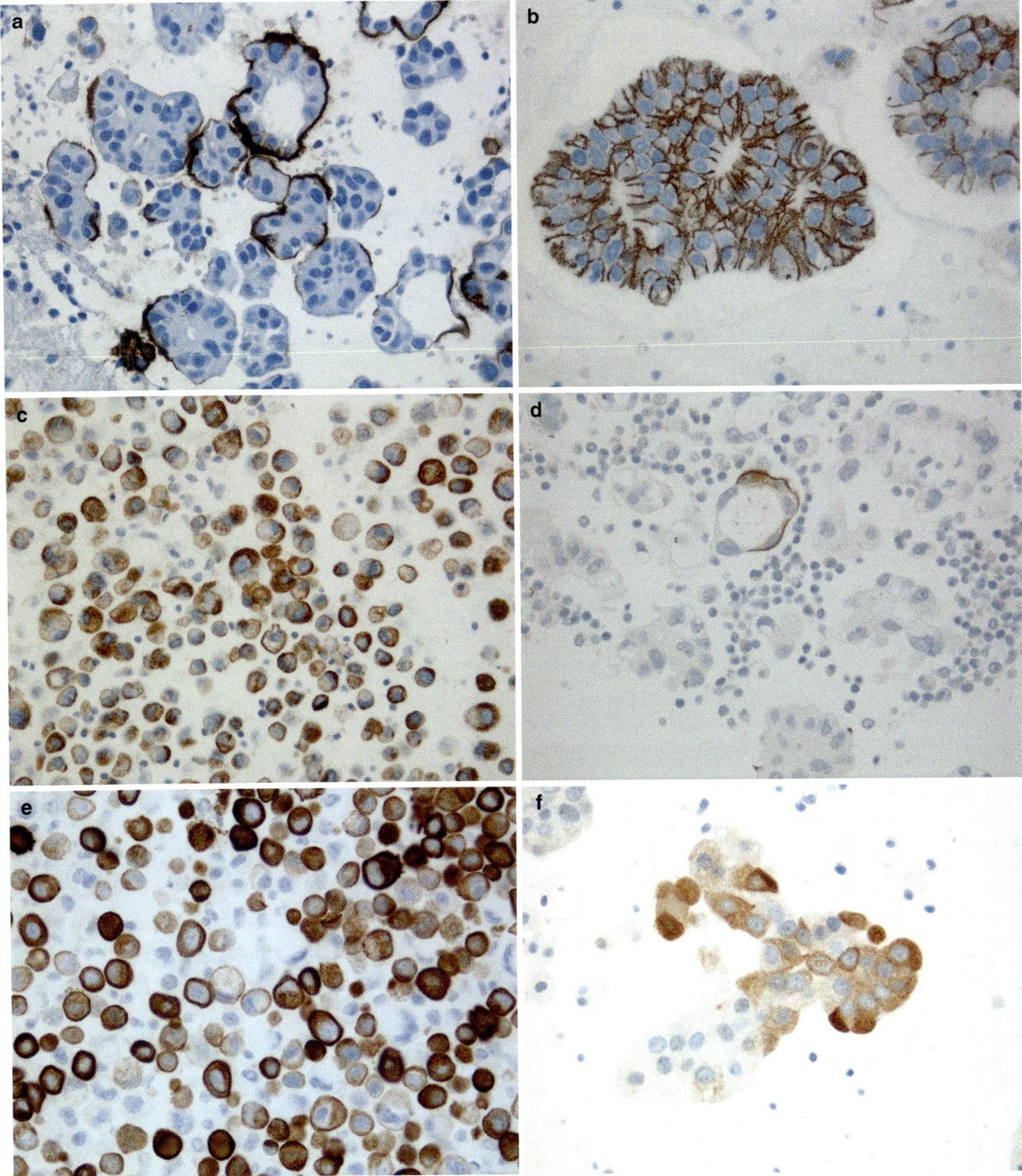

**Fig. 4.9** (**a–j**) Immunohistochemistry. Breast carcinoma cells express B72.3 (**a**), Ber-EP4 (**b**), CK7 (**c**), CEA (**d**), CK5/6 (**e**), GCDFP-15 (**f**), mammaglobin (**g**), GATA-3 (**h**), ER (**i**), PR (**j**), and HER2 (**k**)

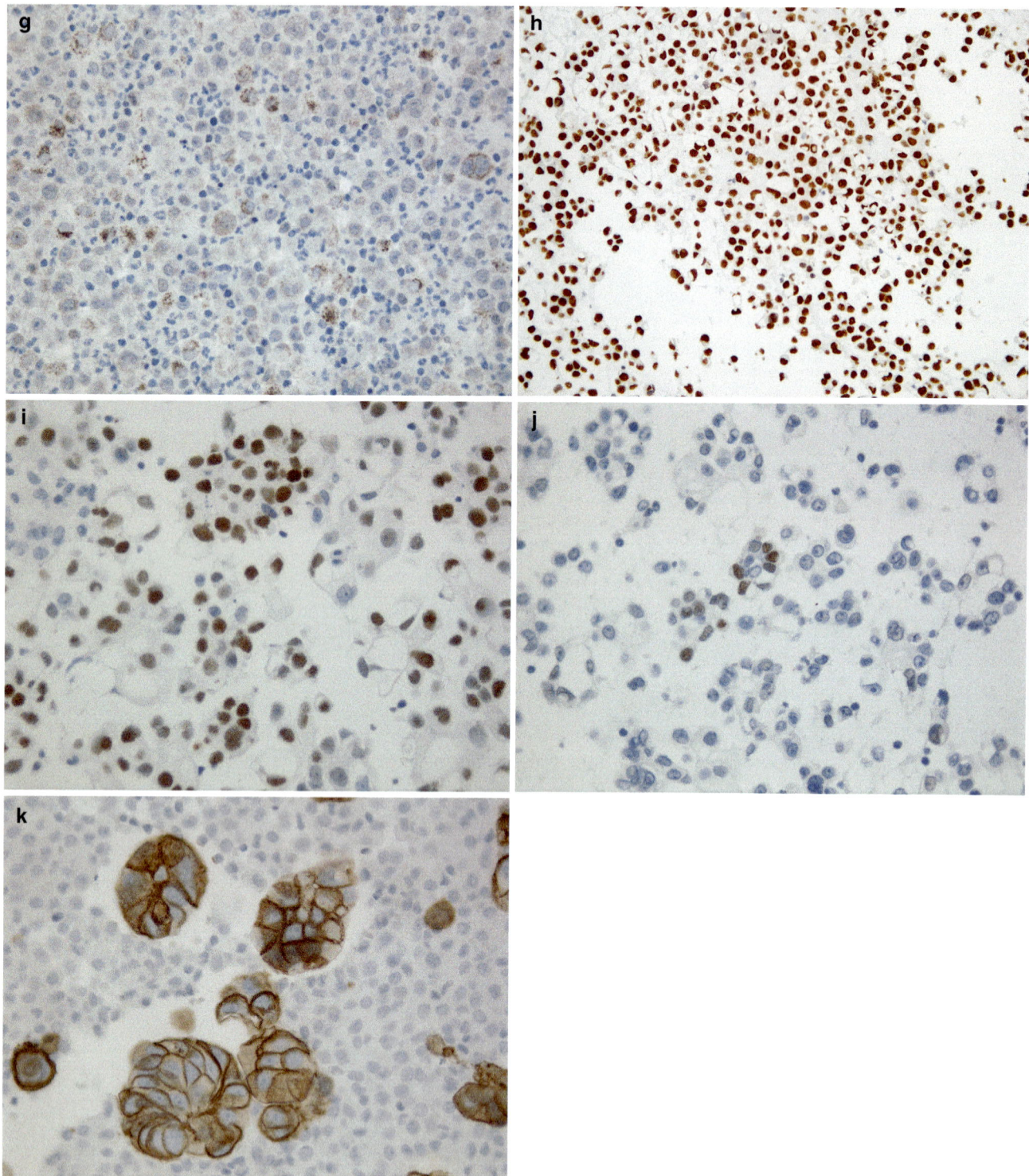

**Fig. 4.9** (continued)

noma in effusions (Fig. 4.9f). GCDFP-15 is a glycoprotein originally isolated from human gross cystic disease fluid that has been used as marker for breast carcinoma. When applied to effusions, GCDFP-15 has shown poor sensitivity (47–56%) [22, 23]. Although considered highly specific, GCDFP-15 can be expressed in a subset of lung adenocarcinoma [24, 25].

Mammaglobin is a 93 amino acid glycoprotein with homology to other secretoglobin-uteroglobin family members. Mammaglobin was originally identified as a breast cancer-restricted biomarker by differential screening, and subsequent studies have focused on further elucidating its function and expression profile [26]. Although data have been accumulating regarding the clinical utility of mammaglobin as a biomarker for diagnostic purposes, few reports have focused on its utility in identifying metastatic breast cancer. Mammaglobin is expressed in 48–72% of breast carcinomas (Fig. 4.9g) but also in 11–39% of endometrial carcinomas, 40% of sweat gland carcinomas, 20% of salivary gland tumors, and rare lung adenocarcinomas [26–28]. A comparative analysis of GCDFP-15 and mammaglobin in tissue sections found the latter more sensitive but less specific than GCDFP-15, staining approximately 8% of non-breast tumors, particularly endometrioid carcinomas [27]. These results suggest that mammaglobin is a valuable diagnostic marker for metastatic carcinoma of breast origin, although endometrial carcinoma should be considered in the differential diagnosis of mammaglobin-positive adenocarcinoma. In body fluids there are two studies examining the value of mammaglobin as a marker for breast carcinoma, showing a sensitivity of 55% and 87% [22, 29].

More recently, GATA-3 was described as a new marker of breast carcinoma origin in metastasis [30–32]. GATA-binding protein 3 (GATA3) is a member of the zinc finger transcription factor family that plays an essential role in regulating mammary gland morphogenesis and normal development of urothelium and a subset of lymphocytes [31]. GATA-3 has recently emerged as a multi-specific but successful marker for breast and urothelial carcinomas in surgical and cytology specimens [32]. GATA3 and estrogen receptor (ER) are involved in a cross regulatory loop and are frequently coexpressed in breast carcinomas. However, there are studies demonstrating that subsets of "triple-negative" breast carcinomas (negative for ER, progesterone receptor [PR], and human epidermal growth factor 2 [HER2]) also stain for GATA3 [31, 33]. This has important implications for confirming metastatic breast carcinoma in patients who have primary and/or metastatic tumors that are negative for ER, PR, and HER2. In pleural effusions, GATA3 is reportedly more sensitive than both GCDFP-15 and mammaglobin as a marker of metastatic breast cancer [30, 31] (Fig. 4.9h). The sensitivity of GATA3 for detecting metastatic breast carcinomas in effusions is around 95% with a specificity of 89%, including for triple-negative carcinomas [31, 32]. However, although GATA3 positivity may be very supportive of the involvement of an effusion by a breast carcinoma, besides urothelial carcinoma, a small percentage of other tumors can exhibit GATA3 positivity, including Mullerian, pancreatobiliary, lung, and gastrointestinal tract primaries [31]. GATA3 should therefore always be used as part of a panel to help rule in or rule out other primary sites. Another word of caution is that GATA3

stains lymphocytes. In cases with rare tumor cells against an inflammatory background, the interpretation of the staining can be challenging [32].

Detection of estrogen receptor (ER) may aid in identifying metastatic breast carcinoma cells in effusions (Fig. 4.9i). However, although mesothelial cells are ER-negative, other malignancies, such as gynecological carcinomas originating in the vulva, vagina, cervix, endometrium, ovary, and fallopian tube, are often ER-positive. ER positivity can be helpful in pointing to a breast or gynecologic origin, but it is important to remember that some pulmonary adenocarcinomas may express ER [34]. Additionally, breast carcinoma cells in effusions are not infrequently hormone receptor-negative. Progesterone receptor (PR) may be expressed (Fig. 4.9j) but is less specific.

Another marker expressed by 15–20% of breast carcinomas is HER2. The overexpression of this tyrosine-kinase receptor detected by immunostaining or the amplification of the gene detected by in situ hybridization can be useful to distinguish breast carcinoma cells from mesothelioma and reactive mesothelial cells (Fig. 4.9k), but other carcinomas may be positive, as, for example, ovarian, gastric, lung, and pancreatic carcinoma. Discrepancies in HER2 expression between the primary breast carcinoma and breast carcinoma effusions have been reported and reinforce the need to analyze the effusion specimen rather than the primary tumor when the former is present, in much the same way as it is done for solid metastases [35–38].

Several cancer-associated molecules have been reported to be highly expressed in breast carcinoma cells in effusions, some of which are upregulated at this anatomic cite compared to primary breast carcinoma ([39–43]; see Chap. 10 of this book). However, none of these molecules appears to have with immediate applicability in the diagnostic setting. More recently, comparative analyses of breast carcinoma and other carcinomas in effusions using high-throughput technology have revealed a larger number of genes and proteins that are differentially expressed among these cancers ([44, 45]; see Chap. 10). It is hoped that some of these markers may be applied to the differential diagnosis between these tumors in effusions in the near future.

## References

1. DeSantis CE, Bray F, Ferlay J, Lortet-Tieulent J, Anderson BO, Jemal A. International variation in female breast cancer incidence and mortality rates. Cancer Epidemiol Biomark Prev. 2015;24:1495–506.
2. Siegel RL, Miller KD, Jemal A. Cancer statistics, 2017. CA Cancer J Clin. 2017;67:7–30.
3. Fentiman IS, Millis R, Sexton S, Hayward JL. Pleural effusion in breast cancer: a review of 105 cases. Cancer. 1981;47:2087–92.
4. Raju RN, Kardinal CG. Pleural effusion in breast carcinoma: analysis of 122 cases. Cancer. 1981;48:2524–7.

5. Wilkes JD, Fidias P, Vaickus L, Perez RP. Malignancy-related pericardial effusion. 127 cases from the Roswell Park Center Institute. Cancer. 1995;76:1377–87.

6. Buck M, Ingle JN, Giuliani ER, Gordon JR, Therneau TM. Pericardial effusion in women with breast cancer. Cancer. 1987;60:263–9.

7. DiBonito L, Falconieri G, Colautti I, Bonifacio D, Dudine S. The positive peritoneal effusion. A retrospective study of cytopathologic diagnoses with autopsy confirmation. Acta Cytol. 1993;37:483–8.

8. Johnston WW. The malignant pleural effusion. A review of cytopathologic diagnoses of 584 specimens from 472 consecutive patients. Cancer. 1985;56:905–9.

9. Pokieser W, Cassik P, Fischer G, Vesely M, Ulrich W, Peters-Engl C. Malignant pleural and pericardial effusion in invasive breast cancer: impact of the site of the primary tumor. Breast Cancer Res Treat. 2004;83:139–42.

10. Kamby C, Vejborg I, Kristensen B, Olsen LO, Mouridsen HT. Metastatic pattern in recurrent breast cancer. Special reference to intrathoracic recurrences. Cancer. 1988;62:2226–33.

11. DeCamp MM Jr, Mentzer SJ, Swanson SJ, Sugarbaker DJ. Malignant effusive disease of the pleura and pericardium. Chest. 1997;112(4 Suppl):291S–5S.

12. Geisinger KR, Stanley MW, Raab SS, Silverman JF, Abati A, editors. Modern cytopathology. Philadelphia: Churchill Livingstone; 2004.

13. Bedrossian CWM, editor. Malignant effusions. A multimodal approach to cytologic diagnosis. New York: Igaku-Shoin; 1994.

14. Shidham VB, Atkinson BF. Cytopathologic diagnosis of serous fluids. London: Elsevier; 2007.

15. Pleural NB. peritoneal and pericardial effusions. In: Bibbo M, Wilbur D, editors. Comprehensive cytopathology. Philadelphia: Elsevier; 2008. p. 515–78.

16. Shidham VB, Falzon M. Serous effusions. In: Gray W, Kocjan G, editors. Diagnostic cytopathology. London: Churchill Livingstone; 2010. p. 115–78.

17. Rappa G, Lorico A. Phenotypic characterization of mammosphere-forming cells from the human MA-11 breast carcinoma cell line. Exp Cell Res. 2010;316:1576–86.

18. Danner DE, Gmelich JTA. comparative study of tumor cells from metastatic carcinoma of the breast in effusions. Acta Cytol. 1975;19:509–18.

19. Goldberg S, Rey G, Luce D, Gilg Soit Ilg A, Rolland P, Brochard P, Imbernon E, Goldberg M. Possible effect of environmental exposure to asbestos on geographical variation in mesothelioma rates. Occup Environ Med. 2010;67:417–21.

20. Pai RK, West RB. MOC-31 exhibits superior reactivity compared with Ber-EP4 in invasive lobular and ductal carcinoma of the breast: a tissue microarray study. Appl Immunohistochem Mol Morphol. 2009;17:202–6.

21. Matos I, Dufloth R, Alvarenga M, Zeferino LC, Schmitt F. p63, cytokeratin 5, and P-cadherin: three molecular markers to distinguish basal phenotype in breast carcinomas. Virchows Arch. 2005;447:688–94.

22. Yan Z, Gidley J, Horton D, Roberson J, Eltoum IE, Chhieng DC. Diagnostic utility of mammaglobin and GCDFP-15 in the identification of metastatic breast carcinoma in fluid specimens. Diagn Cytopathol. 2009;37:475–8.

23. Fiel MI, Cernaianu G, Burstein DE, Batheja N. Value of GCDFP-15 (BRST-2) as a specific immunocytochemical marker for breast carcinoma in cytologic specimens. Acta Cytol. 1996;40:637–41.

24. Wang LJ, Greaves WO, Sabo E, et al. GCDFP-15 positive and TTF-1 negative primary lung neoplasms: a tissue microarray study of 381 primary lung tumors. Appl Immunohistochem Mol Morphol. 2009;17:505–11.

25. Yang M, Nonaka D. A study of immunohistochemical differential expression in pulmonary and mammary carcinomas. Mod Pathol. 2010;23:654–61.

26. Wang Z, Spaulding B, Sienko A, Liang Y, Li H, Nielsen G, Yub Gong G, Ro JY, Jim Zhai Q. Mammaglobin, a valuable diagnostic marker for metastatic breast carcinoma. Int J Clin Exp Pathol. 2009;2:384–9.

27. Barghava R, Beriwal S, Dabbs DJ. Mammaglobin vs GCDFP-15: an immunohistologic validation survey for sensitivity and specificity. Am J Clin Pathol. 2007;127:103–13.

28. Sasaki E, Tsunoda N, Hatanaka Y, Mori N, Iwata H, Yatabe Y. Breast-specific expression of MGB1/mammaglobin: an examination of 480 tumors from various organs and clinicopathologic analysis of MGB1-positive breast cancers. Mod Pathol. 2007;20:208–14.

29. Roncella S, Ferro P, Franceschini MC, Bacigalupo B, Dessanti P, Sivori M, Carletti AM, Fontana V, Canessa PA, Pistillo MP, Fedeli F. Diagnosis and origin determination of malignant pleural effusions through the use of the breast cancer marker mammaglobin. Diagn Mol Pathol. 2010;19:92–8.

30. Shield PW, Papadimos DJ, Walsh MD. GATA3: a promising marker for metastatic breast carcinoma in serous effusion specimens. Cancer Cytopathol. 2014;122:307–12.

31. Lew M, Pang JC, Jing X, Fields KL, Roh MH. Young investigator challenge: the utility of GATA3 immunohistochemistry in the evaluation of metastatic breast carcinomas in malignant effusions. Cancer Cytopathol. 2015;123:576–81.

32. El Hag MI, Ha J, Farag R, El Hag AM, Michael CW. Utility of GATA-3 in the work-up of breast adenocarcinoma and its differential diagnosis in serous effusions: a cell-block microarray study. Diagn Cytopathol. 2016;44:731–6.

33. Albergaria A, Paredes J, Sousa B, Milanezi F, Carneiro V, Bastos J, Costa S, Vieira D, Lopes N, Lam EW, Lunet N, Schmitt F. Expression of FOXA1 and GATA3 in breast cancer: the prognostic significance in hormone receptor-negative tumours. Breast Cancer Res. 2009;11:R40.

34. Dabbs DJ, Landreneau RJ, Liu Y, Raab SS, Maley RH, Tung MY, Silverman JF. Detection of estrogen receptor by immunohistochemistry in pulmonary adenocarcinoma. Ann Thorac Surg. 2002;73:403–5.

35. Shabaik A, Lin G, Peterson M, Hasteh F, Tipps A, Datnow B, Weidner N. Reliability of Her2/neu, estrogen receptor, and progesterone receptor testing by immunohistochemistry on cell block of FNA and serous effusions from patients with primary and metastatic breast carcinoma. Diagn Cytopathol. 2011;39: 328–32.

36. Schlüter B, Gerhards R, Strumberg D, Voigtmann R. Combined detection of HER2/neu gene amplification and protein overexpression in effusions from patients with breast and ovarian cancer. J Cancer Res Clin Oncol. 2010;136:1389–400.

37. Arihiro K, Oda M, Ogawa K Tominaga K, Kaneko Y, Shimizu T, Matsumoto S, Oda M, Kurita Y, Taira Y. Discordant HER2 status between primary breast carcinoma and recurrent/metastatic tumors using fluorescence in situ hybridization on cytological samples. Jpn J Clin Oncol. 2013;43:55–62.

38. Nakayama Y, Nakagomi H, Omori M, Inoue M, Takahashi K, Maruyama M, Takano A, Furuya K, Amemiya K, Ishii E, Oyama T. Benefits of using the cell block method to determine the discordance of the HR/HER2 expression in patients with metastatic breast cancer. Breast Cancer. 2016;23:633–9.

39. Davidson B, Konstantinovsky S, Nielsen S, Dong HP, Berner A, Vyberg M, Reich R. Altered expression of metastasis-associated and regulatory molecules in effusions from breast cancer patients- a novel model for tumor progression. Clin Cancer Res. 2004;10:7335–46.

40. Konstantinovsky S, Smith Y, Zilber S, Tuft Stavnes H, Becker AM, Nesland JM, Reich R, Davidson B. Breast carcinoma cells in primary tumors and effusions have different gene array profiles. J Oncol. 2010;2010:969084.

41. Davidson B, Dong HP, Holth A, Berner A, Risberg B. The chemokine receptor CXCR4 is more frequently expressed in breast compared to other metastatic adenocarcinomas in effusions. Breast J. 2008;14:476–82.

42. Davidson B, Konstantinovsky S, Kleinberg L, Nguyen MTP, Bassarova A, Kvalheim G, Nesland JM, Reich R. The mitogen-activated protein kinases (MAPK) p38 and JNK are markers of tumor progression in breast carcinoma. Gynecol Oncol. 2006;102:453–61.

43. Yuan Y, Leszczynska M, Konstantinovsky S, Tropé CG, Reich R, Davidson B. Netrin 4 is upregulated in breast carcinoma effusions compared to corresponding solid tumors. Diagn Cytopathol. 2011;39:562–6.

44. Davidson B, Stavnes HT, Holth A, Chen X, Yang Y, Shih IM, Wang TL. Gene expression signatures differentiate ovarian/peritoneal serous carcinoma from breast carcinoma in effusions. J Cell Mol Med. 2011;15:535–44.

45. Davidson B, Stavnes HT, Nesland JM, Wohlschlaeger J, Yang Y, Shih IM, Wang TL. Gene expression signatures differentiate adenocarcinoma of lung and breast origin in effusions. Hum Pathol. 2012;43:684–94.

# Malignant Mesothelioma

Claire W. Michael

## Introduction

While malignant mesothelioma is a relatively rare neoplasm, it provokes a lot of anxiety due to its poor prognosis, the litigation that follows such a diagnosis, and the difficulty in establishing the diagnosis itself. Mesothelioma presents with a large serosal effusion in over 90% of patients [1], a fact that situates cytology as the primary mode of evaluation and diagnosis. Previous guidelines by the International Mesothelioma Interest Group (IMIG) for the diagnosis and treatment of mesothelioma shed doubt on the role of cytology in the definitive diagnosis of mesothelioma and hence the need for tissue biopsy despite ample literature to the contrary [2]. However, recent guidelines published by several groups acknowledged that cytology can have a role in this diagnosis, and consequently supplemental guidelines for the cytopathologic diagnosis in effusions were published [3–6].

## Epidemiologic and Mineralogical Aspects

Malignant mesothelioma is one of very few malignancies directly associated with exposure to a natural substance. The reported rate of asbestos exposure in patients with mesothelioma has ranged between 15% and 80%. This wide range is primarily attributed to the methodology of taking history and asking the right questions as well as inaccurate histories sometimes provided by family members. It is now well established that asbestos exposure can be documented in over 80% of cases [1]. Not only direct exposure is implicated in mesothelioma; secondary exposure of family members has been documented as well to cause mesothelioma in the spouses and children of asbestos workers. It is believed that asbestos fibers are carried on their clothes, etc. Despite the

well-documented association of asbestos and mesothelioma, the threshold of exposure is not known yet, in part because of the long latency period between exposure and the development of symptoms (at least 20 years), decades from the exposure, and the far higher prevalence of lung carcinoma with asbestos exposure [7]. In a study by Roggli et al., the authors compared the number of asbestos bodies from patients who died of mesothelioma versus those who died of other diseases and found no correlation with development of the disease [8].

Other causes for mesothelioma have also been reported, albeit very rarely. These include history of radiation and exposure to beryllium, nickel and silica dust, and fiberglass. Few patients may genuinely have no history of exposure [7].

Historically, the use of asbestos has been reported as early as 3000 BC. Its fire-resistant quality made its use very popular for many applications, including incorporation into pottery since antiquity, designing of funeral clothes by the Greeks that would survive cremation of nobility, coating of the feet of victims undergoing trial by fire in the Middle Ages, and manufacturing of purses that safeguard money against fire. While asbestos-related lung disease has also been reported as early as 100 AD, and while rare reports of mesothelioma have been published throughout the last two centuries, malignant mesothelioma as a pleura-based distinct malignancy has only been recognized around the second half of the twentieth century [9].

Asbestos is a general term applied to a group of crystalline hydrated silicates with fibrous geometry defined as having a length three times greater than their width. There are three commonly occurring asbestos varieties: chrysotile, crocidolite, and amosite. Anthophyllite, tremolite, and actinolite occur less commonly and mainly as contaminants. Pleural plaques are strongly dose-dependent, yet the threshold for mesothelioma is unknown. While crocidolite has a more well-established association with mesothelioma than chrysotile, cases with pure exposure to the latter have also been documented [7].

In addition to asbestos, erionite was identified and documented in the villages of Cappadocia, Turkey, as another

C. W. Michael
Department of Pathology, MSPTH 5077, University Hospitals Cleveland Medical Center, Case Western Reserve University, Cleveland, OH, USA
e-mail: Claire.michael@uhhospitals.org

© Springer International Publishing AG, part of Springer Nature 2018
B. Davidson et al. (eds.), *Serous Effusions*, https://doi.org/10.1007/978-3-319-76478-8_5

highly potent mineral that induces mesothelioma. Erionite is a member of the zeolite family, a complex group of silicates found in volcanic ash [10].

## Clinical Presentation

Despite the banning of asbestos products for several decades, the incidence of mesothelioma is reported as 2500 cases in the USA and 5000 cases in Western Europe annually. In fact, it is projected that the incidence worldwide will peak by 2020 [1].

Mesothelioma can occur in any of the body cavities lined with serosal cells. However, it most commonly arises in the pleural, followed by the peritoneal and pericardial cavities. The ratio of pleura to peritoneum ranges from 3:1 to 11:1 according to the literature. Pleural mesothelioma presents mainly as a unilateral disease, although it might be bilateral in rare cases.

Because of the long latency period that may last up to four decades, the age of presentation is generally around 60 years. Patients with history of exposure in their childhood may present earlier. The presenting symptoms tend to be insidious, and it consequently takes between 3 and 6 months before a definitive diagnosis is established. Most patients initially present with shortness of breath that develops due to the large pleural effusion or nonpleuritic chest pain resulting from significant chest wall and diaphragmatic invasion. Other symptoms may include fever, fatigue, dry cough, and weight loss. Pleural effusion tends to be unilateral in about 95% of cases and bilateral in the remaining 5%. The right pleura is affected in 60% of these patients. Pleural mesothelioma is a disease that predominates in males.

Initial workup by chest X-ray detects large pleural effusions in 80–95% of patients, while the remaining patients may have no detectable fluids. Pleural plaques are also detected in patients with asbestos-related lung disease, and focal or diffuse pleural thickening is also detected, although it may initially be obscured by the large effusion. As the disease progresses, the pleural fluid decreases, becomes loculated, and eventually disappears due to fusion of the visceral and parietal surfaces, forming a rind that encases the lung and extends into the fissures. Computed chest tomography with contrast has recently been proven to be more sensitive, especially in the detection of pleural effusions, assessment of the size of hilar and mediastinal lymph nodes, and evaluation of the presence of pleural masses or rind. Magnetic resonance imaging of the chest with contrast is more useful in detecting chest wall invasion and diaphragmatic spread. Positron emission tomography is used to detect contralateral chest involvement and extrathoracic metastatic sites. The latter information is essential for tumor staging and for treatment planning, particularly surgery [1, 11].

## Diagnosis and Treatment

Pleural mesothelioma presents early as small rounded yellow to gray nodules studding the parietal pleura that coalesce as the disease advances to eventually form the characteristic thick pleura otherwise known as "pleural rind." With disease progression, the parietal and visceral pleura fuse and the effusion disappears. Peritoneal mesotheliomas were reported to have a more variable growth pattern and could present as disseminated carcinomatosis-like pattern or as large omental masses and mimic carcinoma [12].

Since most mesotheliomas are associated with large effusions, cytological examination is logically the first line of workup. However, the effectiveness of cytology is a subject of great controversy. Several factors may contribute to this controversy, including the subtle cytological features that are not easily recognized by pathologists, a general lack of pathologists experienced in mesothelioma diagnosis due to the rare occurrence of the disease, and finally, the fact that some effusions are mostly bloody or lack diagnostic cells. It is recommended that a minimum of 100 mL of fluid and preferably the entire volume of aspirated fluid is submitted for cytological examination. Such volume would allow the preparation of a cell block with optimum cellularity for additional ancillary testing [6].

When a definitive diagnosis by cytological examination is not achieved, a pleural biopsy is the next step. CT-guided needle biopsy of a pleural mass can be up to 87% sensitive, while video-assisted thoracoscopy (VATS) allows direct visualization of the chest with aspiration of the pleural fluid, direct biopsies of the pleural mass, and direct injection of talc. This results in up to 95% accuracy and the highest rate of successful pleurodesis. It is important, however, to recognize that seeding of the tumor along the chest tube and the surgical incision tracts, eventually resulting in chest wall invasion, is a possible complication of VATS in up to 20% of patients.

While a diagnosis of malignant mesothelioma can be made by cytology, VATS with extensive pleural biopsies is still recommended to exclude the presence of a sarcomatoid component. Mediastinoscopy to examine the mediastinal lymph nodes is also essential prior to considering the patient for extrapleural pneumonectomy (EPP). This is because, as previously mentioned, patients with either metastatic lymph nodes or sarcomatoid component do not respond to EPP [1, 6, 11, 13].

Untreated, the mean survival rate is about 6 months. With recent treatment regimens including surgery and chemotherapy, survival rate of up to 5 years has been reported, a fact that underscores the significance of early detection and diagnosis of mesothelioma. For pleural mesothelioma, surgical procedures used for either treatment or palliation include VATS with talc pleurodesis, pleurectomy with decortications

(P/D), and EPP. The latter provides the most complete reduction of tumor and is the only method in which long-term survival is documented. Unfortunately, EPP does not control the nonepithelial variant of mesothelioma, and only 10–15% of patients with the epithelial variant, particularly those with negative mediastinal lymph nodes, seem to benefit from this procedure. Chemotherapy with combination of cisplatin and pemetrexed demonstrated significant survival advantage (12 months) and is currently used as first-line treatment, while radiation therapy is only used to control local chest wall invasion such as implants in chest tube or surgical wound tracts [1, 6, 11].

Considering the localized nature of peritoneal mesothelioma, locoregional therapies have been explored [14]. The most accepted therapy at this time is cytoreduction and hyperthermic intraoperative intraperitoneal perfusion with chemotherapy (HIPEC). First, cytoreduction is performed so as to remove all grossly visible tumor. This is followed by HIPEC which distributes the high-dose IP chemotherapy uniformly to all the peritoneal surfaces. Infusing a clinically relevant hyperthermic IP is known to enhance the cytotoxic effect of multiple chemotherapeutic agents. While experience is limited with peritoneal mesotheliomas due to the rarity of the disease and the variability in its biological behavior, it has been noted that patients with smaller tumor burden and female gender had prolonged survival [15–17]. In a review of 83 patients, epithelioid histology, low mitotic count, complete gross cytoreduction, and pathologically negative lymph nodes were identified as independent factors associated with improved survival [18].

## Morphology

### Histological Features

Histologically, malignant mesothelioma is divided into epithelioid (50%), sarcomatoid (16%), or mixed variants (34%) [12]. The epithelioid variant may present with a variety of patterns, most commonly tubulopapillary, acinar, and confluent sheets. Well-differentiated tumors present mainly with papillary and tubular architecture (Fig. 5.1). The papillary structures project into large tubular structures and usually contain fibrous cores. The tubular structures form elongated and complex clefts lined by the malignant cells. Henderson et al. noted that they frequently observed an eruptive organizing granulation tissue layer covering the mesothelioma and eventually entrapping the mesothelial proliferation within a fibrous tissue layer at the interface with the adjacent adipose tissue [19]. Metaplastic changes such as squamous differentiation have been described [20]. Less common patterns include signet ring, small cell [21], clear [22], lipid-rich [23], and microcystic. The sarcomatoid variant may be homolo-

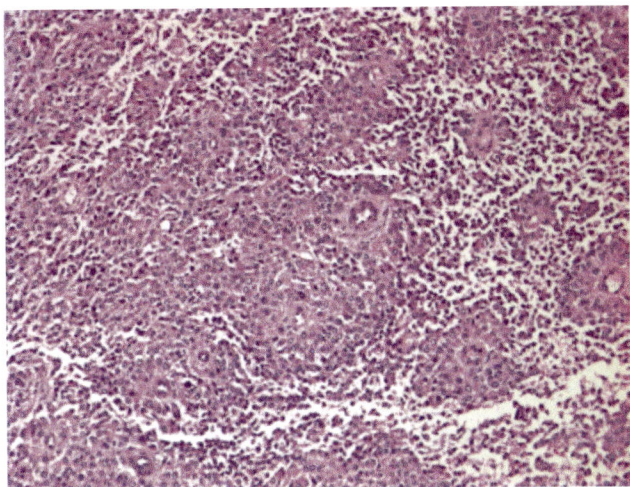

**Fig. 5.1** Well-differentiated epithelioid mesothelioma showing papillary and tubular structures admixed with cellular sheets. Notice the overall monotony of the cells; H&E

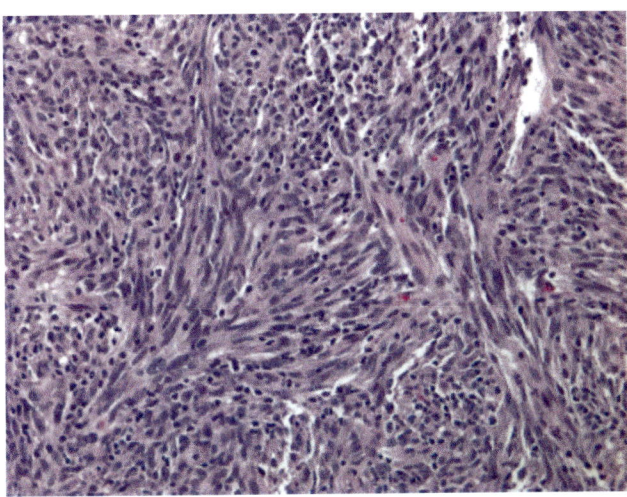

**Fig. 5.2** Sarcomatoid variant of mesothelioma consisting predominantly of fibrosarcoma-like proliferations of spindled cells; H&E

gous, consisting predominantly of a fibrosarcoma-like proliferation (Fig. 5.2), or contain heterologous stroma, such as osteoid, chondroid, rhabdomyoblastic, etc. [24]. The biphasic variant is a mixture of the epithelioid and sarcomatoid patterns (Fig. 5.3). Rare variants include an undifferentiated (Fig. 5.4), desmoplastic [25, 26], lymphohistiocytoid [27, 28], and deciduoid type [29–31]. Desmoplastic mesothelioma is defined as a mesothelioma in which collagenous tissue constitutes more than 50% of the tumor (Fig. 5.5). The majority of these mesotheliomas are of the sarcomatoid variant.

While the rare variants are very infrequently encountered, their features are worth noting because of the differential diagnosis they present.

The small cell variant is characterized by sheets of uniform small cells with open nuclei and prominent nucleoli. In

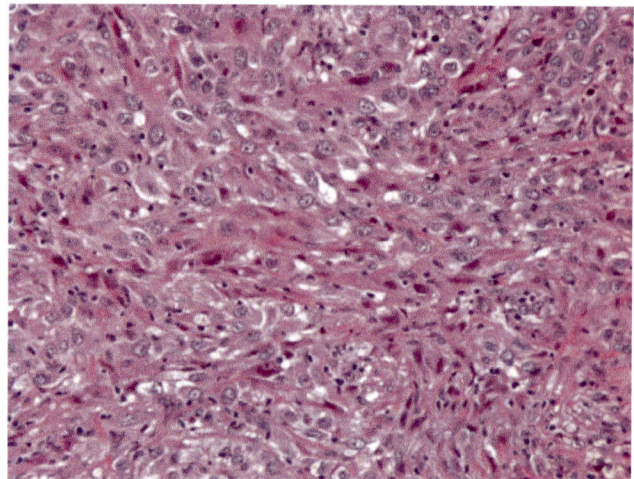

**Fig. 5.3** Biphasic variant of mesothelioma exhibiting both the spindle cell proliferation and the epithelioid-type cells; H&E

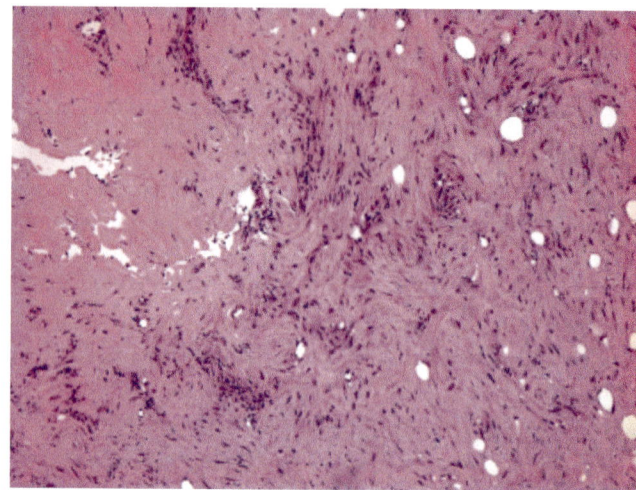

**Fig. 5.5** Desmoplastic mesothelioma showing few abnormal spindled cells infiltrating in a very heavily collagenous connective tissue stroma; H&E

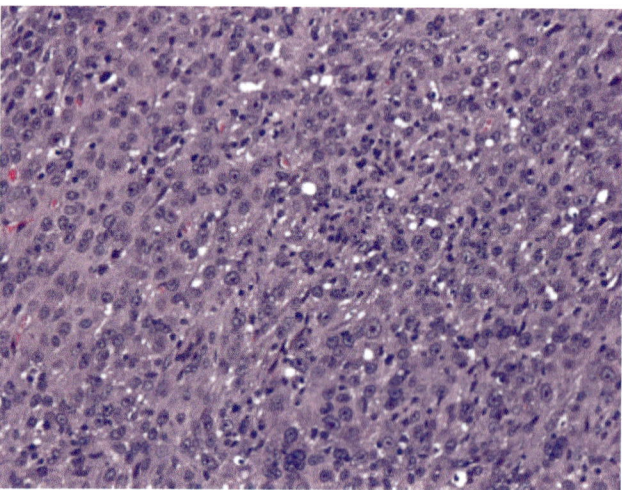

**Fig. 5.4** Poorly differentiated mesothelioma appearing predominantly as solid sheets of malignant cells with no papillary, tubular, nesting, or other previously described features. The cells are not readily identified as mesothelial; H&E

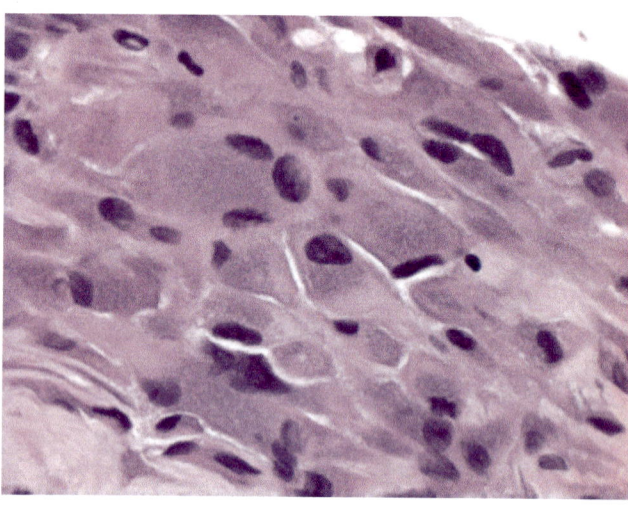

**Fig. 5.6** Deciduoid mesothelioma exhibiting large cells with abundant pink glassy cytoplasm and enlarged obviously abnormal nuclei. The cellular features are closely akin to those of decidual cells; H&E

all reported cases, adequate sectioning of the tumor revealed a component of typical epithelioid or sarcomatoid mesotheliomatous patterns. According to Mayall et al. [21], who reported 13 cases, all cases contained frequent areas of necrosis and lymphatic invasion. In some cases, intralymphatic tumors exhibited a typical mesotheliomatous pattern. Mitotic activity was low in all cases (less than 5 per 10 high-power fields). The classic features of neuroendocrine tumors described by Azzopardi [32], such as pseudo-rosettes, streams, ribbons, or tubular growth patterns, salt-and-pepper hyperchromatic nuclei, nuclear molding, and hematoxyphilia in blood vessels, were all consistently lacking in their cases.

The deciduoid variant is a very rare morphologic phenotype first described in 1985 as a diffuse epithelioid mesothelioma

occurring in the peritoneum of a 13-year-old female with morphologic resemblance to deciduosis [33]. Since then, it has also been described in the pleural surface and in older patients of both genders [29, 31, 34, 35]. Histologically, this variant presents as sheetlike proliferation of large polygonal cells with abundant pink, glassy cytoplasm and well-defined borders (Fig. 5.6). Some cells have a perinuclear cytoplasmic density. The nuclei are round to oval with vesicular chromatin and single prominent nucleoli. Binucleated cells are also present. Mitotic figures are present and may be abnormal but not frequent.

The lymphohistiocytoid variant presents as sheets of histiocyte-like cells with no evidence of differentiation in the form of tubular or papillary architecture (Fig. 5.7). The cells vary from round to spindle in appearance. The

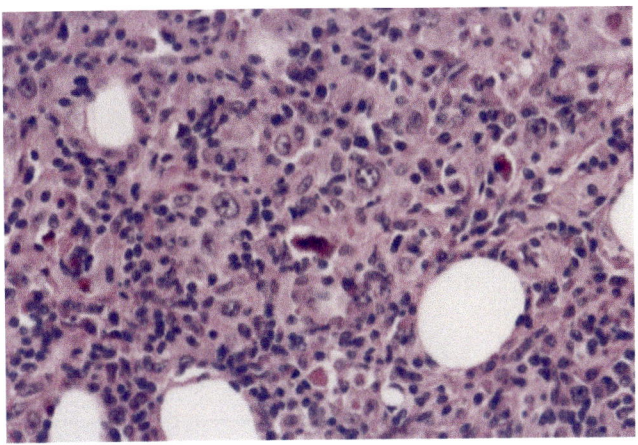

**Fig. 5.7** Lymphohistiocytoid mesothelioma presenting as large histiocyte-like cells with abundant clear cytoplasm admixed with a highly lymphocytic background; H&E

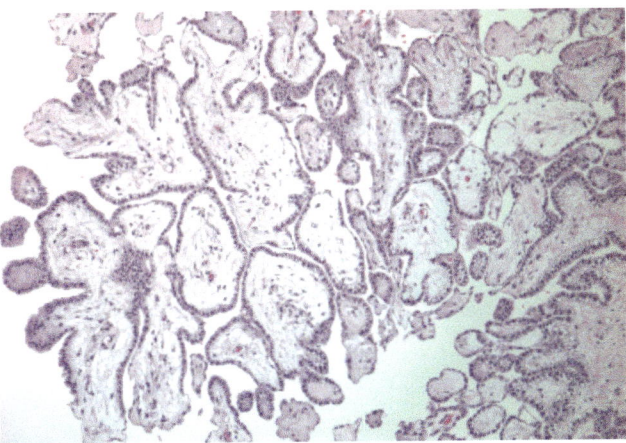

**Fig. 5.8** Well-differentiated localized papillary mesothelioma presenting as well-defined papillary proliferation with thick fibrovascular cores covered by a single layer of mesothelial cells; H&E

nuclei are usually round to oval, are vesicular, and contain prominent nucleoli. The cytoplasm is moderate in amount and eosinophilic. A diffuse lymphoid infiltrate predominantly of T cells is noted. The histiocytoid cells have an immunostaining profile that is similar to epithelioid mesothelioma [28].

Localized well-differentiated papillary mesothelioma is another rare variant that arises in the peritoneum and is frequently discovered incidentally during abdominal and pelvic surgeries. It is believed to have an indolent clinical course and may behave either as a benign neoplasm or have a tendency to recur. Histologically it is a localized proliferation of well-developed papillary structures with thick fibrovascular cores covered by a single layer of mesothelial cells (Fig. 5.8). It is important to distinguish this variant from the well-differentiated diffuse papillary mesothelioma that carries a much worse prognosis.

## Cytological Features

### The Role of Cytology in the Diagnosis of Mesothelioma [3, 36]

The reported sensitivity of cytology for the diagnosis of mesothelioma ranges from 4% to 63%, and many doubt the utility of cytology in establishing this diagnosis [37]. However, the reader should distinguish the probability of establishing the diagnosis by examining serosal effusions from the ability of the pathologist to render the diagnosis from a cellular fluid based on cytological features. In fact, the literature suggests that in experienced hands, mesothelioma diagnosis can be established in up to 50% by cytological evaluation alone and in up to 80% of cases utilizing ancillary techniques [38].

The cytological diagnosis is challenged at two points; the first is that not all malignant mesothelioma effusions contain diagnostic cells. In fact, about 10% of the effusions are bloody and virtually acellular. Sarcomatoid and some of the other rare variants do not exfoliate. In almost all cases, it is the epithelioid component that exfoliates and renders itself to diagnosis. The second challenge was much more significant in the past because of the difficulty in separating mesothelioma from adenocarcinoma. However, with the availability of new immunocytochemical stains, the last decade has witnessed a plethora of literature confirming that mesothelioma can be distinguished from carcinoma with a high degree of accuracy [39, 40]. A more significant morphologic challenge is separating mesothelioma from reactive effusions. Rakha et al. reviewed a total of 154 effusions with histologically proven pleural mesothelioma and were able to either diagnose or suspect mesothelioma in 79 cases, with a sensitivity of 53%. A benign or reactive diagnosis was rendered in 65 cases (42.2%), and 5 cases (3.2%) were considered inadequate for diagnosis. The sarcomatoid variant presented mainly as benign effusion and showed the least sensitivity (20%), with 11/15 cases diagnosed as benign [41]. The lack of exfoliated diagnostic cells in mesothelioma fluids has been attributed to several factors: (1) the tumor could be covered by a thick layer of fibrinous material or fibrosis; (2) the tumor may consist predominantly of fibrous stroma, as in the case of desmoplastic or sarcomatoid tumors [42].

The inability to detect invasion of preexisting tissue (not granulation tissue), a key feature in the definitive histologic diagnosis of mesothelioma, has been used for the last several decades as a supportive evidence against the cytological diagnosis of mesothelioma. However, the latest guidelines recognize that the cytological diagnosis relies on different criteria. The updated statement on mesothelioma from British Thoracic Society (BTS) and the guidelines issued by the Asbestos Disease Research Institute (ADRI) accept the cytological diagnosis as sufficient in some patients when correlated with imaging studies, i.e., utilizing imaging studies as an equivalent to the histologic diagnosis of invasion [5, 6].

It is important to recognize that despite the limitation of diagnosing mesothelioma by cytology, it still plays a major role as the initial and least invasive step in the evaluation of the patient. In fact, a definitive diagnosis may be established in a patient with positive radiological and clinical findings, and further workup may not be necessary if the tumor is unresectable. On the other hand, suspicion of mesothelioma or a negative persistent effusion in a patient with positive clinical findings should be followed up aggressively to avoid further progression of the disease and afford a patient at an early stage of the disease the opportunity for surgical treatment or adjuvant therapy [43].

## Stepwise Review of Effusions [3, 44]

When evaluating an exudative effusion, the pathologist should answer three questions based on the morphologic features:

1. Are the cells mesothelial or epithelial in origin?
2. If mesothelial, are the cells benign or malignant?
3. If epithelial, what is the primary origin?

Features of mesothelial origin have been described in chap. 1. The following is a summary of these features which tend to be subtle in quiescent effusions, easily detected in reactive effusions, and prominent in mesotheliomas.

1. Cell windows seen in mesothelial cords and within clusters (Fig. 5.9).
2. Cellular clasping and pinching (described as pincerlike) (Fig. 5.10).
3. Cell within cell arrangement (Fig. 5.11).
4. Clusters with scalloped borders (Fig. 5.12).

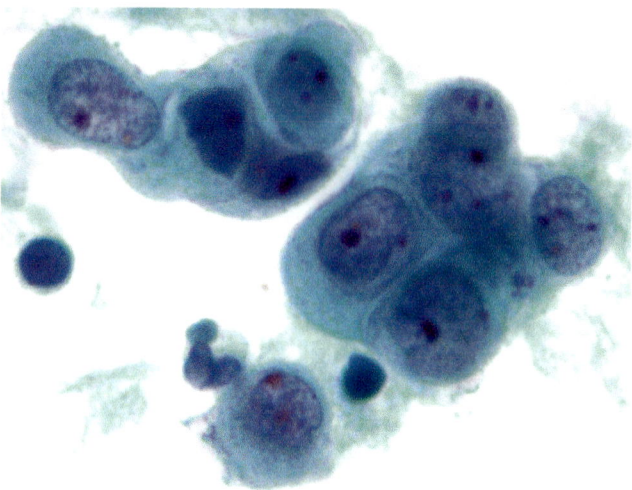

**Fig. 5.10** The cytoplasm of one mesothelial cell wraps around the adjacent cell to form the cellular clasping rather than the windows as seen in the short cord in the *top left*; PAP

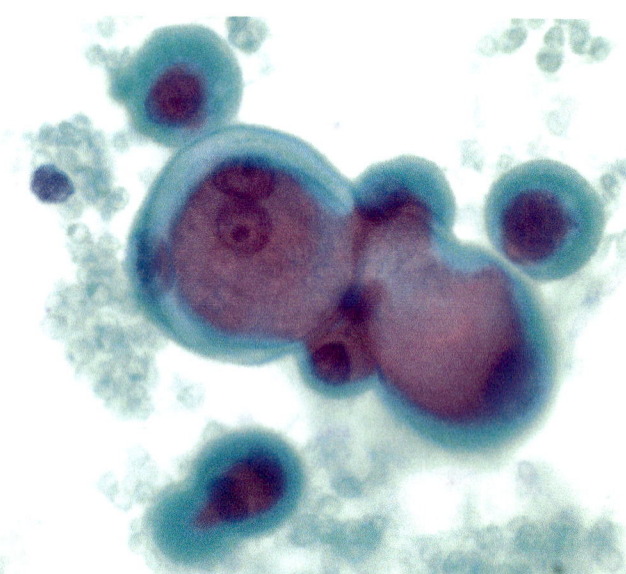

**Fig. 5.11** A mesothelial cell might be situated within the cytoplasm of the other cell like a cup sitting on its plate giving the appearance of "cell within cell"; PAP

5. Cells with two-tone cytoplasm, i.e., endo-ectoplasmic demarcation (Fig. 5.12).
6. Vague cell borders or brush border (Fig. 5.13).
7. Sub-membranous glycogen vacuoles. Yellow glycogen might be detected on fixed smears (Fig. 5.14).
8. Perinuclear small fat vacuoles best detected on Romanowsky stain.

## Cytological Features of Mesothelioma

The cytological features of mesothelioma appeared in sporadic reports since the nineteenth century. However, the first well-illustrated examples were shown by Dr. Papanicolaou

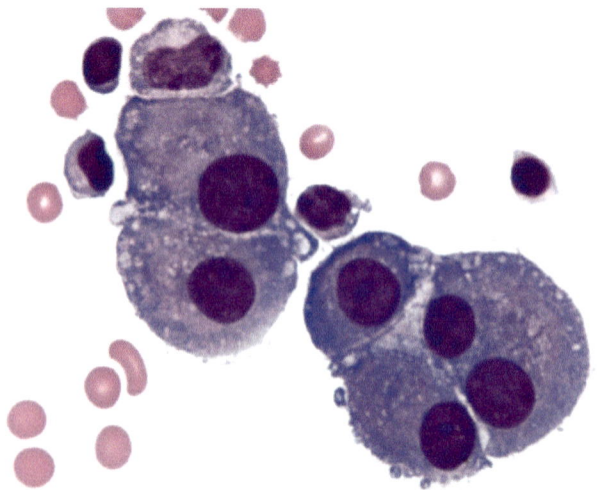

**Fig. 5.9** Mesothelial cells in apposition with windows between the adjacent cells. The cells form short cords and small clusters; Diff-Quik

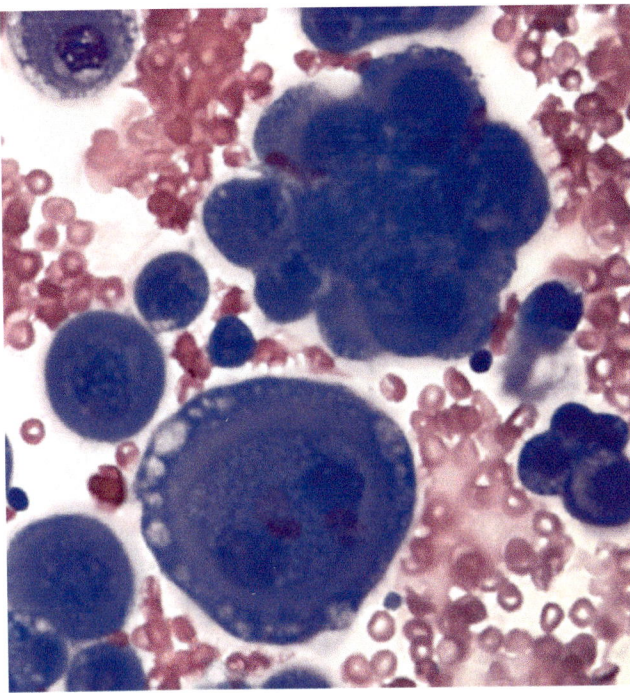

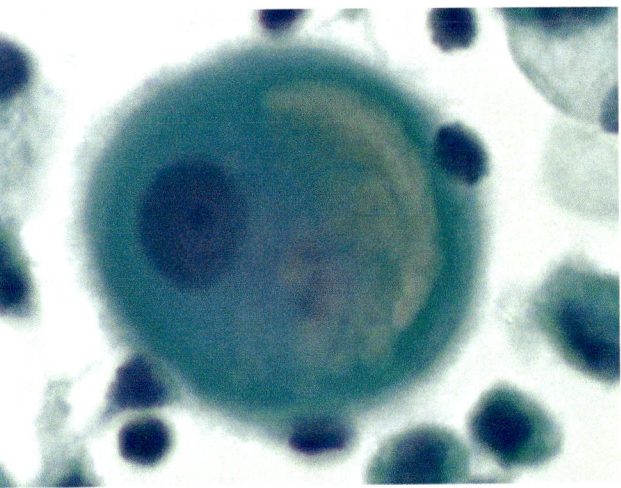

**Fig. 5.14** Large cytoplasmic vacuoles are full of glycogen that is sometimes readily recognized as yellow granular material within these vacuoles; PAP

### Epithelioid Variant (Table 5.1)

The fluids are usually of large volume, although the entire volume may not be submitted to the laboratory. Grossly, the fluid has been described to have a viscous, tar, or honey-like consistency while processing and smearing. The majority of fluids are moderately to highly cellular and can comprise almost exclusively cellular clusters and spheres (cohesive) (Fig. 5.15), single cells (discohesive) (Fig. 5.16), or a mixture of both (Fig. 5.17), with the latter being the most common. The background is usually very bloody or contains a very viscous material. Chronic inflammatory cells may be seen. However, acute inflammation is not characteristic. Once a drain is permanently installed, the fluid will exhibit a considerable acute inflammatory background.

Most mesotheliomas are highly cellular, although some cases are low in cellularity. The individual cells exhibit all the previously described mesothelial features. Mitotic figures may be seen but tend to be inconspicuous, and atypical mitoses are not seen [52]. Examination at scanning magnification reveals a monotonous population of cells that exhibit similar morphologic features yet vary tremendously in size. The cells may vary from the size and shape of benign or reactive mesothelial cells to large or even gigantic cells (Fig. 5.18). Binucleated and trinucleated cells are very frequent and many scattered multinucleated cells can be identified (Fig. 5.19). In fact, the multinucleated cells in mesothelioma have been described to contain between 2 and 50 cells or more nuclei (Fig. 5.20). Despite the obvious nuclear enlargement, the cells retain abundant cytoplasm and consequently have low nuclear-to-cytoplasmic (N/C) ratio.

The nuclei are centrally located and do not exhibit obvious malignant features, contrary to their counterparts in adenocarcinoma and other metastatic epithelial malignancies. Nevertheless, closer examination will reveal nuclear

**Fig. 5.12** Mesothelial cells from a mesothelioma case forming loose clusters with scalloped borders. The adjacent single cell is markedly enlarged with two-tone cytoplasm and well-defined sub-membranous vacuoles; Diff-Quik

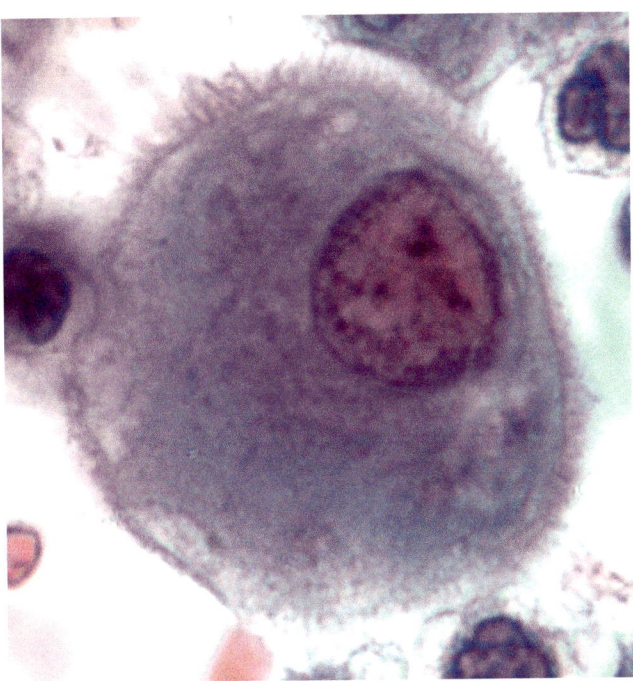

**Fig. 5.13** The mesothelial cell has a poorly defined cell circumference with a brushlike border corresponding to the long slender microvilli seen by electron microscopy; PAP

in 1954 [45]. Following that, many reports describing mesothelioma appeared in the literature [38, 42, 46–51].

**Table 5.1** Features of malignant mesothelioma

| Feature | Description | Comment |
|---|---|---|
| Gross appearance | Thick and viscous fluid<br>Bloody in most cases | Tar- or honey-like consistency |
| Background | Numerous red blood cells<br>Lymphocytosis frequent | Neutrophils are only seen after insertion of drain |
| Cell population | Monotonous single cell population | No alien population identified |
| Pattern | 1. Predominantly cohesive groups | Morules and clusters |
| | 2. Predominantly discohesive cells | |
| | 3. Mixture of clusters and single cells | Most common pattern |
| Clusters | 1. Cohesive tight clusters | Smooth outline, sphere like |
| | 2. Loose clusters | Knobby borders, berrylike |
| Cellular features | | |
| Scanning magnification | Mesothelial characteristics | Small to gigantic; cells are large and may attain the size of a small morule |
| | Wide variation in size | |
| Cytoplasm | Dense with vague brush border | Blebs may also be seen |
| | Endo-ectoplasmic demarcation | Two-tone staining |
| | Sub-membranous vacuoles | Glycogen might be seen |
| | Small perinuclear vacuoles | Fat droplets |
| Nucleus | Centrally located | |
| | Enlarged | |
| | Frequently 2–3 nuclei | May contain up to 50 nuclei |
| | Multinucleation common | |
| Nucleoli | Prominent | Macronucleoli might be seen |
| | One or more | |
| Chromatin | Slightly coarse | May be clumped |
| | Slightly hyperchromatic | |
| Nuclear membrane | Smooth or slightly irregular | Rarely very irregular |
| N/C ratio | Low | May be high in few cells |
| Cytological atypia | Mild to moderate at most | Rare cases are very atypical |

atypia in the form of slightly coarse chromatin, irregular nuclear membranes, and most importantly, prominent nucleoli, and sometimes macronucleoli. The cytoplasm in well-visualized cells has two-tone or endo-ectoplasmic demarcation. The cell circumference tends to be hazy due

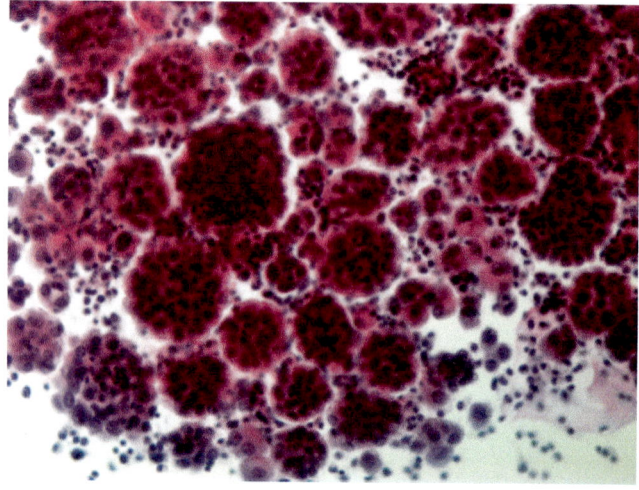

**Fig. 5.15** Highly cellular smear of mesothelioma, consisting mainly of cellular spheres and morules; PAP

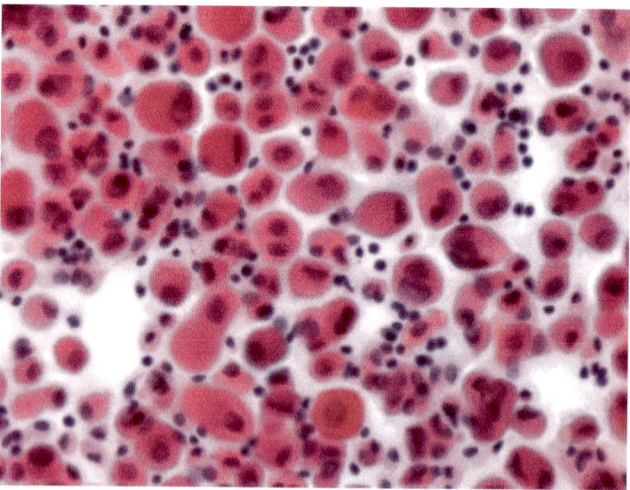

**Fig. 5.16** Highly cellular smear consisting of discohesive single cell population of malignant mesothelial cells; PAP

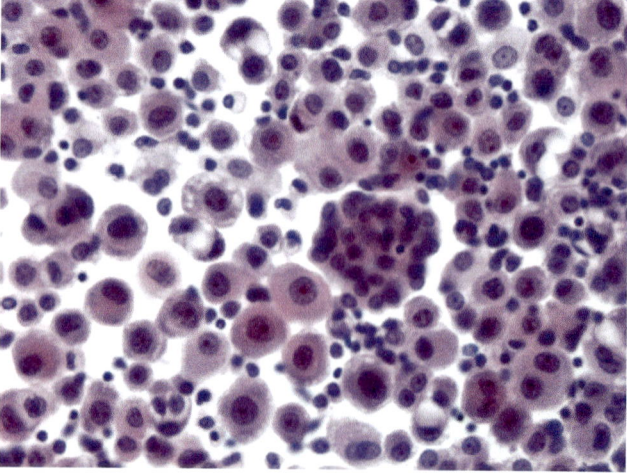

**Fig. 5.17** Mesothelioma presenting with a mixture of cellular morules and numerous discohesive single cells; PAP

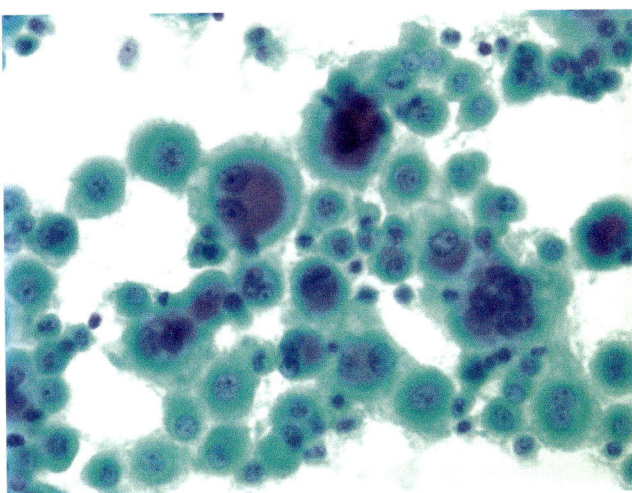

Fig. 5.18 The mesothelioma cells exhibit a wide variation of size ranging from small size similar to those of benign mesothelial cells to very large cells attaining gigantic size. Notice the large cell on the left approaching the same size of the small morule on the right; PAP

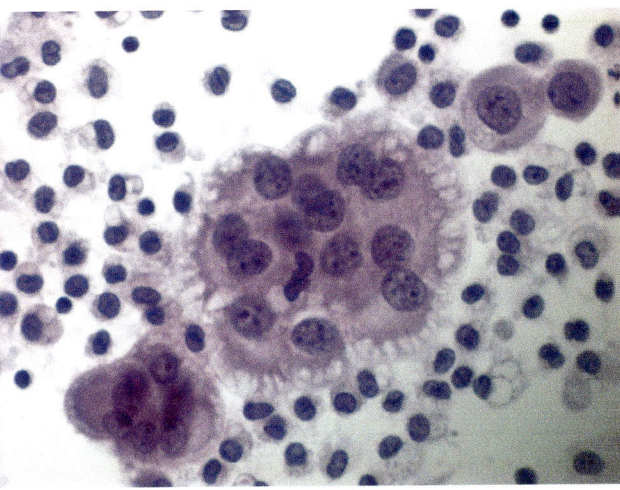

Fig. 5.21 Mesothelioma with high glycogen content appearing as large cytoplasmic vacuoles beneath the cell membrane; PAP

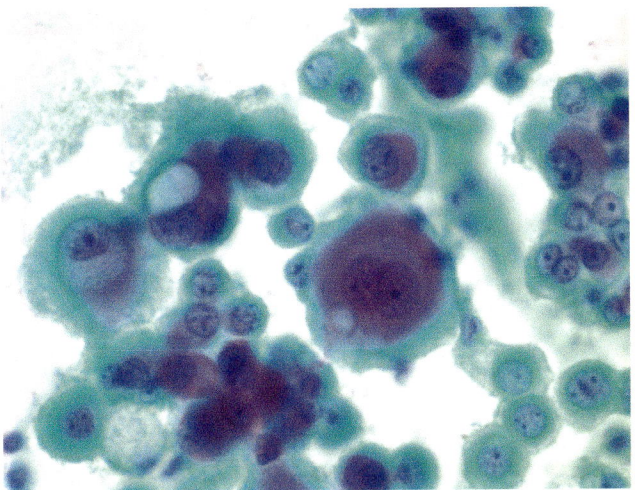

Fig. 5.19 Enlarged mesothelial cells with binucleation and prominent nucleoli; PAP

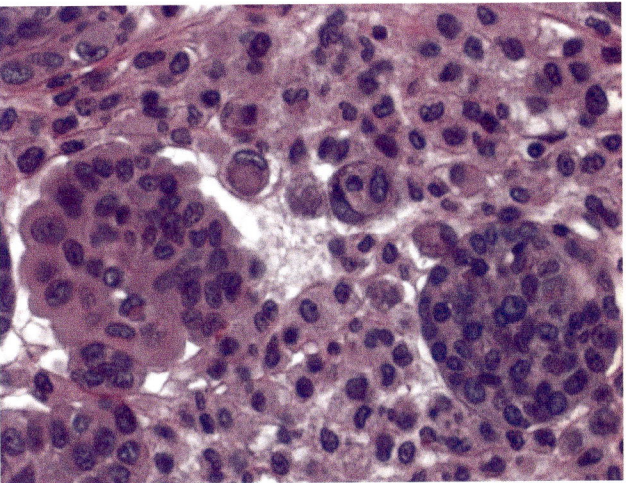

Fig. 5.22 Cell block of a mesothelioma presenting with two types of cellular clusters, the loose cluster having a knobby or scalloped border (berrylike) and the tight spherical group with smooth outline; H&E

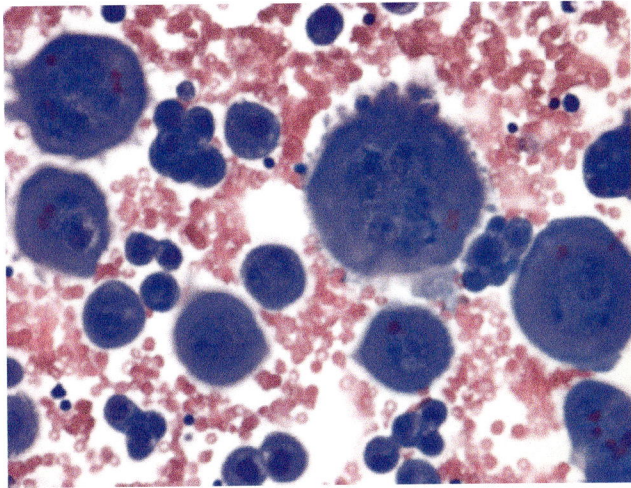

Fig. 5.20 Multinucleation is common in mesothelioma with nuclear number ranging from 2 to 50 or more; Diff-Quik

to the circumferential brush border formed by the long slender microvilli visualized by electron microscopy. Submembranous vacuoles are frequently noted and sometimes coalesce to form long vacuoles, described as sausage links. It is not unusual, especially in the Papanicolaou-stained smears, to see yellow glycogen clumps within these vacuoles (Fig. 5.21).

The cellular clusters are of two types. The first are loose clusters with knobby or scalloped borders, also described as berrylike. The second are tight clusters or spheres with smooth borders also known as morules (Fig. 5.22). In the former type, the crowded cells forming the clusters can be easily visualized and intercellular windows can be identified. The cytoplasm with its characteristic mesothelial features can be visualized, particularly in those cells located at the knobby borders. The cells in the morules are very tightly cohesive and therefore frequently

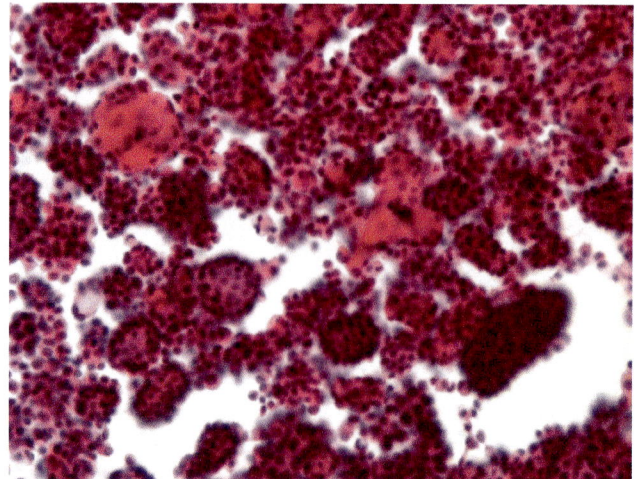

**Fig. 5.23** A well-differentiated mesothelioma with papillary features presenting as highly cellular smear consisting predominantly of papillary groups with complex branching and obvious collagen cores; PAP

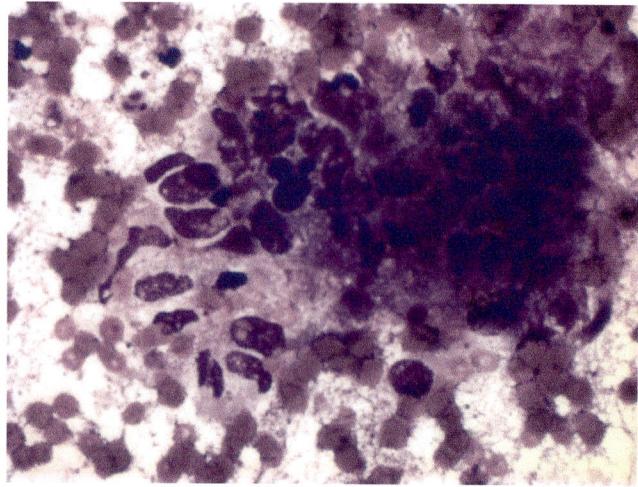

**Fig. 5.25** Sarcomatoid mesothelioma presenting as bloody and sparsely cellular smear with rare clusters of spindled cells; Diff-Quik

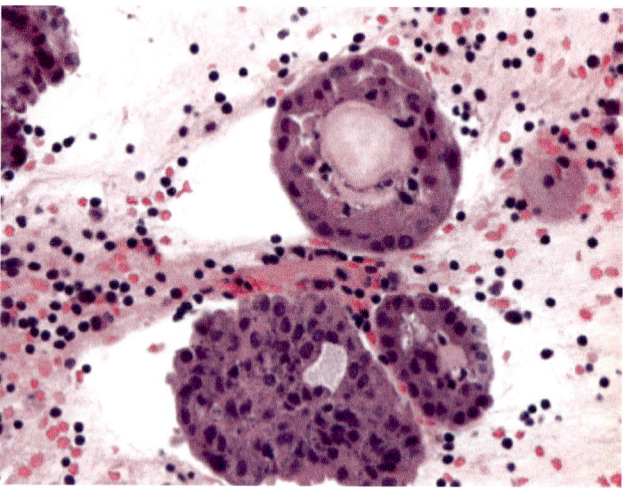

**Fig. 5.24** Cell block of the corresponding papillary mesothelioma showing the papillary groups with central collagenous cores; H&E

difficult to discern. Large branching and papillary clusters may be seen and rarely predominate (Fig. 5.23). The clusters may contain an amorphous eosinophilic core that stains negative with PAS, positive with Van Gieson stains, and bright blue with the Martius Scarlet Blue technique, indicating that it comprises collagen (Fig. 5.24). On electron microscopy, these cores were found to consist of whorls with periodicity of 640 Å, confirming their collagenous origin [53].

Whitaker et al. identified five features to be of particular value in the diagnosis of mesothelioma, namely, the presence of cell aggregates, multinucleation, brushlike borders, close opposition of cell borders, and the characteristic two-tone cytoplasm [39].

## Sarcomatoid and Biphasic Variants

While most of these mesotheliomas present with persistent effusions, they seldom exfoliate the sarcomatoid malignant cells in the fluids. Consequently, the fluids tend to be bloody and virtually acellular. Rarely, very few malignant spindled or highly atypical large cells are seen with diligent search (Fig. 5.25). The biphasic type may exfoliate, but only the epithelioid component is found in the effusion.

## Other Rare Variants

Because of their rarity, very few cases have been reported in the cytology literature and the following features are mainly based on the author's experience. Effusions with the small cell variant have low cellularity. The exfoliated cells are small in size and show the immunophenotypic profile of mesothelioma rather than that of small cell carcinoma (Fig. 5.26a, b). The lymphohistiocytoid variant may present with cellular effusion consisting predominantly of lymphocytes and histiocyte-like cells that stain as mesothelial cells. The deciduoid variant tends to have large and cellular effusions with highly atypical cells that have definitive malignant features, but may not be initially recognized as mesothelial in origin [54–57] (Fig. 5.27a, b). The majority of the reported cases had the immunostaining pattern of mesothelioma.

Localized well-differentiated papillary mesothelioma has mainly been described in peritoneal washes or fine needle aspirates. However, two cases with ascitic fluids were described [58, 59]. Cytological evaluation revealed papillary clusters formed mainly of a collagenous core surrounded by one layer of mesothelial cells.

While most of the cytology literature has focused on pleural effusions, Patel et al. reviewed 49 cases of peritoneal mesothelioma, including 6 peritoneal washes obtained after

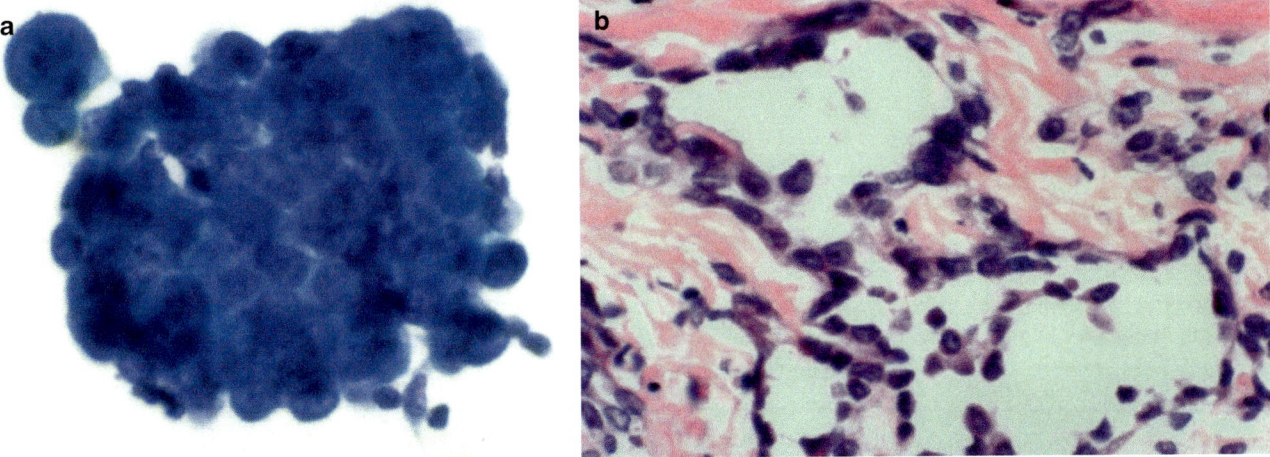

**Fig. 5.26** (**a**) Mesothelioma of the small cell variant presenting as a sparsely cellular smear with few clusters as the one shown. The cells are tightly cohesive and exhibit molding simulating small cell carcinoma; PAP. (**b**) Mesothelioma of small cell variant, corresponding biopsy showing small mesothelial cells invading the fibrous stroma; H&E

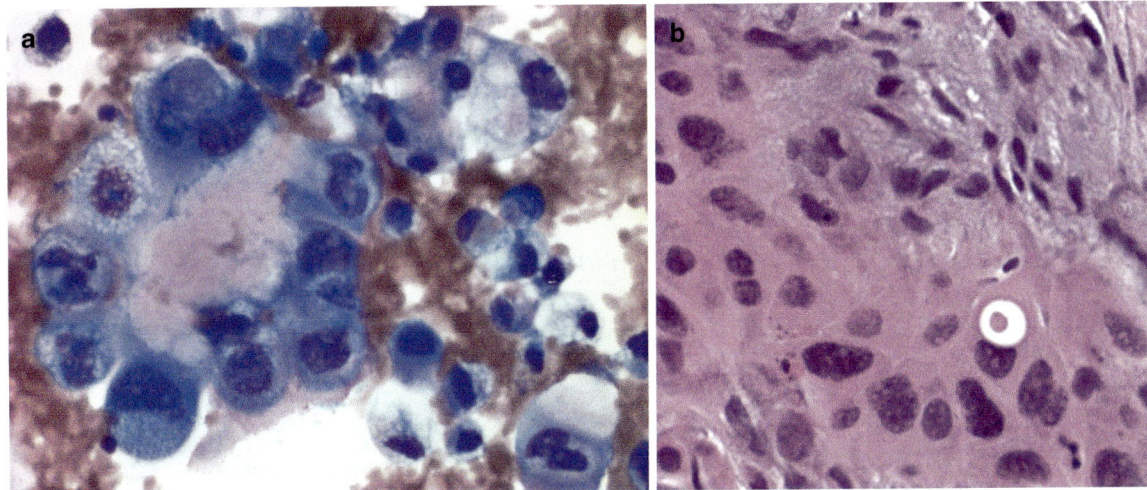

**Fig. 5.27** (**a**) Deciduoid mesothelioma presenting as enlarged highly atypical cells with abundant cytoplasm. While occasional cells show two-tone cytoplasm and sub-membranous vacuoles, the mesothelial ori- gin is difficult to ascertain without the confirmatory immunostains; Diff- Quik. (**b**) Deciduoid mesothelioma, corresponding peritoneal biopsy showing a highly atypical infiltrative mesothelial proliferation; H&E

cytoreduction and HIPEC and reported as negative for resid- ual mesothelioma [52]. The peritoneal fluids ranged from 15 to 1000 mL in volume and were predominantly moderate to highly cellular. The smears were typically bloody or had pro- teinaceous background. The discohesive single cell presenta- tion was uncommon in these cases, but otherwise cytological features similar to those of pleural mesothelioma were described. Mitotic activity was noted in one-third of the cases, but no atypical mitotic figures were identified. Peritoneal washes presented with some different features. When compared to effusions, peritoneal washes were more likely to contain broad, irregular branching sheets, frequently containing several hundreds of malignant cells. Mitotic fig- ures were more readily observed in washes, particularly within the cellular sheets. Peritoneal washes post-HIPEC

were uniformly bloody and generally low in cellularity. Residual malignant cells manifested as few small scattered clusters and small sheets admixed with clusters of reactive mesothelial cells. To address this challenge, the authors rec- ommended comparing these samples with diagnostic mate- rial evaluated prior to therapy.

## Ancillary Tests

### Histochemical Stains

Prior to the recent introduction of the currently available wide array of immunostains, particularly mesothelial mark- ers, histochemical stains used to play a major role in the diagnosis of mesothelioma. At present, these stains do not play such an essential role, with the exception of the rare undifferentiated case that may not express the expected immunostaining profile.

Because of the high glycogen content of mesothelial cells, they stain strongly positive with PAS and convert to negative or weakly positive upon treatment with diastase (PAS-D). Mesothelial cells secrete hyaluronic acid (HA) and acid muco-substances. Consequently, 40–50% of mesotheliomas stain positive with Alcian blue, which converts to negative upon treatment with hyaluronidase. Mayer's Mucicarmine is generally negative in mesothelioma, although rare cases may focally stain positive [60] (Fig. 5.28a). This positive staining will convert to negative with hyaluronidase treatment, confirming a focal nonspecific staining [61].

Measurement of HA in the fluid is believed to be of value. Whitaker et al. measured HA in fluids of reactive mesothelium, mesotheliomas, and metastatic adenocarcinomas. They found that mesothelioma specimens tend to have levels higher than 200 mg/L, and in some cases, levels were as high as 3130 mg/L. The authors noted, however, that some mesotheliomas had levels of less than 90 mg/L and therefore commented that while high HA levels confirm the diagnosis of mesothelioma, low levels do not necessarily exclude it [62]. In a study by Welker et al., the authors reported the cutoff value of 30 mg/L as having maximum diagnostic reliability, with 87% sensitivity and 86% specificity, while a value of 100 mg/L resulted in sensitivity and specificity of 39% and 98%, respectively. The addition of HA measurement to cytology increased the sensitivity from 48% to 71–91%, while only slightly decreasing the specificity to 94–96% [63].

A useful, fast and very affordable yet underutilized stain is Oil Red O to identify the perinuclear fat droplets characteristic of mesothelial cells (Fig. 5.28b) [3].

## Electron Microscopy (EM)

Before the introduction of immunoperoxidase stains, EM was the most conclusive method to document mesothelioma. The following are features described as characteristic of mesothelial origin [50]:

1. Cytoplasm rich in intermediate filaments concentrically arranged and particularly concentrated in a ringlike pattern around the nuclear envelope and in the subplasmalemmal position beneath the cell surface. This phenomenon contributes to the endo-ectoplasmic demarcation noticed on light microscopy.
2. Paucity of organelles and mainly glycogen vacuoles seen near the periphery of the cytoplasm.
3. Cell surface rich with microvilli that are distributed throughout the periphery of the cell. Characteristically, these microvilli are bushy, complex, and frequently branching and very long. The microvilli lack glycocalyceal bodies and filamentous core rootlet at their base and usually contain actin-like filaments along their length.

The role of EM in diagnosing mesothelioma is discussed in more detail in Chap. 11.

## Immunostains

To date, there is no specific marker that can alone separate adenocarcinoma from mesothelioma, and it is important to use a panel of stains including a minimum of two mesothelial markers and two carcinoma markers. Additional markers can follow if the results of the initial panel are not conclusive [3].

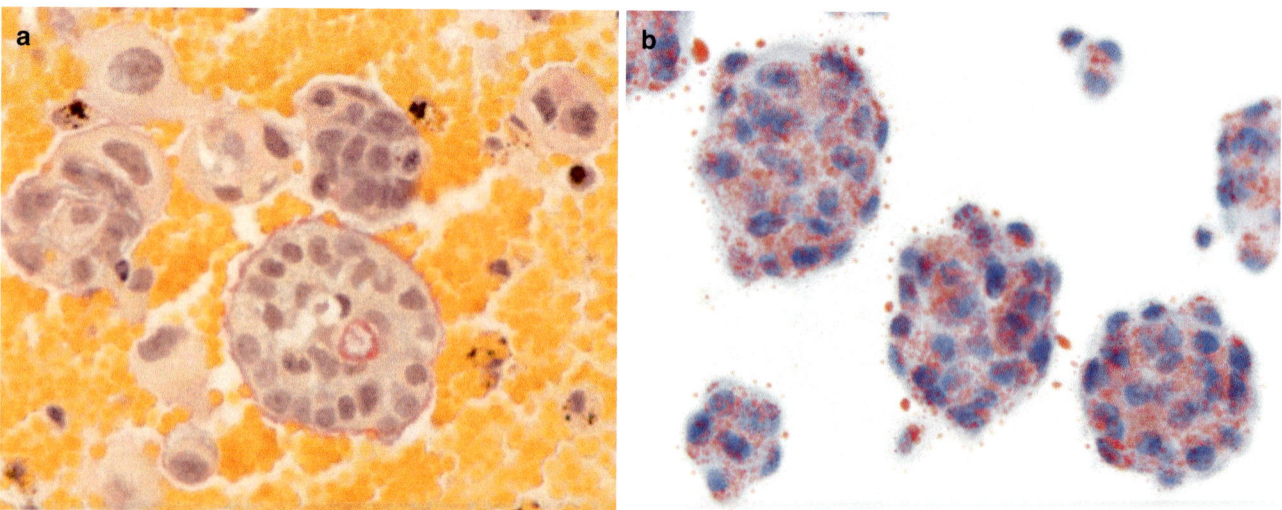

**Fig. 5.28** (a) Mesothelioma showing rare focal positive staining with Mucicarmine stain. (b) Mesothelioma showing distinct perinuclear fat droplets with Oil Red O stain

## Positive Mesothelial Markers [64–66]

*Mesothelin* (Fig. 5.29) was reported to show a diffuse strong staining in up to 100% of mesotheliomas, and some consider a negative stain as strong evidence against mesothelioma. However, it has also been reported to stain a high percentage of adenocarcinomas.

*Calretinin* (Fig. 5.30) is considered as one of the most sensitive stains for mesothelioma. It strongly and diffusely stains both nuclei and cytoplasm, resulting in a "fried egg" appearance. It was reported to stain from 55% to 100% of epithelioid mesotheliomas cases and 30–60% of sarcomatoid mesotheliomas. The wide range of positivity is likely related to the type of antibody used, and the best results were reported with polyclonal antibodies against recombinant human calretinin. It is worth noting that calretinin was

reported to stain carcinomas from various sites of origin including 6–23% of lung ADC, 31–38% of serous carcinomas, 15–74% of breast ADC, 0–10% of renal cell carcinomas, 23–40% of squamous cell carcinomas of the lung, and 41–49% of small cell carcinomas.

*Wilms tumor 1 protein (WT-1)* (Fig. 5.31) is strongly expressed in the nuclei and has been reported to stain 43–100% of epithelioid mesotheliomas. It was also reported to react with 83–100% of serous carcinoma of the ovary and peritoneum. However, it is negative or very weakly positive in adenocarcinoma of the lung and squamous cell carcinoma and therefore useful in this differential diagnosis [67].

*Podoplanin A and D2–40* (Fig. 5.32) are expressed in the cytoplasm of over 90% of epithelioid and 57% of sarcomatoid mesotheliomas. Up to 15% of adenocarcinomas may also show positive staining, though the expression is usually

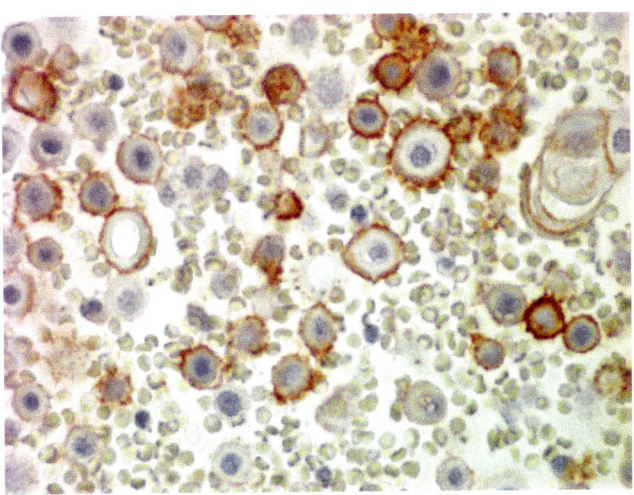

**Fig. 5.29** Mesothelioma with positive membranous reaction to mesothelin

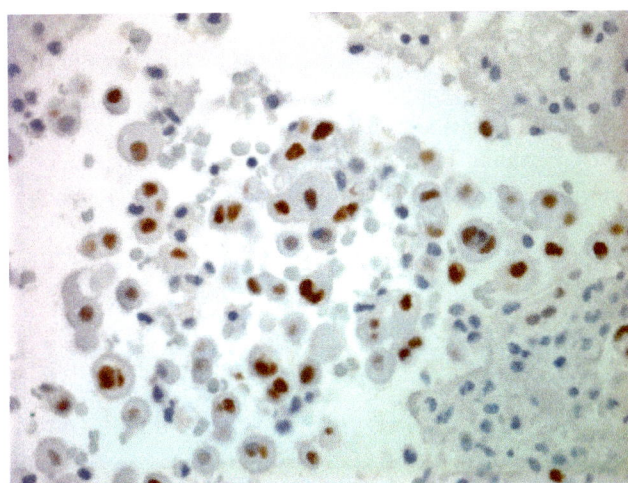

**Fig. 5.31** Mesothelioma with positive nuclear reaction with WT-1 antibody

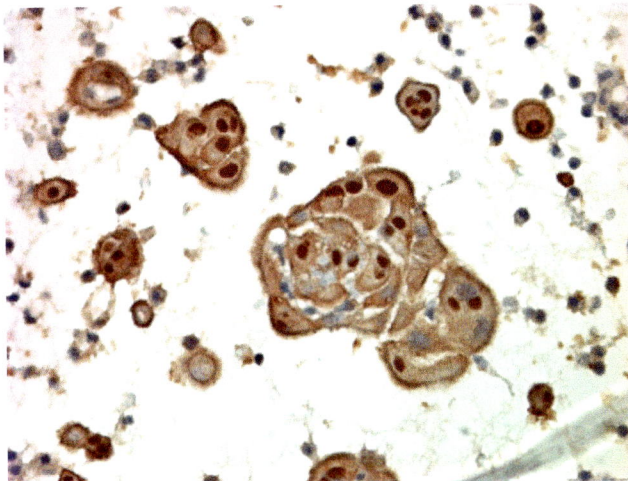

**Fig. 5.30** Mesothelioma with positive nuclear and cytoplasmic reaction (so-called fried egg appearance) to calretinin

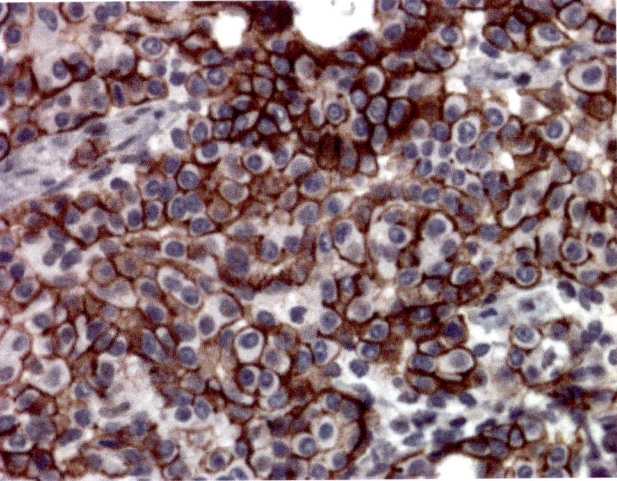

**Fig. 5.32** Mesothelioma with distinct membranous staining for D2–40

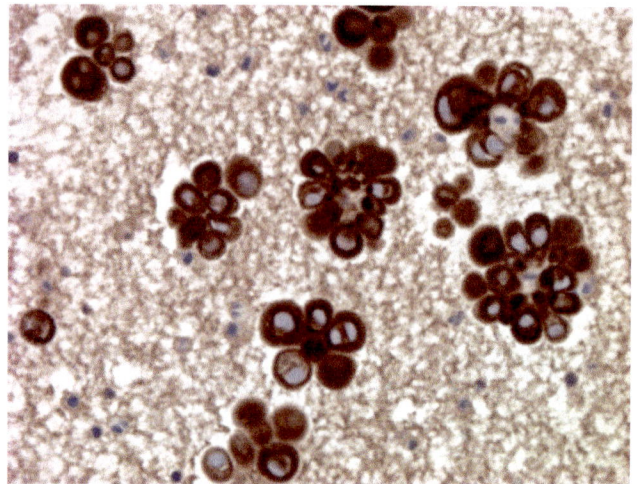

**Fig. 5.33** Mesothelioma with strong cytoplasmic reaction with cyto-keratin 5/6 antibody

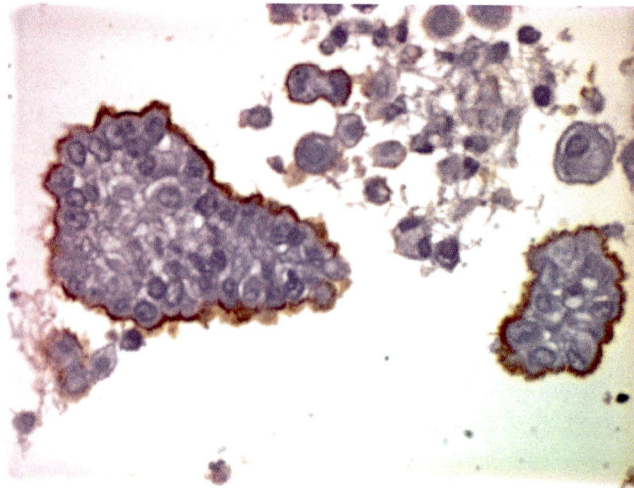

**Fig. 5.34** Mesothelioma expressing HBME-1, highlighting the brush border of the cells

weak [68, 69]. Podoplanin is also expressed in squamous cell carcinoma of the lung and serous carcinomas. Bassarova et al. [70] evaluated the diagnostic role of D2–40 in 290 effusions, including 169 ovarian carcinomas and 32 mesotheliomas, and observed frequent staining in the former tumor, concluding that it performed poorly in this differential diagnosis. Ordonez reported similar performance for these two antibodies in surgical specimens [66].

*Thrombomodulin* stains over 75% of mesotheliomas but was reported to be expressed in up to 25% of adenocarcinomas, although staining is weaker. Staining is also seen in squamous cell carcinoma [71].

*Cytokeratin 5/6* (Fig. 5.33) exhibits strong cytoplasmic staining in 65–100% of epithelioid mesotheliomas and a high percentage of squamous cell carcinomas. It has also been reported to stain a significant percentage of breast and gynecologic adenocarcinomas [67]. However, it is predominantly negative in adenocarcinoma of the lung with only 0–19% reported to express CK5/6, attributed to be likely due to squamous differentiation.

*HBME-1* (Fig. 5.34) is seldom used now because of the significant staining overlap with adenocarcinomas, particularly of ovarian origin. It is expressed with a distinct membranous or brush border staining in mesothelioma [72],

## Negative Mesothelial Markers

*Carcinoembryonic antigen (CEA)* exhibits cytoplasmic staining in 50–90% of adenocarcinomas, particularly breast (80%), gastrointestinal, and lung origin, as well as in 77–86% of squamous cell carcinoma. While the old literature describes up to 30% staining in mesothelioma, newer clones are more specific and are consistently negative. Of note, most ovarian carcinomas, except for mucinous carcinomas, rarely express CEA, and this marker is therefore not useful

by itself in the differential diagnosis between mesothelioma and ovarian carcinoma [73].

*B72.3* identifies the Sialyl-Tn sugar group and stains the membrane and/or cytoplasm in over 80% of adenocarcinomas, 75–85% of lung carcinoma, 70–75% serous carcinoma, and 50–70% of breast carcinoma. It is also reportedly expressed in 45–84% of lung squamous cell carcinoma but negative in mesothelioma.

*CD15 (Leu-M1)* exhibits cytoplasmic staining in a high percentage of adenocarcinomas of various body sites, up to 30% of squamous cell carcinoma and is negative in mesothelioma.

*MOC-31* antibody recognizes the membrane protein EpCAM and exhibits strong and diffuse membrane and/or cytoplasmic staining in most adenocarcinomas and squamous cell carcinoma of the lung. It can be focally expressed in 2–15% of mesotheliomas [67, 74].

*Ber-EP4* is directed against the same epitope as MOC-31 and exhibits a staining pattern similar to the latter. It may be focally positive in 13–26% of mesotheliomas [74].

*BG-8* identifies the Lewis$^y$ sugar group and strongly stains the membrane and/or cytoplasm of over 95% of adenocarcinomas. It can be weakly and focally expressed in 3–9% of mesotheliomas.

*Claudin 4* is a transmembrane protein located in the tight junctions. It is expressed in most epithelial cells but not in mesothelioma. It is expressed in most adenocarcinomas of the lung, breast, ovary, and kidney and most squamous and urothelial carcinomas but predominantly negative in mesotheliomas [75].

*PAX8 stains* as strong nuclear reaction. This stain is essentially negative in mesothelioma and positive in a high percentage of Müllerian tumors, with a sensitivity of 96% and specificity of 100% [76].

*MMP-7* is a member of the matrix metalloproteinases, a family of more than 20 zinc- and calcium-dependent enzymes involved in degrading all components of basement membranes and consequently the physiologic process of tumor progression. Davidson et al. reported that MMP-7 was expressed in 124/307 (40%) of adenocarcinomas and was uniformly negative in all 49 mesotheliomas [77].

## Other Immunostains

*Pancytokeratin* (Fig. 5.35) is usually strongly positive in mesothelioma, squamous cell carcinoma, and adenocarcinoma [78].

*Cytokeratin 7* is strongly positive in mesothelioma and in some adenocarcinomas but is expressed in only 30% of squamous carcinomas [79].

*Cytokeratin 20* (Fig. 5.36) is variably expressed in mesothelioma and therefore should be cautiously evaluated in the differential diagnosis with adenocarcinomas

known to express CK20, such as gastrointestinal tract or urothelial carcinomas that may occasionally mimic mesothelioma [78].

*BRCA1-associated protein 1 (BAP1)* is a tumor suppression gene encoded by the BAP 1 gene at 3p21.1. Recent studies revealed that BAP1 expression is lost in 57–66% of mesothelioma while expressed in reactive mesothelium with a specificity of 100%. This stain is emerging now as the best immunostain to distinguish mesothelioma from reactive mesothelium [80–82].

*Desmin and EMA* (Figs. 5.37 and 5.38) play a role in the differential diagnosis between mesothelioma and reactive mesothelium. Mesothelioma has strong membranous EMA staining in the majority of cases which is rarely present in reactive mesothelium. Desmin is preferentially expressed by benign mesothelium and is lost in mesothelioma. Caution should be exercised when evaluating desmin in mesothelioma, since scattered reactive mesothelium in the background may stain positive [69, 83].

*E-cadherin and N-cadherin* are currently not believed to be of use in the differential diagnosis between mesothelioma and adenocarcinoma. E-cadherin, however, is useful in

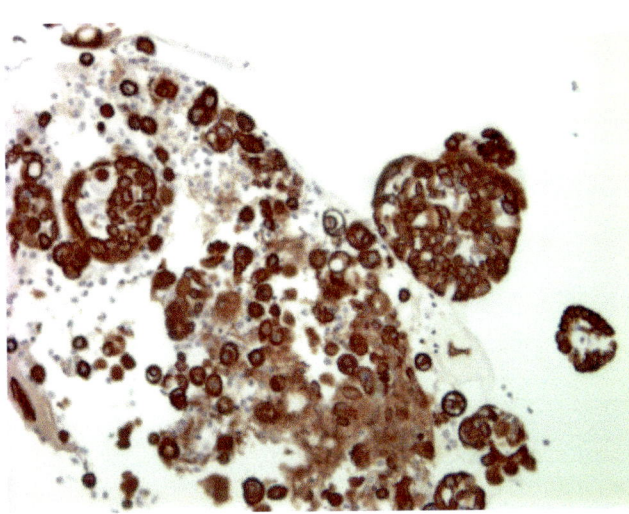

**Fig. 5.35** Mesothelioma with strong cytoplasmic cytokeratin 7 staining

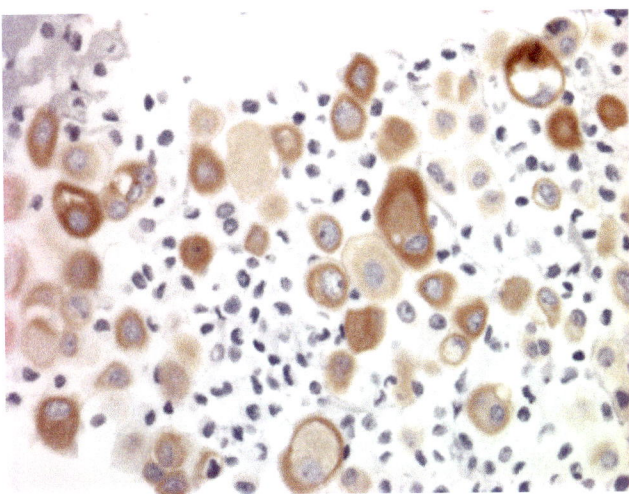

**Fig. 5.36** Mesothelioma showing a rare reaction to cytokeratin 20

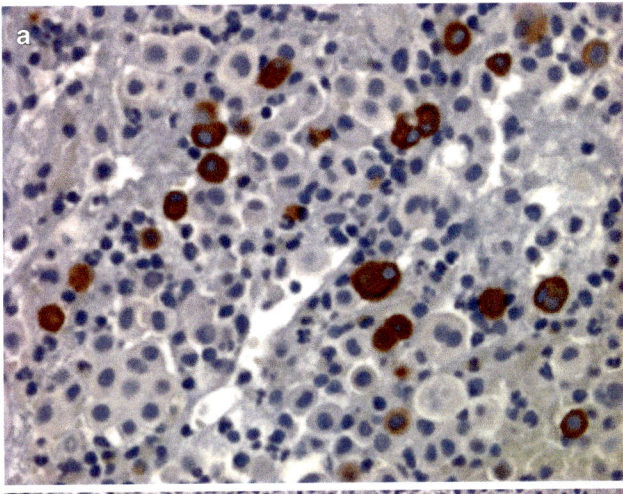

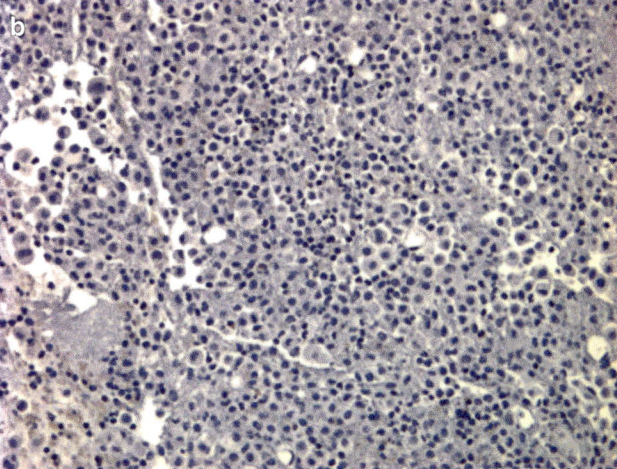

**Fig. 5.37** (**a**) Reactive mesothelium showing positive staining for desmin. (**b**) Reactive mesothelium showing negative reaction to EMA

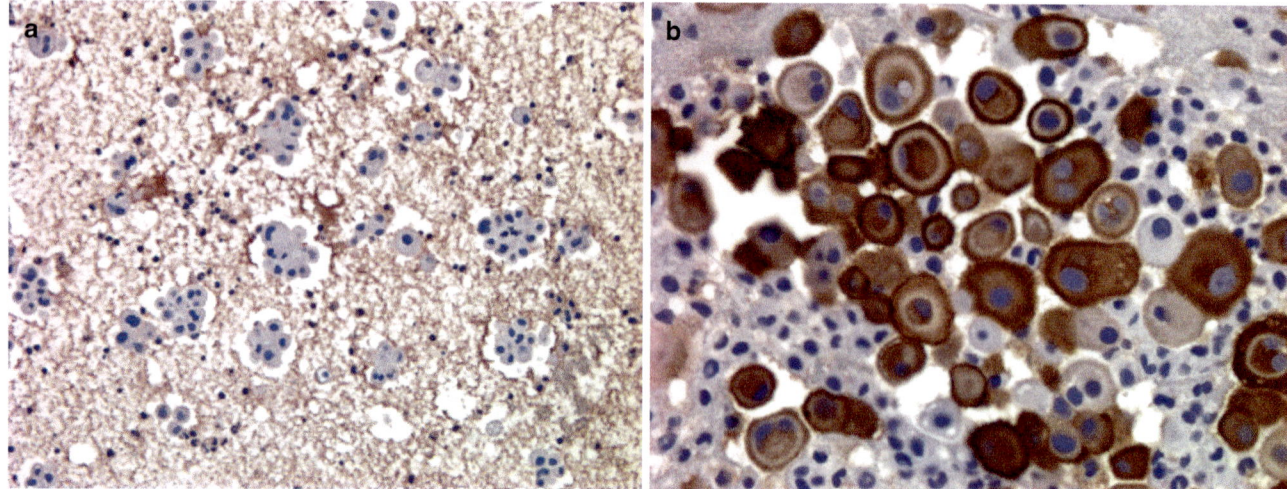

**Fig. 5.38** (**a**) Mesothelioma reacting negatively to desmin. (**b**) Mesothelioma reacting strongly to EMA

separating adenocarcinoma, which tends to be positive, from the negatively reacting benign mesothelium [84, 85].

## Other Methods

Several other methods, including traditional cytogenetics, fluorescent in situ hybridization (FISH), measurement of secreted biomarkers, and high-throughput technology, are discussed in Chap. 11.

## Differential Diagnosis

The differential diagnosis depends on the cytological presentation and degree of atypia recognized. When atypia is subtle, reactive mesothelial hyperplasia is the main differential. When malignancy is identified, it is important to separate mesothelioma from adenocarcinoma of various primary sites.

## Mesothelioma Versus Reactive Mesothelium
(Table 5.2)

When mesothelium is floridly reactive, it may mimic mesothelioma. The cellularity can be high, with an increase in the number of clusters and multinucleated cells. Mitotic figures may be conspicuous and have been reported to reach their peak in mesothelial surfaces reacting to injury within 48 h [86]. In such cases, examination at low magnification cannot be stressed enough. The cells are monotonous in appearance, i.e., mesothelial in origin, and exhibit a small to moderate size with very subtle difference in size except for a few outliers. Nuclei, while enlarged and somewhat atypical, have vesicular

**Table 5.2** Reactive mesothelium versus malignant mesothelioma

| Feature | | Reactive mesothelium | Malignant mesothelioma |
|---|---|---|---|
| Cellularity | | Moderate | Very high |
| Cell size | | Little variation in size and shape | Wide variation in size from benign to gigantic |
| Multinucleated cells | | | |
| | Number | Few scattered cells | Numerous |
| | Nuclei | Rarely exceed 5 nuclei | May contain >50 nuclei |
| | | Benign appearance | Enlarged and atypical |
| Giant cell | | Rare | Characteristic |
| | | | May reach the size of adjacent morules |
| | | | Normal N/C ratio |
| Clusters | | | |
| | Number | More numerous than normal | Innumerable |
| | Morphology | Flat and lack depth | Morules and spheres with depth |
| | Borders | Scalloped | Scalloped or knobby |
| | Cell arrangement | No crowding | Frequently crowded |
| Nuclei | | | |
| | Size | Slightly enlarged | Markedly enlarged |
| | Chromatin | Mostly vesicular | Atypia present but vary from subtle to definitive |
| | Nuclear membrane | Smooth or subtle irregularity at most | Subtle to definitive irregularity |
| | Nucleoli | Slight to moderate enlargement | Markedly enlarged or macronucleoli |
| | Cytoplasm | Moderate | Abundant and very dense |
| | Mitotic activity | Can be conspicuous | May not be increased |

chromatin and smooth chromatin contours even in the multinucleated cells. The nucleoli may be prominent, but no macronucleoli or irregular nucleoli are detected. Clusters tend to be few in most cases and are small with lack of depth, i.e., flat with scalloped borders. Multinucleation is rarely beyond 3–4 nuclei and these appear normal. No gigantic cells are seen. In contrast, malignant mesothelioma will present with numerous morules and single cells. The single cells in malignant mesothelioma may appear monotonous, consistent with their mesothelial origin. However, they may vary tremendously in size from that of normal mesothelium to gigantic cells. In the author's experience, such large cells may attain the size of the small adjacent morules, a feature that has not been seen except in mesothelioma. The cellular clusters also vary in size and have a spherical appearance with depth of focus and berrylike borders. The presence of small orangiophilic squamous-like or parakeratotic-like cells were reported to be highly correlated with malignant mesothelioma while rarely noted in reactive mesothelium [87, 88].

In a study by Kimura et al. [89], the authors devised a scoring system of the cytological features in an attempt to separate reactive from malignant mesothelium. They assigned a total score of 10 points, 1 point each for variation in cell size, sheetlike arrangement, cyanophilic cytoplasm with windows/blebs/brush border, mirror ball-like cell clusters, cannibalism, and nuclear atypia. Two features, acidophilic large nucleoli and multinucleated cells with more than eight nuclei, received 2 points each. Mesotheliomas consistently scored more than 5, while reactive mesothelial hyperplasia and metastatic adenocarcinomas scored less than 3 points. A study by Cakir et al. [90] using logistic regression analysis identified the presence of cell ball formation, cell-in-cell engulfment, and monolayer sheets as variables useful in the separation of reactive mesothelium from mesothelioma, with the latter finding favoring a reactive diagnosis.

The role of ancillary testing in separating reactive from malignant mesothelium is somewhat controversial. While proliferation markers such as Ki-67 and MIB-1 may be useful in some cases where mesotheliomas have higher activity, it has been the author's experience that they play a limited role in the floridly reactive effusions, where mitotic activity is very high, with a sensitivity of 17% and specificity of 91% [83]. The differential staining of desmin and EMA seems to be more helpful. It is well established that benign mesothelium expresses muscle markers, particularly desmin, which is progressively lost as the mesothelium becomes malignant, with a sensitivity of 91% and specificity of 94%. On the other hand, EMA is not expressed by benign mesothelium and is expressed in most malignant mesotheliomas, with a sensitivity of 100% and specificity of 94%. p53 may also be helpful in this differential diagnosis and has been shown to be expressed at much higher levels in mesothelioma, with a sensitivity of 57% and specificity of 98%. In the author's experience, GLUT-1 has less utility in this differential diagnosis, with a sensitivity of only 47% and specificity of 88% [83].

Otherwise, reactive mesothelium expresses all the immunomarkers expressed by mesothelioma, such as HBME-1, calretinin, D2-40, and WT-1.

## Mesothelioma Versus Adenocarcinoma (Table 5.3)

In over 50% of cases, the distinction between adenocarcinoma and mesothelioma is feasible by routine cytological stains once the characteristic mesothelial features are recognized. Generally, at low magnification, the evaluator should recognize an overall monotony in the type of cells with no alien population in mesothelioma while frequently detecting a two-cell population, namely, carcinoma and benign mesothelium, in adenocarcinoma specimens.

Mesothelioma is characterized by a low degree of atypia. Definitive malignant features are rarely present and mitotic activity is inconspicuous. In contrast, adenocarcinoma generally expresses a noticeable degree of pleomorphism with definitive malignant features and high mitotic activity in most cases.

In the study by Cakir et al. [90], the authors identified the presence of giant atypical mesothelial cells, nuclear pleomorphism, and acinar formation as features useful in distin-

Table 5.3 Mesothelioma versus adenocarcinoma

| Feature | Mesothelioma | Adenocarcinoma |
|---|---|---|
| Cellularity | Very high | Variable, frequently high |
| Overall cell features | | |
| Cell type | Monotonous population | Polymorphous population |
| | One cell type, mesothelial | Two cell types |
| Pleomorphism | Minimal atypia | Obviously atypical |
| | Rarely frankly malignant | Rarely subtle atypia |
| Cell size | Vary from small to gigantic | Generally enlarged and of similar size |
| N/C ratio | Low | High |
| Mitotic activity | Inconspicuous | Variable, can be high |
| Cytoplasm | Abundant | Variable but rarely abundant |
| | Two-tone | One-tone in most cases |
| | Sub-membranous vacuoles and brush border | Fine vacuoles throughout or large disfiguring vacuoles |
| Cell clusters | | |
| Shape | Spheres, morules, and loose clusters | Variable, mainly spheres or clusters |
| Circumference | Knobby or berrylike | Mostly smooth |
| | Scalloped borders | |
| | Cytoplasm forming the border | Nuclei forming the border |
| Cell-to-cell relation | Cellular windows | No windows |
| | Cellular clasping | No cell clasping |
| | Cell within cell | Cell within cell |

guishing mesothelioma from adenocarcinoma, with the latter two favoring adenocarcinoma.

In a subgroup of cases, it is truly difficult to distinguish mesothelioma from adenocarcinoma, and immunostains will play a significant role in establishing the diagnosis. As stated above, we recommend using a minimum of two mesothelial markers and two or three carcinoma markers in the initial panel.

While all adenocarcinomas can present a differential with mesothelioma, certain adenocarcinomas should particularly be considered. These include tumors of lung, ovary, and breast origin, since they can present with numerous cell aggregates in a pattern very similar to mesothelioma. Breast carcinoma in particular tends to present as cellular spheres with only a few single cells. However, breast clusters tend to be very large, frequently with irregular contours, and an overall cribriform pattern in contrast to the smaller morules with scalloped borders in mesothelioma. As previously mentioned, in the author's experience, the presence of multinucleated cells with abundant dense cytoplasm and gigantic cells approaching the size of adjacent morules is a feature frequently seen in mesothelioma and rarely encountered in adenocarcinoma. Primary adenocarcinoma of the serosal surface may be difficult to separate from peritoneal mesothelioma. Both present as a primary peritoneal tumor and may overlap with some immunostains. In a study by Ordonez evaluating multiple markers, the best discriminators among the positive markers for mesothelioma were D2–40, podoplanin, and calretinin. The author recommended a panel of Ber-EP4 and MOC-31 in combination with calretinin, and/or D2–40 or podoplanin [91]. However, since Ber-EP4 and MOC-31 are directed against the same epitope, we believe that one of them is sufficient and recommend instead an additional marker such as B72.3, which is highly specific, to be added to the panel [92]. In addition, it is important to remember that mesothelial markers may also be expressed by a subset of ovarian carcinomas. Estrogen (ER) and progesterone (PR) receptor immunostaining is also helpful in the differential diagnosis, with reactivity for ER in up to 88% of ovarian and 86% of primary peritoneal serous carcinomas, and PR staining in up to 60% and 56% of ovarian and peritoneal carcinomas, respectively [93]. As previously mentioned, PAX-8 is very helpful in this differential diagnosis, with negative staining in mesothelioma and frequent reactivity in serous carcinoma [76].

## Mesothelioma Versus Poorly Differentiated Squamous Carcinoma (Sqcc)

Fortunately, this differential is very rare. Poorly differentiated Sqcc may present with cellular spheres and large cells with abundant two-tone cytoplasm. It should always be con-

sidered when a fluid is suspected to be mesothelioma but staining is inconsistent, e.g., positive staining for both calretinin and carcinoma markers. In these cases, staining with WT-1 and p63 or p40 may be valuable. Sqcc expresses p63 in over 90% of cases and is characteristically WT-1-negative. For further discussion, please refer to Chap. 2 in this book.

## References

1. Ismail-Khan R, Robinson LA, Williams CC Jr, Garrett CR, Bepler G, Simon GR. Malignant pleural mesothelioma: a comprehensive review. Cancer Control. 2006;13(4):255–63.
2. Husain AN, Colby TV, Ordonez NG, et al. Guidelines for pathologic diagnosis of malignant mesothelioma: a consensus statement from the International Mesothelioma Interest Group. Arch Pathol Lab Med. Aug 2009;133(8):1317–31.
3. Hjerpe A, Ascoli V, Bedrossian CW, et al. Guidelines for the cytopathologic diagnosis of epithelioid and mixed-type malignant mesothelioma. Complementary statement from the International Mesothelioma Interest Group, also endorsed by the International Academy of Cytology and the Papanicolaou Society of Cytopathology. Acta Cytol. 2015;59(1):2–16.
4. Husain AN, Colby T, Ordonez N, et al. Guidelines for pathologic diagnosis of malignant mesothelioma: 2012 update of the consensus statement from the International Mesothelioma Interest Group. Arch Pathol Lab Med. 2013;137(5):647–67.
5. British Thoracic Society Standards of Care C. BTS statement on malignant mesothelioma in the UK, 2007. Thorax. 2007;62(Suppl 2):ii1–ii19.
6. van Zandwijk N, Clarke C, Henderson D, et al. Guidelines for the diagnosis and treatment of malignant pleural mesothelioma. J Thorac Dis. 2013;5(6):E254–307.
7. Bedrossian CW. Asbestos-related diseases: a historical and mineralogic perspective. Semin Diagn Pathol. 1992;9(2):91–6.
8. Roggli VL, McGavran MH, Subach J, Sybers HD, Greenberg SD. Pulmonary asbestos body counts and electron probe analysis of asbestos body cores in patients with mesothelioma: a study of 25 cases. Cancer. 1982;50(11):2423–32.
9. Mark EJ, Kradin RL. Pathological recognition of diffuse malignant mesothelioma of the pleura: the significance of the historical perspective as regards this signal tumor. Semin Diagn Pathol. 2006;23(1):25–34.
10. Dogan AU, Dogan M, Hoskins JA. Erionite series minerals: mineralogical and carcinogenic properties. Environ Geochem Health. 2008;30(4):367–81.
11. Boylan AM. Mesothelioma: new concepts in diagnosis and management. Curr Opin Pulm Med. 2000;6(2):157–63.
12. Corson JM. Pathology of diffuse malignant pleural mesothelioma. Semin Thorac Cardiovasc Surg. Oct 1997;9(4):347–55.
13. Chirieac LR, Corson JM. Pathologic evaluation of malignant pleural mesothelioma. Semin Thorac Cardiovasc Surg. 2009;21(2):121–4.
14. Alexander HR Jr. Surgical treatment of malignant peritoneal mesothelioma: past, present, and future. Ann Surg Oncol. 2010;17(1):21–2.
15. Kerrigan SA, Turnnir RT, Clement PB, Young RH, Churg A. Diffuse malignant epithelial mesotheliomas of the peritoneum in women: a clinicopathologic study of 25 patients. Cancer. 2002;94(2):378–85.
16. Hassan R, Remaley AT, Sampson ML, et al. Detection and quantitation of serum mesothelin, a tumor marker for patients with mesothelioma and ovarian cancer. Clin Cancer Res. 2006;12(2):447–53.
17. Antman KH, Osteen RT, Klegar KL, et al. Early peritoneal mesothelioma: a treatable malignancy. Lancet. 1985;2(8462):977–81.

18. Baratti D, Kusamura S, Cabras AD, Laterza B, Balestra MR, Deraco M. Lymph node metastases in diffuse malignant peritoneal mesothelioma. Ann Surg Oncol. 2010;17(1):45–53.

19. Henderson DW. Malignant mesothelioma. New York: Hemisphere Publishing Corporation; 1992.

20. Matsuo T, Ito H, Anami M, Ikeda T, Nishihata S. Malignant peritoneal mesothelioma with squamous metaplasia. Cytopathology. 1993;4(6):373–8.

21. Mayall FG, Gibbs AR. The histology and immunohistochemistry of small cell mesothelioma. Histopathology. 1992;20(1):47–51.

22. Ordonez NG. Mesothelioma with clear cell features: an ultrastructural and immunohistochemical study of 20 cases. Hum Pathol. 2005;36(5):465–73.

23. Chang HT, Yantiss RK, Nielsen GP, McKee GT, Mark EJ. Lipid-rich diffuse malignant mesothelioma: a case report. Hum Pathol. 2000;31(7):876–9.

24. Klebe S, Mahar A, Henderson DW, Roggli VL. Malignant mesothelioma with heterologous elements: clinicopathological correlation of 27 cases and literature review. Modern Pathol. 2008;21(9):1084–94.

25. Wilson GE, Hasleton PS, Chatterjee AK. Desmoplastic malignant mesothelioma: a review of 17 cases. J Clin Pathol. Apr 1992;45(4):295–8.

26. Ishikawa R, Kikuchi E, Jin M, et al. Desmoplastic malignant mesothelioma of the pleura: autopsy reveals asbestos exposure. Pathol Int. 2003;53(6):401–6.

27. Yao DX, Shia J, Erlandson RA, Klimstra DS. Lymphohistiocytoid mesothelioma: a clinical, immunohistochemical and ultrastructural study of four cases and literature review. Ultrastruct Pathol. 2004;28(4):213–28.

28. Henderson DW, Attwood HD, Constance TJ, Shilkin KB, Steele RH. Lymphohistiocytoid mesothelioma: a rare lymphomatoid variant of predominantly sarcomatoid mesothelioma. Ultrastruct Pathol. 1988;12(4):367–84.

29. Shia J, Erlandson RA, Klimstra DS. Deciduoid mesothelioma: a report of 5 cases and literature review. Ultrastruct Pathol. 2002;26(6):355–63.

30. Shanks JH, Harris M, Banerjee SS, et al. Mesotheliomas with deciduoid morphology: a morphologic spectrum and a variant not confined to young females. Am J Surg Pathol. 2000;24(2):285–94.

31. Ordonez NG. Epithelial mesothelioma with deciduoid features: report of four cases. Am J Surg Pathol. 2000;24(6):816–23.

32. Azzopardi JG. Oat-cell carcinoma of the bronchus. J Pathol Bacteriol. 1959;78:513–9.

33. Talerman A, Montero JR, Chilcote RR, Okagaki T. Diffuse malignant peritoneal mesothelioma in a 13-year-old girl. Report of a case and review of the literature. Am J Surg Pathol. 1985;9(1):73–80.

34. Henley JD, Loehrer PJ Sr, Ulbright TM. Deciduoid mesothelioma of the pleura after radiation therapy for Hodgkin's disease presenting as a mediastinal mass. Am J Surg Pathol. 2001;25(4):547–8.

35. Serio G, Scattone A, Pennella A, et al. Malignant deciduoid mesothelioma of the pleura: report of two cases with long survival. Histopathology. 2002;40(4):348–52.

36. Paintal A. The evolving role of effusion cytology in the diagnosis of malignant mesothelioma. Cytopathology. 2015;26(3):137–8.

37. Renshaw AA, Dean BR, Antman KH, Sugarbaker DJ, Cibas ES. The role of cytologic evaluation of pleural fluid in the diagnosis of malignant mesothelioma. Chest. 1997;111(1):106–9.

38. Nguyen GK. Cytopathology of pleural mesotheliomas. Am J Clin Pathol. 2000;114(Suppl):S68–81.

39. Fetsch PA, Abati A. Immunocytochemistry in effusion cytology: a contemporary review. Cancer. 2001;93(5):293–308.

40. Westfall DE, Fan X, Marchevsky AM. Evidence-based guidelines to optimize the selection of antibody panels in cytopathology: pleural effusions with malignant epithelioid cells. Diagn Cytopathol. 2010;38(1):9–14.

41. Rakha EA, Patil S, Abdulla K, Abdulkader M, Chaudry Z, Soomro IN. The sensitivity of cytologic evaluation of pleural fluid in the diagnosis of malignant mesothelioma. Diagn Cytopathol. 2010;38(12):874–9.

42. Tao LC. The cytopathology of mesothelioma. Acta Cytol. 1979;23(3):209–13.

43. Hasegawa S, Kondo N, Matsumoto S, et al. Practical approaches to diagnose and treat for T0 malignant pleural mesothelioma: a proposal for diagnostic total parietal pleurectomy. Int J Clin Oncol. 2012;17(1):33–9.

44. Bedrossian CWM. The cytologic diagnosis of malignant mesothelioma. In: Michael CW, Bedrossian CWM, editors. Cytohistology of small tissue samples. Cambridge, UK Kingdom: Cambridge University Press; 2015.

45. Papanicolaou G. Atlas of exfoliative cytology. Cambridge, MA: harvard University Press; 1956.

46. Naylor B. The exfoliative cytology of diffuse malignant mesothelioma. J Pathol Bacteriol. 1963;86:293–8.

47. Roberts GH, Campbell GM. Exfoliative cytology of diffuse mesothelioma. J Clin Pathol. 1972;25(7):577–82.

48. Whitaker D, Shilkin KB. The cytology of malignant mesothelioma in Western Australia. Acta Cytol. 1978;22(2):67–70.

49. Ehya H. The cytologic diagnosis of mesothelioma. Semin Diagn Pathol. 1986;3(3):196–203.

50. Bedrossian CW, Bonsib S, Moran C. Differential diagnosis between mesothelioma and adenocarcinoma: a multimodal approach based on ultrastructure and immunocytochemistry. Semin Diagn Pathol. 1992;9(2):124–40.

51. Kho-Duffin J, Tao LC, Cramer H, Catellier MJ, Irons D, Ng P. Cytologic diagnosis of malignant mesothelioma, with particular emphasis on the epithelial noncohesive cell type. Diagn Cytopathol. 1999;20(2):57–62.

52. Patel NP, Taylor CA, Levine EA, Trupiano JK, Geisinger KR. Cytomorphologic features of primary peritoneal mesothelioma in effusion, washing, and fine-needle aspiration biopsy specimens: examination of 49 cases at one institution, including post-intraperitoneal hyperthermic chemotherapy findings. Am J Clin Pathol. 2007;128(3):414–22.

53. Whitaker D. Cell aggregates in malignant mesothelioma. Acta Cytol. 1977;21(2):236–9.

54. Gillespie FR, van der Walt JD, Derias N, Kenney A. Deciduoid peritoneal mesothelioma. A report of the cytological appearances. Cytopathology. 2001;12(1):57–61.

55. Huang CC, Michael CW. Deciduoid mesothelioma: cytologic presentation and diagnostic pitfalls. Diagn Cytopathol. 2013;41(7):629–35.

56. Ustun H, Astarci HM, Sungu N, Ozdemir A, Ekinci C. Primary malignant deciduoid peritoneal mesothelioma: a report of the cytohistological and immunohistochemical appearances. Diagn Cytopathol. 2011;39(6):402–8.

57. Reis-Filho JS, Pope LZ, Milanezi F, Balderrama CM, Serapiao MJ, Schmitt FC. Primary epithelial malignant mesothelioma of the pericardium with deciduoid features: cytohistologic and immunohistochemical study. Diagn Cytopathol. 2002;26(2):117–22.

58. Ikeda K, Suzuki T, Tate G, Mitsuya T. Cytomorphologic features of well-differentiated papillary mesothelioma in peritoneal effusion: a case report. Diagn Cytopathol. 2008;36(7):512–5.

59. Hejmadi R, Ganesan R, Kamal NG. Malignant transformation of a well-differentiated peritoneal papillary mesothelioma. Acta Cytol. 2003;47(3):517–8.

60. Cook DS, Attanoos RL, Jalloh SS, Gibbs AR. 'Mucin-positive' epithelial mesothelioma of the peritoneum: an unusual diagnostic pitfall. Histopathology. 2000;37(1):33–6.

61. Triol JH, Conston AS, Chandler SV. Malignant mesothelioma. Cytopathology of 75 cases seen in a New Jersey community hospital. Acta Cytol. 1984;28(1):37–45.

62. Whitaker D, Shilkin KB. Diagnosis of pleural malignant mesothelioma in life—a practical approach. J Pathol. 1984;143(3):147–75.

63. Welker L, Muller M, Holz O, Vollmer E, Magnussen H, Jorres RA. Cytological diagnosis of malignant mesothelioma—improvement by additional analysis of hyaluronic acid in pleural effusions. Virch Arch. 2007;450(4):455–61.

64. Ordonez NG. Application of immunohistochemistry in the diagnosis of epithelioid mesothelioma: a review and update. Hum Pathol. 2013;44(1):1–19.

65. Beasley MB. Immunohistochemistry of pulmonary and pleural neoplasia. Arch Pathol Lab Med. 2008;132(7):1062–72.

66. Ordonez NG. What are the current best immunohistochemical markers for the diagnosis of epithelioid mesothelioma? A review and update. Hum Pathol. 2007;38(1):1–16.

67. Pu RT, Pang Y, Michael CW. Utility of WT-1, p63, MOC31, mesothelin, and cytokeratin (K903 and CK5/6) immunostains in differentiating adenocarcinoma, squamous cell carcinoma, and malignant mesothelioma in effusions. Diagn Cytopathol. 2008;36(1):20–5.

68. Hanna A, Pang Y, Bedrossian CW, Dejmek A, Michael CW. Podoplanin is a useful marker for identifying mesothelioma in malignant effusions. Diagn Cytopathol. 2010;38(4):264–9.

69. Saad RS, Cho P, Liu YL, Silverman JF. The value of epithelial membrane antigen expression in separating benign mesothelial proliferation from malignant mesothelioma: a comparative study. Diagn Cytopathol. 2005;32(3):156–9.

70. Bassarova AV, Nesland JM, Davidson B. D2-40 is not a specific marker for cells of mesothelial origin in serous effusions. Am J Surg Pathol. 2006;30(7):878–82.

71. Ascoli V, Scalzo CC, Taccogna S, Nardi F. The diagnostic value of thrombomodulin immunolocalization in serous effusions. Arch Pathol Lab Med. 1995;119(12):1136–40.

72. Fetsch PA, Abati A, Hijazi YM. Utility of the antibodies CA 19-9, HBME-1, and thrombomodulin in the diagnosis of malignant mesothelioma and adenocarcinoma in cytology. Cancer. 1998;84(2):101–8.

73. Mimura T, Ito A, Sakuma T, et al. Novel marker D2-40, combined with calretinin, CEA, and TTF-1: an optimal set of immunodiagnostic markers for pleural mesothelioma. Cancer. 2007;109(5):933–8.

74. Lozano MD, Panizo A, Toledo GR, Sola JJ, Pardo-Mindan J. Immunocytochemistry in the differential diagnosis of serous effusions: a comparative evaluation of eight monoclonal antibodies in Papanicolaou stained smears. Cancer. 2001;93(1):68–72.

75. Jo VY, Cibas ES, Pinkus GS. Claudin-4 immunohistochemistry is highly effective in distinguishing adenocarcinoma from malignant mesothelioma in effusion cytology. Cancer Cytopathol. 2014;122(4):299–306.

76. Wiseman W, Michael CW, Roh MH. Diagnostic utility of PAX8 and PAX2 immunohistochemistry in the identification of metastatic Mullerian carcinoma in effusions. Diagn Cytopathol. 2011;39(9):651–6.

77. Davidson B, Stavnes HT, Hellesylt E, et al. MMP-7 is a highly specific negative marker for benign and malignant mesothelial cells in serous effusions. Hum Pathol. 2016;47(1):104–8.

78. Sack MJ, Roberts SA. Cytokeratins 20 and 7 in the differential diagnosis of metastatic carcinoma in cytologic specimens. Diagn Cytopathol. 1997;16(2):132–6.

79. Ordonez NG. The diagnostic utility of immunohistochemistry in distinguishing between epithelioid mesotheliomas and squamous carcinomas of the lung: a comparative study. Modern Pathol. 2006;19(3):417–28.

80. Hwang HC, Sheffield BS, Rodriguez S, et al. Utility of BAP1 immunohistochemistry and p16 (CDKN2A) FISH in the diagnosis of malignant mesothelioma in effusion cytology specimens. Am J Surg Pathol. 2016;40(1):120–6.

81. Cigognetti M, Lonardi S, Fisogni S, et al. BAP1 (BRCA1-associated protein 1) is a highly specific marker for differentiating mesothelioma from reactive mesothelial proliferations. Modern Pathol. 2015;28(8):1043–57.

82. Andrici J, Sheen A, Sioson L, et al. Loss of expression of BAP1 is a useful adjunct, which strongly supports the diagnosis of mesothelioma in effusion cytology. Modern Pathol. 2015;28(10):1360–8.

83. Hasteh F, Lin GY, Weidner N, Michael CW. The use of immunohistochemistry to distinguish reactive mesothelial cells from malignant mesothelioma in cytologic effusions. Cancer Cytopathol. 2010;118(2):90–6.

84. Sivertsen S, Berner A, Michael CW, Bedrossian C, Davidson B. Cadherin expression in ovarian carcinoma and malignant mesothelioma cell effusions. Acta Cytol. 2006;50(6):603–7.

85. Simsir A, Fetsch P, Mehta D, Zakowski M, Abati A. E-cadherin, N-cadherin, and calretinin in pleural effusions: the good, the bad, the worthless. Diagn Cytopathol. 1999;20(3):125–30.

86. Mutsaers SE. The mesothelial cell. Int J Biochem Cell Biology. 2004;36(1):9–16.

87. Chen L, Caldero SG, Gmitro S, Smith ML, De Petris G, Zarka MA. Small orangiophilic squamous-like cells: an underrecognized and useful morphological feature for the diagnosis of malignant mesothelioma in pleural effusion cytology. Cancer Cytopathol. 2014;122(1):70–5.

88. Gao L, Reeves W, Demay RM. Parakeratotic-like cells in effusions—a clue to diagnosis of malignant mesothelioma. Cytojournal. 2012;9:18.

89. Kimura N, Dota K, Araya Y, Ishidate T, Ishizaka M. Scoring system for differential diagnosis of malignant mesothelioma and reactive mesothelial cells on cytology specimens. Diagn Cytopathol. 2009;37(12):885–90.

90. Cakir E, Demirag F, Aydin M, Unsal E. Cytopathologic differential diagnosis of malignant mesothelioma, adenocarcinoma and reactive mesothelial cells: a logistic regression analysis. Diagn Cytopathol. 2009;37(1):4–10.

91. Ordonez NG. Value of immunohistochemistry in distinguishing peritoneal mesothelioma from serous carcinoma of the ovary and peritoneum: a review and update. Adv Anat Pathol. 2006;13(1):16–25.

92. Davidson B, Risberg B, Kristensen G, et al. Detection of cancer cells in effusions from patients diagnosed with gynaecological malignancies. Evaluation of five epithelial markers. Virch Arch. 1999;435(1):43–9.

93. Ordonez NG. Value of estrogen and progesterone receptor immunostaining in distinguishing between peritoneal mesotheliomas and serous carcinomas. Hum Pathol. 2005;36(11):1163–7.

# Hematologic and Lymphoid Neoplasia

**6**

Anne Tierens and William Geddie

## Introduction

Serous effusions occur in lymphomas, in about 20–30% of cases, and are less frequently seen with myeloid malignancy [1, 2]. In children, effusions are more commonly associated with lymphoma and leukemia than with other malignancies [3]. Most effusions are secondary and are caused by direct infiltration with leukemia or lymphoma from adjacent disease infiltrates, by obstruction of the lymphatic system draining the body cavity, or by infection secondary to immune depression due to extensive marrow involvement or treatment of lymphoma or leukemia. In addition, effusions may also be caused by inflammation following direct damage by radiation, chemotherapy, and tyrosine kinase inhibitors such as dasatinib or by graft versus host disease in the case of bone marrow transplantation for the malignancy [4–6]. In this section, only serous effusions due to direct lymphoma or leukemia infiltration of a body cavity will be discussed.

Primary involvement of serous cavities by lymphoma is rare, and only three disease entities are recognized by the WHO classification of lymphoid neoplasm: primary effusion lymphoma (PEL), diffuse large B-cell lymphoma (DLBCL) associated with chronic inflammation (DLBCL-CI), and breast implant-associated anaplastic large-cell lymphoma (BI-ALCL) which is a new provisional entity in the 2016 revised WHO classification [7, 8]. In addition, effusion-based HHV8-negative large-cell lymphoma (HHV8-EBL) associated with fluid overload conditions likely represent a distinct disease entity [9]. Other lymphomas such as extranodal marginal zone lymphoma, nasal-type NK/T-cell lymphoma, and adult T-cell lymphoma/leukemia may occasionally manifest in body cavities [10–13].

Secondary infiltration of body cavities with lymphoma is more common than primary lymphoma involvement and can virtually be seen with any lymphoma type [1, 2]. Secondary infiltration of body cavities with leukemia is also seen but is less common than other causes of effusions in those diseases such as those associated with infections or therapy.

## Lymphoma and Leukemia Diagnosis in Effusions

The diagnosis of lymphoma and leukemia in effusions involves primary cytomorphological examination combined with immunophenotypical examination. Serous fluid samples may be sent to both cytology and hematopathology laboratories for examination, and coordination is required to ensure that appropriate preparations are made for morphologic examination and available sample is aliquoted for necessary ancillary investigations. Samples sent to cytology laboratories are often examined by alcoholic fixation and Papanicolaou staining alone, which is suboptimal for examination of lymphoid or myeloid populations. A history or clinical suspicion of lymphoma should trigger the cytology laboratory to make air-dried and Romanowsky-stained preparations for review, and a cell block should also be prepared to allow immunohistochemical stains and in situ hybridization for Epstein-Barr virus (EBV)-encoded small RNA (EBER) to be performed.

Flow cytometry is an especially helpful technique for establishing a final diagnosis [14, 15]. In those cases, where the effusion is the primary localization and the first sample taken for diagnostic purposes, the diagnosis can be supplemented by fluorescent in situ hybridization (FISH) and/or polymerase chain reaction (PCR) analysis for demonstration of immunoglobulin heavy chain (IGH) or T-cell receptor (TCR) rearrangements [16–18]. Analysis of antigen receptor gene rearrangements is most useful in cases suspi-

A. Tierens (✉)
Laboratory Medicine Program, Hematopathology, University Health Network, Toronto, Canada
e-mail: anne.tierens@uhn.ca

W. Geddie
Laboratory Medicine Program, Cytopathology, University Health Network, Toronto, Canada

© Springer International Publishing AG, part of Springer Nature 2018
B. Davidson et al. (eds.), *Serous Effusions*, https://doi.org/10.1007/978-3-319-76478-8_6

cious for lymphomatous involvement in which restricted expression of immunoglobulin light chains or an abnormal immunophenotype cannot be detected [19]. The results of these analyses should always be integrated with the other examinations and the clinical history since both false-positive and false-negative results may occur. Clonal rearrangements, especially of TCR genes, can be seen in inflammatory conditions. Therefore, a positive or negative result can never be used as the only argument in favor or against a lymphoma diagnosis [19]. In addition, examination of a histological specimen, if feasible, is recommended when the effusion is likely a secondary disease infiltrate and the lymphoma has not yet previously been diagnosed. Histological examination allows for the integration of cyto-morphology, immunophenotype, and architecture of the lesion, all of which are often necessary for precise classification of the disease. Grading of follicular lymphomas, typing of T-cell lymphoma with a mature immunophenotype, and resolution of difficult differential diagnoses such as primary mediastinal large B-cell lymphoma versus Hodgkin's lymphoma may not be possible without histologic examination. Some series have reported an excellent correlation between cytological examination and histological examination with regard to correct lymphoma typing but were either too small for statistical relevance, did not include all lymphoma types, or did not report a correlation with regard to lymphoma diagnosis according to the current WHO classification [20–22].

## Primary Lymphomas of Body Cavities

### Primary Effusion Lymphoma

Primary effusion lymphoma is a rare large B-cell lymphoma presenting as serous effusions only, affecting the pleural and less frequently the peritoneal and pericardial cavities, and is usually restricted to one cavity [23–27]. Not all PELs present as effusions. Although rare, extra-cavitary variants also called EC-PEL may involve lymph nodes and extranodal sites such as the gastrointestinal tract, lung, skin, and CNS [28, 29]. In addition, cases occurring in peripheral blood, CSF, and the space surrounding breast implants have been reported [30, 31].

PEL belongs to the wide spectrum of Kaposi sarcoma herpesvirus (KSHV)/human herpesvirus 8 (HHV8)-positive lymphoproliferative disorders which also encompass multi-centric Castleman disease (MCD), HHV8-positive DLBCL, not otherwise specified (HHV8+, DLBCL, NOS), and germi-notropic lymphoproliferative disorder (GLPD) [30]. Coinfection with Epstein-Barr virus is often found, especially in HIV-positive patients. PEL tends to arise in severely immune-compromised HIV-positive patients, but it may also affect elderly individuals or patients that are immunocompromised due to organ transplantation [31–33].

Cytocentrifuge or direct smear preparation of the effusion fluid reveals large cells with features of immunoblasts, plasmablasts, and infrequent anaplastic cells resembling Hodgkin cells. The variably dark basophilic cytoplasm and the presence of a perinuclear hof suggest plasma cell differentiation (Fig. 6.1a, b).

The lymphoma cells are positive for CD45 but do not express pan-B-cell antigens such as CD19, CD20, CD79a, or PAX5. Instead, they are positive for plasma cell differentiation antigens CD138, multiple myeloma oncogene 1 (MUM1)/interferon regulatory factor 4 (IRF4), BLIMP1 also known as PR domain zinc finger protein 1 (*PRDM1*), and the activation markers CD38, CD30, and HLA-DR antigens (Fig. 6.2) [34]. Aberrant expression of T-cell antigens is detected in rare cases [30, 36]. The lymphoma invariably stains for the KSHV latency-associated nuclear antigen (LANA-1 or ORF 73) and also EBV by in situ hybridization for EBER in about 75% of AIDS patients (Fig. 6.1c) [34, 35]. Molecular analysis of the immunoglobulin heavy chain gene reveals clonal rearrangements and somatic hypermutations in the majority of cases [37]. The immunophenotypic and genetic features including a gene expression profile sharing features of germinal center B-cells as well as of plasma cells indicate that PEL is derived from terminally differentiated B-cells [38, 39].

Although few recurrent structural aberrancies have been reported, conventional cytogenetic analysis has revealed complex karyotypes [40]. Differential diagnoses include lymphomas with morphologic features similar to PEL including effusion-based HHV8-DLBCL, Burkitt's lymphoma with plasmacytoid differentiation, plasmablastic lymphoma, and anaplastic large-cell lymphoma. The absence of the HHV8 antigen and differences in the antigenic profiles readily distinguish the latter lymphomas from PEL.

Little is known about the pathogenesis of PEL. Although many of the KSHV-associated proteins are oncogenic, their expression in KSHV-infected *in-vitro* cell lines is not sufficient for malignant transformation [34]. Likewise, the contribution of coinfection with EBV in the development of PEL is not known either. Recently, it was reported that the hepatocyte growth factor (HGF)/c-MET pathway is highly activated by KSHV in PEL cell lines and in patients infected with KSHV as shown by the high levels of HGF [41]. The molecular mechanism, however, underlying the activation of this pathway, is not known since no single nucleotide variants in the c-MET genomic regions are demonstrated [42]. HGF is the only known ligand for the *Met* proto-oncogene which encodes a receptor tyrosine kinase, also known as c-MET. The HGF/c-Met pathway induces myriad biological responses including increased cell proliferation and survival,

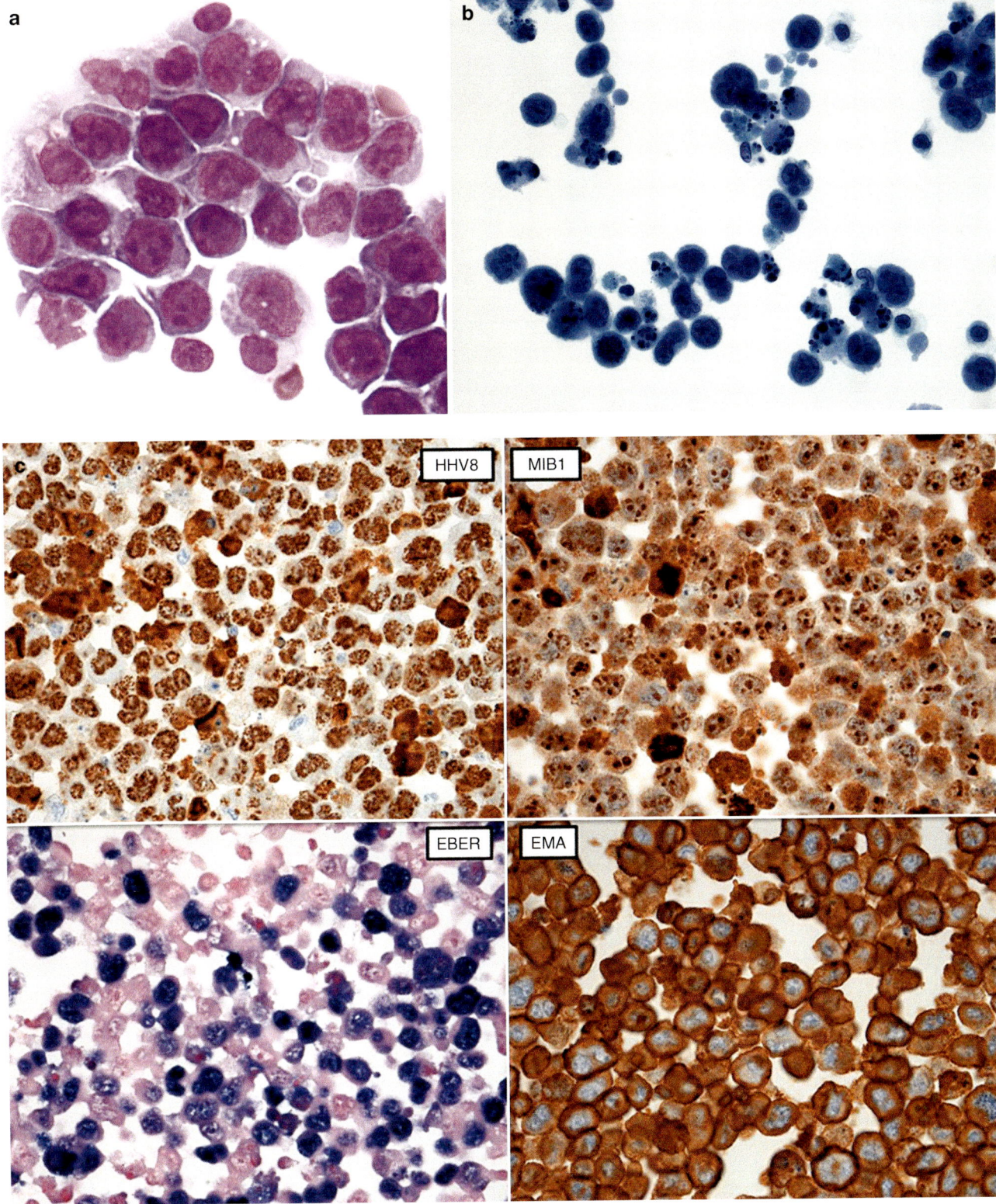

**Fig. 6.1** Cytology of primary effusion lymphoma (PEL). (**a**) May Grunwald Giemsa (MGG) staining, 60× objective. The lymphoma cells exhibit the morphology of large immunoblasts or plasmablasts. They have large round to irregular nuclei with prominent nucleoli and abundant, often dark blue cytoplasm. (**b**) ThinPrep, Papanicolaou stain, 63× objective. In Papanicolaou-stained preparations nuclear pleomorphism, mitoses and apoptosis are easily seen, but chromatin texture and cytoplasmic basophilia are not as apparent. (**c**) Cell block immunohistochemistry, 40× objective. Immunohistochemical stains required for subtyping can be performed on cell block paraffin sections provided validated fixation protocols are adhered. Composite photograph showing HHV8, MIB-1, EBER, and EMA

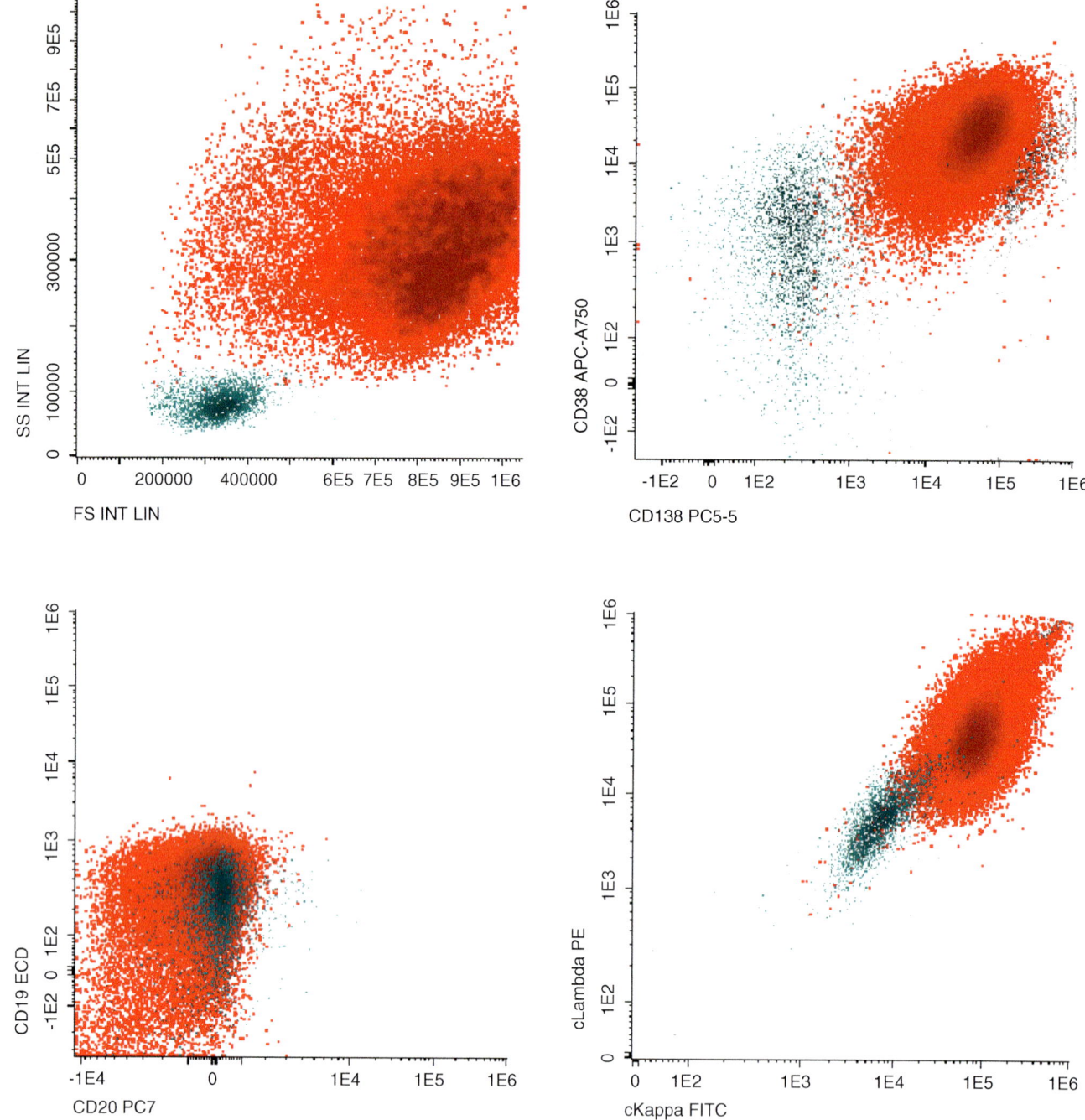

**Fig. 6.2** Immunophenotypic characteristics of PEL. Bivariate dot plots of the typical immunophenotype of PEL. The lymphoma cells are shown as red dots, whereas residual small lymphocytes are represented as green dots. The lymphoma cells exhibit a high forward and side scat- ter and are positive for the plasma cell-related and activation antigens CD138 and CD38. In contrast, they are negative for B-cell antigens CD19, CD20, and immunoglobulin light chains

migration, metastasis, and angiogenesis. Molecules integral to the HGF/c-MET pathway may be potential novel targets in cancer treatment. Indeed, a selective c-Met inhibitor induced apoptosis of the PEL through cell cycle arrest and DNA damage and reduced tumor progression in xenograft models [41]. The ribonucleoside-diphosphate reductase sub-unit-2 (RRM2) controlled by c-Met was also significantly downregulated and may be therefore another potential thera-peutic target.

PEL is an aggressive disease, with a median survival of less than 6 months using conventional chemotherapy regi-mens [43]. Clinical trials are urgently needed to confirm the antitumor effects of the small molecules targeting RRM2 and c-Met in PEL [42].

## Diffuse Large B-Cell Lymphoma Associated with Chronic Inflammation

The best characterized diffuse large B-cell lymphoma associated with chronic inflammation is pyothorax-associated lymphoma (PAL) occurring in patients with long-standing pyothorax resulting from artificial pneumothorax for the treatment of pulmonary or pleural tuberculosis. It was first described in Japan in 1987 where more than 200 PAL have been documented [44]. Rare cases of PAL have also been described in other Asian countries and in the West [45–47]. The interval between the onset of chronic inflammation and presentation of PAL usually exceeds 20 years, with a median clinical history of 37 years. The median age of presentation is 70 years. PAL is far more common in men than women. PAL shows a strong association with EBV with positivity for EBER and the strong diffuse expression of EBV nuclear antigen (EBNA-2) and/or late membrane protein-1 (LMP-1) in the majority of cases [48]. The chronic inflammation likely exposes the EBV-transformed B-cells to oxidative stress signals impairing DNA damage responses and enables them to escape immune surveillance through cytokines such as IL-6 providing autocrine growth signals and IL-10 mediating immune suppression [49].

PAL presents as a large pleural tumor mass comprised of large cells with centroblastic or immunoblastic morphology and prominent single or multiple nucleoli. Areas of necrosis and an angiocentric growth pattern are frequently present [45, 46]. The lymphoma cells are typically positive for B-cell antigens CD19, CD20, and CD79a and often also express MUM1/IRF4 and are infrequently positive for CD138 [45]. Monotypic expression of immunoglobulin light chain expression can be detected in a subset. Occasionally, expression of one or more T-cell antigens is detected together with the expression of CD20 and CD79a [46]. BCL-6 and CD10 are negative, indicating derivation from post-germinal center B-cells. The gene expression profile of PAL differs from nodal DLBCL [45, 49]. The most differentially expressed genes involve interferon-inducible (IFI) protein 27 that is induced in B-cells stimulated by interferon-α and HLA class I molecules that are downregulated. PAL is further characterized by a high frequency of *TP53* mutations and *MYC* amplifications explaining its aggressive behavior and a 5-year overall survival of 20–35% [45, 50]. With the discontinuation of artificial pneumothorax, PAL has become rare, but other DLBCL-CI associated with chronic osteomyelitis, metallic implants, and chronic skin ulcers have been described.

The recently reported fibrin-associated EBV-positive B-cell lymphoma has also been included in this category in the WHO classification. The fibrin-associated EBV-positive B-cell lymphomas present as small lesions in pseudocysts, chronic epidural hematomas, or hematomas associated with prior vascular surgery, prosthetic cardiac valves, and atrial myxomas [51]. Despite similarities with PAL and DLBCL-CI, fibrin-associated EBV-positive B-cell lymphomas have distinct pathologic and clinical features. In contrast to DLBCL-CI, clusters or sheets of large B-cells are identified in a background of fibrin with variable signs of chronic inflammation, the latter more prominent in pseudocysts and chronic hematomas. Furthermore, they show low expression of *MYC* and *TP53* unlike DLBCL-CI. Also the absence of a long history of chronic inflammation and the indolent course of these lymphoproliferations, especially the cases occurring in pseudocysts which are often cured by surgery only, distinguish fibrin-associated EBV-positive B-cell lymphomas from DLBLC-CI.

## Breast Implant-Associated Anaplastic Large-Cell Lymphoma (Figures 6.3 and 6.4)

Breast implant-associated anaplastic large-cell lymphoma is a rare T-cell lymphoma occurring in women with breast implants [52, 53]. It most commonly presents as a peri-implant seroma fluid confined within a fibrous capsule and more seldom as a breast tumor with or without involvement of adjacent lymph nodes [54–56]. According to the Ann Arbor lymphoma staging system, 83–84% of patients with BI-ALCL present with stage1E, 10–16% of patients with stage IIE, and 1–7% patients with stage IV [57, 58]. A tumor (T), lymph node (N), and metastasis (M) staging system for BI-ALCL was proposed by MD Anderson (MDA) [58]. In the MDA TNM staging system, stage I disease was divided in three subgroups IA, IB, and IC which are, respectively, characterized by effusion only, early capsule invasion, and a mass confined to capsule. Locally infiltrative disease without involvement of adjacent lymph nodes or localized disease with involvement by one lymph node is classified as stage IIA and IIB, respectively. Advanced local disease with one or more affected lymph nodes and metastasized diseases are grouped as stage III and stage IV, respectively.

The median age ranges from 52 to 61 years, and the median time interval between the breast implant to the diagnosis of BI-ALCL is 8–9 years [54–56]. Although the odds ratio for BI-ALCL is increased in patients with breast implants, especially in those with textured implants, the risk remains very low (0.1–0.3 per 100,000 women with prostheses) [56, 59]. A chronic inflammatory and/or immunologic response is suggested to contribute to the pathogenesis of BI-ALCL, in keeping with its origin from activated cytotoxic T-cells. Recently, mutations in the Janus kinase (*JAK*)/signal transducer and activator or transcription (*STAT*) signaling pathway genes such as gain-of-function mutations in *JAK1* and *STAT3* and loss of function mutations in suppressor of cytokine signaling 1 (*SOCS1*) have been detected in two of five BI-ALCL cases using whole exome sequencing [60, 61]. Similarly, *STAT3* activation due to *STAT3* mutations or translocations involving dual specificity 22 (*DUSP22*) locus has been reported in 18% of ALK-negative ALCL and 5% of cutaneous ALCL [62]. Taken together, constitutive activation of *JAK/STAT* signaling may contribute to the development of a subset of BI-ALCL and systemic ALK-negative and cutaneous ALCL. Whereas *SOCS1* and *STAT3* may be co-mutated in the same tumor, only one case of BI-ALCL harbored a nonsense mutation in *DNTM3A* [60]. *DNTM3A* is a DNA methyltransferase required for genome-wide de novo methylation. *DNTM3A* mutations impairing its catalytic activity are frequent in myeloid neoplasms and early T-cell precursor acute lymphoblastic leukemia but have also been detected in 33% of peripheral T-cell lymphomas [63].

An aspiration of peri-prosthetic fluid collections should be submitted with appropriate history for cytologic and immunophenotypic examination. A discrete mass amenable to core or excisional biopsy is rarely present, and examination of tissue frequently requires removal of the implant with surrounding fibrous tissue capsule. Because these cases require special procedures, direct contact with the responsible pathologist is advisable.

The lymphoma cells are large and pleomorphic and have abundant cytoplasm and irregular nuclear contours with dispersed chromatin and occasional prominent nucleoli (Fig. 6.3). Occasionally, hallmark cells with horseshoe or kidney-shaped nuclei may be detected in the effusion confined to the capsule. However, they are more frequent in the infiltrative variant. The cells typically express CD30, are variably positive for T-cell antigens, of which CD4 is most frequently positive, and are negative for anaplastic lymphoma kinase (ALK) [54–56]. Bright expression of CD25 and HLA-DR, as well as weak expres-

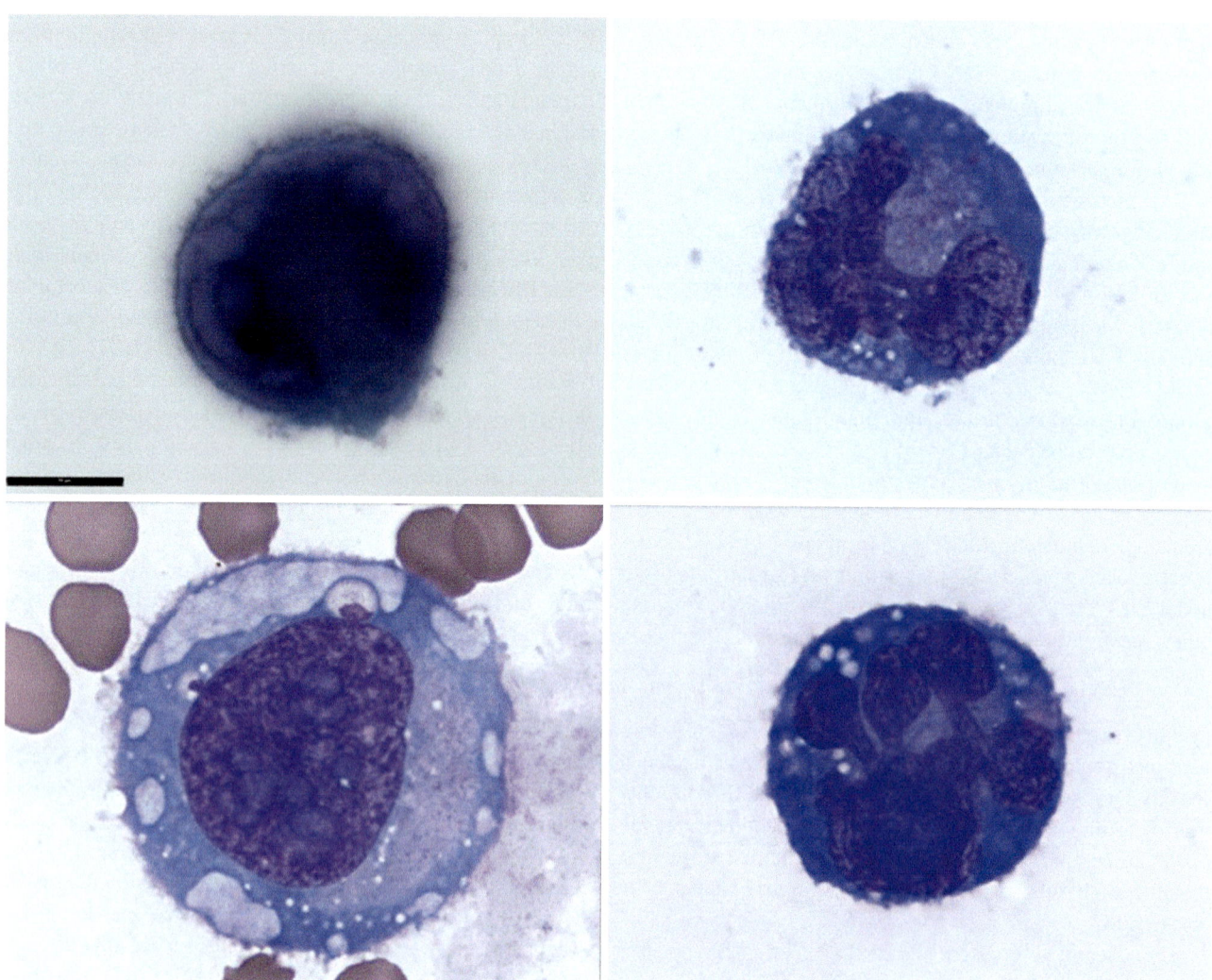

**Fig. 6.3** Late seroma adjacent to breast implant: Upper left: ThinPrep, Papanicolaou stain (size bar 40 μm)—hallmark cell with horseshoe-shaped nucleus. The thickness of cells fixed in an alcoholic solution makes it difficult to resolve detail. Upper right and bottom panel: Cytospin slide, MGG stain—The cells of anaplastic large-cell lymphoma display great pleomorphism

sion of CD95 and CD40, may further characterize the lymphoma cells (Fig. 6.4) [64, 65]. Staining by immunohistochemistry may reveal positivity for epithelial membrane antigen and nuclear expression of pSTAT3 [56]. Clonal rearrangement of T-cell receptor (TCR) γ chain gene is demonstrated in the majority of cases [56, 66]. In 50% of cases, the TCR β chain is clonally rearranged [56]. Differential diagnoses include poorly differentiated carcinoma, systemic ALK-negative or locally invasive cutaneous ALCL, and classical Hodgkin lymphoma. Once a diagnosis of ALCL is confirmed, integration of all pathology findings with clinical history and imaging results confirms the diagnosis of BI-ALCL.

BI-ALCL is an indolent disease with overall survival at 3 and 5 years of 94% and 91%, respectively [67]. Surgery alone is sufficient to cure most of the patients with BI-ALCL confined to the capsule [56, 58]. However, locally invasive BI-ALCL and lymph node involvement requires additional chemotherapy in addition to the surgical excision of the lesion [56, 58].

## Effusion-Based HHV8-Negative Diffuse Large B-Cell Lymphoma

Effusion-based HHV8-negative large-cell lymphoma (EBL) arises in elderly patients with underlying conditions leading to fluid overload including cirrhosis which is often associated with hepatitis C infection, cardiac problems, or protein-losing enteropathy [9, 68]. These patients are not immunosuppressed and are usually not HIV-positive. Pleural effusions are the most common and, in contrast to PEL, may present bilaterally. The neoplastic cells may be immunoblastic, plasmablastic, or pleomorphic, similar to PEL, but they are defined by pan-B-cell antigen and cytoplasmic immunoglobulin expression in keeping with the clonal immunoglobulin heavy chain rearrangements documented in most cases. Rare cases may be of T-cell lineage. EBV is detected in about one third of the patients. Often, HHV8-negative EBL carries a complex karyotype.

The pathogenesis is not known, but the coinfection with HCV, identified in one third of the patients with

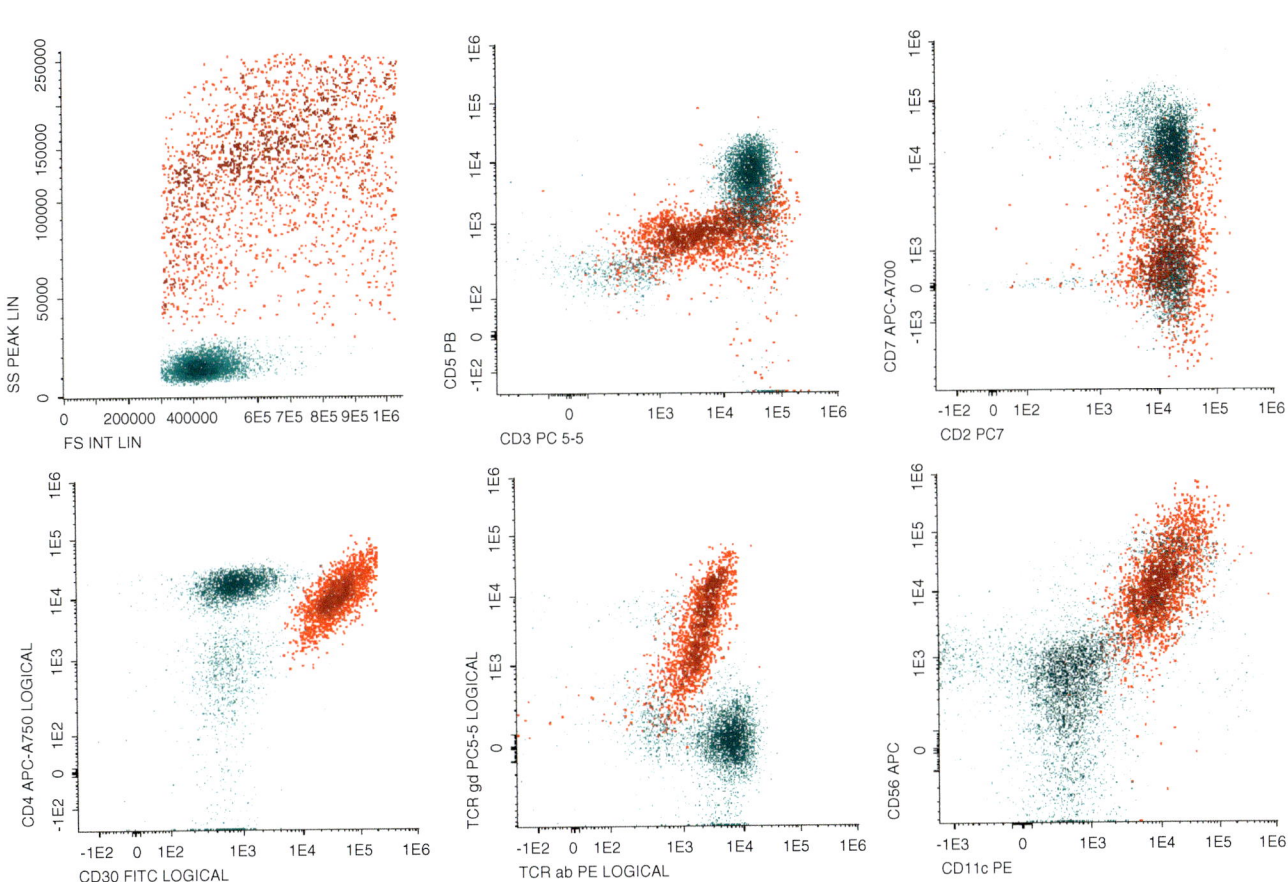

**Fig. 6.4** Flow cytometry findings in breast implant-associated anaplastic large cell lymphoma. Bivariate dot plots of the light scatter features and antigen profile of BI-ALCL. The anaplastic lymphoma cells are shown in red dots, whereas residual lymphocytes are represented as green dots. The lymphoma cells typically show heterogeneous light scatter signals consistent with their pleomorphism. They are positive for CD2, CD4, and CD30 and negative for CD5. They exhibit bimodal expression of CD3 and CD7. Expression of CD56 and CD11c is demonstrated

HHV8-negative EBL, may suggest a causative role of HCV in triggering a B-cell proliferation. It is also postulated that long-standing pre-existing effusions with chronic serosal stimulation may predispose to lymphoma [9].

HHV8-EBL appears to have a more favorable prognosis than PEL with complete or partial remission of 70% and 82% with aspiration only or chemotherapy [9].

## Secondary Lymphoma Infiltration in Body Cavities

Effusions are a common complication of Hodgkin as well as non-Hodgkin lymphomas (Figs. 6.5 and 6.7). Pleural effusions are the most common and have been reported with variable frequency between 6.7% and 48% of all cases, depending on the publication series [1, 2]. Ascites and peri-

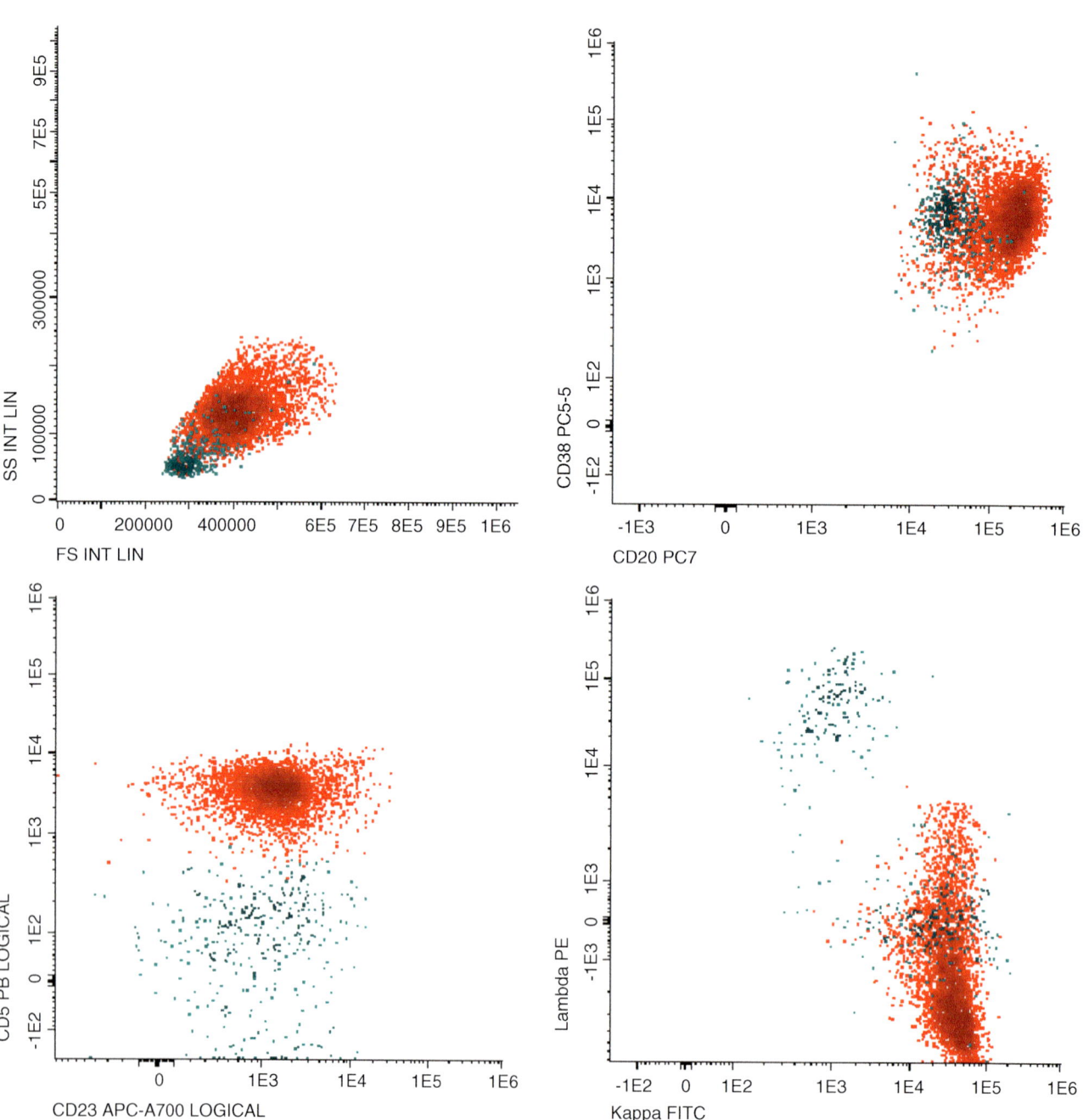

**Fig. 6.5** Pleural fluid with secondary infiltration by mantle cell lymphoma. Bivariate dot plots of the immunophenotypic features of mantle cell lymphoma. Mantle cell lymphoma cells are represented as red dots and poly-typic B-cells as green dots. The mantle cell lymphoma cells are monotypic for immunoglobulin light chain kappa and show bright expression of CD20 and CD38 and are positive for CD5 but negative for CD23

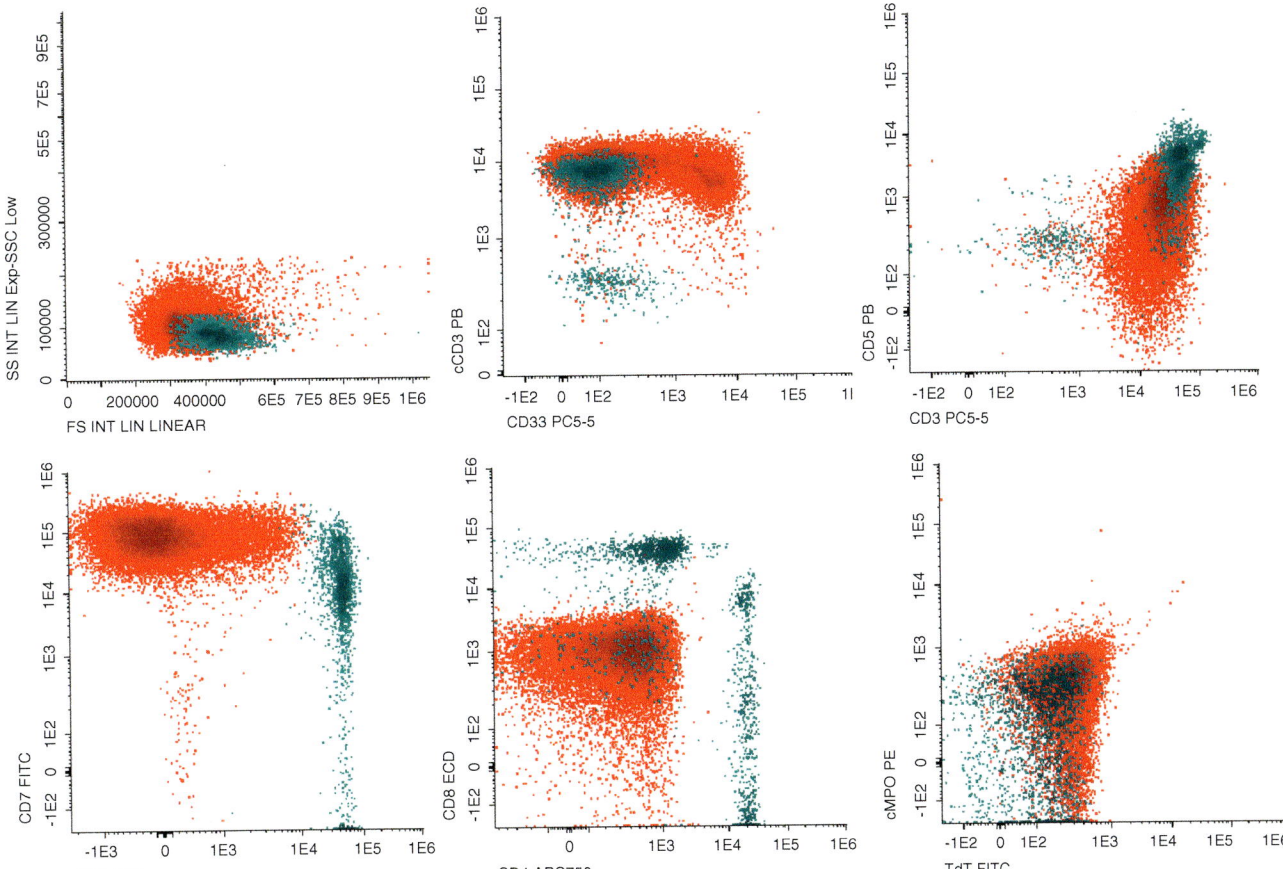

**Fig. 6.6** Pleural fluid with secondary infiltration by T-lymphoblastic lymphoma/leukemia. Bivariate dot plots of a T-ALL. The T-lymphoblasts are shown as red dots, whereas mature lymphocytes are represented as green dots. The lymphoblasts are positive for surface and cytoplasmic (c) CD3, show bright expression of CD7, but are only partially positive for CD5 and CD2. They are negative for CD4, CD8, cytoplasmic myeloperoxidase (cMPO), and Tdt. A subset of the lymphoblasts is positive for the myeloid antigen CD33

cardial effusions are uncommon. Pleural and pericardial effusions are mostly associated with lymphoma localization in the mediastinum. Lymphoblastic lymphoma, Burkitt's lymphoma, and T-cell lymphomas are associated with pleural effusions at a higher frequency than other lymphoma types (Figs. 6.6 and 6.8). Although malignant cells can be detected by cytological examination in many cases, and although immunophenotyping by flow cytometry is helpful in corroborating the diagnosis, a tissue biopsy is recommended for final classification of the lymphoma. A biopsy is usually not necessary when the effusion occurs at the time of lymphoma relapse. In those instances, cytological examination followed by flow cytometry suffices.

## Myeloid Leukemia Infiltration in Body Cavities

Myeloid leukemic effusions are rare. These have mostly been reported in chronic myelomonocytic leukemia and in chronic myeloid leukemia in accelerated phase or blast crisis. Leukemic effusions do also occur in other myeloproliferative neoplasms in blastic transformation. The effusions are usually hemorrhagic and show a mixture of immature and mature myeloid cells as well as a variable number of myeloblasts. The diagnosis can readily be established by cytologic examination followed by flow cytometry.

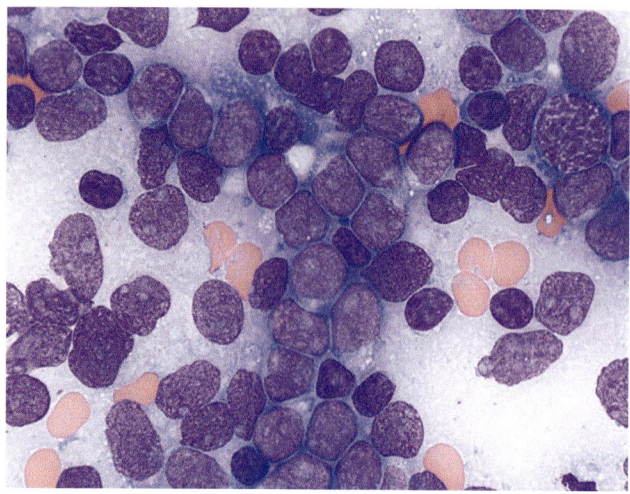

**Fig. 6.7** Mantle cell lymphoma, pleomorphic variant (MGG, 63× objective). The lymphoma cells display round to slightly cleaved nuclei with coarse chromatin and no apparent nucleoli

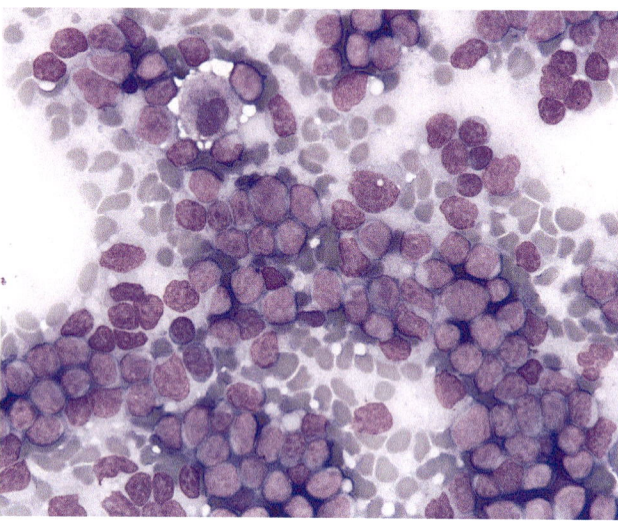

**Fig. 6.8** T-lymphoblasts (MGG, 63× objective). The lymphoblasts are identified by their high N/C ratio, fine chromatin pattern, and distinct nucleolus (i)

## References

1. Alexandrakis MG, Passam FH, Kyriakou DS, Bouros D. Pleural effusions in hematologic malignancies. Chest. 2004;125:1546–55.
2. Das DK. Serous effusions in malignant lymphomas: a review. Diagn Cytopathol. 2006;34:335–47.
3. Wong JW, Pitlik D, Abdul-Karim FW. Cytology of pleural, peritoneal and pericardial fluids in children. A 40-year summary. Acta Cytol. 1997;41:467–73.
4. Van Renterghem DM, Pauwels RA. Chylothorax and pleural effusion as late complications of thoracic irradiation. Chest. 1995;108:886–7.
5. Brixey AG, Light RW. Pleural effusions due to dasatinib. Curr Opin Pulm Med. 2010;16:351–65.
6. Seber A, Khan SP, Kersey JH. Unexplained effusions: association with allogeneic bone marrow transplantation and acute or chronic graft-versus-host disease. Bone Marrow Transplant. 1996;17:207–11.
7. Swerdlow SH, Campo E, Pileri SA, Harris NL, Stein H, Siebert R, Advani R, Ghielmini M, Salles GA, Zelenetz AD, Jaffe ES. The 2016 revision of the World Health Organization classification of lymphoid neoplasms. Blood. 2016;127:2375–90.
8. Thompson PA, Lade S, Webster H, Ryan G, Prince HM. Effusion-associated anaplastic large cell lymphoma of the breast: time for it to be defined as a distinct clinico-pathological entity. Haematologica. 2010;95:1977–9.
9. Alexanian S, Said J, Lones M, Puliarkat ST. KSHV/HHV8-negative Effusion-based lymphoma, a distinct entity with fluid overload states. Am J Surg Pathol. 2013;37:241–9.
10. Mitchell A, Meunier C, Ouellette D, Colby T. Extranodal marginal zone lymphoma of mucosa-associated lymphoid tissue with initial presentation in the pleura. Chest. 2006;129:791–4.
11. Motta G, Conticello C, Amato G, Moschetti G, Colarossi C, Cosentino S, Ippolito M, Giustolisi R, Di Raimondo F. Pleuric presentation of extranodal marginal zone lymphoma of mucosa-associated lymphoid tissue: a case report and a review of the literature. Int J Hematol. 2010;92:369–73.
12. Pullarkat VA, Medeiros LJ, Brynes RK. Body cavity-based presentation of natural killer cell lymphoma. Leuk Lymphoma. 2005;46:293–6.
13. Chaves FP, Quillen K, Xu D. Pericardial effusion: a rare presentation of adult T-cell leukemia/lymphoma. Am J Hematol. 2004;77:381–3.
14. Czader M, Ali SZ. Flow cytometry as an adjunct to cytomorphologic analysis of serous effusions. Diagn Cytopathol. 2003;29:74–8.
15. Bangerter M, Brudler O, Heinrich B, Griesshammer M. Fine needle aspiration cytology and flow cytometry in the diagnosis and subclassification of non-Hodgkin's lymphoma based on the World Health Organization classification. Acta Cytol. 2007;51:390–8.
16. Evans PA, Pott C, Groenen PJ, Salles G, Davi F, Berger F, Garcia JF, van Krieken JH, Pals S, Kluin P, Schuuring E, Spaargaren M, Boone E, González D, Martinez B, Villuendas R, Gameiro P, Diss TC, Mills K, Morgan GJ, Carter GI, Milner BJ, Pearson D, Hummel M, Jung W, Ott M, Canioni D, Beldjord K, Bastard C, Delfau-Larue MH, van Dongen JJ, Molina TJ, Cabeçadas J. Significantly improved PCR-based clonality testing in B-cell malignancies by use of multiple immunoglobulin gene targets. Report of the BIOMED-2 Concerted Action BHM4-CT98-3936. Leukemia. 2007;21:207–14.
17. Brüggemann M, White H, Gaulard P, Garcia-Sanz R, Gameiro P, Oeschger S, Jasani B, Ott M, Delsol G, Orfao A, Tiemann M, Herbst H, Langerak AW, Spaargaren M, Moreau E, Groenen PJ, Sambade C, Foroni L, Carter GI, Hummel M, Bastard C, Davi F, Delfau-Larue MH, Kneba M, van Dongen JJ, Beldjord K, Molina TJ. Powerful strategy for polymerase chain reaction-based clonality assessment in T-cell malignancies. Report of the BIOMED-2 Concerted Action BHM4 CT98-3936. Leukemia. 2007;21:215–21.
18. Tong LC, Ko HM, Saig MA, Boerner S, Geddie WR, da Cunha Santos G. Subclassification of lymphoproliferative disorders in serous effusions: a 10 year experience. Cancer Cytopathol. 2013;121:261–70.
19. Langerak AW, Molina TJ, Lavender FL, Pearson D, Flohr T, Sambade C, Schuuring E, Al Saati T, van Dongen JJ, van Krieken JH. Polymerase chain reaction-based clonality testing in tissue samples with reactive lymphoproliferations: usefulness and pitfalls. A report of the BIOMED-2 Concerted Action BMH4-CT98-3936. Leukemia. 2007;21:222–9.
20. Mann G, Attarbaschi A, Steiner M, Simonitsch I, Strobl H, Urban C, Meister B, Haas O, Dworzak M, Gadner H. Austrian Berlin-Frankfurt-Münster (BFM) Group. Early and reliable diagnosis of

non-Hodgkin lymphoma in childhood and adolescence: contribution of cytomorphology and flow cytometric immunophenotyping. Pediatr Hematol Oncol. 2006;2:167–76.

21. Mathiot C, Decaudin D, Klijanienko J, Couturier J, Salomon A, Dumont J, Vielh P. Fine-needle aspiration cytology combined with flow cytometry immunophenotyping is a rapid and accurate approach for the evaluation of suspicious superficial lymphoid lesions. Diagn Cytopathol. 2006;34:472–8.

22. Mathur S, Dawar R, Diagnosis VK. Grading of non-Hodgkin's lymphomas on fine needle aspiration cytology. Indian J Pathol Microbiol. 2007;50:46–50.

23. Knowles DM, Inghirami G, Ubriaco A, Dalla-Favera R. Molecular genetic analysis of three AIDS-associated neoplasms of uncertain lineage demonstrated their B-cell derivation and the possible pathogenetic role of the Epstein Bar virus. Blood. 1989;108:792–9.

24. Walts AE, Shintaku IP, Said JW. Diagnosis of malignant lymphoma in effusions from patients with AIDS by gene rearrangements. Am J Clin Pathol. 1990;94:170–5.

25. Chadburn A, Cesarman E, Jagirdar J, Subar M, Mir RN, Knowles DM. CD30 (Ki-1) positive anaplastic large cell lymphomas in individuals infected with the human immunodeficiency virus. Cancer. 1993;72:3078–90.

26. Green I, Espiritu E, Ladanyi M, Chaponda R, Wieczorek R, Gallo L, Feiner H. Primary lymphomatous effusions in AIDS: a morphological, immunophenotypic, and molecular study. Mod Pathol. 1995;8:39–45.

27. Nador RG, Cesarman E, Chadburn A, Dawson DB, Ansari MQ, Said J, Knowles DM. Primary effusion lymphoma: a distinct clinicopathologic entity associated with the Kaposi's sarcoma-associated herpes virus. Blood. 1996;88:645–56.

28. Chadburn A, Hyjek E, Mathew S, Cesarman E, Said J, Knowles DM. KSHV-positive solid lymphomas represent an extra-cavitary variant of primary effusion lymphoma. Am J Surg Pathol. 2004;28:1401–16.

29. DePond W, Said JW, Tasaka T, de Vos S, Kahn D, Cesarman E, Knowles DM, Koeffler HP. Kaposi's sarcoma-associated herpesvirus and human herpesvirus 8 (KSHV/HHV8)-associated lymphoma of the bowel. Report of two cases in HIV-positive men with secondary effusion lymphomas. Am J Surg Pathol. 1997;21:719–24.

30. Chadburn A, Said J, Gratzinger D, Chan JKC, de Jong DE, Jaffe E, Natkunam Y, Goodlad JR. HHV8/KSHV-positive lymphoproliferative disorders and the spectrum of plasmablastic cell neoplasms. Am J Clin Pathol. 2017;147:171–87.

31. Carbone A, Gloghini A, Vaccher E, Marchetti G, Gaidano G, Tirelli U. KSHV/HHV-8 associated lymph node based lymphomas in HIV seronegative subjects: report of two cases with anaplastic large cell morphology and plasmablastic immunophenotype. J Clin Pathol. 2005;58:1039–45.

32. Jones D, Ballestas ME, Kaye KM, Gulizia JM, Winters GL, Fletcher J, Scadden DT, Aster JC. Primary-effusion lymphoma and Kaposi's sarcoma in a cardiac-transplant recipient. N Engl J Med. 1998;339:444–9.

33. Dotti G, Fiocchi R, Motta T, Facchinetti B, Chiodini B, Borleri GM, Gavazzeni G, Barbui T, Rambaldi A. Primary effusion lymphoma after heart transplantation: a new entity associated with human herpesvirus-8. Leukemia. 1999;13:664–70.

34. Du MQ, Bacon CM, Isaacson PG. Kaposi sarcoma-associated herpesvirus/human herpesvirus 8 and lymphoproliferative disorders. J Clin Pathol. 2007;60:1350–7.

35. Chang Y, Cesarman E, Pessin MS, Lee F, Culpepper J, Knowles DM, Moore PS. Identification of herpesvirus-like DNA sequences in AIDS-associated Kaposi's sarcoma. Science. 1994;266:1865–9.

36. Polskj JM, Evans HL, Grosso LE, Popovic WJ, Taylor L, Dunphy CH. CD7 and CD56-positive primary effusion lymphoma in a human immunodeficiency virus-negative host. Leuk Lymphoma. 2000;39:633–9.

37. Matolcsy A, Nador RG, Cesarman E, Knowles DM. Immunoglobulin VH gene mutation analysis suggests that primary effusions derive from different stages of B cell maturation. Am J Pathol. 1998;153:1609–14.

38. Kelin U, Gloghini A, Gaidano G, Chadburn A, Cesarman E, Dalla-Favera R, Carbone A. gene expression profile analysis of AIDS-rleated primary effusions lymphoma (PEL) suggests a plasmablastic derivation and identifies PEL-specific transcripts. Blood. 2003;101:4115–21.

39. Jenner RG, Mailland K, Catttini N, Weiss RA, Boshoff C, Wooster R, Kellam P. Kaposi's sarcoma-associated herpesvirus-infected primary effusion lymphoma has a plasma cell gene expression profile. Proc Natl Acad Sci U S A. 2003;100:10399–404.

40. Wilson KS, McKenna RW, Kroft SH, Dawson DB, Ansari Q, Schneider NR. Primary effusion lymphomas exhibit complex and recurrent cytogenetic abnormalities. Br J Haematol. 2002;116:113–21.

41. Dai L, Trillo-Tinoco J, Cao Y, Bonstaff K, Doyle L, Del Valle L, Whitby D, Parsons C, Reiss K, Zableta J, Qin Z. Targeting HGF/c-MET induces cell cycle arrest, DNA damage, and apoptosis for primary effusion lymphoma. Blood. 2015;126:2821–31.

42. Lam BQ, Dai L, LI L, Qiao J, Lin Z, Qin Z. Molecular mechanisms of activating c-MET in KSHV+ primary effusion lymphoma. Oncotarget. 2017;8:18373–80.

43. Chen YB, Rahemtullah A, Hochberg E. Primary effusion lymphoma. Oncologist. 2007;12:569–76.

44. Iuchi K, Ichimiya A, Akashi A, Mizuta T, Lee YE, Tada H, Mori T, Sawamura K, Lee YS, Furuse K, Yamamoto S, Aozasa K. Non-Hodgkin's lymphoma of the pleural cavity developing from long-standing pyothorax. Cancer. 1987;60:1771–5.

45. Aozasa K. Pyothorax-associated lymphoma. J Clin Exp Hematop. 2006;46:5–10. Review

46. Petitjean B, Jardin F, Joly B, Martin-Garcia N, Tilly H, Picquenot JM, Briere J, Danel C, Mehaut S, Abd-Al-Samad I, Copie-Bergman C, Delfau-Larue MH, Gaulard P. Pyothorax-associated lymphoma. A peculiar clinicopathologic entity derived from B cells at late stage of differentiation and with occasional aberrant dual B- and T- cell phenotype. Am J Surg Pathol. 2002;26:724–32.

47. Nakatsuka S, Yao M, Hoshida Y, Yamamoto S, Iuchi K, Aozasa K. Pyothorax-associated lymphoma: a review of 106 cases. J Clin Oncol. 2002;20:4255–60.

48. Fukayama M, Ibuka T, Hayashi Y, Ooba T, Koike M, Mizutani S. Epstein-Barr virus in pyothorax-associated pleural lymphoma. Am J Pathol. 1993;143:1044–9.

49. Aosaza K, Takkuwa T, Nakatsuka S. Pyothorax-associated lymphoma. A lymphoma developing in chronic inflammation. Adv Anat Pathol. 2005;12:324–31. Review

50. Hongyo T, Kurooka M, Taniguchi E, Iuchi K, Nakajima Y, Aozasa K, Nomura T. Frequent p53 mutations at dipyrimidine sites in patients with pyothorax-associated lymphoma. Cancer Res. 1998;58:1105–57.

51. Boyer D, Mc Kelvie PA, de Leval L, Edlefsen KL, Ko YH, Aberman ZA, Kovach AE, Masih A, Nishino HT, Weiss LM, Meeker AK, Nardi V, Palisoc M, Shao L, Pittalagu S, Ferry JA, Harris NL, Sohani AR. Fibrin-associated EBV-positive B-cell lymphoma. An indolent neoplasm with features distinct from diffuse large B-cell lymphoma associated with chronic inflammation. Am J Surg Pathol. 2017;41:299–312.

52. Keech JA, Creech BJ. Anaplastic T-cell lymphoma in proximity to a saline-filled breast implant. Plast Reconstr Surg. 1997;100:554–5.

53. Gaudet G, Friedberg JW, Weng A, Pinkus GS, Freedman AS. Breast lymphoma associated with breast implants: two case-reports and a review of the literature. Leuk Lymphoma. 2002;43:115–9.

54. de Jong D, Vasmel WL, de Boer JP, Verhave G, Barbé E, Casparie MK, van Leeuwen FE. Anaplastic large-cell lymphoma in women with breast implants. JAMA. 2008;300:2030–5.

55. Xu J, Wei S. Breast-implant-associated anaplastic large cell lymphoma. Review of a distinct clinicopathologic entity. Arch Pathol Lab Med. 2014;138:842–6.

56. Laurent C, Delas A, Gaulard P, Haioun C, Moreau A, Xerri L, Traverse-Glehen A, Rousset T, Quintin-Roue I, Petrella T, Emile JF, Amara N, Rochaix P, Chenard-Neu MP, Tasei AM, Menet E, Chomarat H, Costes V, Andrac-Meyer L, Michiels JF, Chassagne-Clement C, de Leval L, Brousset P, Delsol G, Lamant L. Breast implant associated anaplastic large cell lymphoma: two distinct clinicopathological variants with different outcomes. Ann Oncol. 2016;27:306–14.

57. Miranda RN, Aladily TN, Prince HM, Kanagal-Shamanna R, de Jong D, Fayad LE, Amin MB, Haideri N, Bhagat G, Brooks GS, Shifrin DA, O'Malley DP, Cheah CY, Bacchi CE, Gualco G, Li S, Keech JA Jr, Hochberg EP, Carty MJ, Hanson SE, Mustafa E, Sanchez S, Manning JT Jr, Xu-Monette ZY, Miranda AR, Fox P, Bassett RL, Castillo JJ, Beltran BE, de Boer JP, Chakhachiro Z, Ye D, Clark D, Young KH, Medeiros LJ. Breast implant-associated anaplastic large cell lymphoma: long term follow-up of 60 patients. J Clin Oncol. 2014;32:2375–90.

58. Clemens MW, Medeiros LJ, Butler CE, Hunt KK, Fanale MA, Horwitz S, Weisenburger DD, Liu J, Morgan EA, Kanagal-Shamanna R, Parkash V, Ning J, Sohani AR, Ferry JA, Mehta-Shah N, Dogan A, Liu H, Thormann N, Di Naopli A, Lade S, Piccolini J, Reyes R, Williams T, McCarthy CM, Hanson SE, Nastoupil LJ, Gaur R, Oki Y, Young KH, Miranda RN. Complete surgical excision is essential for the management of patients with brest implant-associated anaplastic large cell lymphoma. J Clin Oncol. 2016;34:160–8.

59. Lipworth L, Tarone RE, McLaughlin JK. Breast implants and lymphoma risk: a review of the epidemiologic evidence through 2008. Plast Reconstr Surg. 2009;123:790–3.

60. Di Napoli A, Jain P, Duranti E, Margolskee E, Arancio W, Fachetti F, Alobeid B, di Pompeo FS, Mansukhani M, Bhagat G. Targeted next generation sequencing of breast implant-associated anaplastic large cell lymphoma reveals mutations in *JAK/STAT* signaling pathway genes, *TP53* and *DNMT3A*. Br J Haematol. 2016. https://doi.org/10.1111/bjh.14431.

61. Blombery P, Thompson E, Jones K, Mir Arnau MG, Lade S, Markham JE, Li J, Deva A, Johnstone RW, Khot A, Prince HM, Westerman D. Whole exome sequencing reveals activating JAK1 and STAT3 mutations in breast implant-associated anaplastic large cell lymphoma. Haematologica. 2016;101:e387–90.

62. Crescenzo R, Abate F, Lasorsa E, Tabbo F, Gaudiano M, Chiesa N, Di Giacomo F, Spaccarotella E, Barbarossa L, Ercole E, Todaro M, Boi M, Acquaviva A, Ficarro E, Novero D, Rinaldi A, Tousseyn T, Rosenwald A, Kenner L, Cerroni L, Tzankov A, Pnozoni M, Paulli M, weisenburger D, Chan WC, Iqbal J, Piris MA, Zamo A, Ciardullo C, Rossi D, Gaidano G, Pileri S, Tiacci E, Falini B, Schultz LD, Mevellec L, Vialard JE, Piva R, Bertoni F, Rabadan R, Inghirami G. Convergent mutations and kinase fusions lead to oncogenic STAT3 activation in anaplastic large cell lymphoma. Cancer Cell. 2015;27:516–32.

63. Yang L, Rau R, Goodell MA. DNMT3A in hematological malignancies. Nat Rev Cancer. 2015;15:152–65.

64. Wu D, Allen CT, Fromm JR. Flow cytometry of ALK-negative anaplastic large cell lymphoma of breast implant-associated effusion and capsular tissue. Cytometry B. 2015;88B:58–63.

65. Montgomery-Goecker C, Fuda F, Krueger JE, Chen W. Immunophenotypic characteristics of breast implant-associated anaplastic large cell lymphoma by flow cytometry. Cytometry B. 2015;88B:291–3.

66. Roden AC, Macon WR, Keeney GL, Myeres JL, Feldman AL, Dogan A. Seroma-associated primary anaplastic large cell lymphoma adjacent to breast implants: an indolent T-cell lymphoproliferative disorder. Mod Pathol. 2008;21:455–63.

67. Clemens MW, Horwitz SM. NCCN Consensus guidelines for the diagnosis and management of breast implant-associated anaplastic large cell lymphoma. Aesth Reconstr Surg. 2017;139:1029–39.

68. Ichinohasama R, Miura I, Kobayashi N, Saitoh Y, DeCoteau JF, Saiki Y, Mori S, Kadin ME, Ooya K. Herpes virus type 8-negative primary effusion lymphoma associated with PAX-5 gene rearrangement and hepatitis C virus: a case report and review of the literature. Am J Surg Pathol. 1998;22:1528–37.

# Cancer of Other Origin

Ben Davidson, Claire Michael, and Pınar Fırat

## Introduction

The list of malignant tumors that may affect the serosal cavities in the form of malignant effusions is essentially as long as the list of existing cancers, as almost any type of malignancy has been described at this anatomic site. There are, however, considerable variations in terms of incidence that must be taken into account. The previous chapters in this section focused on five of the more commonly diagnosed entities in effusion diagnosis—breast, lung, and ovarian carcinoma, malignant mesothelioma, and hematological cancers. The frequency with which one may diagnose any of the remaining cancers depends on the type of institution and diagnostic service one works in, as well as on geographic factors. Nevertheless, the most frequently encountered tumors among those discussed in this chapter are undoubtedly those originating from the gastrointestinal tract, followed by metastases from uterine (endometrial and cervical) carcinomas, with the remaining entities ranging from infrequent to exceedingly rare. It should be noted that papers cited in this chapter are limited to those in which unequivocal presence of tumor cells has been documented in the effusion based on cytological evaluation. Reports in which effusions have been described as "malig-

B. Davidson, M.D., Ph.D. (✉)
Department of Pathology, The Norwegian Radium Hospital, Oslo University Hospital, Oslo, Norway

Faculty of Medicine, Institute of Clinical Medicine, University of Oslo, Oslo, Norway
e-mail: bend@medisin.uio.no; bdd@ous-hf.no

C. Michael, M.D.
UH Cleveland Medical Center, Case Western Reserve University, Cleveland, OH, USA

P. Fırat, M.D.
Department of Pathology, School of Medicine, Koc University, Istanbul, Turkey

[Previously] Department of Pathology, Istanbul Faculty of Medicine, Istanbul University, Istanbul, Turkey
e-mail: pfirat@kuh.ku.edu.tr; pfirat@istanbul.edu.tr

nant" based on the fact that the patient had documented metastasis to the same anatomic compartment that has been diagnosed in biopsy material have not been included in this discussion.

## Gastrointestinal Cancers

The most common gastrointestinal organs of origin for metastases in effusions are the stomach, pancreas, liver, colon and rectum, and esophagus. In addition, dissemination from a primary in the appendix, and less frequently from a colonic, ovarian, or other origin, in the form of pseudomyxoma peritonei deserves discussion, as it represents a distinct clinical entity.

The clinical and morphological characteristics of these tumors will be discussed separately, followed by a joint discussion on their immunohistochemical profile and the differential diagnosis, as several markers are expressed by the majority or all of these cancers.

## Gastric Carcinoma

Globally, gastric cancer, constituting predominantly of adenocarcinoma, is the fourth and fifth most commonly diagnosed cancer in men and women, respectively, and ranks third and fifth in cancer-associated mortality in the two genders, making it a major health problem [1]. Considerable geographic variation exists, with highest disease incidence in Eastern Europe, Asia, and Central and South America [2]. *Helicobacter pylori* is a major causative agent. Mass screening for gastric cancer in Japan and South Korea has led to detection of smaller tumors at an earlier disease stage, resulting in improved survival. However, screening has not been implemented in the majority of countries, resulting frequently in late diagnosis, with 5-year survival at 25–30% for all stages [2]. Malignant ascites is present in 10% of gastric cancer patients and is associated with poor outcome [3].

© Springer International Publishing AG, part of Springer Nature 2018
B. Davidson et al. (eds.), *Serous Effusions*, https://doi.org/10.1007/978-3-319-76478-8_7

Surgery at early stage remains the only curative approach. However, treatment is multidisciplinary, with combination of surgery with chemotherapy or chemoradiotherapy in patients with resectable disease or the use of the latter modalities in the non-resectable setting. Intraabdominal chemotherapy has been assessed as therapeutic modality, with generally disappointing results. Targeted therapy using trastuzumab is used in patients with HER2-overexpressing tumors, and several other therapeutic targets are currently being assessed in clinical trials [2]. Analysis of 72 patient-matched primary and metastatic gastric carcinomas, including 15 effusions, showed good agreement with respect to HER2 status by both FISH (98.5%) and IHC (94.9%) [4]. The feasibility of assessing HER2 status in effusion specimens was confirmed in a more recent study of 46 gastric carcinoma effusions [5].

Gastric carcinoma effusions are often highly cellular (Fig. 7.1a). Tumor cells in effusions most often originate from diffuse infiltrating carcinomas and consequently tend to disseminate in the form of single cells (Fig. 7.1b, c), although more cohesive groups, occasionally with acinar form, may be seen (Fig. 7.1d). Tumor cells have variable size but are generally medium-sized, with high n/c ratio, markedly atypical nuclei with coarse chromatin, and conspicuous nucleoli (Fig. 7.1e, f). Signet ring morphology is common and intracytoplasmic vacuoles are easily detected (Fig. 7.1e–g). Binucleate or multinucleate cells may be seen (Fig. 7.1h). Mitotic figures are easily found (Fig. 7.1g, i).

Cells that have spread from gastric carcinomas of intestinal type tend to be more cylindrical and less atypical and form more cohesive groups [6].

## Pancreatic Carcinoma

Pancreatic cancer, predominantly adenocarcinoma, is a highly lethal malignancy which is more prevalent in developed countries, in which it is the ninth and eighth most commonly diagnosed cancer in men and women, respectively. The aggressiveness of pancreatic cancer is clearly reflected in the fact that it ranks fifth and fourth in cancer-associated mortality in the two genders, with 5-year survival for all stages at 8%. The disease is predicted to become the second most common cancer by 2030 [1, 7].

Pancreatic cancer usually presents as locally advanced or metastatic disease, with only 15–20% of patients deemed eligible for upfront surgery [8]. For the remaining patients, chemotherapy is the mainstay of treatment. However, few patients achieve long-term survival, and data from trials applying targeted therapy have generally been disappointing to date [7].

Individuals with family history of pancreatic cancer are at increased risk of developing the disease, as are those with genetic syndromes, including hereditary pancreatitis, famil-

ial atypical mole and multiple melanoma, Peutz-Jeghers syndrome, Lynch syndrome, and Li-Fraumeni syndrome, as well as those carrying *BRCA* mutations [9]. Effective screening is unavailable to date [9, 10].

The presence of malignant ascites, either at diagnosis or at new onset, is associated with extremely poor survival [11–13]. In a recent study of 180 patients, median survival after development of ascites was 1.8 months [14]. Therapeutic approaches that have been considered in this setting are administration of paclitaxel after failed treatment with gemcitabine, the drug of choice in treating pancreatic cancer [15], and combined regimen of 5-FU and cisplatin [16], the latter with disappointing results.

Warshaw analyzed peritoneal washings from 40 patients diagnosed with pancreatic carcinoma of the head (*n* = 35) or body (=5). Tumor cells were found in 12 cases (30%), and their presence was associated with the presence of non-resectable tumors and shorter survival [17]. In contrast, only three positive specimens were found in analysis of peritoneal washings and ascites specimens from 36 patients with biopsy-proven pancreatic carcinoma, all three from patients with peritoneal carcinomatosis [18].

The morphology of pancreatic carcinoma in effusions depends on the histological type of the primary tumor (serous vs. mucinous) and the degree of differentiation. Di Bonito et al. studied 26 effusions from 20 patients with pancreatic carcinoma of ductal type, of which 18 were peritoneal and 8 pleural. The authors found Indian file formation with nuclear molding to be the most prominent morphological feature. Other non-specific features included eccentric hyperchromatic nuclei, abundant vacuolated cytoplasm, and a reactive background [19].

Spieler and Gloor describe two types of cells in well-differentiated pancreatic and biliary duct carcinoma-small cylindrical cells forming smooth, round, or papilliform clusters and larger cells with abundant vacuolated cytoplasm. Less differentiated cells were difficult to distinguish from adenocarcinomas of other origin [6].

Cases seen by the authors of this chapter encompass a fairly wide morphological spectrum. Pancreatic carcinoma cells may form papillary groups that are indistinguishable from serous carcinoma of the ovary or peritoneum (Fig. 7.2a–c). Vacuolization may be prominent (Fig. 7.2a, d), occasionally encroaching on the nucleus (Fig. 7.2e). Acinar structures may be seen, with nuclear molding (Fig. 7.2f), as well as nondescript groups of various size (Fig. 7.2g, h). Cells have variable n/c ratio and degree of atypia, but the latter may be pronounced (Fig. 7.2i), occasionally with the formation of giant cells, both mononucleated and multinucleated (Fig. 7.2j, k). Tumors with dissociated cells, occasionally with intracytoplasmic vacuoles, which are indistinguishable from gastric carcinoma or lobular breast carcinoma, may be seen (Fig. 7.2m).

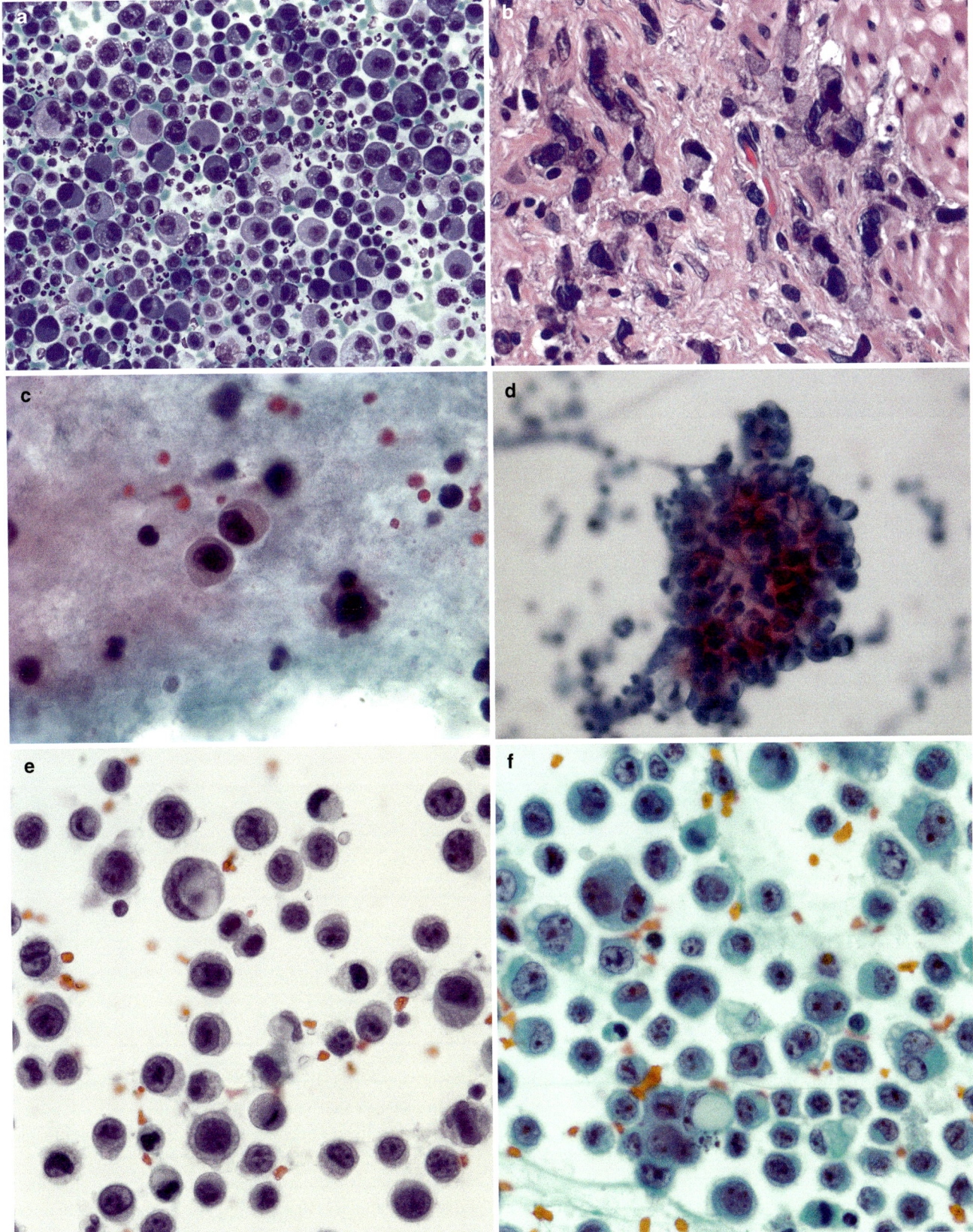

**Fig. 7.1** Gastric carcinoma: (**a**) highly cellular specimen with dissociated tumor cells; (**b** and **c**), matched effusion (**b**) and gastric resection (**c**) from a patient with adenocarcinoma of the diffuse infiltrating type; (**d**) cohesive cell group; (**e** and **f**) prominent atypia; (**g**) signet ring cells; (**h**) binucleation; (**i**) mitosis. (**a**) MGG/Diff-Quik; (**b**) H&E; (**c**–**i**) PAP

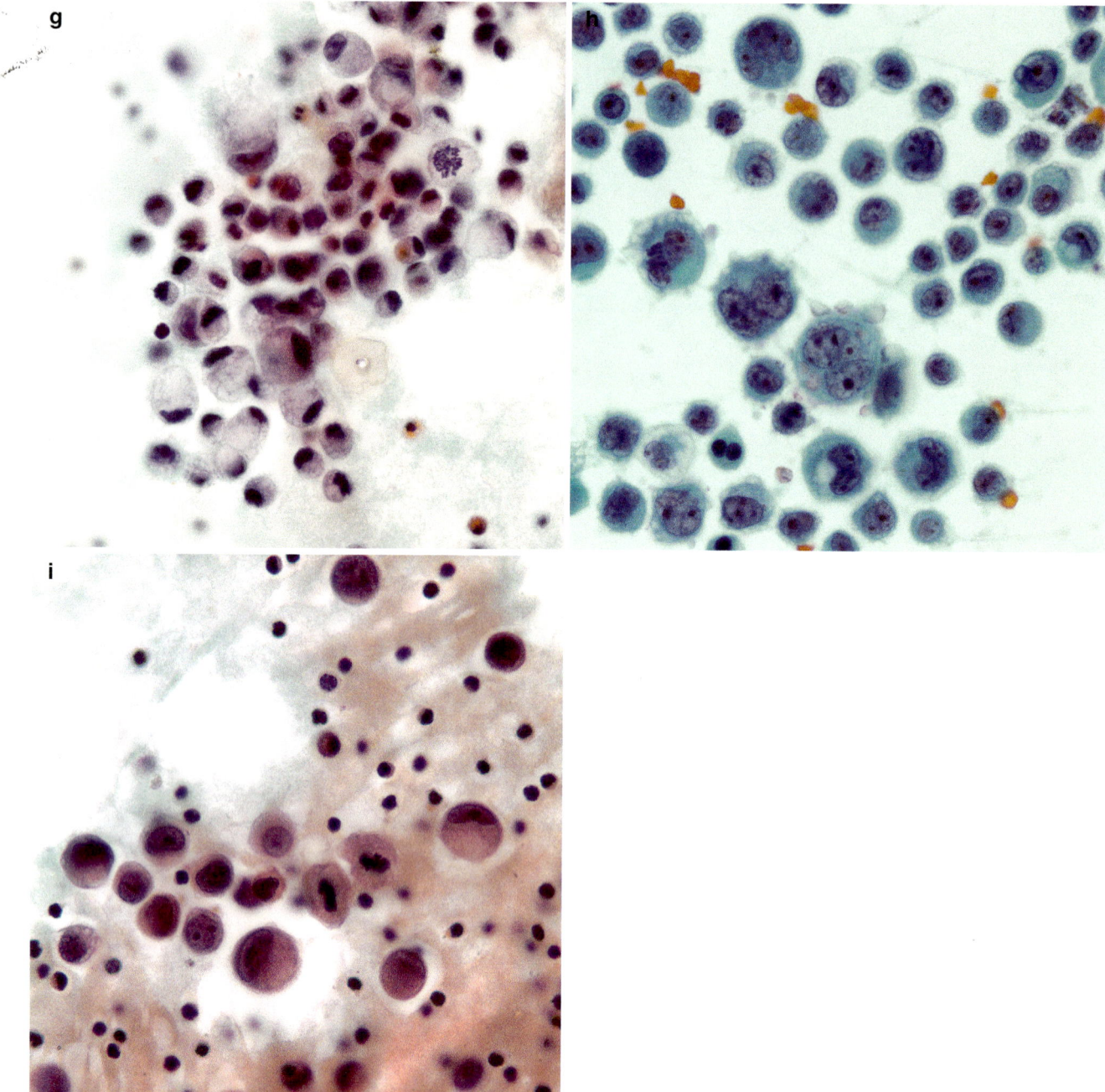

**Fig. 7.1** (continued)

## Colon Carcinoma, Tumors of the Appendix, and Pseudomyxoma Peritonei

Colorectal cancer (CRC), constituting for all practical purposes of adenocarcinomas, is the third most common malignancy in men worldwide, ranking second in women. It is the fourth and third most common cause of cancer-associated deaths in the two genders [1]. Unlike gastric and pancreatic cancer, effective screening available for this disease has led to reduced mortality. Metastatic disease in treated by chemotherapy, to which in recent years targeted therapy has been added, predominantly aimed at inhibition of epidermal growth factor receptor (EGFR) and vascular endothelial growth factor (VEGF) [20].

Colon carcinoma may occasionally be found in effusion specimens, most frequently in the peritoneal cavity. Tumor cells are usually columnar and large, forming glandular, acinar, or papillary structures (Fig. 7.3a–d), but may be smaller and in more tightly arranged groups (Fig. 7.3e). Intracytoplasmic mucous vacuoles of various size may be evident (Fig. 7.3f–h). Nuclear palisading, nuclear membrane irregularities with indentations and lobulations, and apical cytoplasmic densities have been described as characteristic for adenocarcinomas of colonic origin [6, 21]. As in other

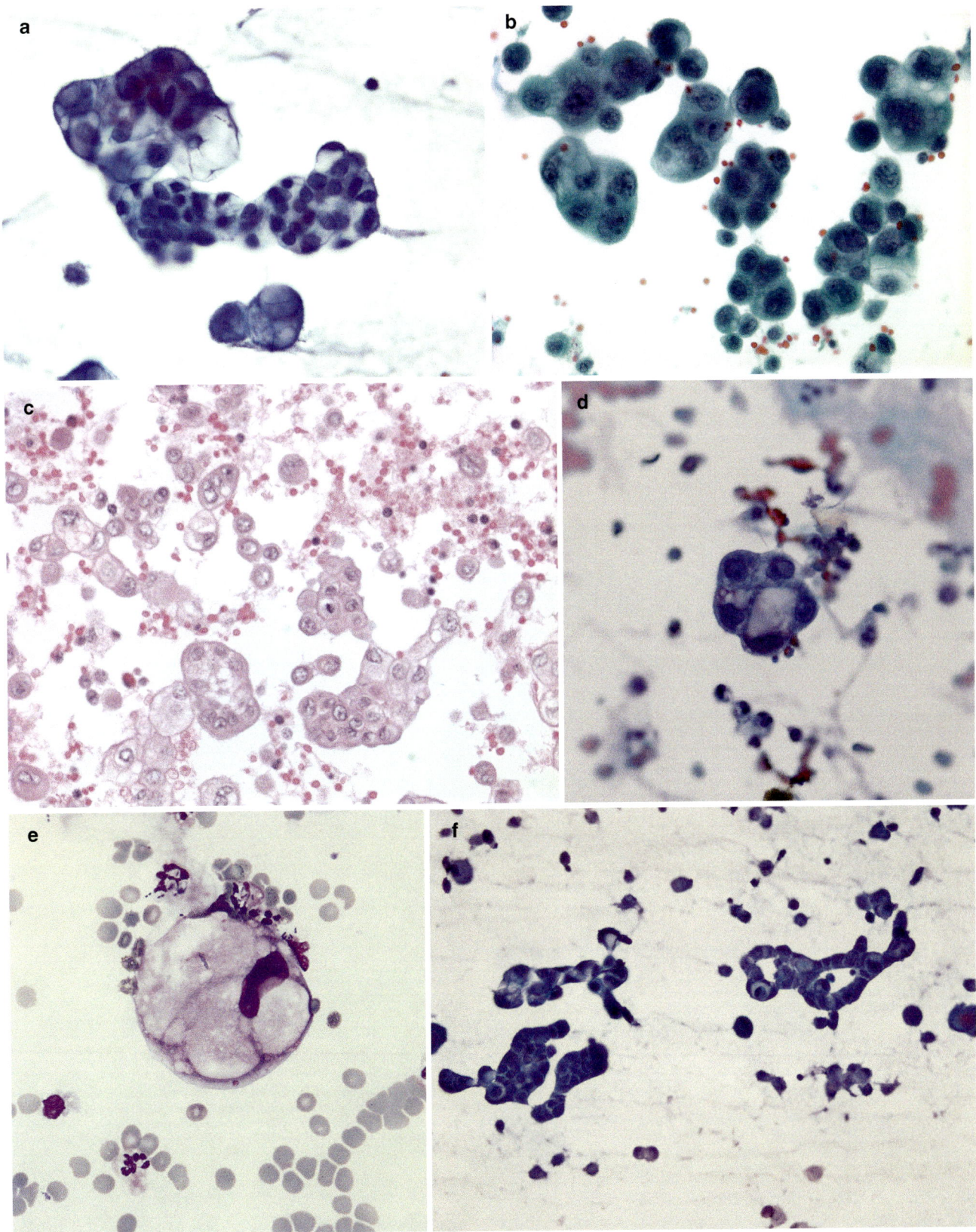

**Fig. 7.2** Pancreatic carcinoma: (**a–c**) papillary groups; (**d, e**) vacuolated cells; (**f**) acinar groups; (**g**) small cohesive group; (**h**) tumor showing both dissociated cells and cohesive groups; (**i**) pronounced atypia; (**j, k**) pleomorphic cells; (**l**) dissociated poorly differentiated carcinoma. (**a, b, d, f**) PAP; (**c, j**) H&E; (**e, g–i, k, l**) MGG/Diff-Quik

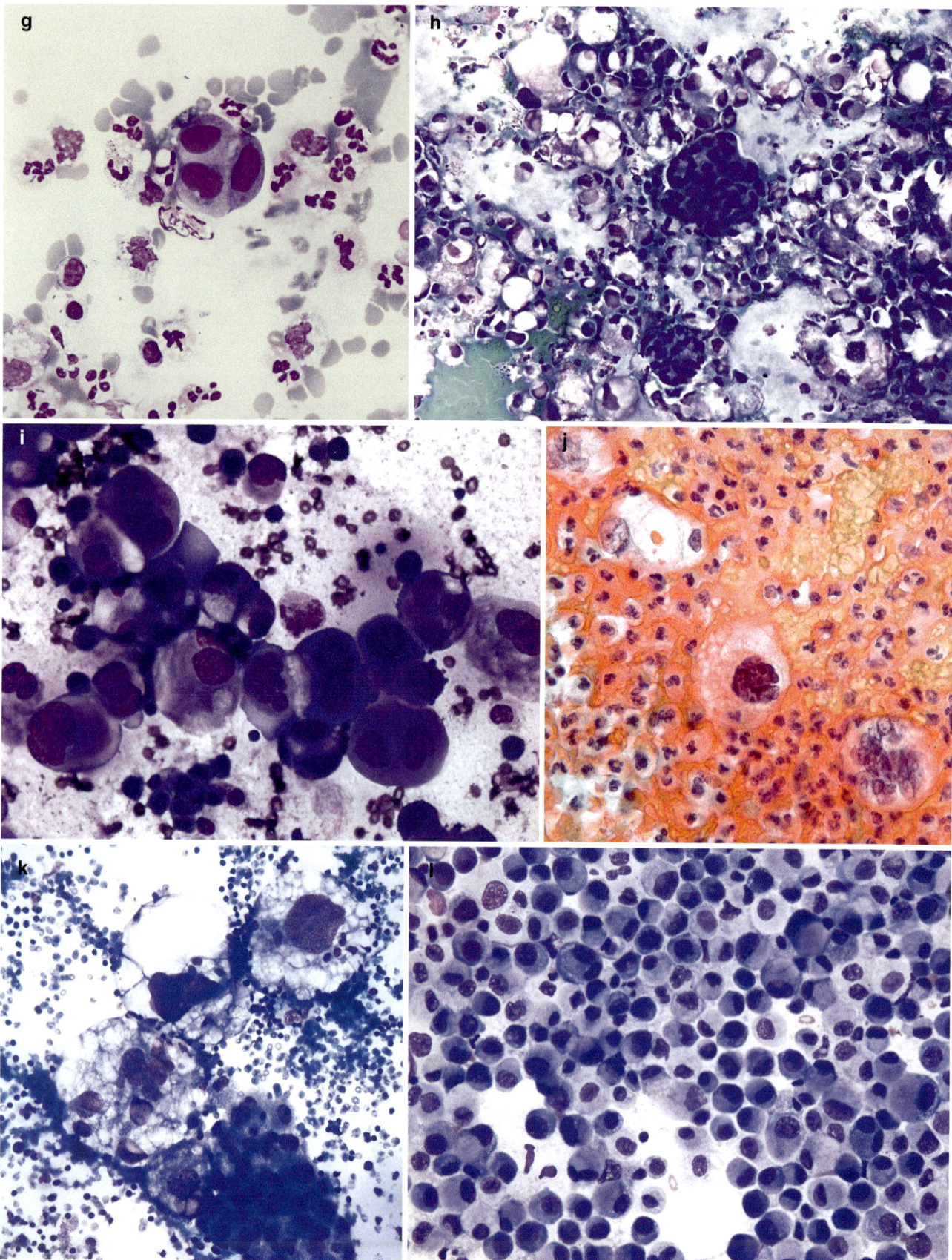

**Fig. 7.2** (continued)

gastrointestinal tumors, pleomorphic cells, signet ring morphology, or dissociated poorly differentiated cells may be encountered in less differentiated tumors (Fig. 7.3f–j).

Pseudomyxoma peritonei (PMP) is characterized by the presence of mucinous ascites and diffuse peritoneal involvement in the form of mucin-containing nodules of variable size. While some foci may contain only mucin and host cells (fibroblasts, mesothelial cells, leukocytes), the majority contain neoplastic mucinous epithelium with a variable degree of atypia. The primary tumor is localized in the appendix in the majority of cases, although dissemination from other primary sites, mainly the ovary and colon, is occasionally seen. Ronnett et al. divided these cases into diffuse peritoneal adenomucinosis (DPAM) and peritoneal mucinous carcinomatosis (PMCA) based on the diagnosis of the primary appendiceal tumor (adenoma vs. carcinoma) and the abundance of epithelial elements, degree of atypia, and mitotic activity in the peritoneal lesions [22]. Differences in survival between these two groups were seen in this report, as well as in subsequent studies [22, 23]. New guidelines for classification and reporting of this tumor were recently published [24]. Among the changes in this document, low-grade and high-grade mucinous carcinoma peritonei were accepted as alternatives to the adenomucinosis and carcinomatosis terms, respectively, and PMP was defined as malignant disease [24].

In the largest study of cytological specimens to date, Jackson et al. reviewed 67 peritoneal washing specimens from PMP patients [25]. Epithelial elements were found in 63 specimens, whereas the remaining 4 contained only mucin. Good agreement was seen between the histological and cytological specimens in differentiating DPAM from PMCA.

In the Jackson series, tumor cells in DPAM cases were characterized by cohesive clusters or monolayered (honeycomb) sheets of cells with discrete cell borders; uniform small, round nuclei with smooth nuclear membranes and inconspicuous nucleoli; and absence of mitotic figures and single tumor cells. In PMCA specimens, tumor cells were found as single cells, small three-dimensional clusters, or irregular sheets. Cells were enlarged and had overlapping nuclei with irregular nuclear membranes, irregular chromatin, and variably sized nucleoli. Signet ring cells and mitotic figures were occasionally found [25].

In a recent report, tumor cells were found in cytological specimens from 18/21 patients, and the presence of higher cellularity was associated with more aggressive disease [26]. A PMP specimen from one of the authors' archive is shown in Fig. 7.3k.

A more rare diagnosis is the finding of a goblet cell carcinoid (adenocarcinoid) in effusion specimens. Only isolated reports of this entity have been published in the literature [27–31], and one of the authors diagnosed an additional specimen in a pleural effusion. These are aggressive tumors which combine the morphological features and immunohistochemical profile of carcinoid and mucinous carcinoma. Wojcik and Selvaggi observed clusters of uniform small cells containing nuclei with finely granular chromatin, small prominent nucleoli, and scant cytoplasm admixed with signet ring cells [27]. Others observed coarse hyperchromasia and nuclear overlap and molding [28] or the additional presence of larger cells with abundant granular cytoplasm, bean-shaped to round nuclei, and prominent eosinophilic nucleoli. Gland-like formations were found, some with eosinophilic material [29]. A tumor with predominant signet ring cell morphology and aggressive clinical behavior was recently described [31]. Our specimen consisted of cohesive groups of variable size, with cells that had vacuolated and eosinophilic cytoplasm, nuclei with relatively little atypia, but with rather conspicuous nucleoli (Fig. 7.3l, m).

Rare reports of dissemination from other non-pulmonary neuroendocrine tumors have been published, including metastasis from a thymic carcinoid in pleural effusion [32] and positive peritoneal cytology from two patients with non-functioning pancreatic endocrine tumors and one with ileal carcinoid [33]. In the latter paper, the cytological features were not described.

## Hepatocellular Carcinoma (HCC)

HCC is the sixth most common and ranks third as cause of death worldwide, with more than 700,000 cases diagnosed in 2008. Considerable geographic variation exists, with the majority of cases diagnosed in Asia or in sub-Saharan Africa. Etiological factors include infection with hepatitis B and C viruses, alcoholism, and aflatoxin B1 exposure, as well as diabetes. HCC is a highly aggressive cancer developing most frequently in the context of pre-existing cirrhosis. Prognosis is extremely poor, especially in the presence of extrahepatic disease, and has not been significantly improved by chemotherapy. However, follow-up of individuals at risk by ultrasonography allows for diagnosis at earlier stages, in which surgery may be curative. Sorafenib, inhibitor of Raf kinase and receptor tyrosine kinases, has been shown to prolong survival in advanced disease [34].

The diagnostic yield of ascites from patients with liver disease was shown to be low.

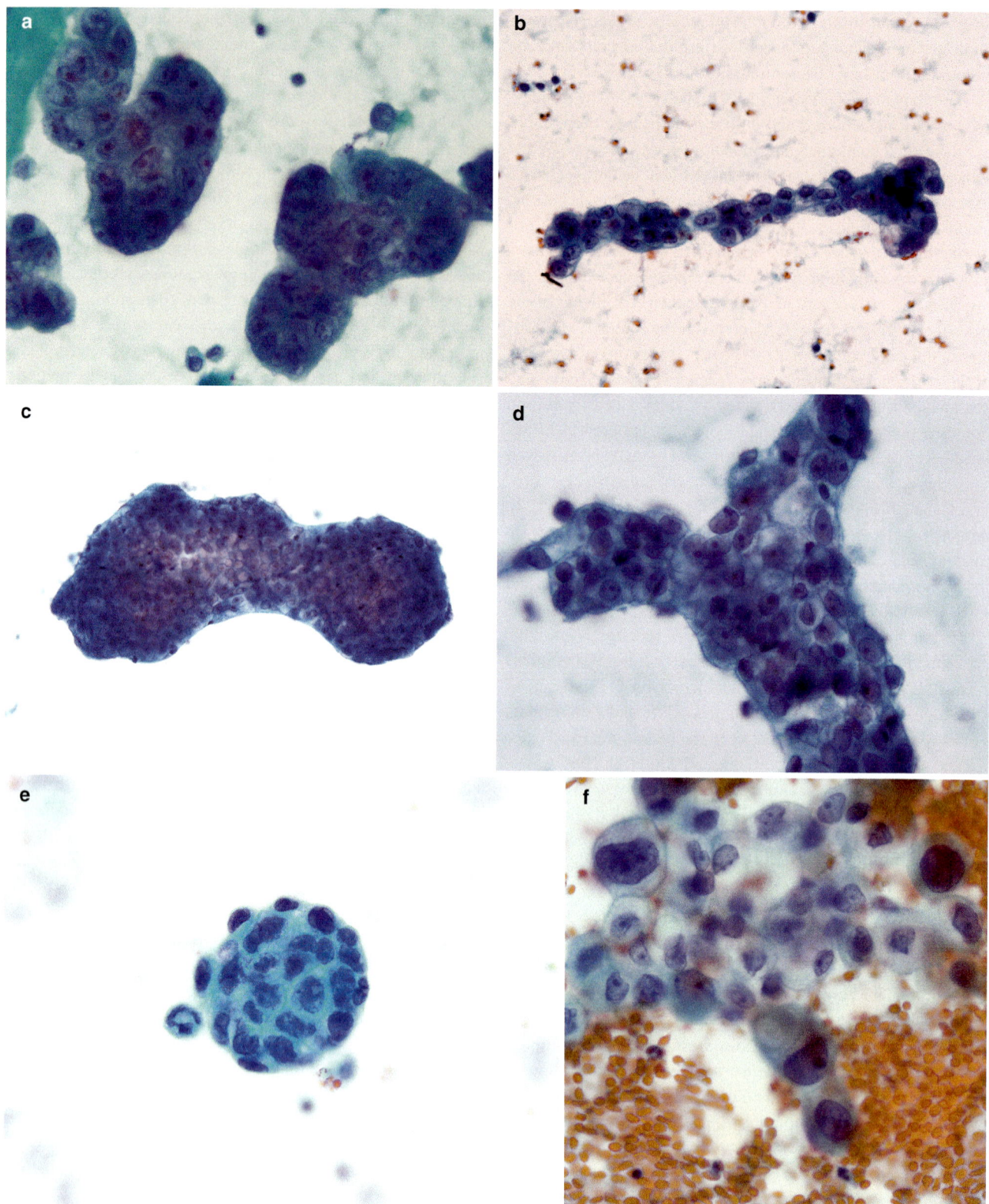

**Fig. 7.3** Colon carcinoma: (**a**–**e**) glandular, acinar, papillary, or tight groups; (**f**–**h**) vacuolated cells; (**i**) pronounced atypia; (**j**) dissociated poorly differentiated carcinoma; (**k**) pseudomyxoma peritonei with copious mucin; (**l**, **m**) goblet cell carcinoid showing papillary group (**l**) and vacuolated cells with neuroendocrine features (**m**). (**a**–**f**, **j**, **l**) pap; (**g**, **i**, **k**) MGG/Diff-Quik; (**h**, **m**) H&E

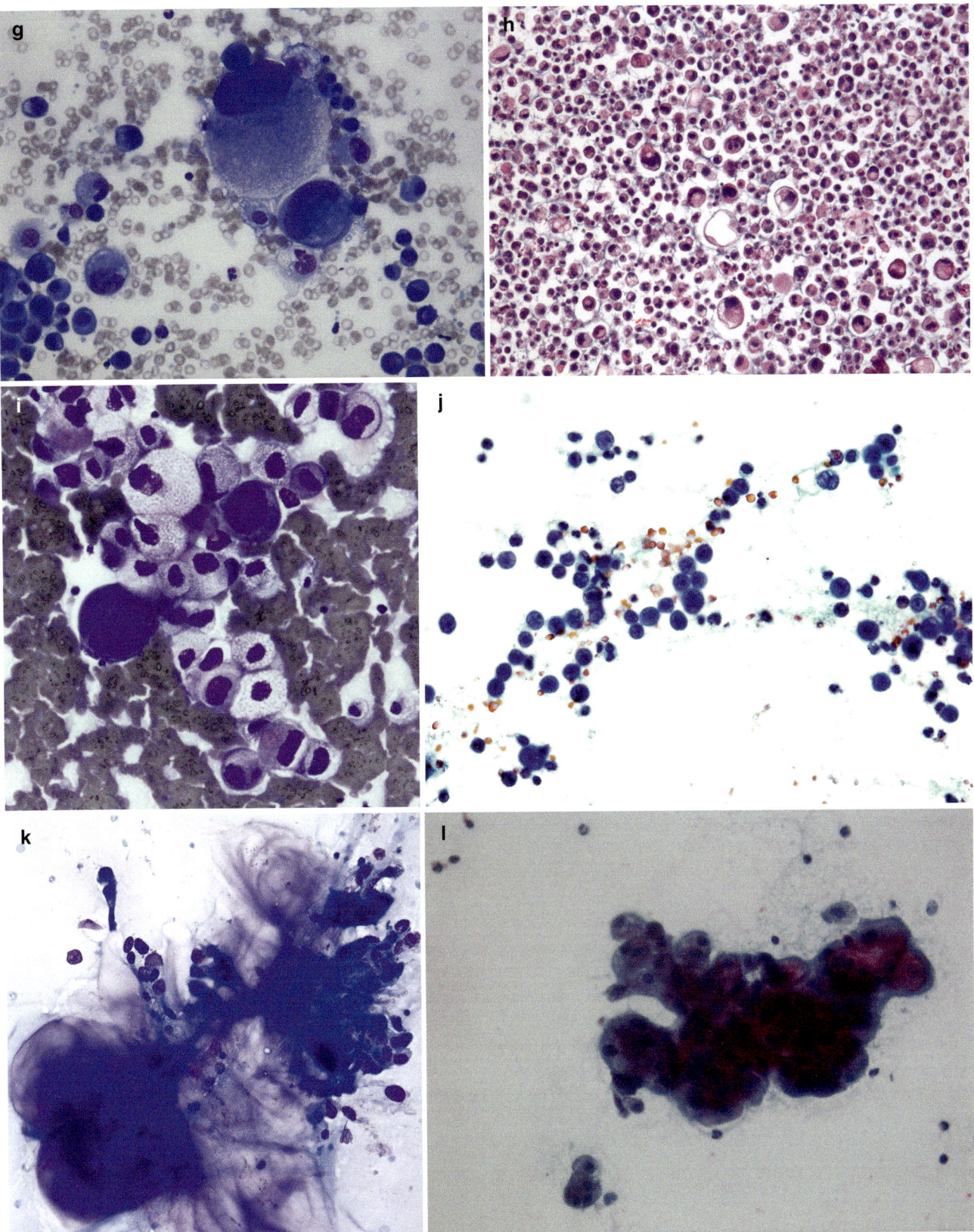

**Fig. 7.3** (continued)

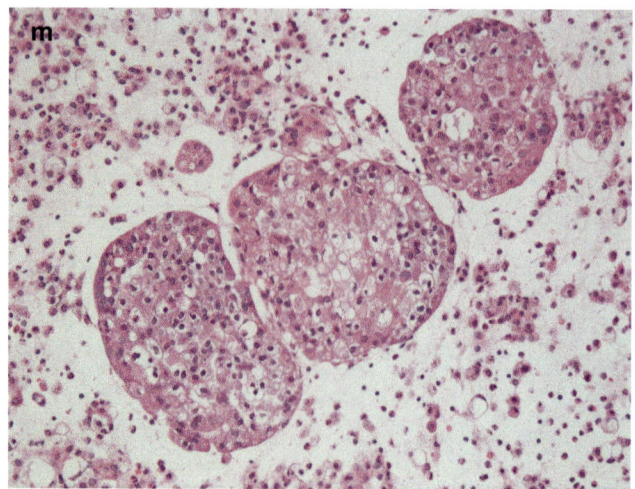

**Fig. 7.3** (continued)

Analysis of 167 specimens from 133 patients, including 17 with suspected HCC and 2 in which this diagnosis was previously made, resulted in no positive specimens [35].

Falconieri et al. reviewed smears from 106 patients with autopsy-proven HCC, of which 11 were positive. These had variable cellularity, with round or linear aggregates of polygonal cells with hyperchromatic or vesicular nuclei and inconspicuous nucleoli. Reactive changes were frequent [36]. Other authors noted a more frequent presence of neutrophils in the absence of superinfection in HCC ascites compared to specimens from patients with cirrhosis [37]. Two cases of sarcomatous HCC were reported [38]. Metastasis from a poorly differentiated HCC was diagnosed by one of the authors. In this effusion, the tumor consisted of large, highly atypical cells with irregular nuclear contours. Cells had variable n/c ratio, chromatin texture, and nucleolar size (Fig. 7.4a–d).

A case of cholangiocarcinoma effusion consisting of tumor cells with high n/c ratio, large nucleoli, and intracytoplasmic vacuoles, lying singly or in small groups, is shown in Fig. 7.4e, f. Another specimen, with immunostains, is shown in Fig. 7.4g–j.

A case of hepatoblastoma, the most common malignant liver tumor in children, was recently diagnosed by one of the authors. Tumor cells had epithelial morphology and nuclei with coarse chromatin and prominent nucleoli and was positive for Hep-Par1 (Fig. 7.4k–m).

## Esophageal Carcinoma

Esophageal cancer, another highly aggressive gastrointestinal cancer, ranks as the ninth most common and sixth cause of death worldwide. Squamous cell carcinoma, which affects primarily the upper and middle two-thirds of the esophagus, is the most common histological type world-

wide, whereas adenocarcinoma, which affects the middle and distal two-thirds of the organ, is the most common one in the USA and Europe. The proportion of the latter has been on the rise in recent years. Both entities are more common in men. Squamous cell carcinomas are strongly related to environmental factors, including smoking, alcohol consumption, exposure to very hot beverages, nitrosamines, and vitamin and mineral deficiency. Consumption of red meat increases disease risk, while fruit and vegetables have a protective effect. Adenocarcinomas are strongly related to gastroesophageal reflux and the presence of Barrett's esophagus, as well as to obesity, whereas consumption of fruit and vegetables and *Helicobacter pylori* infection are protective [39].

Malignant effusions due to metastatic esophageal carcinoma are infrequent. In a series of 85 patients with malignant pleural effusion, only 1 patient had a primary tumor of the esophagus [40].

Renshaw et al. reviewed 70 effusion specimens from 45 patients with biopsy-proven esophageal carcinoma [41]. Only 1 of 17 specimens from patients with squamous cell carcinoma contained tumor cells, compared to 21 of 53 effusions from adenocarcinoma cases. The latter were morphologically similar to adenocarcinomas of other origin, although some specimens were hypocellular, with few carcinoma cells.

The morphology of esophageal adenocarcinoma in effusions is as variable as it is in metastases from other organs. Cells may form cohesive groups with cells having irregular nuclei with vesicular chromatin and prominent nucleoli (Fig. 7.5a). Larger, more dissociated cells with mucin vacuoles of variable size may be seen (Fig. 7.5b), as well as areas with extracellular mucin (Fig. 7.5c). The primary tumor in this case was a well-differentiated adenocarcinoma (Fig. 7.5d). Other specimens consist of small cell groups or dissociated cells with high n/c ratio and very prominent nucleoli (Fig. 7.5e, f).

The squamous cell carcinoma case described by Renshaw had only three malignant cell groups, in which tumor cells had scant eosinophilic cytoplasm, high n/c ratio, and large hyperchromatic and irregular nuclei [41].

## Differential Diagnosis

The majority of metastatic adenocarcinomas of gastrointestinal origin present with easily identifiable malignant cells, making the possibility of a reactive effusion improbable, whereas a minority contain fewer tumor cells. Notably, reactive mesothelial cells in several conditions related to gastrointestinal malignancy, such as cirrhosis, may be extremely atypical, as are mesothelial cells exposed to chemotherapy and radiation. The previously discussed guidelines related to

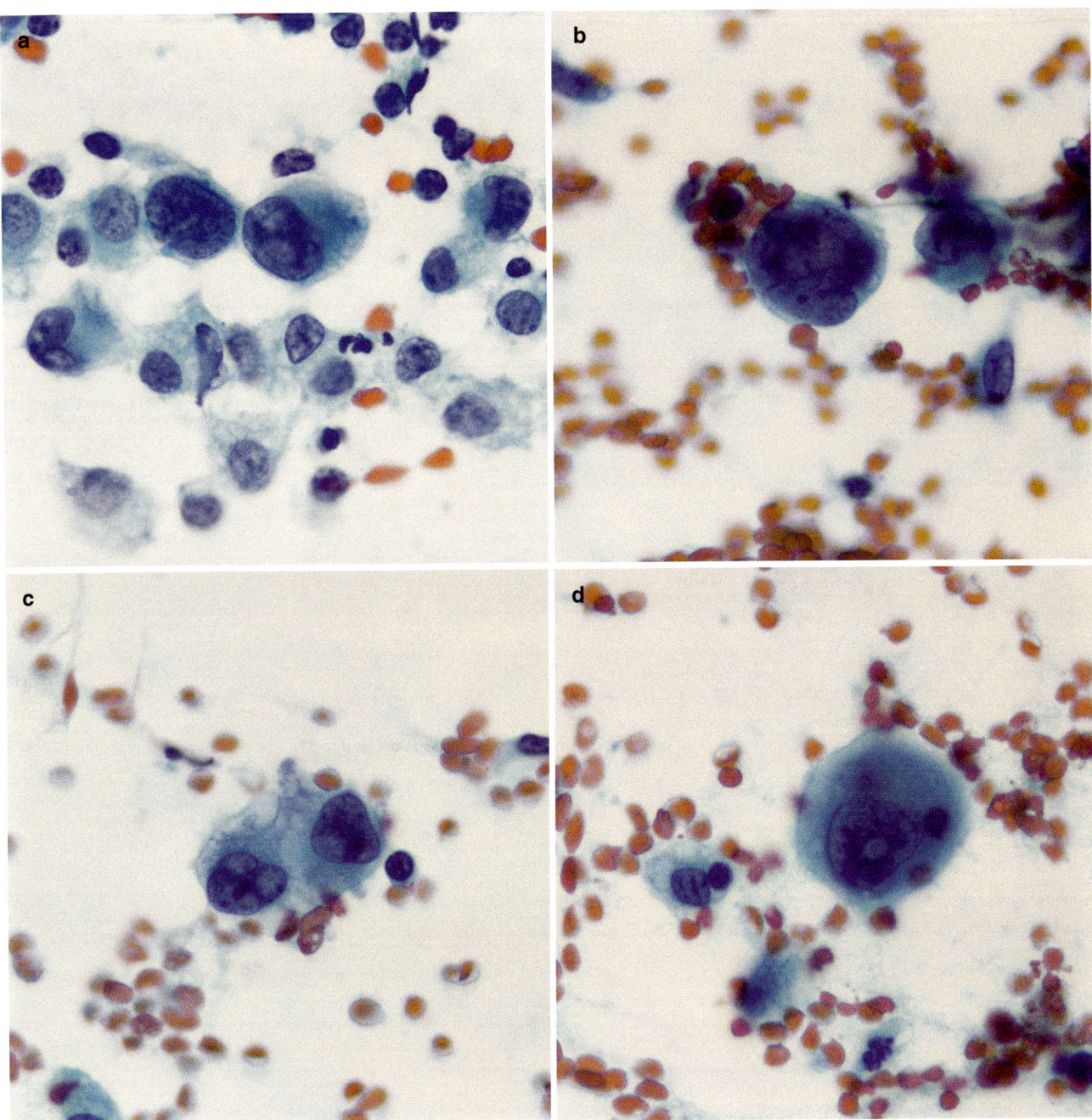

**Fig. 7.4** Liver carcinoma: (**a–d**) *hepatocellular carcinoma*. Large and overtly atypical cells, lying singly or in small groups, with variable amount of lacy, occasionally vacuolated cytoplasm, some with very high n/c ratio. (**e–j**) *cholangiocarcinoma*, consisting of smaller cells with intracytoplasmic vacuoles pushing the nuclei. The latter are a clue for the true nature of the cells, despite the presence of doublets that may mimic mesothelial cells (**f**). (**a–g**) PAP; (**h**) MGG/Diff-Quik; (**i**) Ber-EP4; (**j**) B72.3. (**k–m**) *hepatoblastoma*. Tumor cells have epithelial morphology and nuclei with coarse chromatin and prominent nucleoli. (**k**) PAP; (**l**) H&E; (**m**) Hep-Par1

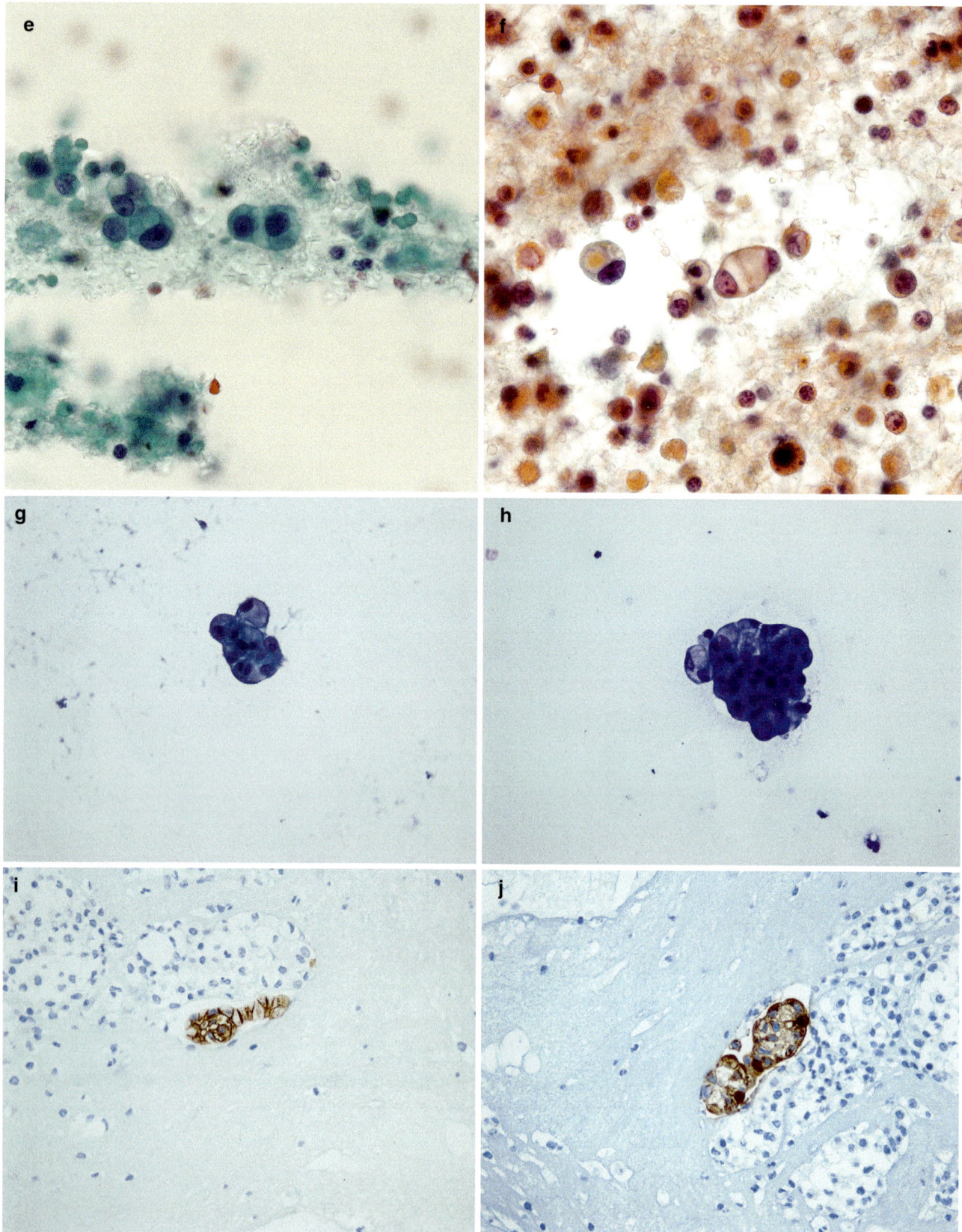

**Fig. 7.4** (continued)

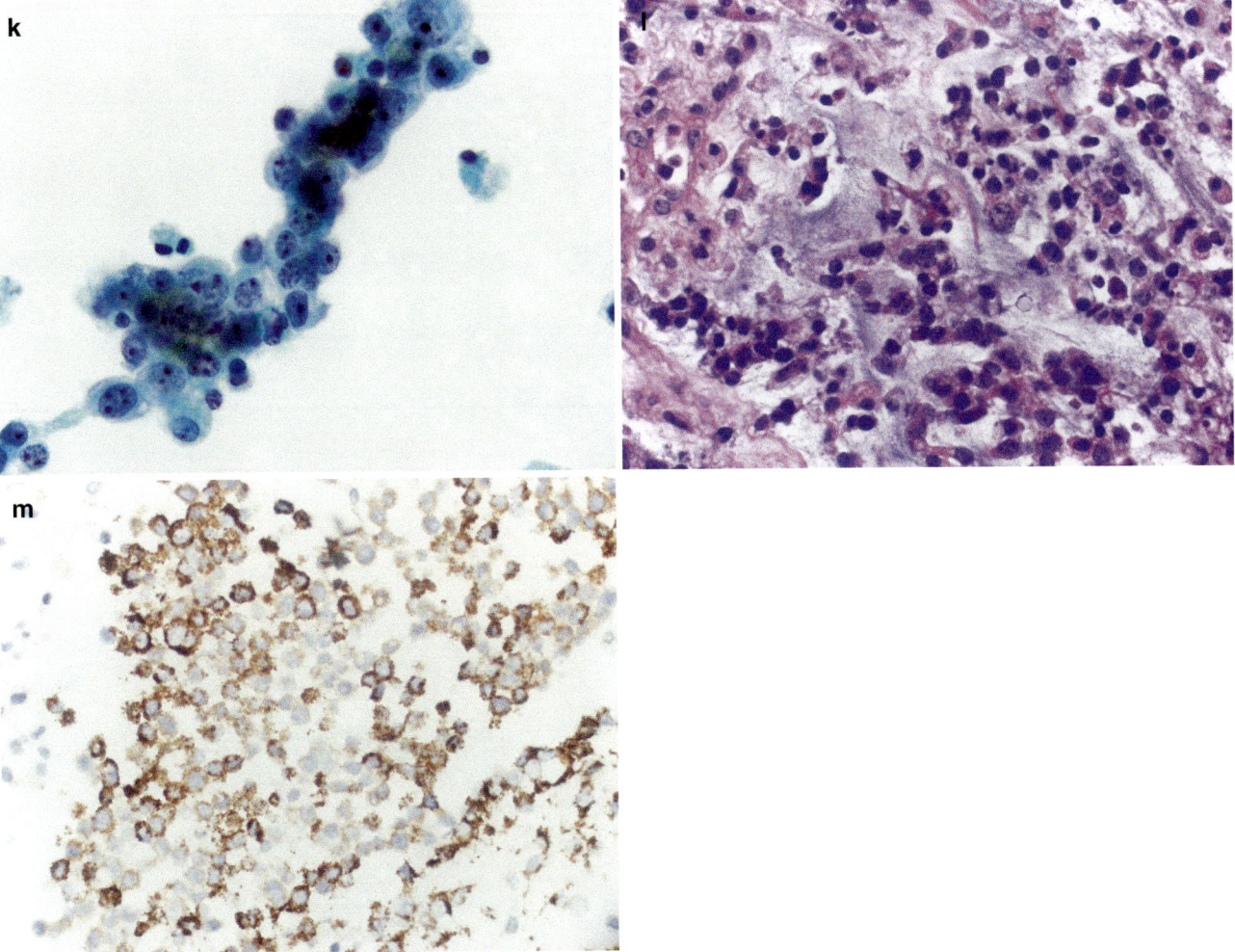

**Fig. 7.4** (continued)

identification of foreign cell population and pattern recognition apply to the diagnosis of these tumors in the same manner they are relevant for the diagnosis of other metastases. The immunohistochemical panels used for diagnosing effusions as adenocarcinoma are presented in the **Appendix** of **Part I**. Mucin stains may also be helpful (Fig. 7.6a).

Well- and moderately differentiated tumors that are recognized as adenocarcinoma need to be differentiated from metastases from other organs, primarily from gastrointestinal tumors of other origin, as well as lung, breast, and ovarian carcinoma. Poorly differentiated tumors, especially with single-lying tumor cells, must be differentiated from any malignant tumor, including carcinoma, mesothelioma, hematological malignancies, germ cell or stromal sex-cord tumors of the ovary, sarcoma, and melanoma. The choice of immunohistochemical panel should be directly influenced by the likelihood that a given tumor is *not* an adenocarcinoma. Markers expressed by tumors of gastrointestinal origin are CDX-2, Villin, CEA, and mucins

(Fig. 7.6b–e), as well as SATB2 in colon carcinoma. None of these is entirely specific, although strong expression of CDX-2 in the nuclei of all tumor cells is strongly suggestive of gastrointestinal origin. These markers are additionally poorly informative with respect to which organ along the gastrointestinal tract is the primary tumor site, as esophageal, gastric, pancreatic, and intestinal tumors have overlapping expression profiles. CK7/CK20 immunostaining may aid in localizing the primary tumor to the colon, as the majority of colonic adenocarcinomas are CK7-negative and CK20-positive (Fig. 7.6f). However, gastric, pancreatic, biliary, and esophageal carcinomas, as well as ovarian mucinous carcinomas, may have similar profile, with diffuse CK7 expression and focal or negative CK20 expression. HCC presents a distinct entity, as it expresses tumor markers shared by few other cancers, such as α-feto protein, glypican-3, Hep-Par1, and arginase-1 (see also Chap. 12). The above-discussed hepatoblastoma similarly expressed Hep-Par1 (Fig. 7.4m).

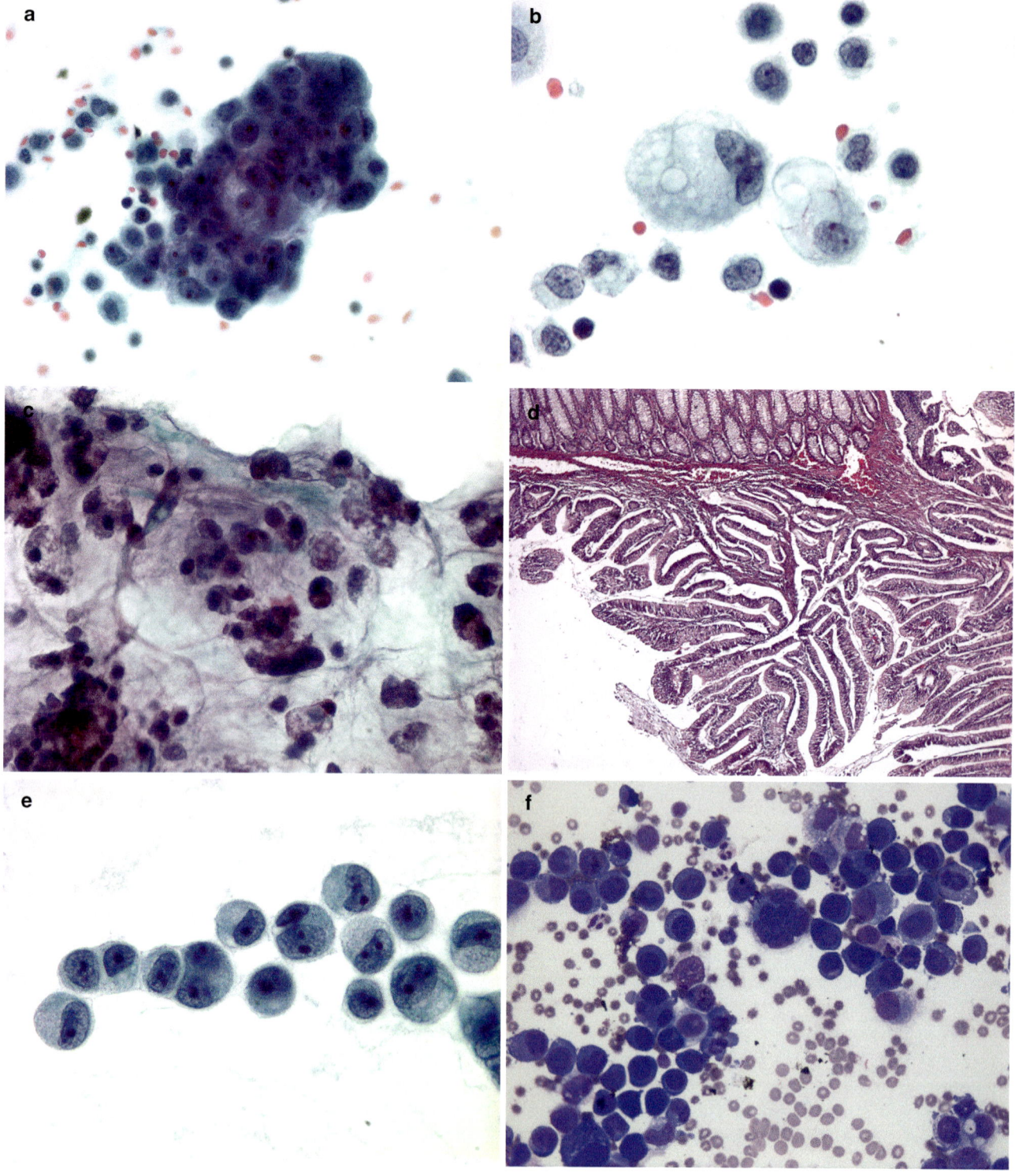

**Fig. 7.5** Esophageal carcinoma: (**a**) cohesive group; (**b**) single cells of variable size, some vacuolated; (**c**) mucin with embedded tumor cells; (**d**) the primary well-differentiated esophageal adenocarcinoma; (**e**) carcinoma cells with pronounced atypia; (**f**) dissociated poorly differentiated carcinoma. (**a**–**c**, **e**) PAP; (**d**) H&E; (**f**) Diff-Quik

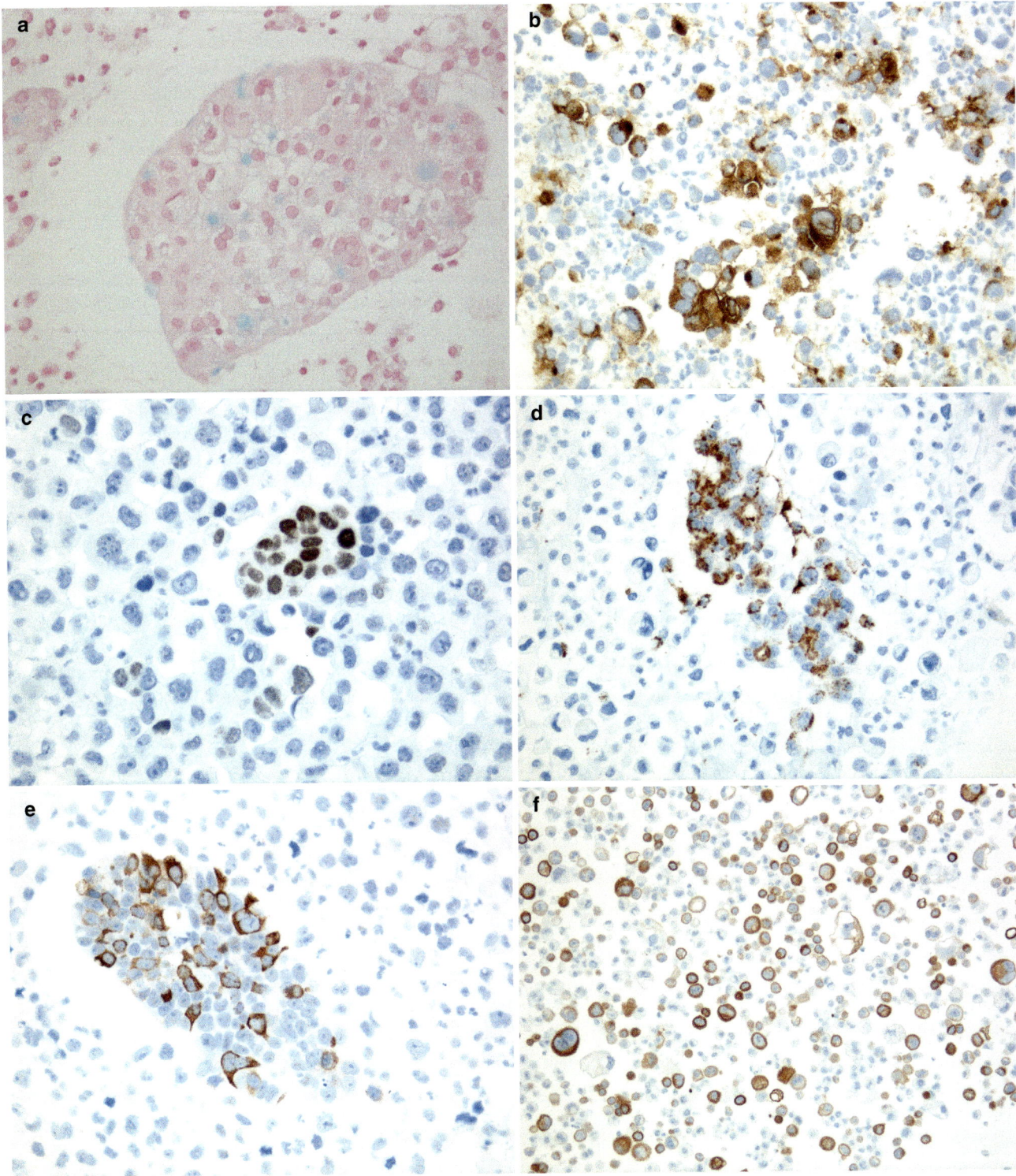

**Fig. 7.6** Histochemistry and immunohistochemistry in gastrointestinal cancers: (**a**) alcian blue stain in goblet cell carcinoid; (**b**) CEA in gastric carcinoma; (**c**) CDX-2 in esophageal adenocarcinoma; (**d**) MUC5AC in gastric carcinoma; (**e**) MUC2 in esophageal carcinoma; (**f**) CK20 in colon carcinoma

Negative markers that may be helpful in excluding gastrointestinal origin are lung carcinoma markers, including TTF-1, surfactant, and Napsin A; breast carcinoma markers such as GATA3, AP-15 (GCDFP-15), and mammaglobin; female genital carcinoma markers, including PAX8, WT-1, and Napsin A; renal cell carcinoma markers such as PAX8, RCC, and CA IX; and urothelial carcinoma markers such as GATA3 and Uro-II (see other chapters and **Appendix** in this section). Staining for hormone receptors may be helpful but should be interpreted cautiously, as some non-gynecologic tumors may express estrogen or progesterone receptor.

The rare squamous cell carcinomas of esophageal origin in effusion need to be differentiated from the more common tumors of pulmonary origin and rare metastases from head and neck and uterine cervix carcinoma. Relevant clinical information is usually available in such cases.

## Carcinomas of the Uterine Cervix and Corpus

Uterine cervix and uterine corpus cancer, consisting predominantly of carcinomas, are both common, ranking fourth and sixth in incidence in women worldwide. However, whereas cervical cancer is the fourth in causing cancer-related deaths, uterine corpus is not among the ten most common causes of cancer mortality globally and ranks tenth in developed countries [1]. This difference reflects both geographic variation and the biology and clinical behavior of these tumors. Cervical cancer is more common in developing countries, where both screening and treatment are sub-optimal, whereas uterine corpus cancer more often affects women in developing countries, where access to medical treatment is better [1]. Additionally, most uterine corpus carcinomas are diagnosed at earlier stage and consist of grade 1–2 endometrioid carcinomas, tumors that are less aggressive compared to carcinomas in other organs.

Metastatic spread from carcinoma of the uterine corpus or cervix to the serosal cavities is less common than in ovarian carcinoma, but is by no means a rare event, especially in the former cancer. Tumors of both origins are most frequently diagnosed in peritoneal effusions or washings, but dissemination to the pleural, and less frequently to the pericardial cavity, has been reported [42–51]. A case of metastatic cervical squamous cell carcinoma in a pericardial effusion was seen by one of the authors (Fig. 7.7a–c).

The vast majority of adenocarcinomas of the uterine corpus that are diagnosed in effusions originate from type II tumors, i.e., serous, clear cell, or poorly differentiated (grade 3) endometrioid carcinomas, although metastasis from type I carcinomas infrequently occurs. These tumors are morphologically impossible to differentiate from their counterparts of ovarian origin (see **Part I**, Chap. 3) (Fig. 7.7d-g).

Metastasis from cervical carcinoma more frequently originates from adenocarcinomas. The morphology of these tumors is usually nondescript and does not differ from that of other adenocarcinomas in effusions (Fig. 7.7h, i). Clinical data are therefore central to establishing the cervix as site of origin. Immunohistochemistry may be helpful, as discussed below.

Squamous cell carcinomas of cervical origin similarly resemble their counterparts in other organs (Fig. 7.7j–l). They may be of keratinizing or non-keratinizing type. Single cells or clusters of variable size are seen, as well as intercellular windows and cell-within-cell arrangement that may cause confusion with reactive mesothelial cells [42].

Rare reports describing the presence of other types of cervical carcinoma in effusions have been published. Metastasis from a mesonephric carcinoma in pleural effusion was reported [52]. Two cases of small cell neuroendocrine cervical carcinoma, of which one was in ascites and one in a pleural effusion, were described. The tumor presented with single cells with little molding, morphologically resembling lymphoma [53]. A primary cervical clear cell carcinoma with metastasis in ascites was reported [54], as well as recurrence of a primary cervical serous carcinoma in ascites [55]. One of the authors diagnosed a metastasis from a mucinous cervical carcinoma in a peritoneal effusion (Fig. 7.7m, n), as well as ascites with metastasis from a cervical adenocarcinoma with neuroendocrine differentiation (Fig. 7.7o, p).

### Differential Diagnosis

The majority of grade 1–2 endometrioid adenocarcinomas of the uterine corpus stain immunohistochemically positive for hormone receptors, PAX8, and vimentin, stain in a patchy pattern for p16, have wild-type p53 staining pattern, and show loss of PTEN and occasionally of ARID1A. They may be positive for HNF1β. Grade 3 endometrioid adenocarcinomas more often have aberrant (strongly and diffusely positive or completely absent) p53 expression and stain diffusely and strongly for p16, as do serous carcinomas. Clear cell carcinomas express Napsin A and HNF1β and may have loss of ARID1A. They are usually negative for hormone receptors, with variable p16 and p53 pattern. None of these features is particularly helpful in differentiating these tumors from their counterparts in the ovary/tube/peritoneum, although WT1 tends to be less expressed in serous carcinomas of uterine corpus origin compared to their adnexal or peritoneal counterparts. These stains may nonetheless help in excluding adenocarcinomas of other origin.

Both squamous cell carcinoma and adenocarcinoma of the cervix are often positive for CEA, p16, and CK7, and squamous cell carcinomas additionally express CK5/6, p63, and p40, while adenocarcinomas are positive for CK8 and

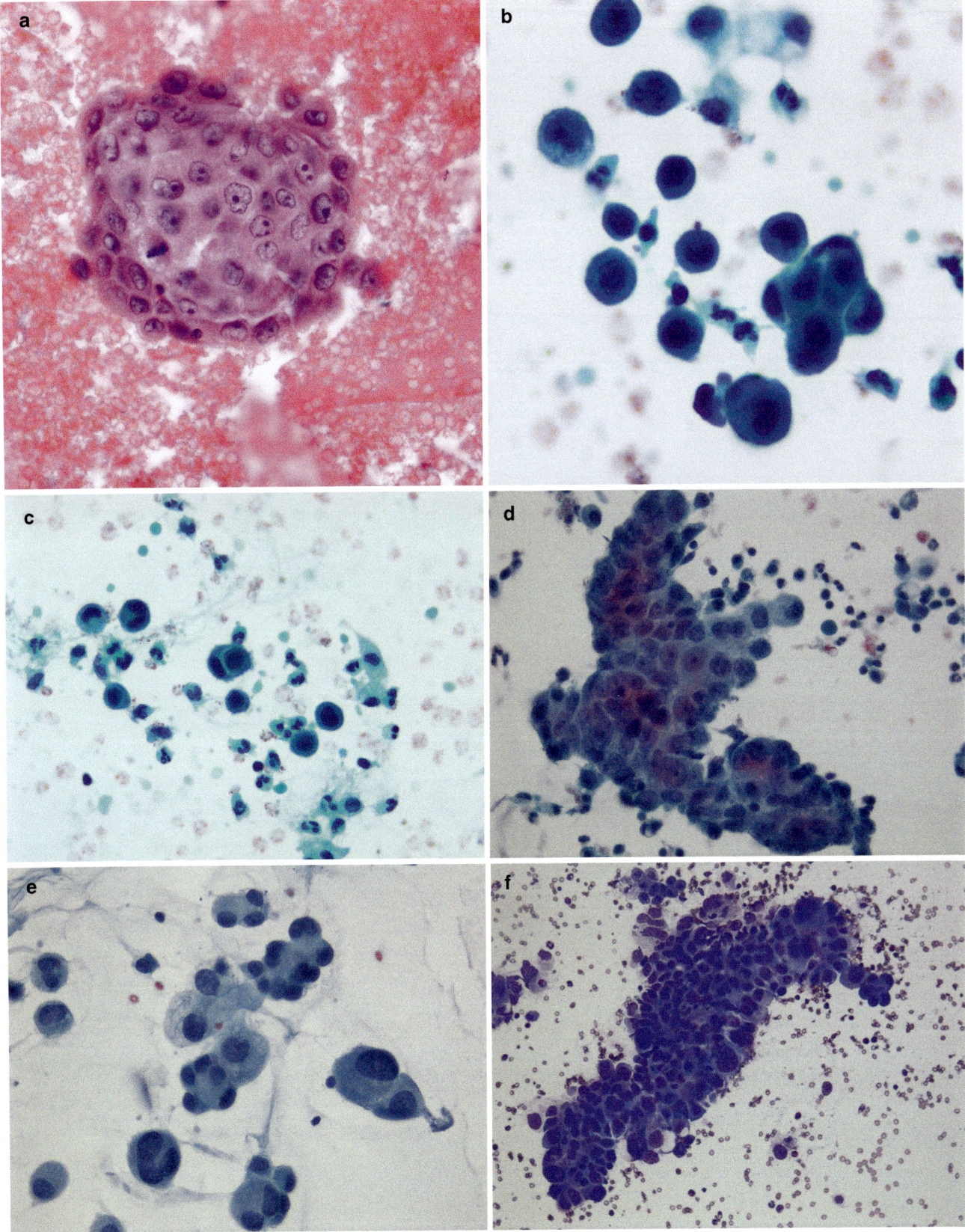

**Fig. 7.7** Cervical and endometrial carcinoma: (**a–c**) cervix squamous cell carcinoma in pericardial effusion. Note cell-in-cell arrangement in **c**; (**d**) serous carcinoma of the endometrium; (**e**) clear cell carcinoma of the endometrium; (**f, g**) Endometrial carcinosarcoma metastasizing as serous adenocarcinoma; (**h, i**) cervical adenocarcinoma; (**j–l**) cervical squamous cell carcinoma in a peritoneal effusion; (**m, n**) cervical muci-nous carcinoma; (**o**) cervical adenocarcinoma with neuroendocrine differentiation. (**a, g, i, k, n, o**) H&E; (**b–e, j, m**) PAP; (**f, h, l**) Diff-Quik. *Immunohistochemistry*: (**p**) synaptophysin in cervical adenocarcinoma with neuroendocrine differentiation; (**q–s**) cervical adenocarcinoma staining for Ber-EP4 (**q**), CEA (**r**), and p16 (**s**); (**t**) p63-positive in cervix squamous cell carcinoma in pericardial effusion

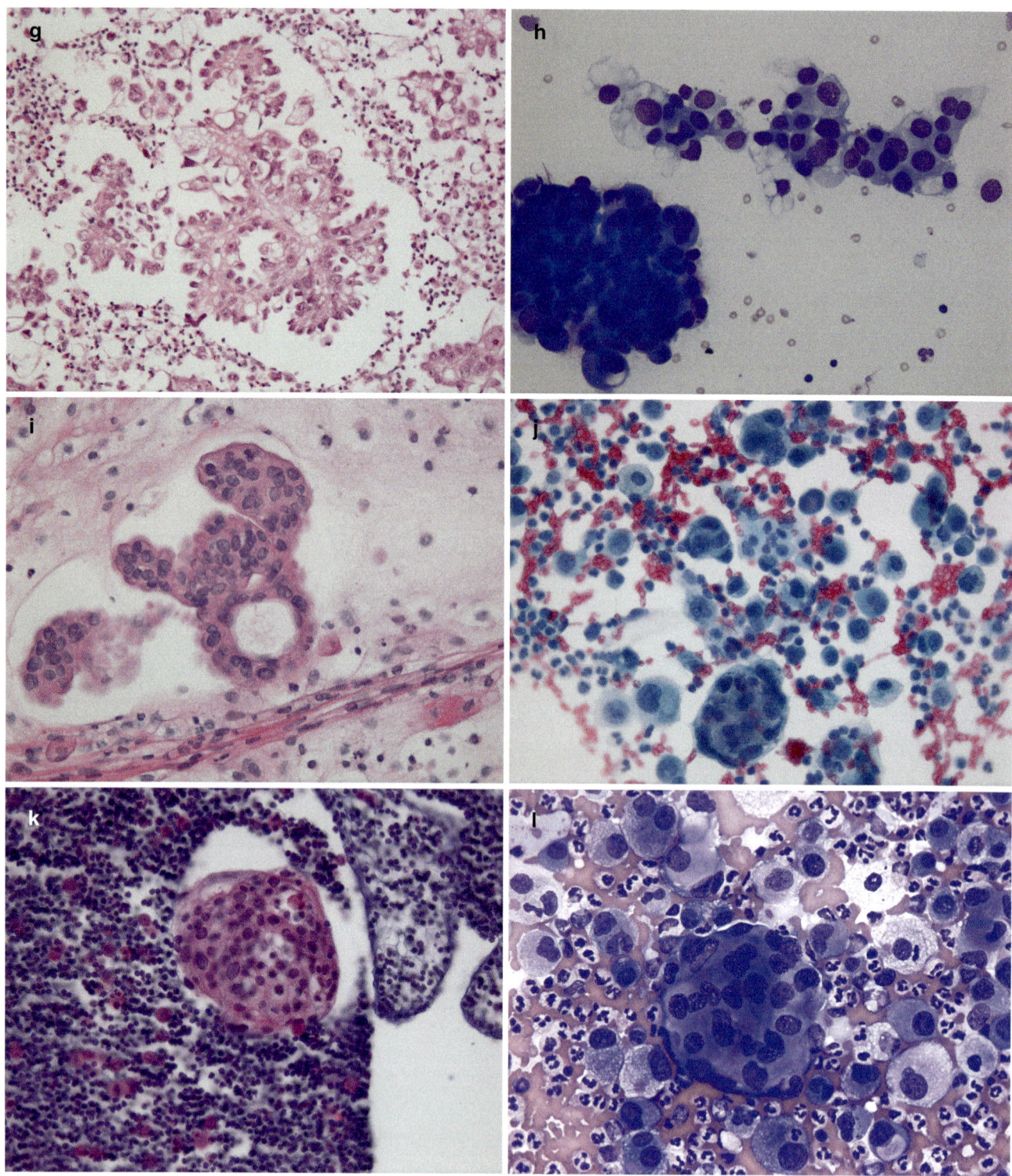

**Fig. 7.7** (continued)

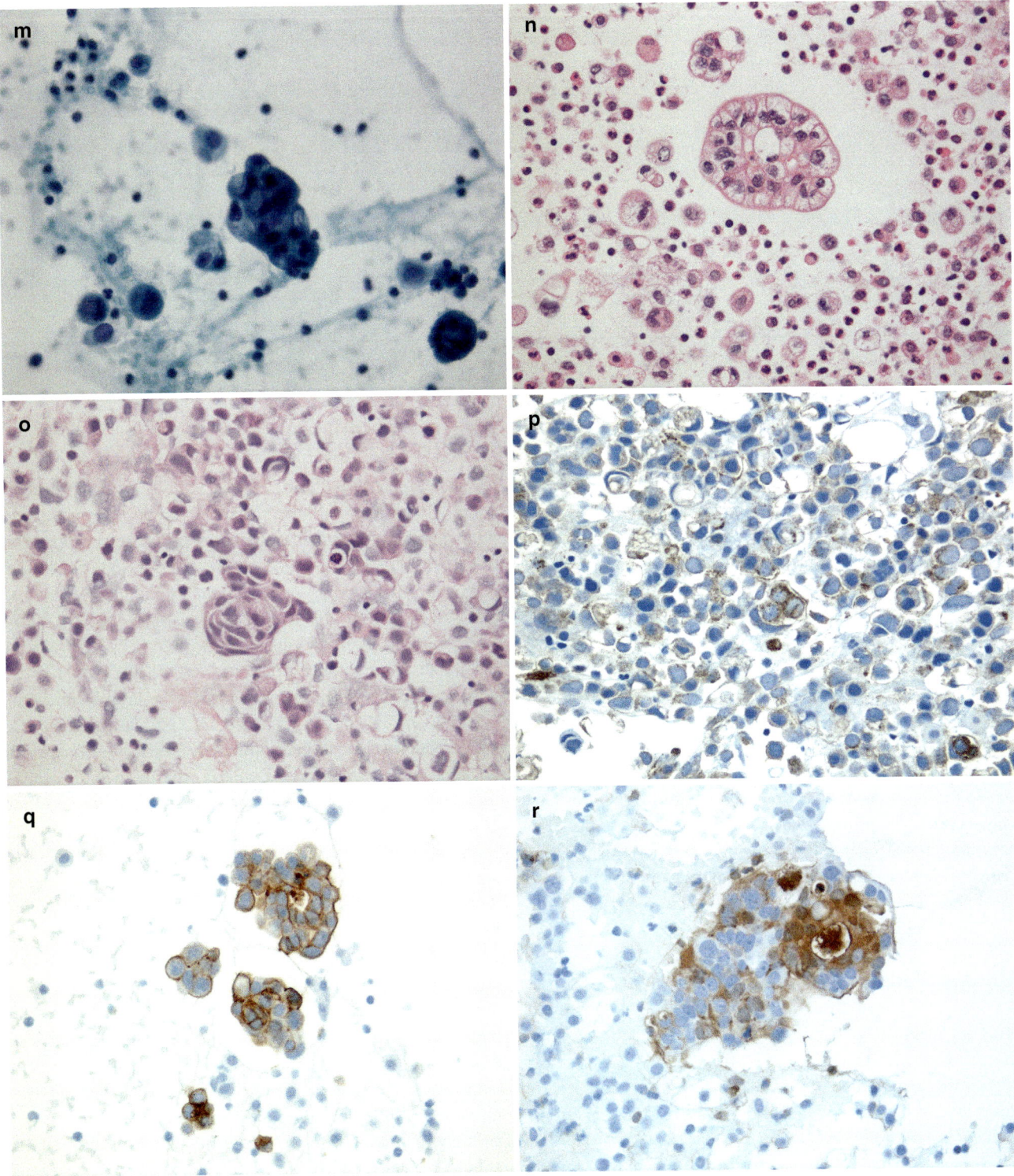

**Fig. 7.7** (continued)

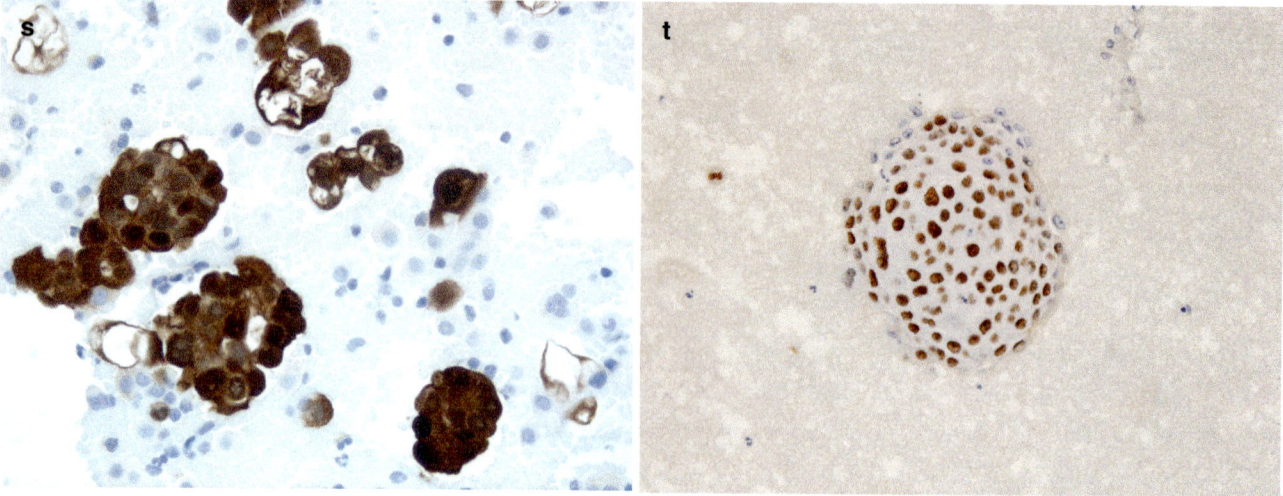

**Fig. 7.7** (continued)

Ber-EP4 (Fig. 7.7q–t). Overlaps in the staining pattern between these entities are not infrequent. Molecular genotyping for HPV may be of considerable help in establishing the cervical origin of a squamous cell carcinoma or adenocarcinoma.

## Genitourinary Carcinomas

Involvement of the serosal cavities by metastatic carcinomas originating in the urinary tract is an infrequent but well-documented entity. In a series of 472 malignant pleural effusions, 6% of metastases in males were from genitourinary organs [56]. The primary tumor may involve any of the genitourinary tract organs, including the kidney, prostate, and urinary bladder. All three serosal cavities may be involved, with pericardial involvement being the least common.

## Urinary Bladder Carcinoma

Tumors originating from the urinary bladder are usually transitional cell carcinomas [57–60], although two cases of signet ring cell carcinoma of bladder origin in ascites were described [61, 62], as well as metastasis from a transitional cell carcinoma of the renal pelvis [63].

Transitional cells carcinoma (TCC) may have variable morphologic features. Renshaw reviewed eight pleural effusions from five patients. Tumor cells had squamous or glandular morphology. Eosinophilic inclusions (Melamed-Wolinska bodies), which have been frequently observed in urine specimens and fine needle aspirates, were generally few, and their absence did not exclude the diagnosis of TCC [58]. McGrath et al. reported a case with numerous pleomor-

phic malignant cells, lying as single cells or in groups, in which numerous intracytoplasmic eosinophilic inclusions with clear halo were found. Few signet ring cells were additionally observed [57]. In the case reported by Fabozzi, tumor cells were found singly or in aggregates and had hyperchromatic nuclei of variable size with abundant cytoplasm. Only one cell had a large cytoplasmic vacuole [59]. Xiao found mostly dispersed tumor cells, as well as occasional small loose clusters, with moderate cellular pleomorphism, binucleation, and cell-in-cell arrangement. Cytoplasmic vacuoles and pseudo-windows were observed. Nuclei were centrally or paracentrally located and enlarged, with coarse chromatin, irregular nuclear membranes, and prominent eosinophilic nucleoli. Mitoses were rare [60].

A specimen with plasmacytoid morphology and another with pseudomesotheliomatous morphology were described [64, 65].

The largest series published to date, analyzed by one of the authors, included 25 specimens (15 pleural, 8 peritoneal, and 2 pericardial effusions) from 20 patients with urothelial carcinoma [66]. The predominant morphological pattern was of a single cell population with or without clusters or short cords, frequently with "cell wrapping." Nuclear enlargement with increased n/c ratio, irregular nuclear membranes, hyperchromatic coarse chromatin, and prominent nucleoli were observed, as were double or multinucleated cells, cells with vacuolated cytoplasm, or signet ring cells. These morphological characteristics were deemed non-specific, emphasizing the importance of patient history and ancillary techniques.

In selected specimens shown in this chapter, cells were predominantly found in clusters of variable size, including papillary structures and looser aggregates (Fig. 7.8a–c). Indian file-like arrangement was seen in one case

(Fig. 7.8d). Nuclei were enlarged, hyperchromatic, and overtly atypical. Nucleoli were prominent and mitoses were readily found (Fig. 7.8e). Distinct cell borders, cytoplasmic vacuolization, and a possible attempt to form eosinophilic vacuoles were additionally seen (Fig. 7.8f). Cell-in-cell arrangement was seen in another specimen (Fig. 7.8g). The degree of atypia appeared somewhat milder in the H&E-stained cell blocks in one case, but mitoses were evident there as well (Fig. 7.8h).

TCC express CK7, CK20, and CEA, as well as high-molecular-weight-keratin 34βE12 and more organ-specific markers such as GATA3, uroplakin II and III, and carbonic anhydrase IX. The combination of CK7, CK20, and CEA generally excludes many of the carcinomas that enter this differential diagnosis (e.g., breast, lung, and colon adenocarcinoma), although exceptions occur, but does not exclude adenocarcinomas of the upper gastrointestinal tract or ovarian mucinous carcinoma. Consequently, the more specific markers are often used to establish urothelial origin. The case shown in Fig. 7.8e, f, h expressed CK7, CK20, and high-molecular-weight keratin 34βE12 (Fig. 7.8i–k) but was negative for CEA and uroplakin III. A tumor with uroplakin II expression is shown in Fig. 7.8l.

## Prostate Carcinoma

Prostate carcinoma metastases most frequently involve the pleural cavity [67, 68]. However, Saif reported a case in which malignant ascites was the only manifestation of metastatic disease [69], and a subsequent review of the literature in the years 1969–2005 revealed 12 patients with malignant ascites due to prostate carcinoma, either at diagnosis or at disease recurrence [70]. As with bladder carcinoma, an ascites specimen with signet ring cell morphology was reported [71].

Mai et al. reviewed 50 cytological specimens, including 6 pleural effusions. Tumor cells formed clusters with overlapping nuclei or sheets of cells. The cytoplasm varied from filmy to dense with indistinct cytoplasmic borders. Nuclei were usually round or oval, uniform, and hyperchromatic with a single nucleolus. Multinucleated tumor cells were not seen [67].

Renshaw reviewed 14 pleural effusions from ten patients. Specimens contained isolated tumor cells or small loosely cohesive groups. Cells had scant cytoplasm, round to oval nuclei, irregular nuclear borders, and prominent nucleoli. Three patients had small cell carcinoma, and these metastases were morphologically different [68]. Specimens seen by the authors had comparable morphology to that described in these two series (Fig. 7.9a–d), although mitoses, distinct cell borders, and cytoplasmic clearing were seen in one

specimen (Fig. 7.9e). Another tumor had open acinar structures in addition to the more common solid groups (Fig. 7.9f).

Prostate carcinomas express prostate-specific antigen (PSA), p504s (AMACR), prostate-specific acid phosphatase (PAP), prostate-specific membrane antigen (PSMA), and p501S (prostein) [72]. However, negative staining for some of these markers can be seen in adenocarcinoma, particularly metastatic ones. It is therefore advisable to use several markers. One of the above-illustrated cases did express PSA, p504s, and PAP (Fig. 7.9g–i), while others were negative for one or two of these three markers.

## Renal Carcinoma

The diagnosis of renal cell carcinoma (RCC) in serous effusions is a relatively rare one. In the series by Sears and Hajdu, 19/812 malignant pleural and 3/456 malignant peritoneal effusions originated from renal adenocarcinomas [73]. In the study by Spieler and Gloor, only 2/448 specimens were from patients with RCC [6].

Renshaw et al. studied eight RCC effusions, consisting of both clear cell and papillary carcinomas, and were able to differentiate these histological types in effusion only when well-defined papillae were present. Specimens had variable cellularity. Tumor cells were single or in clusters and had abundant clear to granular and vacuolated cytoplasm, large nuclei, vesicular or clumped chromatin, and large nucleoli [74]. Gupta et al. recently reported two cases, consisting of one clear cell and one papillary RCC, with emphasis on the occasionally bland morphology of this tumor which may be overlooked [75].

Specimens seen by two of the authors consisted of large cells with ample clear, foamy, or eosinophilic cytoplasm, vesicular nuclei with coarse chromatin, and large nucleoli, lying singly or in groups of variable size (Fig. 7.10a–h).

Several of the less common variants of renal carcinoma, including two cases of chromophobe RCC [76, 77], two cases of medullary carcinoma [78], and two cases of collecting duct carcinoma [79], have been diagnosed in effusions. Drut diagnosed a renal rhabdoid tumor in a 4-month-old patient who later developed malignant pleural effusion [80].

RCC expresses several immunohistochemical markers, including vimentin (Fig. 7.10i), EMA (Fig. 7.10j), PAX8 (Fig. 7.10k), CD10 (Fig. 7.10l), PAX2, and carbonic anhydrase IX (CA IX) (Fig. 7.10m). Chute and co-workers recently analyzed 11 RCC effusions, of which 6 were clear cell carcinomas, 3 papillary, and 2 RCC, not otherwise specified. CD10 and RCC antigen were expressed in 10/11 and 5/11 cases, respectively. PAX2 staining was negative or

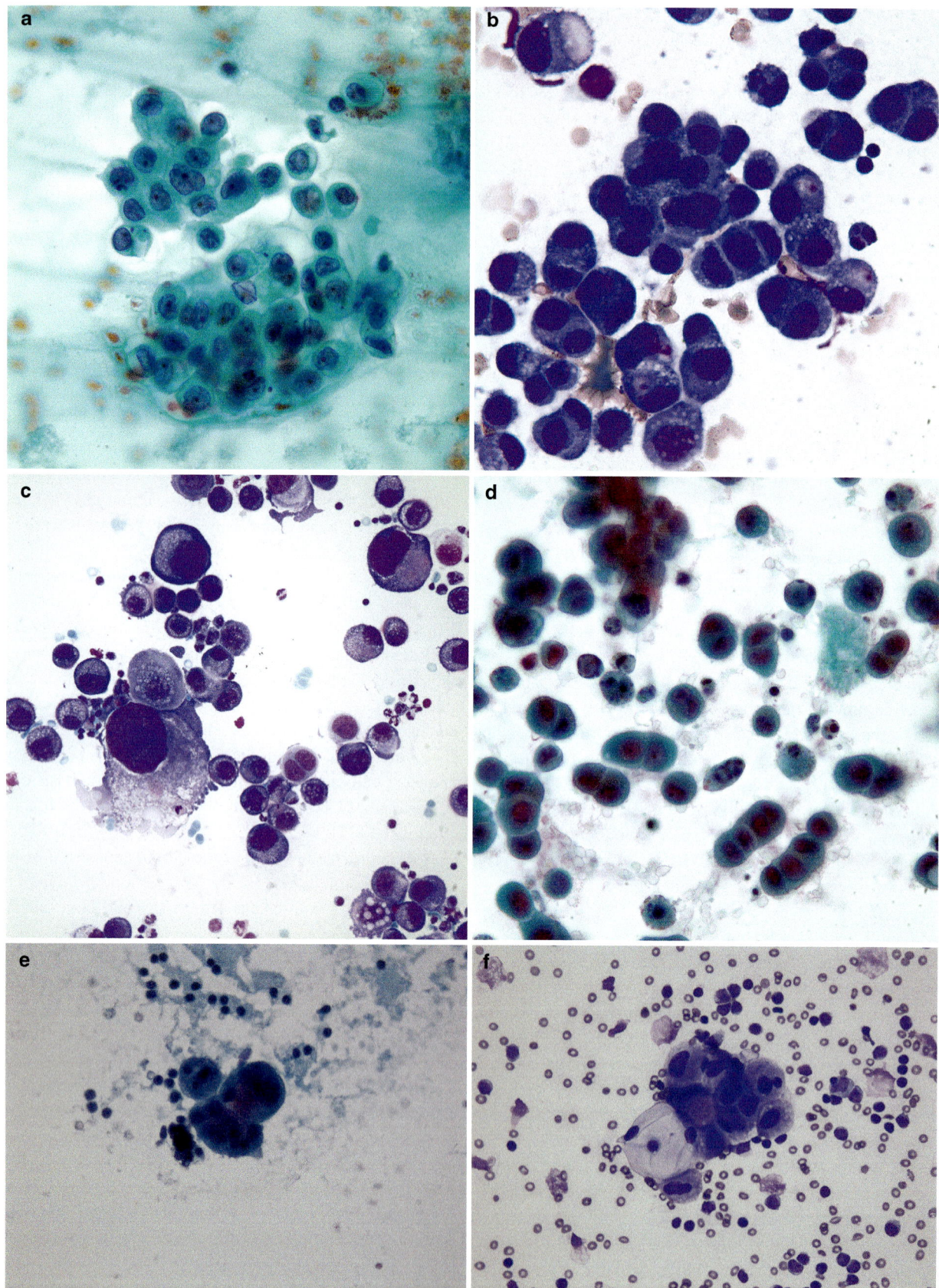

**Fig. 7.8** Transitional cell carcinoma: (**a**, **b**) papillary groups; (**c**) vacu-olated pleomorphic cells; (**d**–**f**) overtly atypical cells dissociated, in short cords and in small tight clusters. Note attempt to form eosino-philic core in **d**, **e**; (**g**) cell-in-cell arrangement; (**h**) two mitotic figures in a cell group with relatively mild atypia. (**a**, **d**, **e**, **g**) PAP; (**b**, **c**, **f**) MGG/Diff-Quik; (**h**) H&E. *Immunohistochemistry*: staining for CK7 (**i**), CK20 (**j**), and 34βE12 (**k**) in the case shown in **h**. Uroplakin II stain is shown in **l**

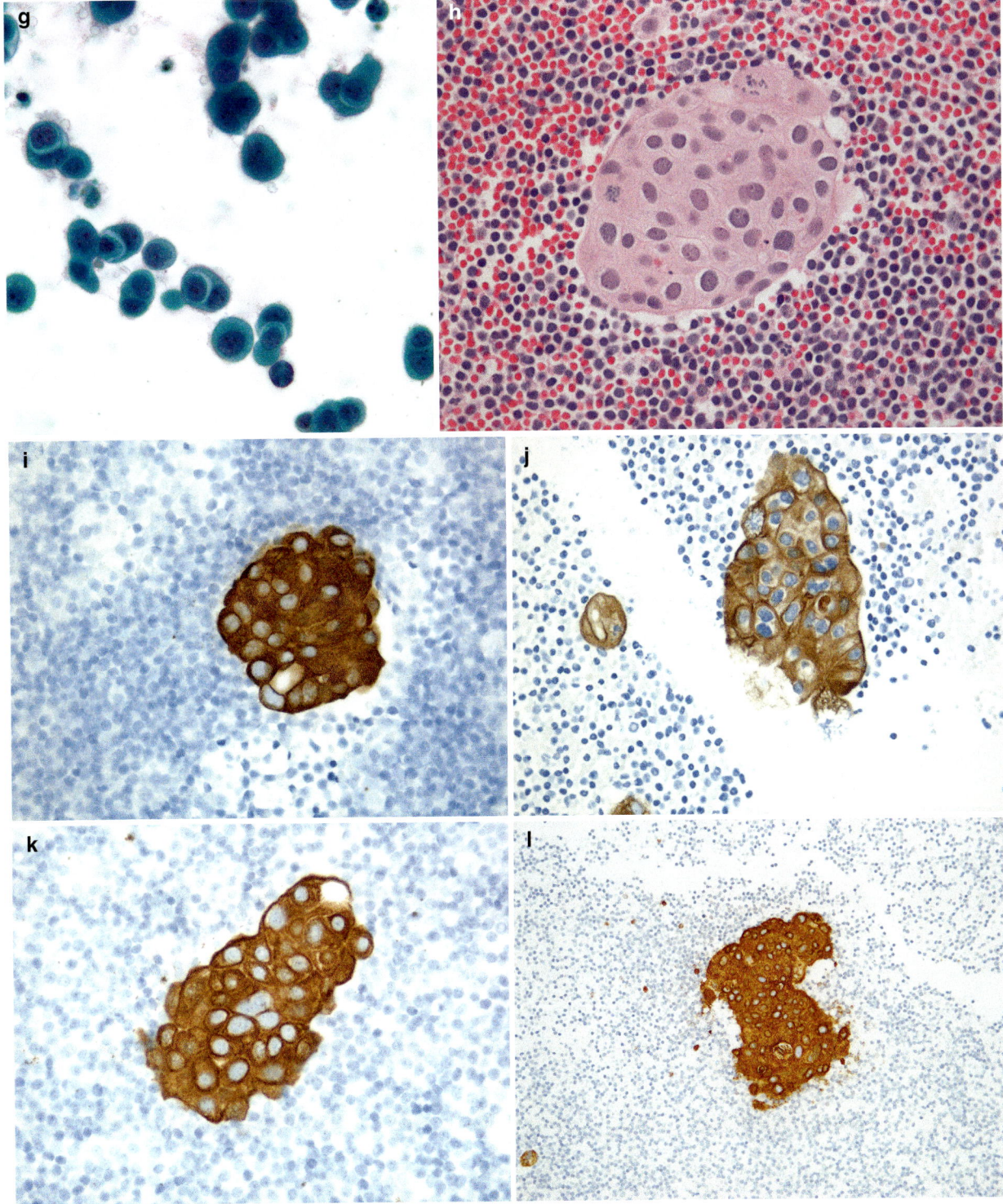

**Fig. 7.8** (continued)

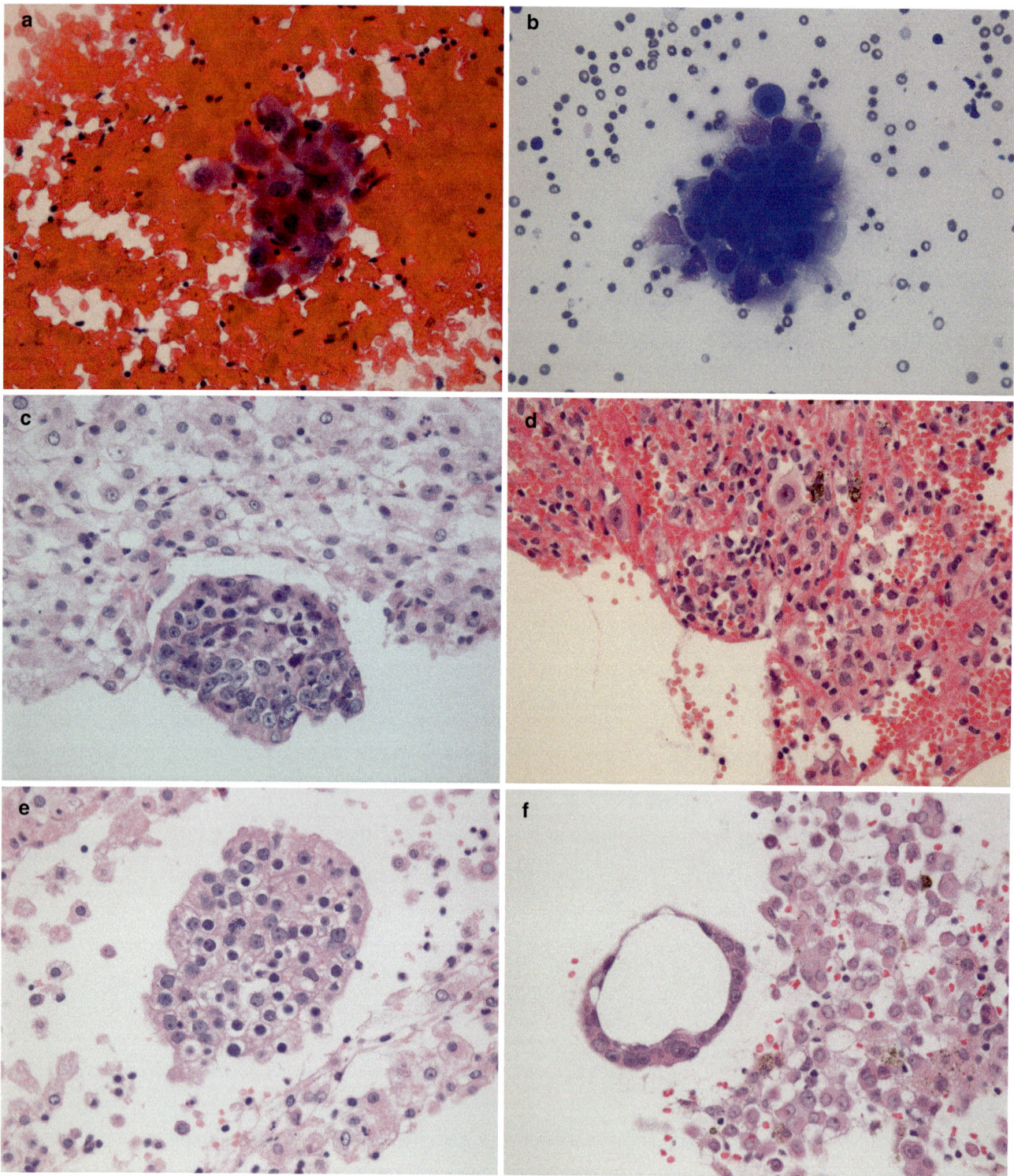

**Fig. 7.9** Prostate carcinoma: (**a–c**) cohesive groups with atypical tumor cells having prominent nucleoli; (**d**) single-lying tumor cells; (**e**) mitosis; (**f**) open acinar form. (**a**) PAP; (**b**) Diff-Quik; (**c–f**) H&E.

*Immunohistochemistry*: staining for PSA (**g**), p504s (**h**), and 34βE12 (**i**) in the case shown in **f**

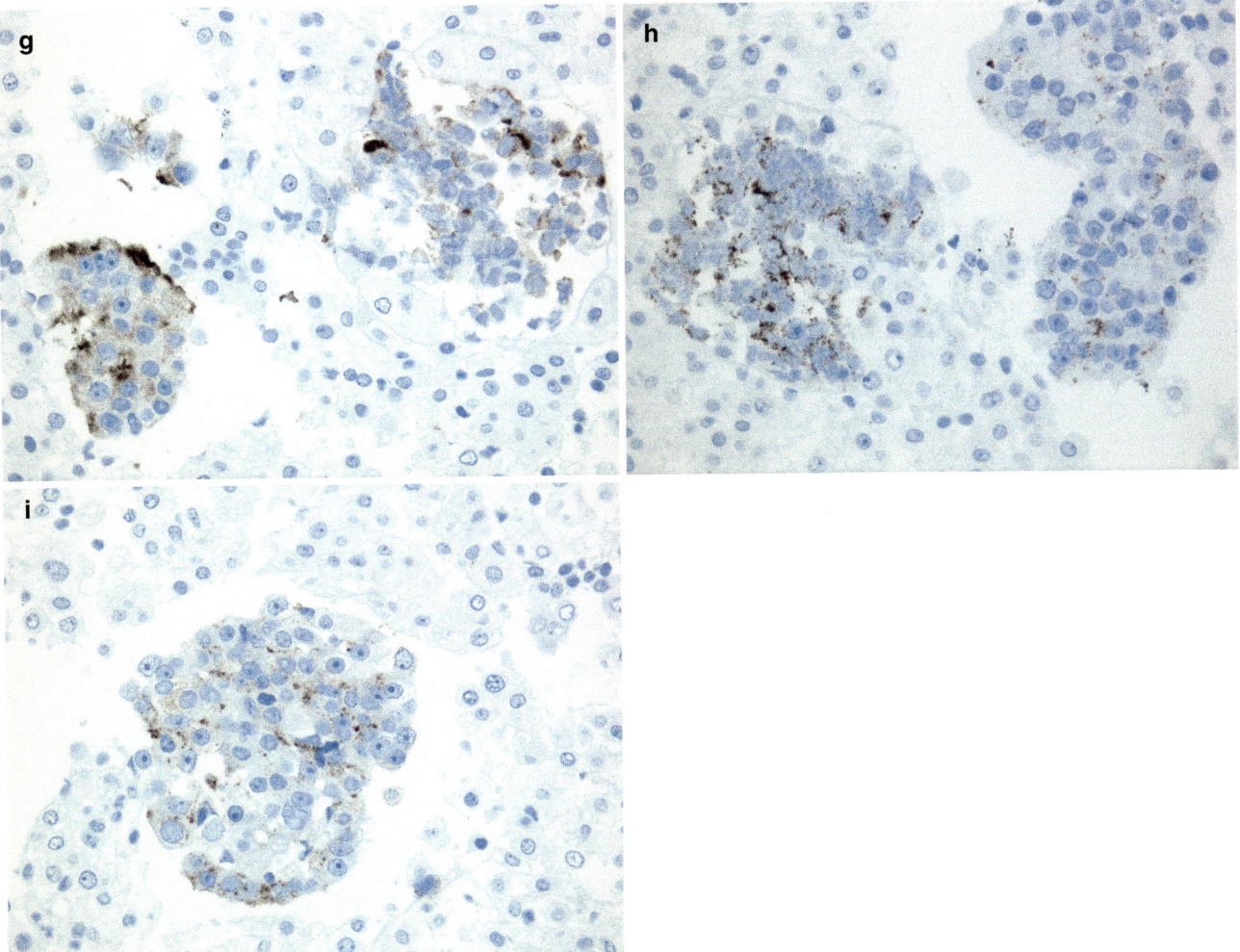

**Fig. 7.9** (continued)

equivocal in RCC cells, whereas reactive mesothelial cells had strong cytoplasmic staining [81]. In contrast, in analysis of 24 cytological RCC specimens, including 4 effusions, both PAX2 and PAX8 were found to be sensitive markers, expressed in 83% and 88% of cases, respectively [82]. In the series of Waters et al., all tumors (eight and nine RCC effusions analyzed for PAX2 and PAX8 expression, respectively) were positive for both markers [83]. The single RCC in the series of Wiseman and co-workers expressed PAX8 and was negative for PAX2 [84], and the single RCC in the Tong series was similarly PAX8-positive [85].

## Other Cancers

### Germ Cell Tumors

Spreading of germ cell tumors to effusions is well-recognized and has been documented in both large series and case reports [86–96]. The majority of these tumors had their primary site in the ovary, although metastasis from other organs, mainly from the testis, has been reported. The series of Hajdu and Nolan included a total of 58 positive effusions from patients with germ cell tumors, including 26 pleural, 30 peri-

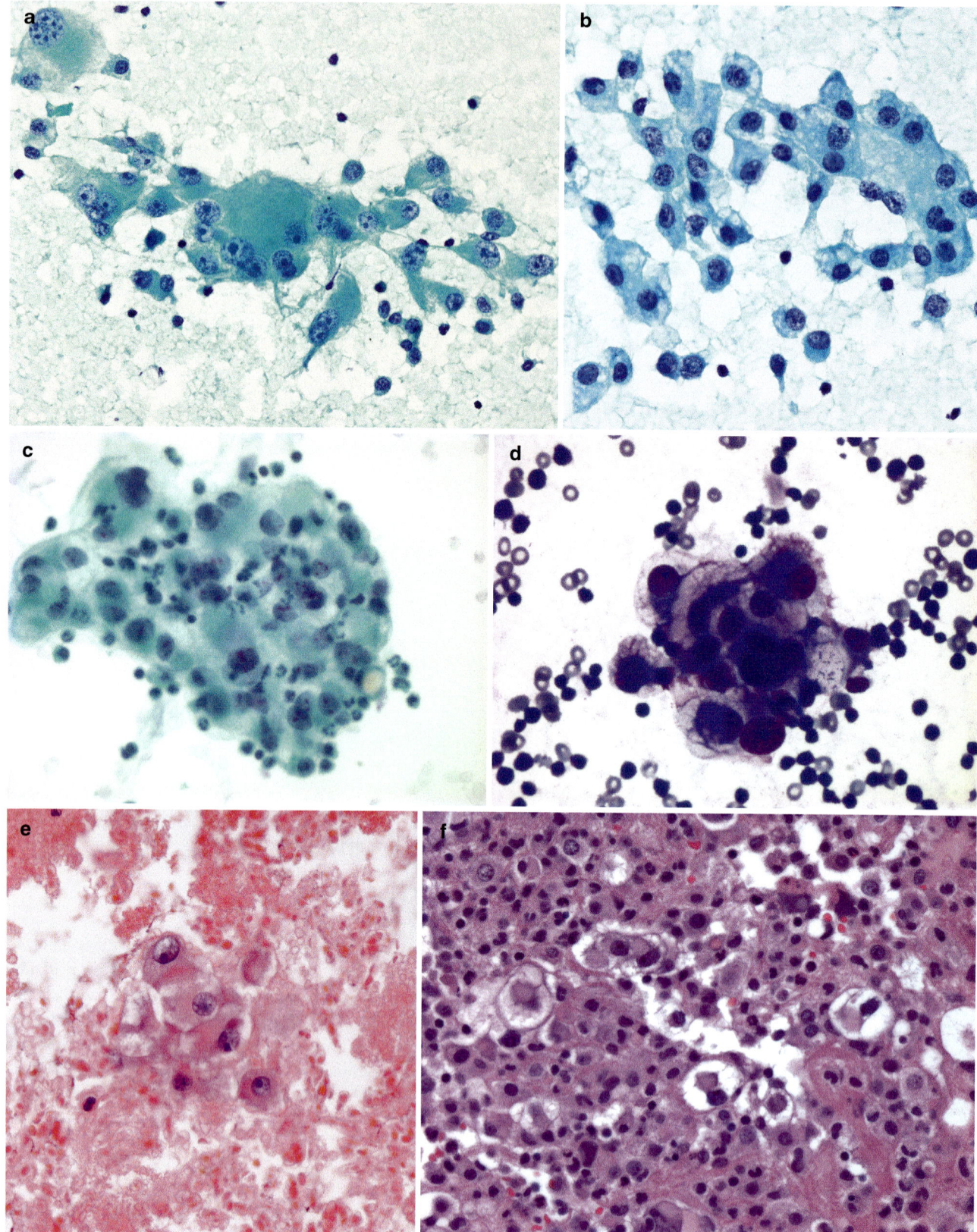

**Fig. 7.10** Renal cell carcinoma: (**a–h**) atypical tumor cells with clear or eosinophilic cytoplasm in loose groups, doublets, or singly. (**a–c, h**) PAP; (**d, g**) Diff-Quik; (**e, f**) H&E. *Immunohistochemistry*: staining for vimentin (**i**), EMA (**j**), PAX8 (**k**), CD10 (**l**), and CA IX (**m**)

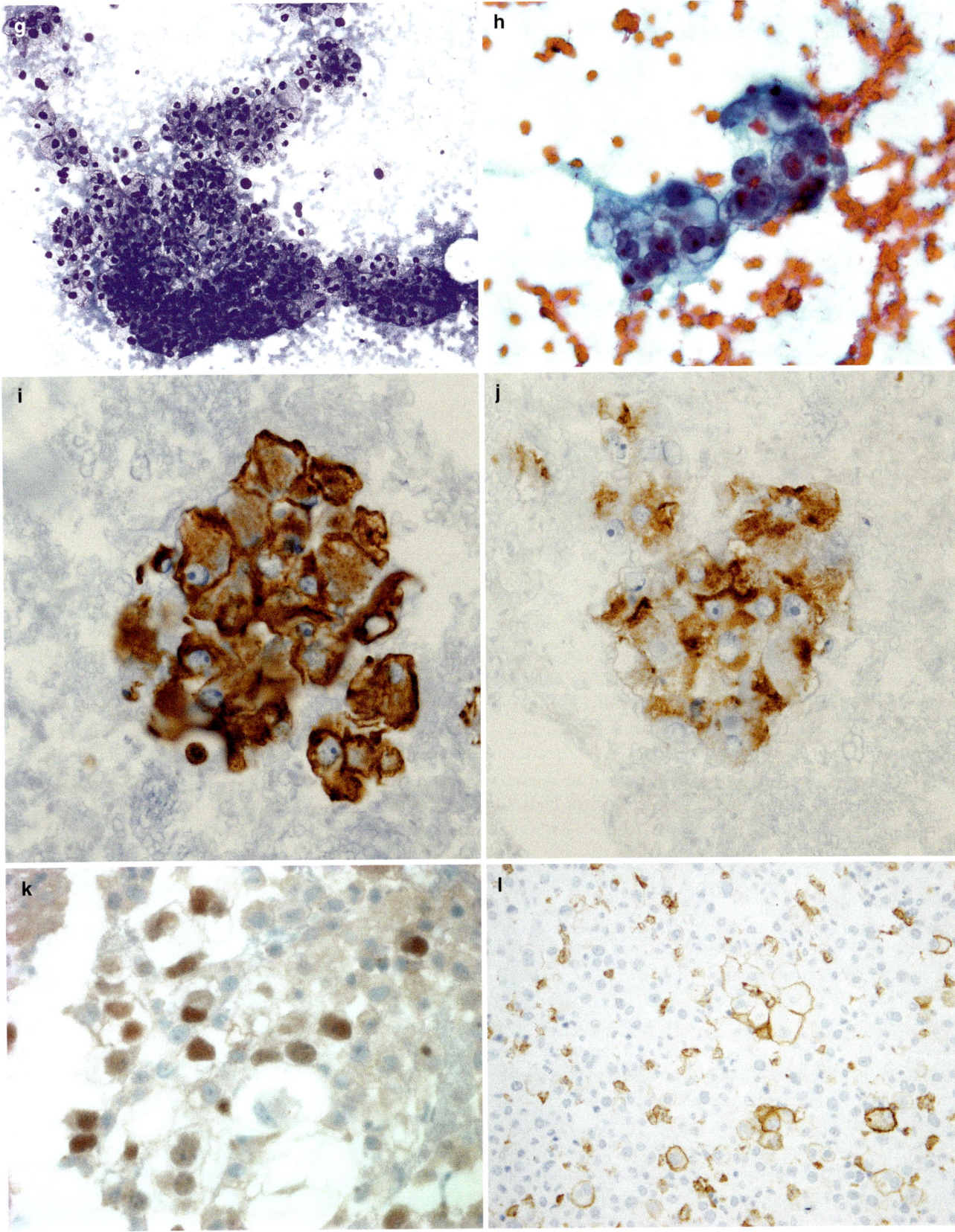

**Fig. 7.10** (continued)

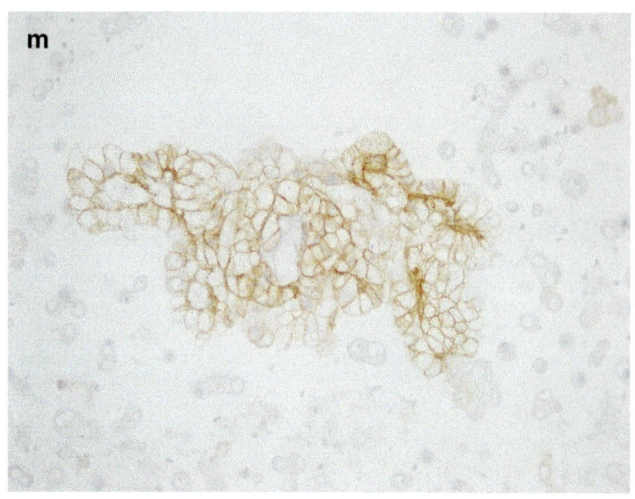

**Fig. 7.10** (continued)

toneal, and 2 pericardial specimens [86]. Geisinger et al. reviewed 780 exfoliative cytology specimens from 144 patients younger than 17 years of age with nonlymphoreticular neoplasms. Among the 120 malignant pleural and peritoneal effusions reviewed, 12 were metastases from germ cell tumors [87]. Germ cell tumors constituted 8% of 88 malignant effusions in the series of Wong et al. [88].

Seminoma and dysgerminoma cells are uniform, with variable cytoplasm, and large oval or round centrally located nuclei with fine chromatin and prominent nucleoli. Cells are observed mostly as single-lying or in pairs [86, 87, 92]. Abe observed atypical cells with hyperchromatic nuclei and high nucleus/cytoplasm ratio in a metastatic testicular seminoma [94]. The dysgerminoma case seen by one of the authors similarly consisted of overtly atypical cells with high n/c ratio and large nucleoli, lying singly or in small groups (Fig. 7.11a, b).

Cells originating from Yolk sac tumors (endodermal sinus tumors) were described as small, dark, and cuboidal, lying in clusters [86]. Roncalli et al. observed loosely arranged irregular or papillary groups consisting of cells with ill-defined microvaculated cytoplasm, high n/c ratio, and prominent nucleoli. In cell block sections, tubular and microcystic structures were seen, as well PAS- and AFP-positive hyaline globules [90]. Comparable findings were described by Valente [92] and seen by one of the authors. In the latter case, the hyaline material was evident in the MGG-stained smears (Fig. 7.11c, d).

Embryonal carcinoma cells in effusions were described as relatively small pleomorphic cells with hyperchromatic nuclei and pale or poorly preserved cytoplasm. Cells were observed singly, in nondescript clusters or in glandular structures [87].

Rare reports of immature teratomas in effusion specimens have been published [87, 91, 93, 95]. Geisinger reported a case in an 11-year-old patient with a large grade III ovarian teratoma, in which the cells in pleural effusions resembled neuroblastoma [87]. Selvaggi reported two cases, of which one consisted of ependymal elements, and the second one of neuroepithelial elements [91, 93]. In the case reported by Ikeda, immature neuroepithelial cells forming rosette-like structures were admixed with keratinized squamous cells, squamoid metaplastic cells, and immature glial-appearing cells [95]. A specimen seen by one of the authors is shown in Fig. 7.11e–g.

The presence of choriocarcinoma in cytological specimens was reported [86] but is probably a very rare event. An effusion specimen with choriocarcinoma metastasis was seen by one of the authors (Fig. 7.11h).

The presence of mature teratoma elements, consisting of fat, keratin, and hair, in effusions does not constitute true metastasis and is observed in the event of spontaneous or iatrogenic spillage of mature teratoma elements (Fig. 7.11i, j). One should nevertheless be familiar with the morphological picture of this condition.

Germ cell tumors should be suspected when a malignant effusion is found in a child or young adult, although they may also occur later in life. The differential diagnosis of germ cell tumors in effusions depends on their type. Yolk sac tumors and embryonal carcinomas need to be differentiated from metastatic carcinomas. For the former tumor, this primarily includes clear cell carcinomas, as well as secretory endometrioid carcinomas and mucinous carcinomas.

Seminomas should be differentiated from carcinomas, as well as all other tumors that present with dissociated malignant cells. Germ cell tumors express to a varying degree embryonic markers such as SALL4, OCT4, SOX2, and Nanog. Yolk sac tumors additionally stain for AFP, whereas embryonal carcinomas are CD30-positive. Dysgerminomas stain for placental alkaline phosphatase (PLAP), c-Kit (CD117), and D2–40. Glypican-3 stains germ cell tumors, particularly yolk sac tumor, but is expressed in many carcinomas, and its presence should therefore be interpreted in the context of a broader panel of markers.

In young patients, the neuroepithelial cells in immature teratomas need to be differentiated from Wilms' tumor, neuroblastoma, embryonal rhabdomyosarcoma, Ewing sarcoma, and non-Hodgkin lymphoma [87, 39], which may be achieved based on morphology, immunohistochemistry, and for some of these entities, molecular analysis (see below).

## Malignant Melanoma

The diagnosis of malignant melanoma in effusion specimens is an infrequent, though not a rare one, reflecting the ability of this tumor to metastasize to practically any organ. In the

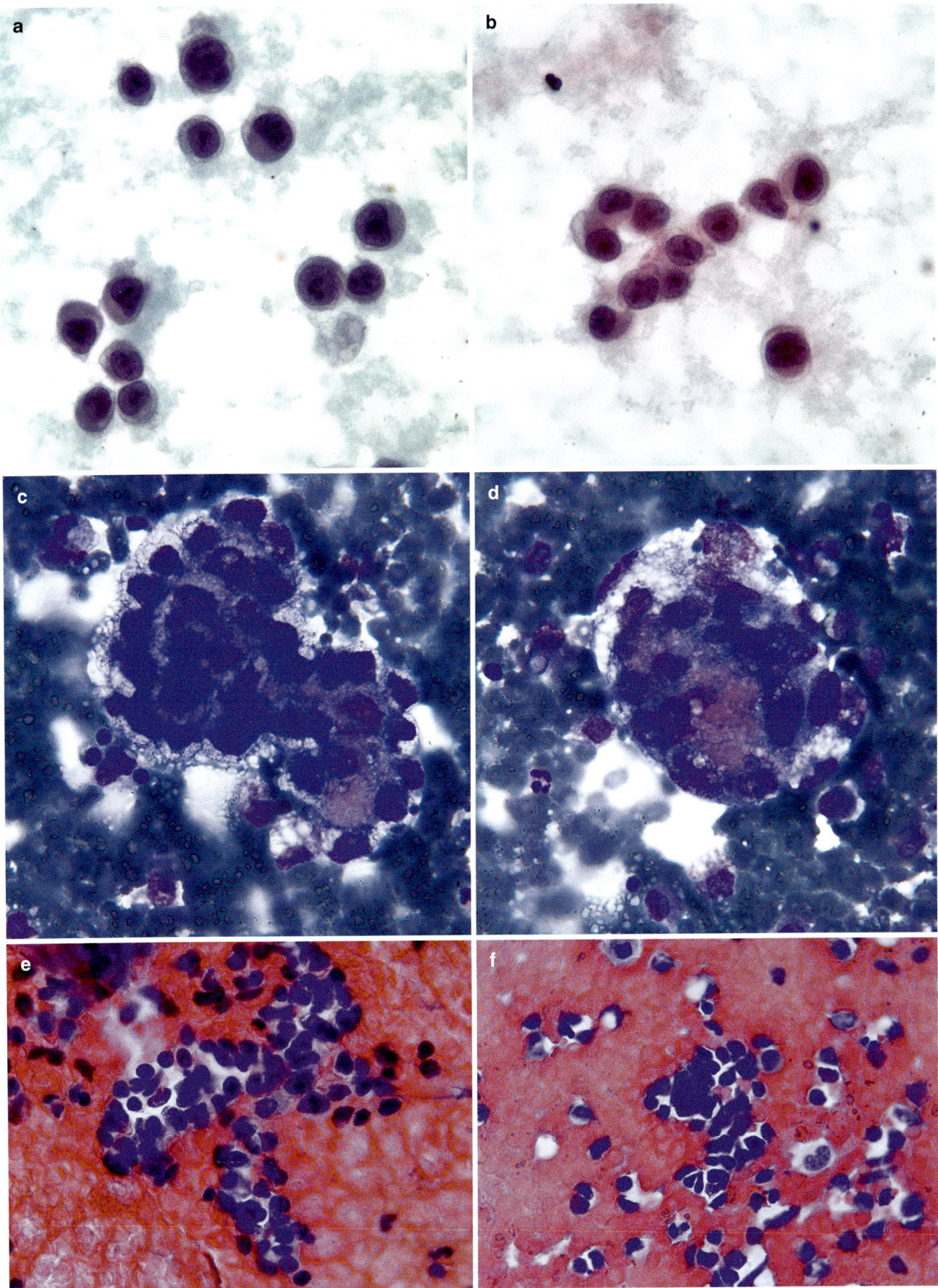

**Fig. 7.11** Germ cell tumors: (**a**, **b**) dysgerminoma. Small cells with high n/c ratio, lying in short cords or singly. (**c**, **d**) Yolk sac tumor. Vacuolated cells and formation of metachromatic extracellular sub- stance; (**e**–**g**) immature teratoma; (**h**) choriocarcinoma; (**i**, **j**) material from mature teratoma. (**a**, **b**, **j**) PAP; (**c**–**i**) MGG/Diff-Quik

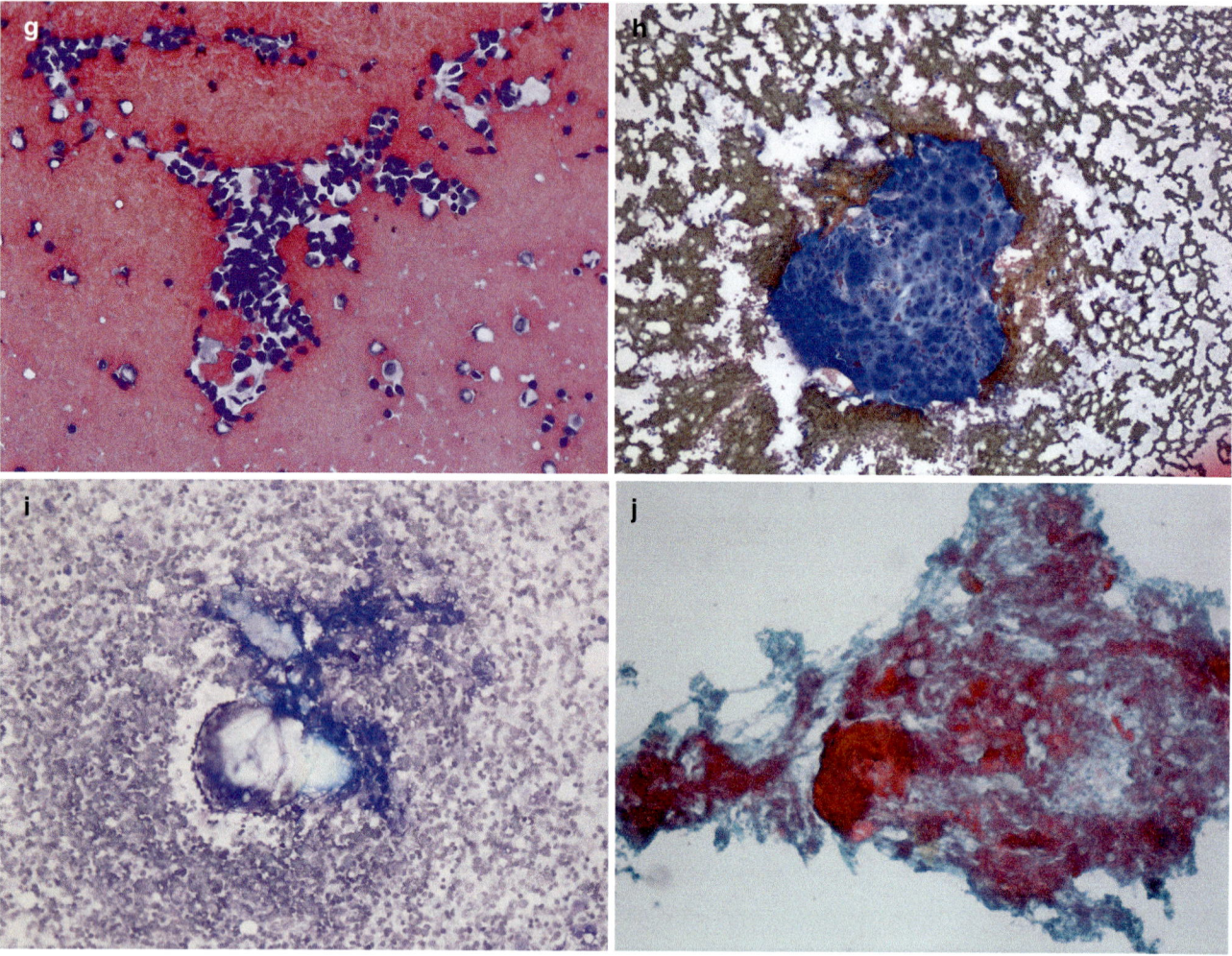

**Fig. 7.11** (continued)

series by Johnston [56], malignant melanoma was the primary tumor in 10/472 patients with malignant pleural effusion, whereas Sears and Hajdu reported the presence of metastatic melanoma in 17/812 and 7/423 malignant pleural and peritoneal effusions, respectively [73].

The primary site is most frequently exposed skin, but metastasis from a primary tumor in the vulva was reported [97]. A primary pulmonary/pleural melanoma in a 13-year-old girl was recently described [98].

Melanoma metastases in effusions may be melanotic or amelanotic. Specimen cellularity is variable but may be very high (Fig. 7.12a, b). Cells may lie singly or in groups of variable size (Fig. 7.12a–d). The cytoplasm is generally abundant, with variable n/c ratio. Intracytoplasmic vacuoles are evident (Fig. 7.12a). Nuclei are large, overtly atypical, round or vesicular, and eccentrically placed, with coarse chromatin and one or multiple large nucleoli (Fig. 7.12e–h). The presence of pigment is strongly supportive of a melanoma diagnosis.

Longatto-Filho et al. reviewed 21 peritoneal and pleural melanoma effusions and found the majority to consist of single cells. Characteristic morphological features consisted of cytoplasmic pigment, perinuclear halos, cell cannibalism, and the presence of intranuclear inclusions, atypical mitoses, multinucleation, and prominent nucleoli [99]. Similar findings were reported in two other series [100, 101]. A case of melanoma with signet ring cells in a peritoneal effusion was reported [102].

The diagnosis of malignant melanoma in effusions is best supported by ancillary methods, especially when the primary site is unknown and/or the tumor is amelanotic. The Masson-Fontana silver stain detects melanin (Fig. 7.12i), but as in other areas of effusion cytology, immunohistochemistry is currently the most widely used method. In 1985, Pinto reported immunoreactivity of melanoma cells to S-100 in 4/7 melanomas [103]. Since then, several other markers, including HMB45, MART-1 (Melan-A), and SOX10, have been added to the panel

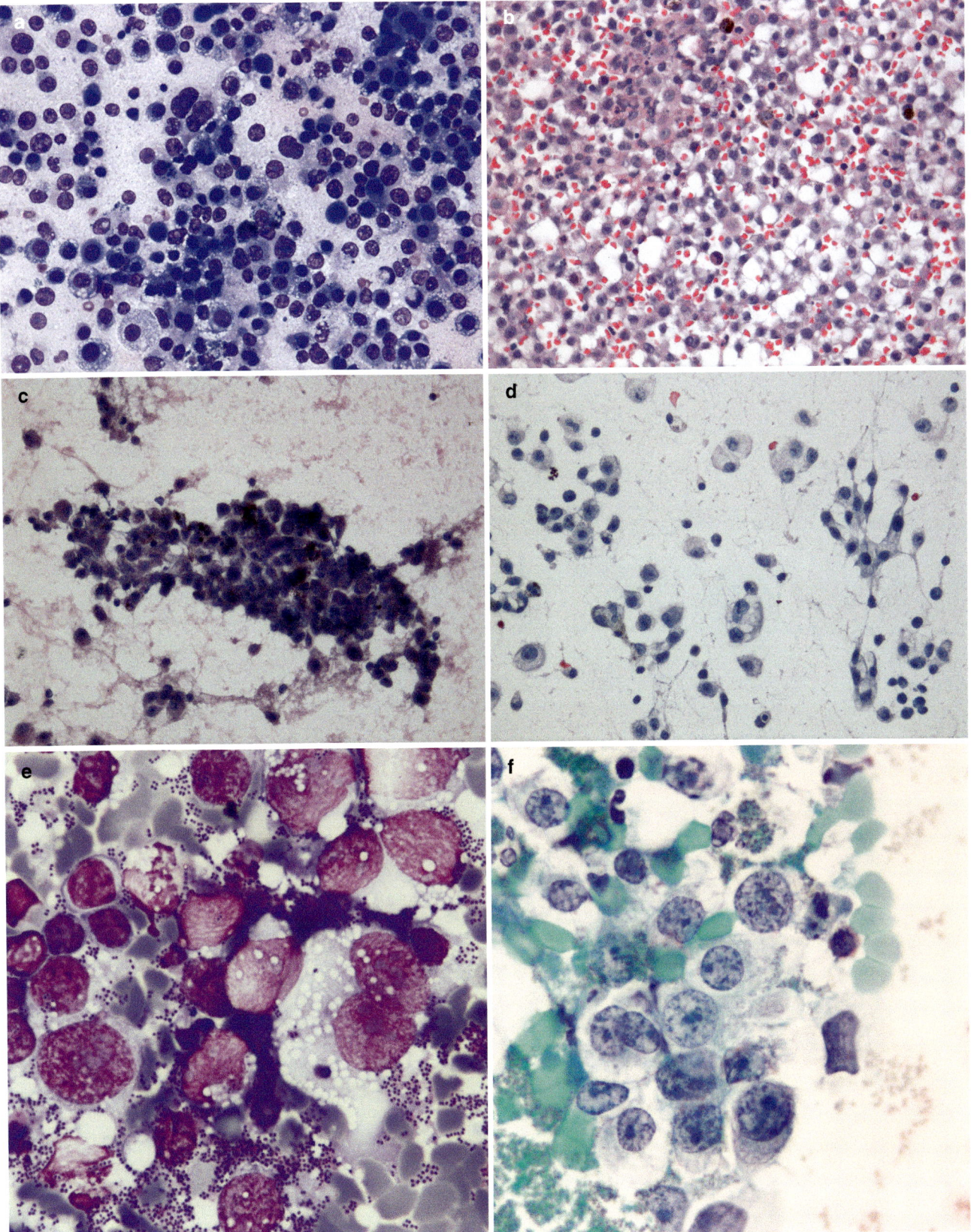

**Fig. 7.12** Malignant melanoma: (**a**, **b**) numerous dissociated tumor cells; (**c**) cohesive group; (**d**) small loose groups and single cells. Melanin is seen in all four figures; (**e–h**) tumor cells with pronounced atypia. Note vacuolization and melanin granules in **e**. (**a, e, h**) MGG/ Diff-Quik; (**c, d, f, g**) PAP; (**b**) H&E. *Histochemistry and immunohistochemistry*: (**i**) Masson-Fontana stain for melanin; (**j**) Melan-A (MART-1); (**k, l**) HMB-45; (**m**) vimentin

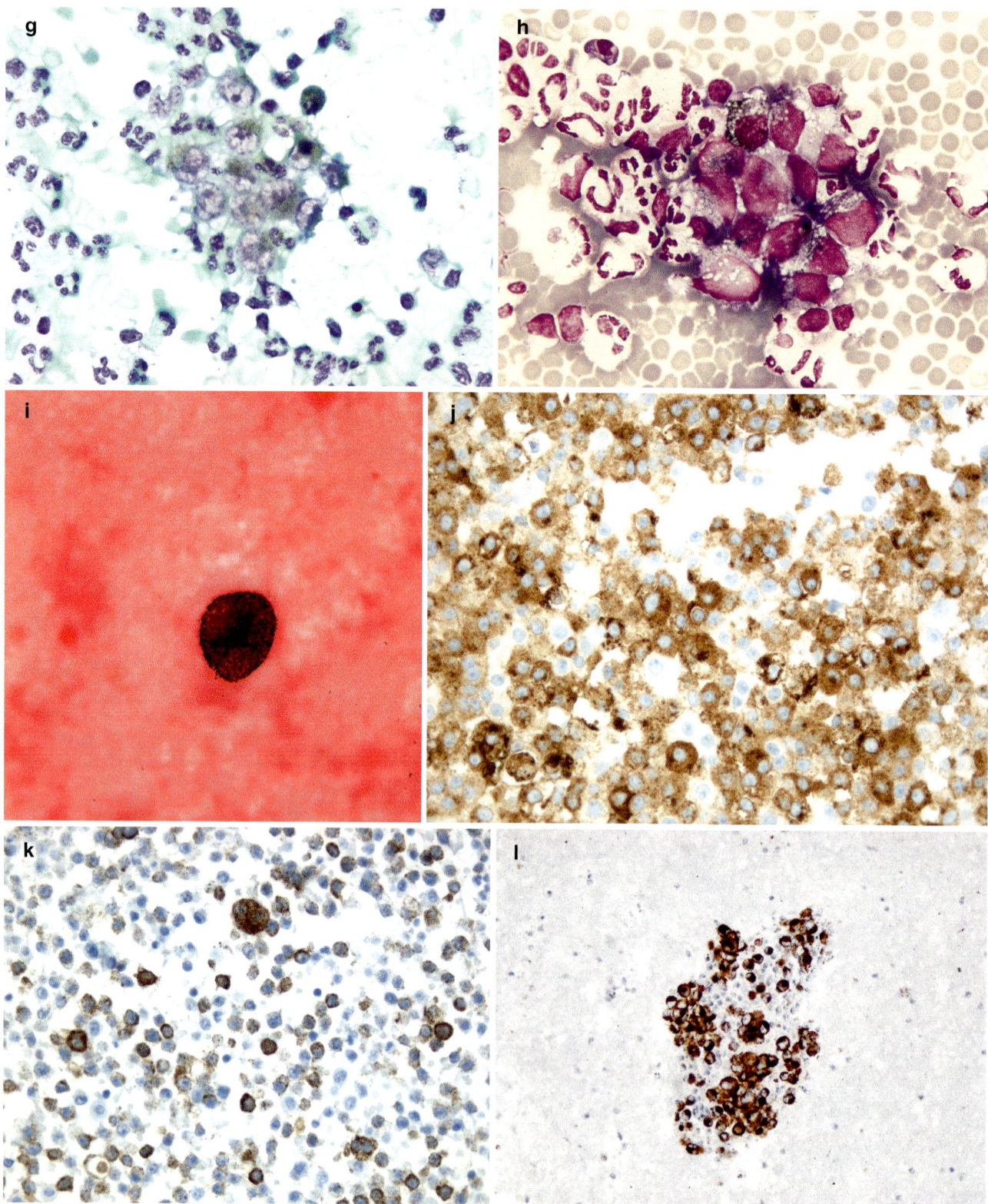

**Fig. 7.12** (continued)

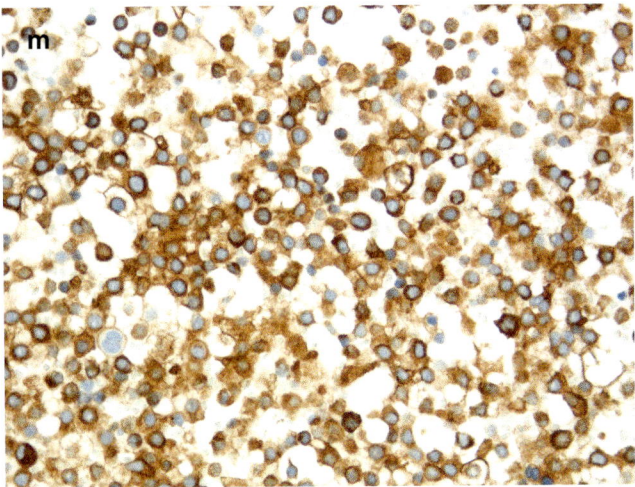

**Fig. 7.12**  (continued)

of melanoma markers. HMB45 and Melan-A are often expressed in melanoma effusions (Fig. 7.12j–l), with sensitivity of 80% in the two largest series published to date [99, 100]. Vimentin is additionally expressed in this tumor (Fig. 7.12m) but is considerably less specific. The use of double-staining for WT1 and pan-cytokeratin AE1/AE3 was suggested to aid in the differential diagnosis between metastatic melanoma, metastatic carcinoma, and benign or malignant mesothelial cells in effusions, with melanomas (n = 17) usually displaying cytoplasmic WT1 expression and negative AE1/AE3 staining [104].

Merkel cell tumor, a skin tumor with neuroendocrine differentiation, may rarely affect the serosal cavities [105–107]. In the most recent report, tumor cells were seen singly, single-file or in clusters, and had round-to-oval nuclei, irregular nuclear borders, stippled chromatin, inconspicuous nucleoli, scant cytoplasm, and occasional nuclear molding [107].

Merkel cell tumor metastatic to effusion was recently seen by one of the authors. Tumor cells were immunhistochemically positive for CK20, synaptophysin, and chromogranin A, negative for TTF1 (Fig. 7.13a–e).

## Sarcomas

Sarcoma metastasis to effusions is an infrequent event in adults but represents a considerable part of the diagnostic spectrum of malignant effusions in children and adolescents.

Practically every type of sarcoma has been described at this anatomic site. Disease presentation as effusion is uncommon but has been described [108].

In the Geisinger series of pediatric patients, 43/80 malignant pleural effusions and 4/40 malignant peritoneal effusions were sarcomas [87], whereas Wong et al. reported that 7% of 88 malignant effusions were diagnosed as sarcoma [88]. A study of 24 sarcomas by Abadi and Zakowski included 8 malignant fibrous histiocytomas, 5 leiomyosarcomas, 3 rhabdomyosarcomas, 3 liposarcomas, 2 high-grade sarcomas, 1 osteogenic sarcoma, 1 synovial sarcoma, 1 one chondrosarcoma [109]. In another report, 28 of 154 effusions from sarcoma patients were positive and 6 were suspicious [110].

General characteristics of sarcomas in effusions described by Abadi included single cell arrangement, indistinct cell borders, nuclear pleomorphism, multinucleation, and the presence of a proteinaceous background with lysed blood [109].

In a recent series of 40 small round cell tumor effusions, including 14 Ewing sarcoma/primitive neuroectodermal tumor (PNET) specimens, 5 synovial sarcomas, and 6 rhabdomyosarcomas, no morphologic differentiators between these entities were observed [111]. In another series of 183 effusions from pediatric patients, 40 specimens were malignant, of which 9 were rhabdomyosarcomas, constituting the most common diagnostic entity [112].

Embryonal rhabdomyosarcomas consist of single-lying or loose groups of small cells with high n/c ratio. Nuclei have variable chromatin pattern and one or more conspicuous nucleoli (Fig. 7.14a–d). Geisinger described the presence of small notches in the nuclear membrane. Although the cytoplasm is scanty, as in all small round blue cell tumors, it was more voluminous than in neuroblastoma [87]. A specimen studied for DNA content using flow cytometry was shown to be aneuploid [113]. Metastasis from a testicular tumor with pleomorphic cells was described [114]. Uncommon primary sites for rhabdomyosarcomas which have been described are the ovary (two cases) [115], the prostate [116], and the breast [117]. A case of malignant pleural effusion from a rhabdomyosarcoma that developed in a mixed germ cell tumor of the testis was reported [118].

The diagnosis of rhabdomyosarcoma requires ancillary tests. Immunostaining for muscle markers, such as desmin and actin, and skeletal muscle markers such as myogenin (Fig. 7.14e) [119] and MYF-4 is helpful, as is electron microscopy showing muscle filaments. Embryonal rhabdo-

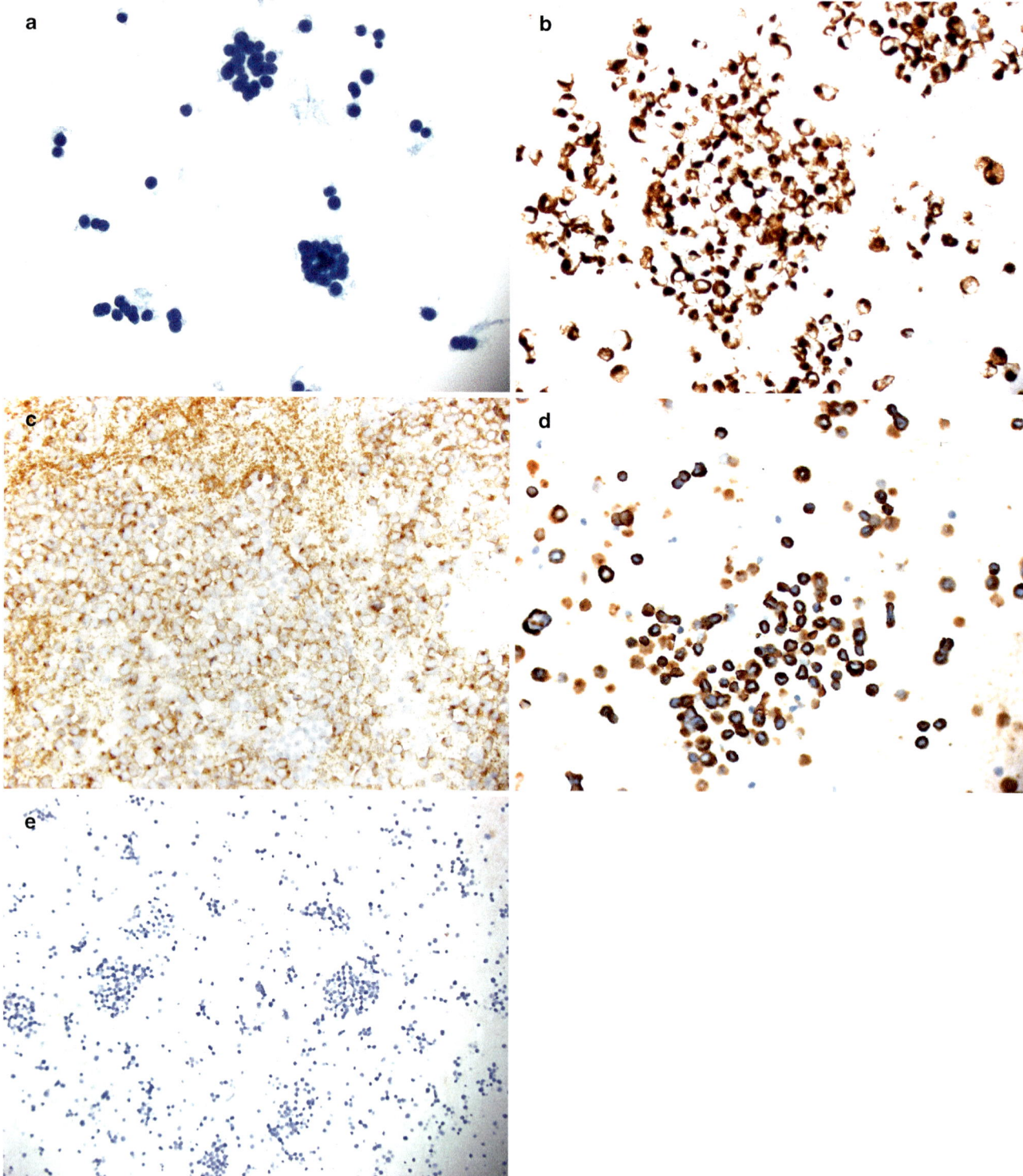

**Fig. 7.13** Merkel cell tumor: (**a**) PAP stain showing tumor cells lying singly or in small groups. *Immunohistochemistry*: (**b**) CK20; (**c**) synapto-physin; (**d**) chromogranin A; (**e**) TTF1

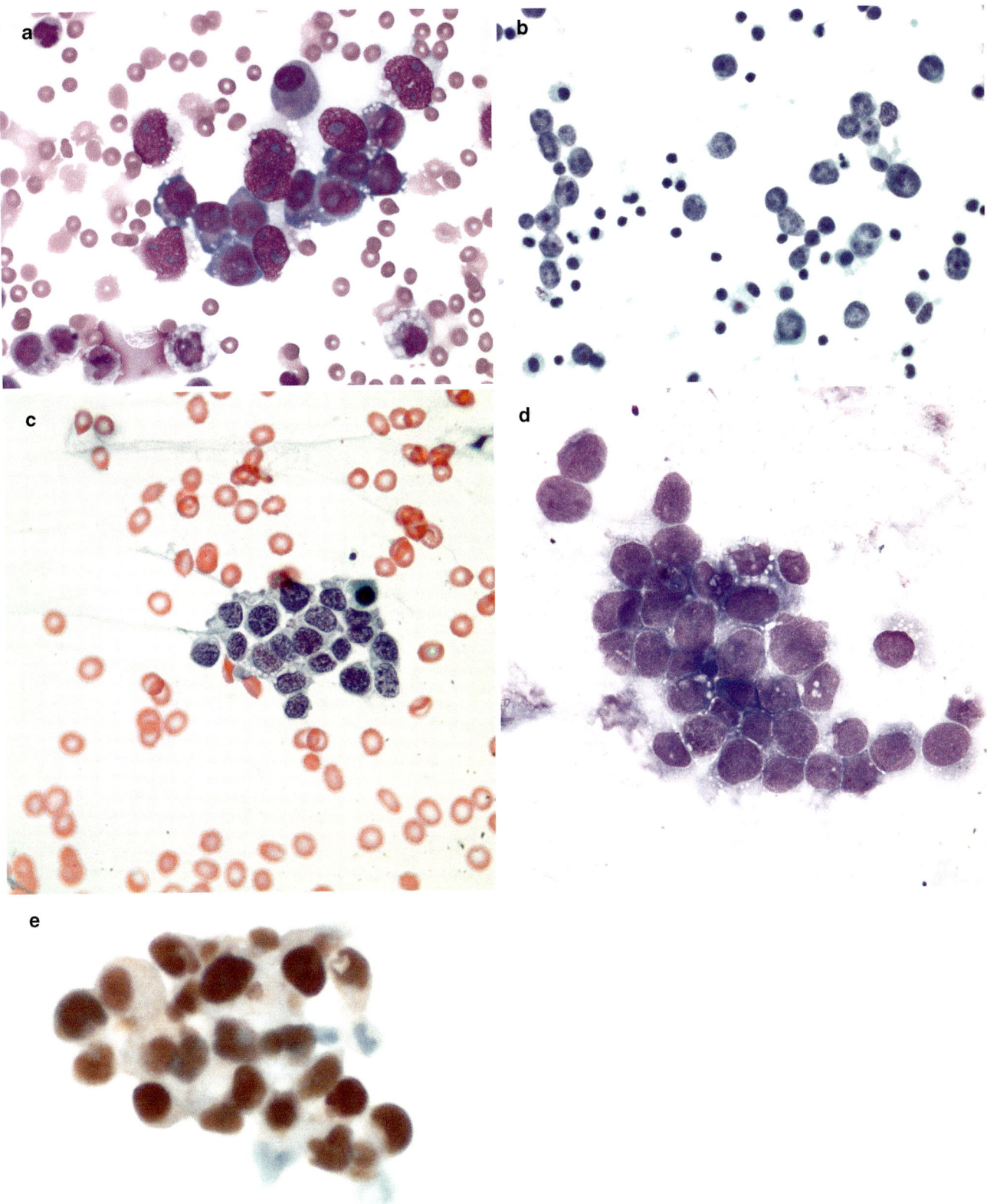

**Fig. 7.14** Rhabdomyosarcoma: (**a–d**) small cells with high n/c ratio, dissociated or in small clusters; (**a, d**) MGG/Diff-Quik; (**b, c**) PAP. (**e**) immunostaining for myogenin in the specimen shown in **a, b**

myosarcomas have a specific translocation at t(2;13) (q35;q14) creating the PAX3-FKHR gene fusion that can be showed using FISH [120–122].

Ewing sarcoma is an obvious differential diagnosis to rhabdomyosarcoma. Geisinger studied nine pleural specimens and describes small malignant cells with very high n/c ratio, occasionally with no discernible cytoplasm, lying singly or in small loosely cohesive groups. Nuclei were irregular and jagged [87]. Similar morphological findings were observed in a case diagnosed by one of the authors (Fig. 7.15a, b).

In more recent studies, Ewing sarcoma cells in effusion were shown to have the characteristic t(11;22)(q24;q12) translocation creating the EWS/FLI1 fusion transcript, also shown in the case illustrated in this chapter, as well as additional aberrations (48, XY, i(1)(q11), +10), in one report [123, 124]. Ewing sarcoma cells are immunohistochemically positive for CD99 (Fig. 7.15c), vimentin, and neuron-specific antigen (NSE) [124].

Several cases of desmoplastic small round cell tumor in effusion have been reported [125–128]. In one of these studies, tumor cells expressed vimentin, desmin, cytokeratin, EMA, NSE, and CD57 (Leu-7) and exhibited the pathognomonic t(11;22)(p13;q12) translocation [126].

In a recently described case of a 30-year-old man, tumor cells in the pleural effusion had cell spheres without cores mimicking carcinoma or mesothelioma. The diagnosis was confirmed by immunohistochemistry and FISH, the latter showing *EWSR1* rearrangement [127]. In another report, cells in pleural effusion had a "floating island" pattern, characteristic of hepatocellular carcinoma, renal cell carcinoma, and adrenocortical carcinoma in effusions [128].

Several reports of angiosarcoma in effusions have been published [129–132]. Berry et al. studied three cases. Numerous single tumor cells and small loose clusters were seen. The malignant cells had delicate, finely vacuolated cytoplasm with distinct borders. Nuclei were irregular with indentations and had prominent nuclei and coarse chromatin.

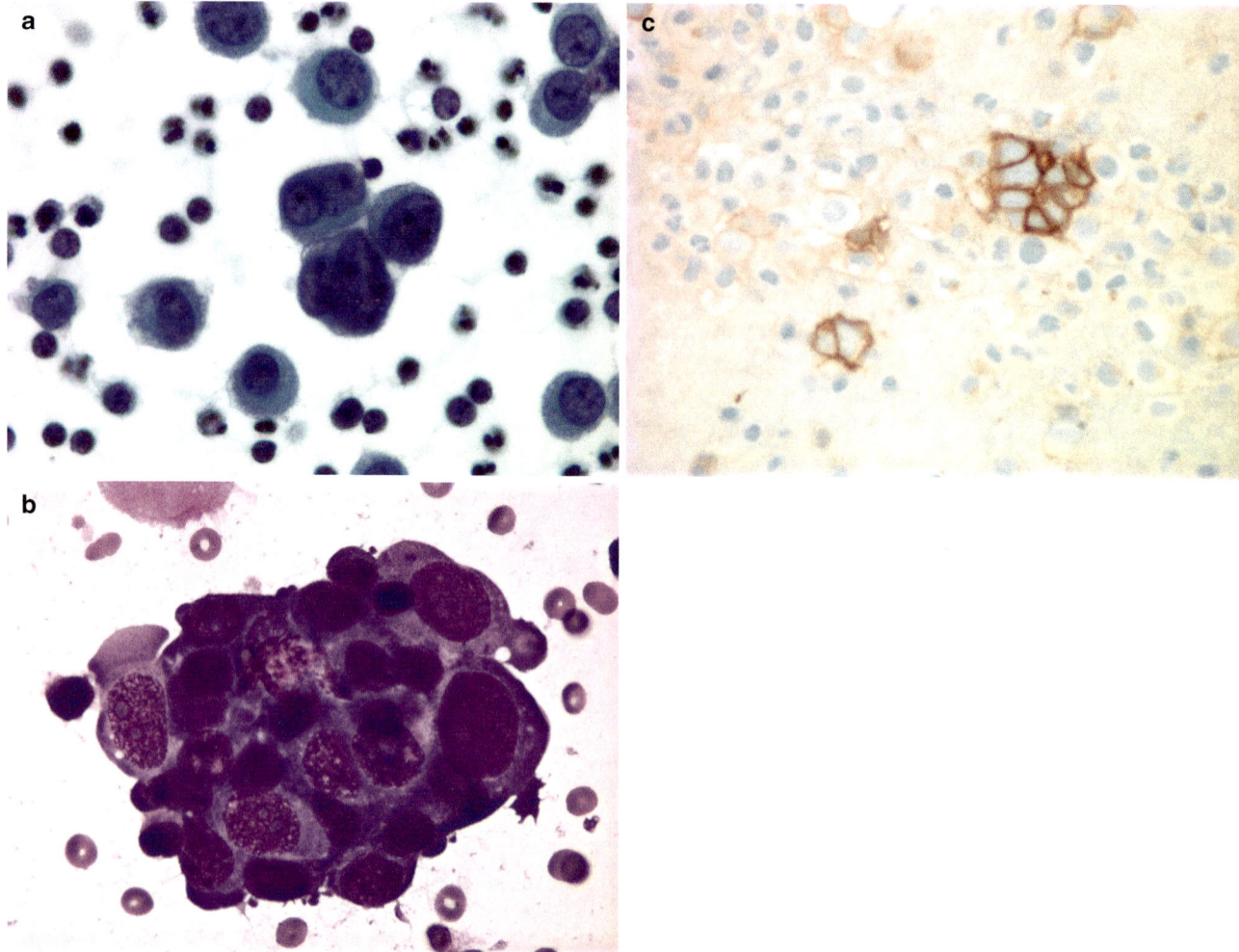

**Fig. 7.15** Ewing sarcoma: (**a**, **b**), cell clusters of variable size with very high n/c ratio and large nucleoli; (**a**) PAP, (**b**) MGG/Diff-Quik. (**c**) immunostaining for CD99

Binucleate forms were occasionally seen [129]. An ovarian angiosarcoma metastasis in peritoneal effusion diagnosed by one of the authors consisted of cell groups of variable size, some with papillary architecture, with large poorly defined cells with overlapping nuclei, high n/c ratio, and large nucleoli, findings which may easily mimic adenocarcinoma (Fig. 7.16a–c) [131].

Alderman et al. had one angiosarcoma effusion in their series [119]. Angiosarcomas express vascular markers, including CD31, CD34 (Fig. 7.16d), and factor VIII.

Few cases of epithelioid hemangioendothelioma in pleural effusion have been described [133–136], in which tumor cells expressed vascular markers [133, 135, 136] or were shown to have Weibel-Palade bodies by electron microscopy [134]. A specimen diagnosed by one of the authors, positive for CD31, is shown in Fig. 7.16e–h.

Osteosarcoma was one of the commonly found tumors in the Geisinger series, with 22 positive specimens, of which 21 were pleural and 1 peritoneal. Cells were described as highly pleomorphic, with round, oval, or spindle-shaped form, relatively abundant eosinophilic cytoplasm, and nuclei which appeared to be pyknotic or were coarsely granular, with large nucleoli [87]. A case metastatic to ascites with poor outcome was described [137]. Two specimens seen by the authors consisted of highly atypical cells of variable form, with vacuolated cytoplasm, high-grade nuclei with large nucleoli and formation of osteoid (Fig. 7.17a–d).

A report of two pleomorphic liposarcomas that metastasized to pleural effusion was published, in which electron microscopy aided in establishing the diagnosis [138]. Abadi and Zakowski reported three specimens, in which cells had a pale and delicate cytoplasm and irregular nuclei with fine and even chromatin and small nucleoli [109]. A pleural effusion specimen with tumor cells in papillary structures mimicking carcinoma was described [139]. A specimen seen by one of

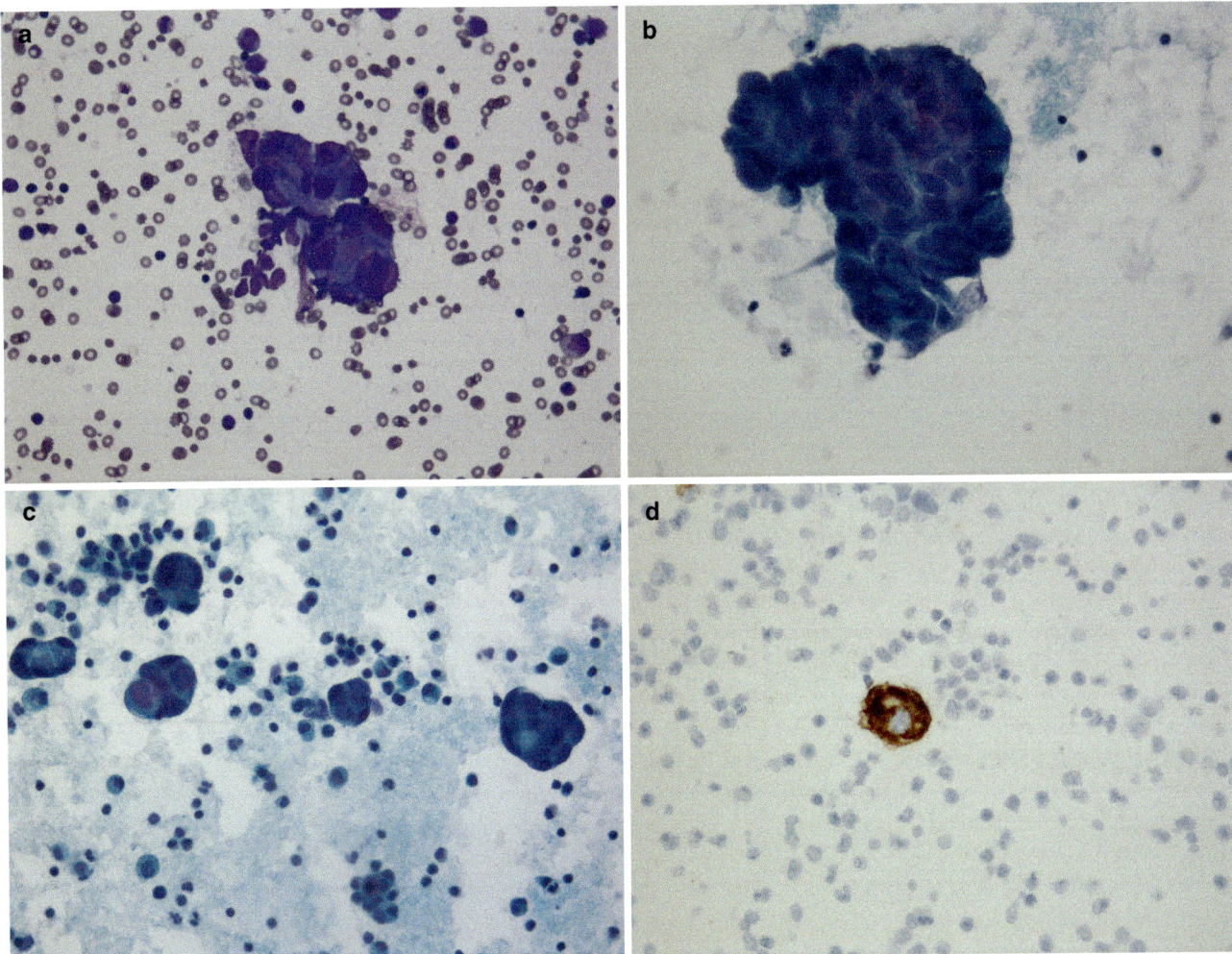

**Fig. 7.16** Angiosarcoma: (**a–c**) tumor cell groups of variable size, some with papillary architecture which mimics adenocarcinoma. Cells are large and atypical; (**a**), MGG/Diff-Quik; (**b, c**) PAP. (**d**) CD34 immunostain. Hemangioendothelioma (**e–g**) tumor cells with epithelioid morphology. Cells have delicate chromatin and easily discernible nucleoli; (**e, f**) MGG/Diff-Quik; (**g**) PAP. (**h**) CD31 immunostain

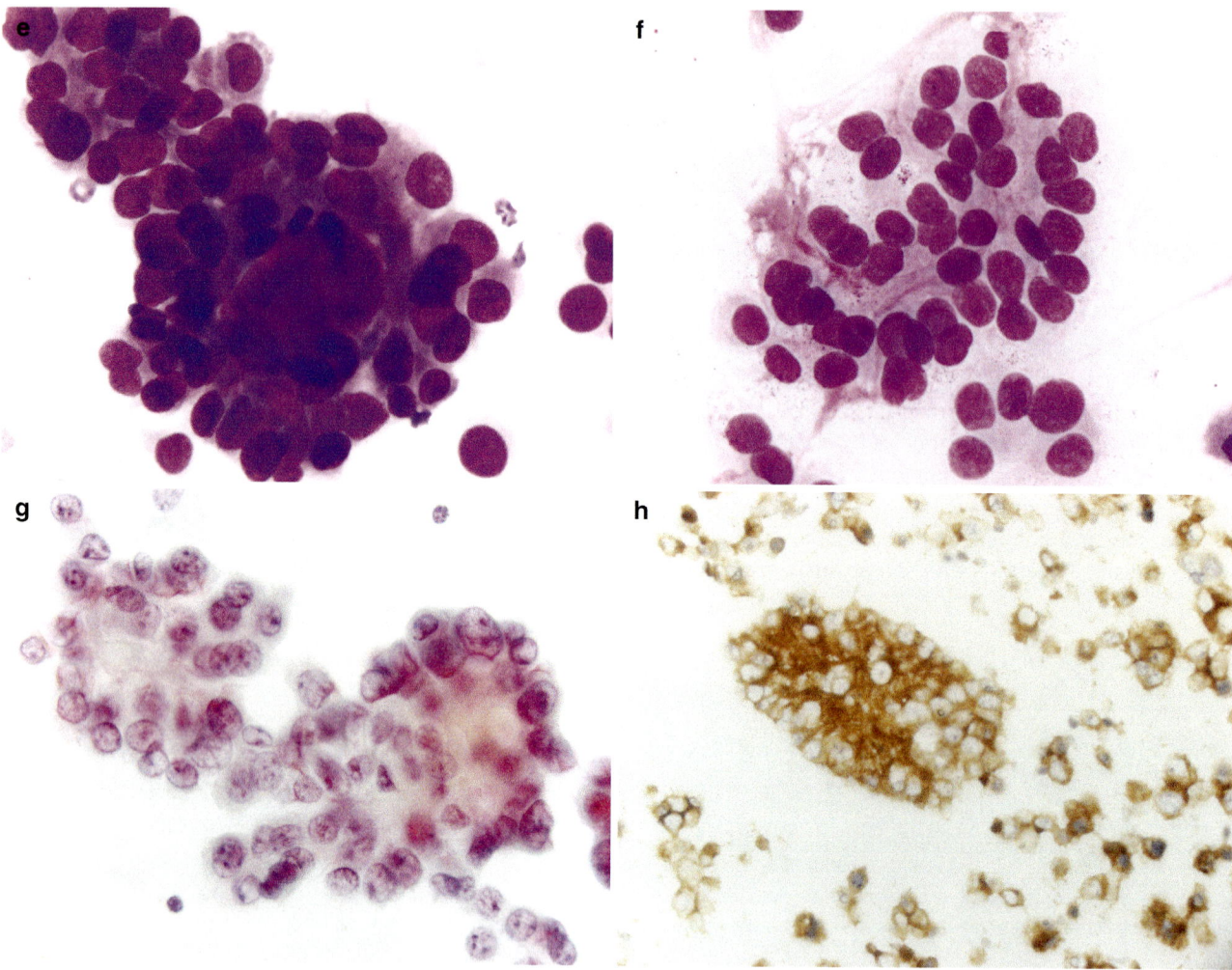

**Fig. 7.16** (continued)

the authors consisted of large lipoblasts with vesicular nuclei containing one or two large nucleoli. Tumor cells stained for vimentin and MDM-2 (Fig. 7.18a–c).

Metastases from a dedifferentiated chondrosarcoma of the femur and from a primary chondrosarcoma of the urinary bladder were described [140, 141]. A myxoid chondrosarcoma in pleural effusion was described, consisting of cells that had exclusively epithelioid morphology, with a potential to be misdiagnosed as carcinoma [142]. A case of myxoid chondrosarcoma seen by one of the authors consisted of spindle cells with cartilaginous material in the background (Fig. 7.19a–c).

Metastasis from a sclerosing fibrosarcoma of the buttock in a pleural effusion was reported [143], in which tumor cells were arranged in medium-sized epithelioid clusters. Tumor cells had pleomorphic nuclei with occasional multinucle-

ation, with fine chromatin and small nucleoli. Recently, positive pleural effusion in a 63-year-old female patient diagnosed with cardiac myxofibrosarcoma was reported [144]. Tumor cells were medium to large in size, occasionally multinucleated, and had round nuclei with fine chromatin and prominent nucleoli, and pale and lace-like cytoplasm. A case seen by one of the authors consisted of more monomorphic spindle cells (Fig. 7.19d).

The presence of synovial sarcoma in serous effusions was reported in several studies [87, 109, 111, 145, 146], of which the former three displayed a biphasic pattern and the fourth was monophasic, with a spindle cell component. Expression of cytokeratins, vimentin, and EMA, as well as the pathognomonic t(X;18)(p11;q11) translocation, was seen in one of the specimens, which was characterized as a newly established cell line [146].

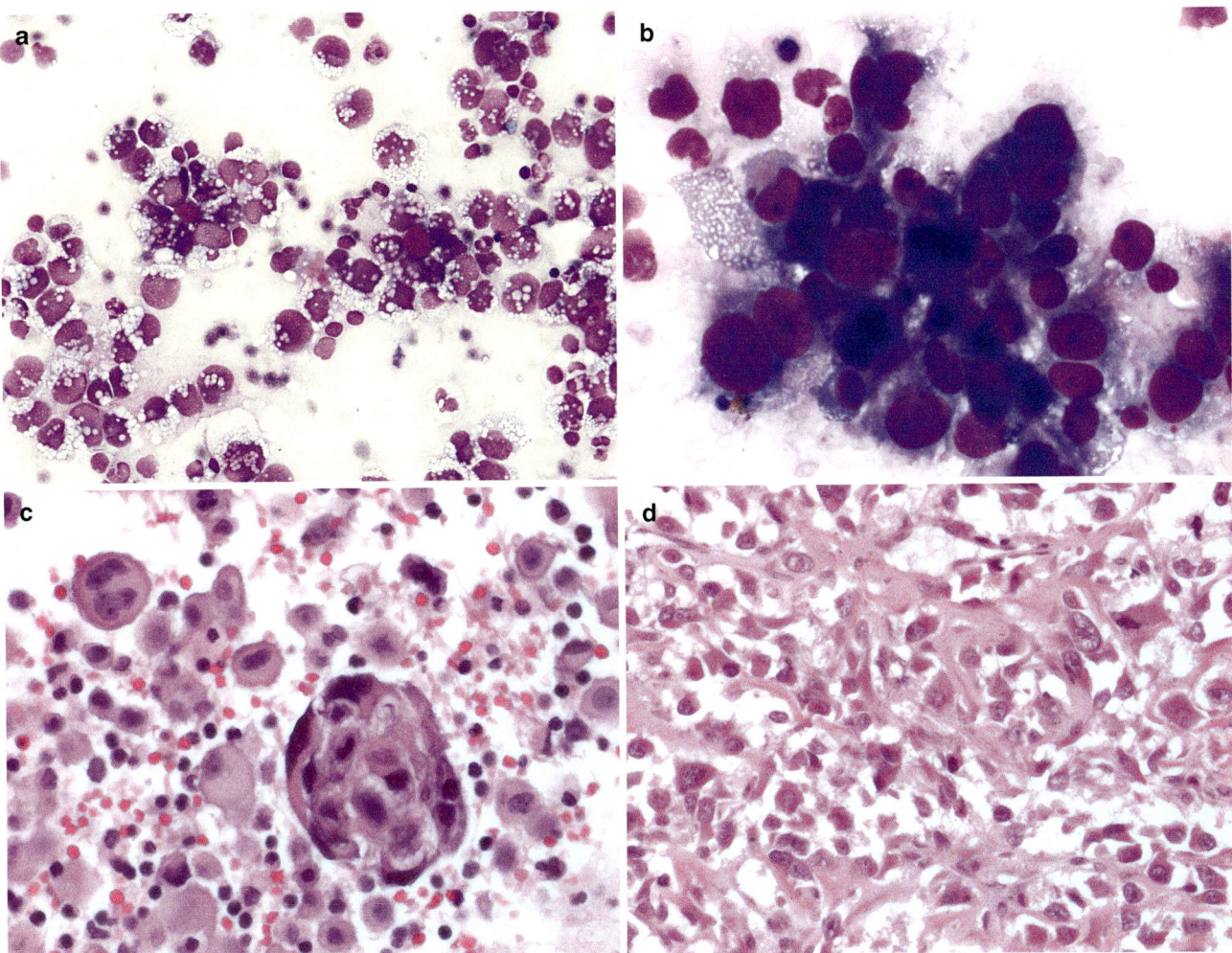

**Fig. 7.17** Osteosarcoma: (**a–d**) large and highly atypical tumor cells in groups of variable size and form, some dissociated. Extracellular osteoid is evident. (**a**, **b**) MGG/Diff-Quik; (**c**, **d**) H&E

Eight malignant fibrous histiocytomas, five leiomyosarcomas, and two high-grade sarcomas were characterized in the Abadi series [109]. These had single-lying pleomorphic cells, in agreement with their histological properties. A case of myxoid leiomyosarcoma in a peritoneal washing specimen was reported, in which cells had epithelioid and spindle cell morphology [147]. A case of inflammatory malignant fibrous histiocytoma was recently described [148]. A high-grade leiomyosarcoma was seen by one of the authors (Fig. 7.20a, b).

Other sarcomas or other soft tissue tumors diagnosed in effusions are uterine sarcoma with rhabdoid features [149], ovarian adenosarcoma [150], clear cell sarcoma (malignant melanoma of soft parts) [151], and melanotic schwannoma [152].

A series of six cytological specimens, including three effusions, from five patients diagnosed with the new entity epithelioid inflammatory myofibroblastic sarcoma was recently published [153].

Tumor cells in effusion specimens were fewer than in FNA specimens, and consisted of large degenerated epithelioid cells with eccentrically located nuclei. Tumors were ALK-positive by immunohistochemistry and had *ALK* rearrangement by FISH.

While not a true sarcoma, the possibility of a carcinosarcoma metastasizing in the form of sarcomatous elements should be kept in mind, although this is a very rare event [154].

Small round blue cell tumors other than the ones discussed above, including neuroblastoma and Wilms' tumor, are an important differential diagnosis in effusion cytology in the pediatric or young adult population.

The series of Farr and Hajdu consisted of 51 malignant effusions from patients with neuroblastoma, including 48 pleural and 3 peritoneal specimens. Effusions were moderately cellular, with small, round, or polygonal cells with

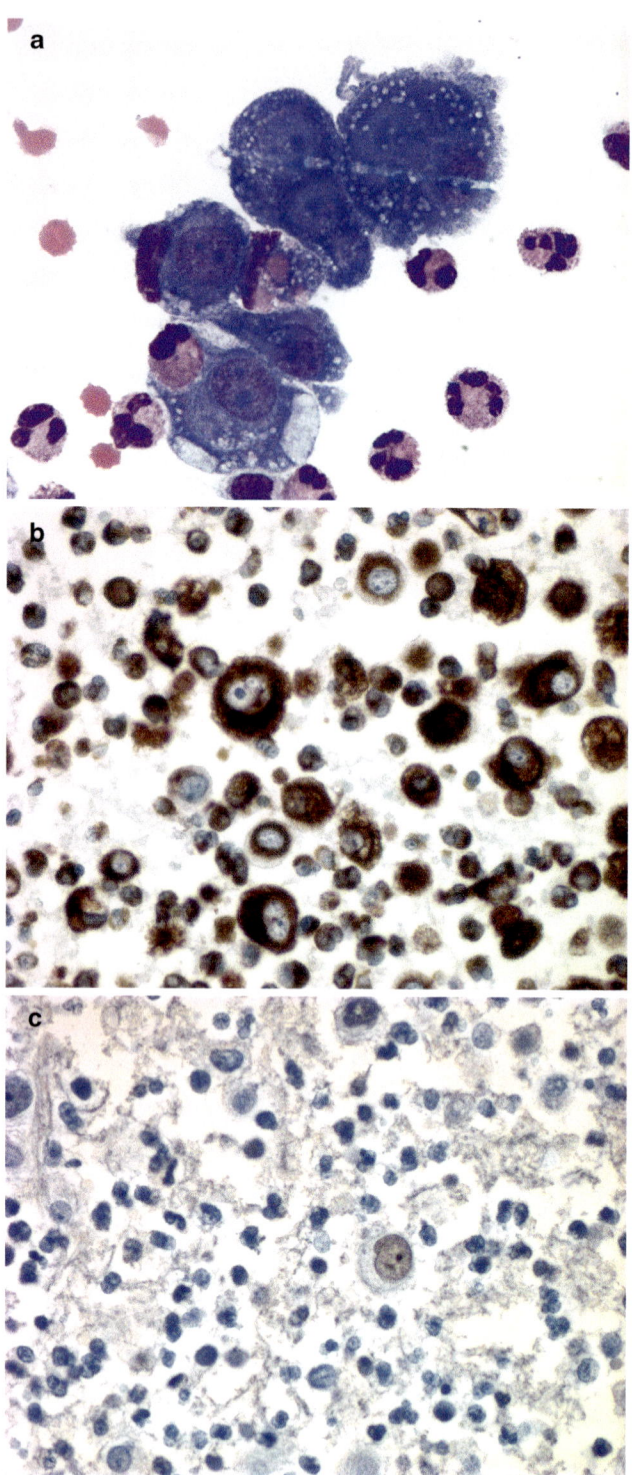

**Fig. 7.18** Liposarcoma: (**a**) large atypical lipoblasts, MGG/Diff-Quik; (**b, c**) immunostaining for vimentin (**b**) and MDM-2 (**c**)

round or oval hyperchromatic nuclei, one or two round nucleoli, and scant cytoplasm. Rosette formation was seen in the majority of specimens [155]. Geisinger described the presence of large flat plaques, short chains with molding, and

rosettes in 23 studied specimens. Rare specimens from patients with medulloblastoma, pinealoblastoma, and retino-blastoma were morphologically indistinguishable from neu-roblastomas [87].

Cells in Wilms' tumor lie singly or in pairs and organ-oid structures are rarely found. A biphasic cell population consisting of round or polygonal cells and plump spindle cells was described, both with hyperchromatic nuclei, even chromatin distribution, prominent nucleoli, and sparse cyto-plasm [87]. The role of effusion cytology in correctly stag-ing these patients was emphasized in a case report by Baliga et al. [156].

Examples of neuroblastoma, Wilms' tumor, and PNET effusions are shown in Fig. 7.21a–f.

## Head and Neck Cancers

Metastasis from a primary tumor at this anatomic region is uncommon in effusion cytology but has been reported. Spreading from nasopharyngeal carcinoma has been reported in two series [73, 87]. Metastasis from a squamous cell car-cinoma, e.g., from laryngeal carcinoma (Fig. 7.22a, b), may be observed and needs to be differentiated from a primary tumor of the lung or other origin.

Thyroid carcinoma of various histological type, includ-ing papillary carcinoma (Fig. 7.22c–h) [157–159] and its follicular variant [160], Hürthle cell carcinoma [161] and medullary carcinoma [162] (Fig. 7.22i, j) may be detected in serous effusions. A case of malignant pleural effusion as the site of recurrence for a sclerosing mucoepidermoid carci-noma of the thyroid with eosinophilia was additionally reported [163].

Three relatively large series of this rare entity were pub-lished in recent years [164–166]. Olson et al. found in their archives six metastatic thyroid carcinomas in effusions, all in the pleural cavity, in a period of 26 years, including four pap-illary carcinomas and two anaplastic carcinomas. Four speci-mens available for morphological assessment had variable degrees of cellularity, lymphocytic infiltration, nuclear fea-tures of papillary carcinoma, single tumor cells, and frag-ments [164]. Lew and co-workers published a series of five cases of metastatic papillary thyroid carcinoma, all within the pleural cavity. Tumor cells had characteristic nuclear features of this entity, as well as cytoplasmic vacuolization [165]. The series of Vyas and Harigopal similarly included five pleural effusions with metastatic papillary thyroid carcinoma [166].

The diagnosis of thyroid carcinoma is supported by posi-tive immunostaining for thyroglobulin (Fig. 7.22k), PAX8, and TTF-1, although the latter two markers are far more commonly observed in gynecological and lung adenocarci-noma effusions, respectively, in everyday practice.

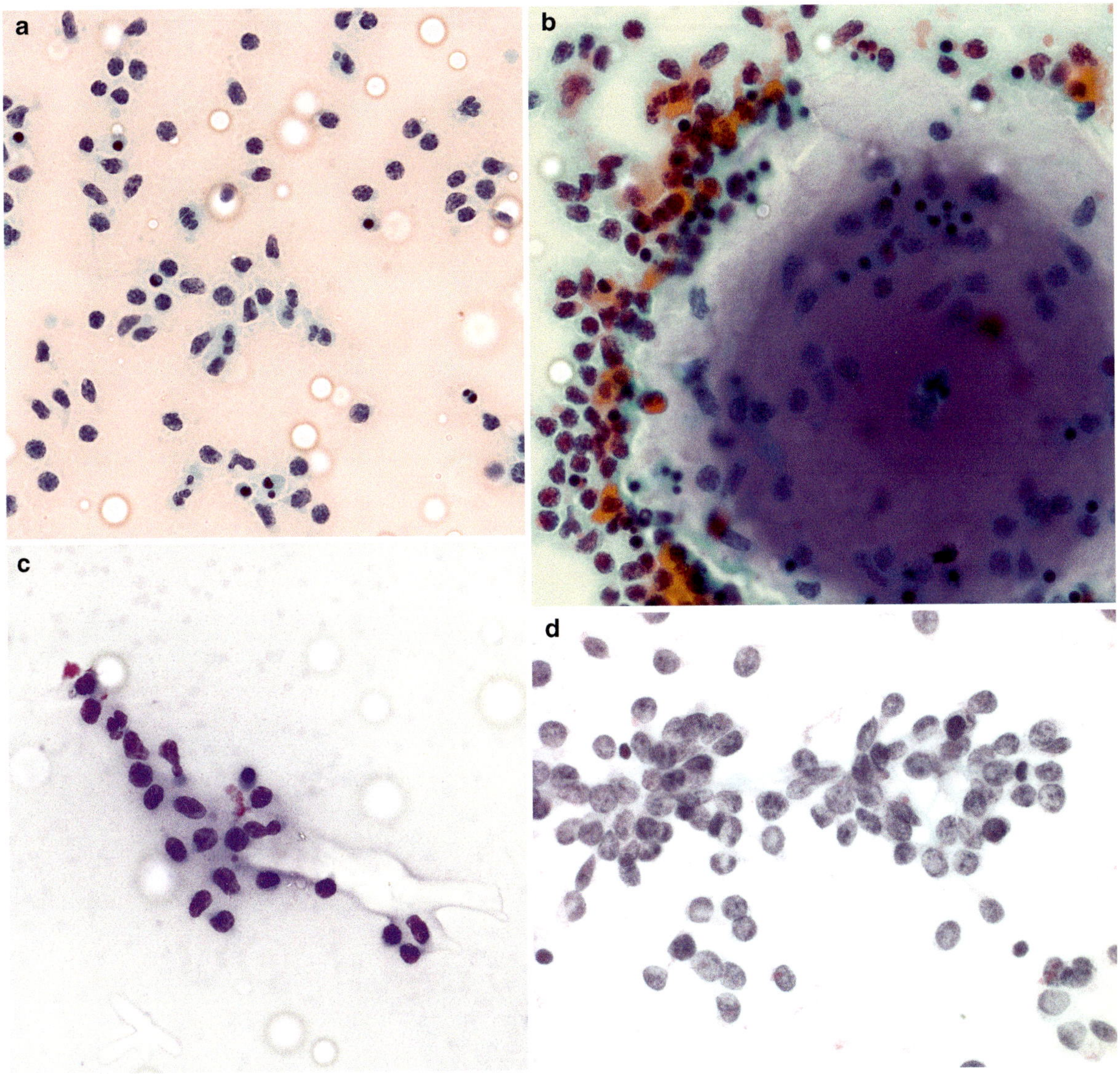

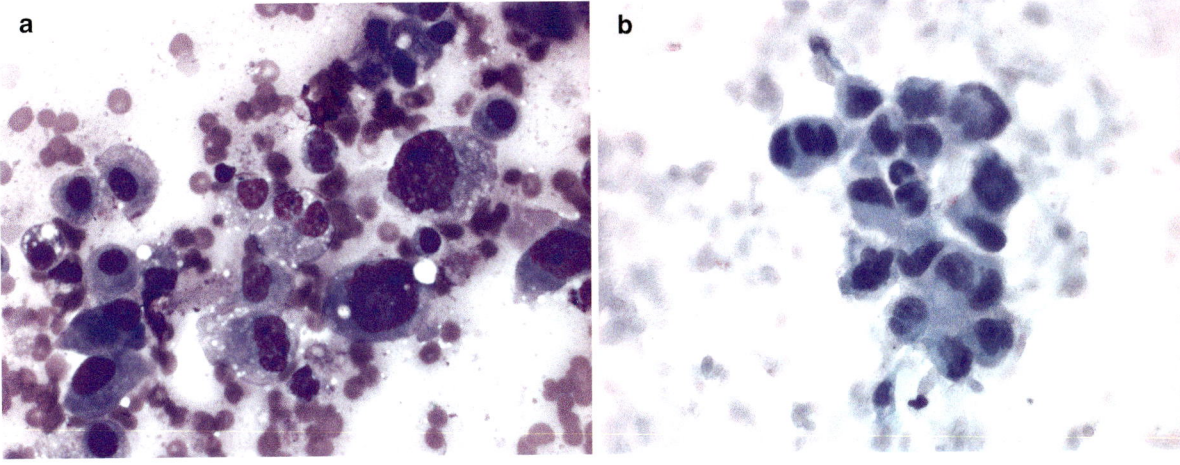

**Fig. 7.19** Chondrosarcoma: (**a–c**), relatively small spindle-shaped tumor cells lying singly or in loose branching groups. Note cartilaginous material in **b**. (**a, b**) PAP; (**c**) MGG. Fibrosarcoma (**d**) relatively small spindle-shaped tumor cells lying singly or in loose branching groups. PAP

**Fig. 7.20** Leiomyosarcoma: High-grade tumor with markedly atypical cells. (**a**) Diff-Quik; (**b**) PAP

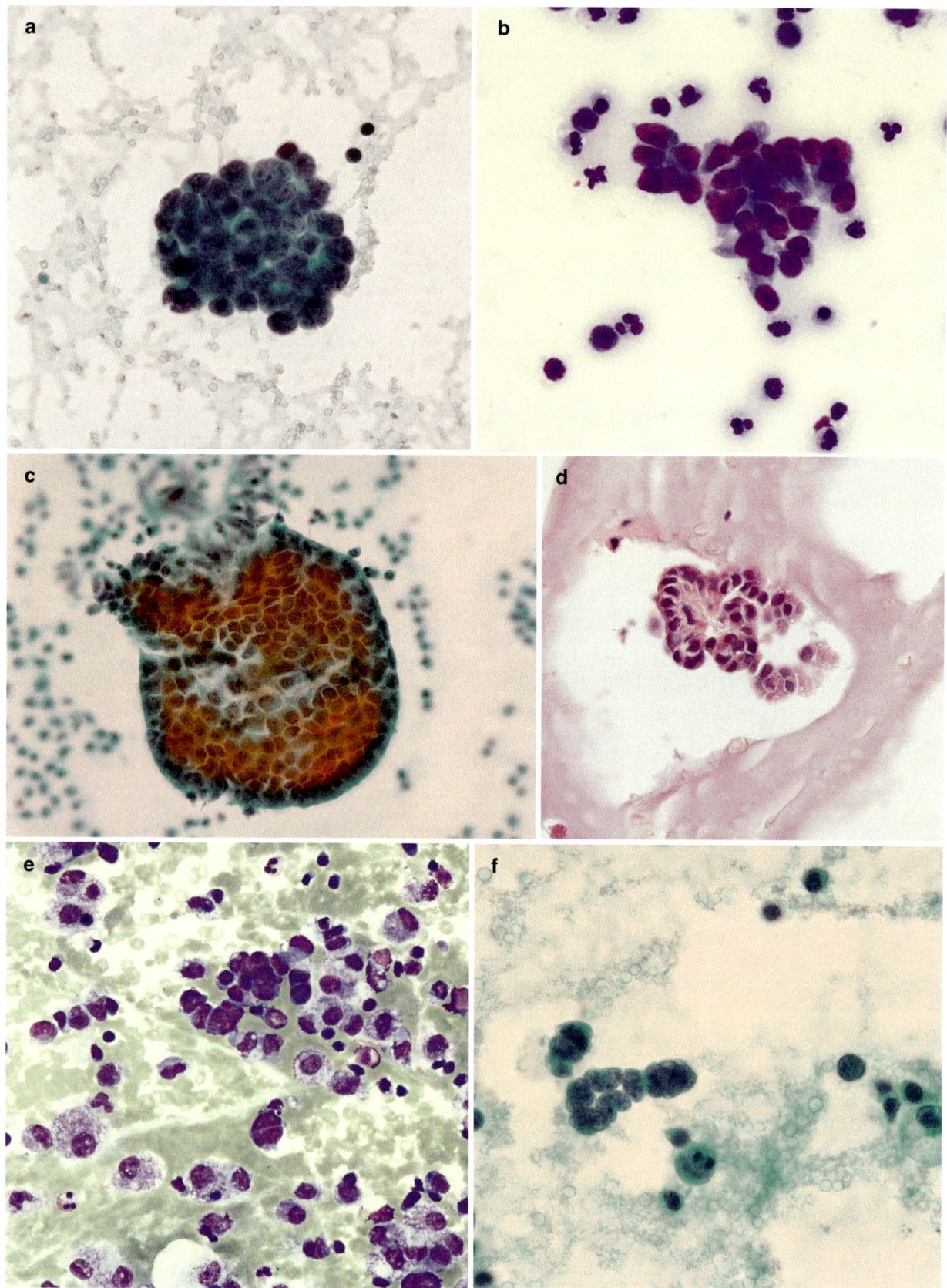

**Fig. 7.21** Primitive neuroectodermal and small round blue cell tumors: (**a**) *neuroblastoma*. Tight cluster of atypical cells with high n/c ratio, coarse chromatin, and distinct nucleoli; (**b–d**) *Wilms' tumor*. Small tumor cells with moderate atypia and distinct nucleoli forming primitive structures. (**e**, **f**) *PNET*. Tumor cells with high n/c ratio, some poorly preserved, with molding and cytoplasmic vacuolization (**e**) or chain formation (**f**). (**a, c, f**) PAP; (**b, e**) MGG; (**d**) H&E

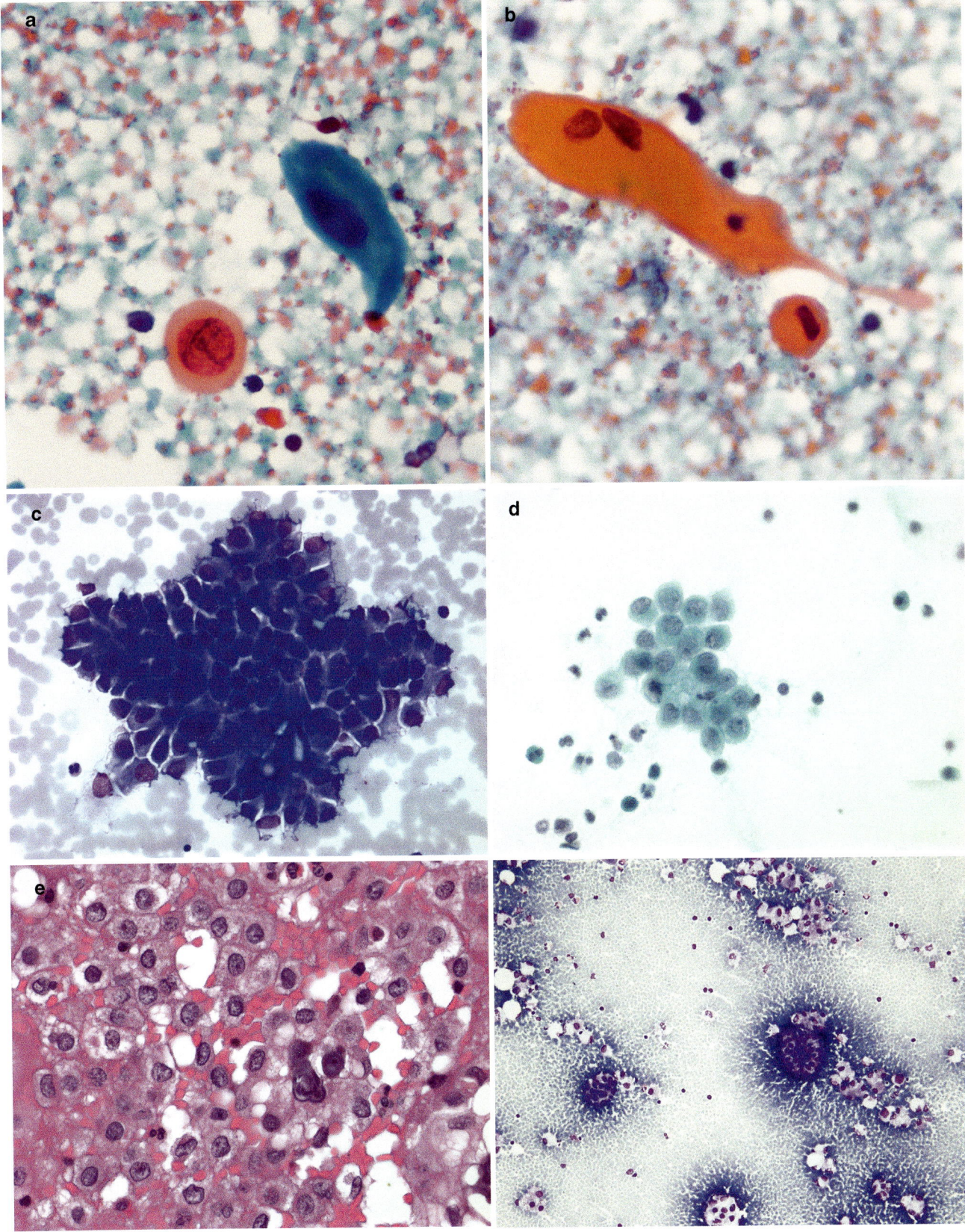

**Fig. 7.22** Head and neck tumors. *Larynx*: (**a**, **b**) squamous cell carcinoma of the larynx. *Thyroid*: (**c**–**h**) two papillary thyroid carcinomas. Calcifications are evident in both cases. (**i**, **j**) medullary carcinoma of the thyroid. Dissociated cells of variable size, some spindle-shaped. (**a**, **b**, **d**, **g**, **i**) PAP; (**c**, **f**, **h**, **j**) MGG/Diff-Quik; (**e**) H&E. (**k**) thyroglobulin immunostaining in the specimen seen in **c** to **e**; *Parotid*: (**l**–**n**) metastatic carcinoma of parotid gland origin. Dissociated tumor cells are seen in **l**, **m**, MGG/Diff-Quik; (**n**) androgen receptor immunostaining

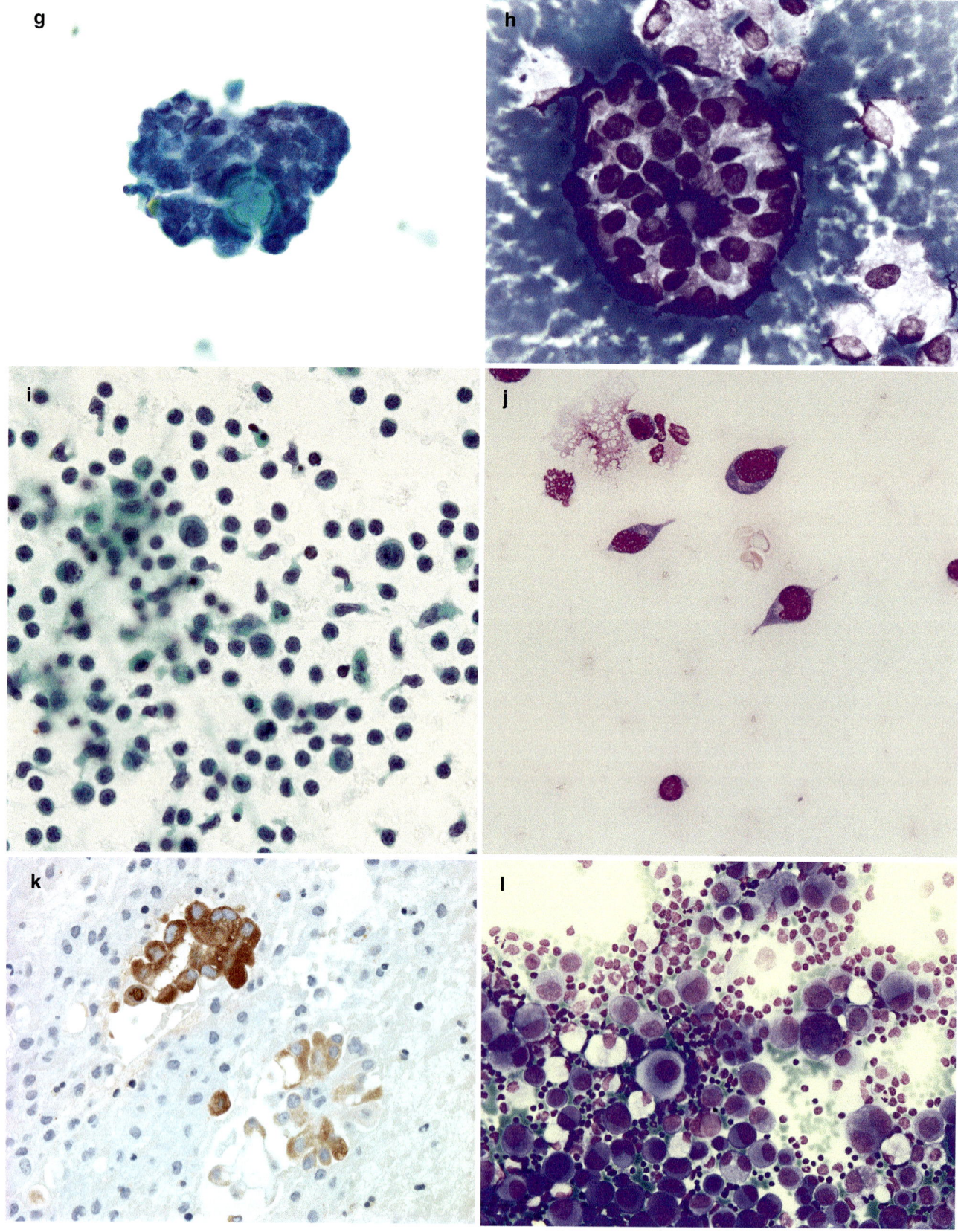

**Fig. 7.22** (continued)

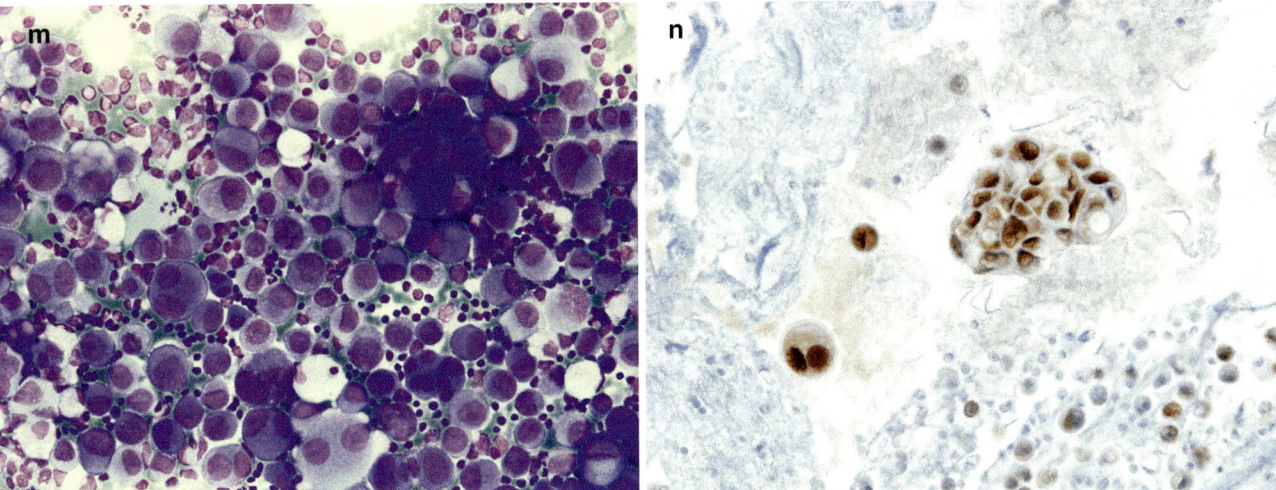

**Fig. 7.22** (continued)

Rare reports of malignant effusions with non-thyroidal head and neck tumors have been published, including metastasis from a lymphoepithelial carcinoma in the pleural cavity [167] and metastasis from an adenoid cystic carcinoma [168]. Metastasis from the latter entity was also described from a primary cutaneous tumor [169].

Metastatic carcinoma of parotid gland origin was diagnosed by one of the authors. Tumor cells expressed androgen receptor (Fig. 7.22l–n).

## Concluding Remarks

The breadth of differential diagnosis of cancer in serous effusions is evident from the above-discussed entities, as well as from the other chapters in this section. As is true for all pathology specimens, clinical data may resolve much of the difficulty. Their absence requires careful prioritizing of the most plausible differential diagnoses based on the morphological findings and patient age and gender. This may aid in directing the ancillary tests in a cost-effective direction. Nevertheless, some undifferentiated tumors require inclusion of all major cancer types in the differential diagnosis. In these cases, the use of selected antibodies that identify carcinoma, melanoma, sarcoma, and hematological tumors is mandated, followed by a second panel which should be more focused on the tentative diagnosis. Our suggestions for antibody panels that are relevant in the diagnostic algorithm for effusion work-up, with focus on epithelial and mesothelial cells, are presented in the **Appendix** of this section. Molecular testing is rapidly becoming central in classifying some of the malignancies affecting the serosal cavities, including in soft tissue and bone tumors, pediatric cancers, and hematological malignancies, but as carcinomas outnumber all other cancers, the majority of cases can still be resolved using immunohistochemistry. High-throughput technology, particularly next-generation sequencing, is likely to play a growing role in the setting of targeted therapy for these tumors in coming years.

## References

1. Torre LA, Bray F, Siegel RL, Ferlay J, Lortet-Tieulent J, Jemal A. Global cancer statistics, 2012. CA Cancer J Clin. 2015;65:87–108.
2. Ajani JA, Lee J, Sano T, Janjigian YY, Fan D, Song S. Gastric adenocarcinoma. Nat Rev Dis Primers. 2017;3:17036.
3. Maeda H, Kobayashi M, Sakamoto J. Evaluation and treatment of malignant ascites secondary to gastric cancer. World J Gastroenterol. 2015;21:10936–47.
4. Bozzetti C, Negri FV, Lagrasta CA, Crafa P, Bassano C, Tamagnini I, Gardini G, Nizzoli R, Leonardi F, Gasparro D, Camisa R, Cavalli S, Silini EM, Ardizzoni A. Comparison of HER2 status in primary and paired metastatic sites of gastric carcinoma. Br J Cancer. 2011;104:1372–6.
5. Wong DD, de Boer WB, Platten MA, Jo VY, Cibas ES, Kumarasinghe MP. HER2 testing in malignant effusions of metastatic gastric carcinoma: is it feasible? Diagn Cytopathol. 2015;43:80–5.
6. Spieler P, Gloor F. Identification of types and primary sites of malignant tumors by examination of exfoliated tumor cells in serous fluids. Comparison with the diagnostic accuracy on small histologic biopsies. Acta Cytol. 1985;29:753–67.
7. Chiaravalli M, Reni M, O'Reilly EM. Pancreatic ductal adenocarcinoma: State-of-the-art 2017 and new therapeutic strategies. Cancer Treat Rev. 2017;60:32–43.
8. Conroy T, Bachet JB, Ayav A, Huguet F, Lambert A, Caramella C, Maréchal R, Van Laethem JL, Ducreux M. Current standards and new innovative approaches for treatment of pancreatic cancer. Eur J Cancer. 2016;57:10–22.
9. Das KK, Early D. Pancreatic cancer screening. Curr Treat Options Gastroenterol. 2017;15:562–75.
10. Kamisawa T, Wood LD, Itoi T, Takaori K. Pancreatic cancer. Lancet. 2016;388:73–85.
11. DeWitt J, Yu M, Al-Haddad MA, Sherman S, McHenry L, Leblanc JK. Survival in patients with pancreatic cancer after the diagnosis

of malignant ascites or liver metastases by EUS-FNA. Gastrointest Endosc. 2010;71:260–5.

12. Zervos EE, Osborne D, Boe BA, Luzardo G, Goldin SB, Rosemurgy AS. Prognostic significance of new onset ascites in patients with pancreatic cancer. World J Surg Oncol. 2006;4:16.

13. Nakata B, Nishino H, Ogawa Y, Yokomatsu H, Kawasaki F, Kosaka K, Wada T, Suto R, Montani A, Hirakawa K. Prognostic predictive value of endoscopic ultrasound findings for invasive ductal carcinomas of pancreatic head. Pancreas. 2005;30:200–5.

14. Hicks AM, Chou J, Capanu M, Lowery MA, Yu KH, O'Reilly EM. Pancreas adenocarcinoma: ascites, clinical manifestations, and management implications. Clin Colorectal Cancer. 2016;15(4):360–8.

15. Shukuya T, Yasui H, Boku N, Onozawa Y, Fukutomi A, Yamazaki K, Taku K, Kojima T, Machida N. Weekly Paclitaxel after failure of gemcitabine in pancreatic cancer patients with malignant ascites: a retrospective study. Jpn J Clin Oncol. 2010;40:1135–8.

16. Yonemori K, Okusaka T, Ueno H, Morizane C, Takesako Y, Ikeda M. FP therapy for controlling malignant ascites in advanced pancreatic cancer patients. Hepato-Gastroenterology. 2007;54:2383–6.

17. Warshaw AL. Implications of peritoneal cytology for staging of early pancreatic cancer. Am J Surg. 1991;161:26–9. Discussion 29–30

18. Lei S, Kini J, Kim K, Howard JM. Pancreatic cancer. Cytologic study of peritoneal washings. Arch Surg. 1994;129:639–42.

19. Di Bonito L, Dudine S, Falconieri G. Cytopathology of exocrine pancreatic carcinoma in effusions. Acta Cytol. 1991;35:311–4.

20. Dienstmann R, Vermeulen L, Guinney J, Kopetz S, Tejpar S, Tabernero J. Consensus molecular subtypes and the evolution of precision medicine in colorectal cancer. Nat Rev Cancer. 2017;17:79–92.

21. DeMay RM, editor. The art & science of cytopathology. Chicago: ASCP Press; 1996. p. 257–325.

22. Ronnett BM, Zahn CM, Kurman RJ, Kass ME, Sugarbaker PH, Shmookler BM. Disseminated peritoneal adenomucinosis and peritoneal mucinous carcinomatosis. A clinicopathologic analysis of 109 cases with emphasis on distinguishing pathologic features, site of origin, prognosis, and relationship to "pseudomyxoma peritonei". Am J Surg Pathol. 1995;19: 1390–408.

23. Bradley RF, Stewart JH 4th, Russell GB, Levine EA, Geisinger KR. Pseudomyxoma peritonei of appendiceal origin: a clinicopathologic analysis of 101 patients uniformly treated at a single institution, with literature review. Am J Surg Pathol. 2006;30: 551–9.

24. Carr NJ, Cecil TD, Mohamed F, Sobin LH, Sugarbaker PH, González-Moreno S, Taflampas P, Chapman S, Moran BJ, Peritoneal Surface Oncology Group International. A consensus for classification and pathologic reporting of pseudomyxoma peritonei and associated appendiceal neoplasia: the results of the Peritoneal Surface Oncology Group International (PSOGI) modified Delphi process. Am J Surg Pathol. 2016;40:14–26.

25. Jackson SL, Fleming RA, Loggie BW, Geisinger KR. Gelatinous ascites: a cytohistologic study of pseudomyxoma peritonei in 67 patients. Mod Pathol. 2001;14:664–71.

26. Badyal RK, Khairwa A, Rajwanshi A, Nijhawan R, Radhika S, Gupta N, Dey P. Significance of epithelial cell clusters in pseudomyxoma peritonei. Cytopathology. 2016;27:418–26.

27. Wojcik EM, Selvaggi SM. Goblet-cell carcinoid tumor in peritoneal fluid: a case report. Diagn Cytopathol. 1991;7:155–7.

28. Kobayashi TK, Ueda M, Nishino T, Tamagaki T, Watanabe S, Kushima R. Malignant pleural effusions due to adeno-endocrine-cell carcinoma of the appendix: a case report. Diagn Cytopathol. 1997;16:522–5.

29. Zafar S, Chen H, Sun W, Das K. Cytology of metastatic appendiceal goblet cell carcinoid in pleural effusion fluid: a case report. Diagn Cytopathol. 2008;36:894–8.

30. Gupta A, Patel T, Dargar P, Shah M. Metastatic appendiceal goblet cell carcinoid masquerading as mucinous adenocarcinoma in effusion cytology: a diagnostic pitfall. J Cytol. 2013;30:136–8.

31. Tonooka A, Oda K, Hayashi M, Sakazume K, Tanaka H, Kaburaki KH, Uekusa T. Cytological findings of appendiceal mixed adenoneuroendocrine carcinoma in pleural effusion: morphological changes evident after metastasis. Diagn Cytopathol. 2015;43: 577–80.

32. Cameron SE, Alsharif M, McKeon D, Pambuccian SE. Cytology of metastatic thymic well-differentiated neuroendocrine carcinoma (thymic carcinoid) in pleural fluid: report of a case. Diagn Cytopathol. 2008;36:333–7.

33. Vasseur B, Cadiot G, Zins M, Fléjou JF, Belghiti J, Marmuse JP, Vilgrain V, Bernades P, Mignon M, Ruszniewski P. Peritoneal carcinomatosis in patients with digestive endocrine tumors. Cancer. 1996;78:1686–92.

34. Forner A, Llovet JM, Bruix J. Hepatocellular carcinoma. Lancet. 2012;379:1245–55.

35. Thrall MJ, Giampoli EJ. Routine review of ascites fluid from patients with cirrhosis or hepatocellular carcinoma is a low-yield procedure: an observational study. Cytojournal. 2009;6:16.

36. Falconieri G, Zanconati F, Colautti I, Dudine S, Bonifacio-Gori D, Di Bonito L. Effusion cytology of hepatocellular carcinoma. Acta Cytol. 1995;39:893–7.

37. Colli A, Cocciolo M, Riva C, Marcassoli L, Pirola M, Di Gregorio P, Buccino G. Ascitic fluid analysis in hepatocellular carcinoma. Cancer. 1993;72:677–82.

38. Morishita Y, Etori F, Sawada K, Kachi H, Yamada T, Kawamori T, Tanaka T. Sarcomatous hepatocellular carcinoma with malignant ascites. A report of two cases. Acta Cytol. 1998;42:759–64.

39. Lagergren J, Smyth E, Cunningham D, Lagergren P. Oesophageal cancer. Lancet. 2017;390:2383–96.

40. Ozyurtkan MO, Balci AE, Cakmak M. Predictors of mortality within three months in the patients with malignant pleural effusion. Eur J Intern Med. 2010;21:30–4.

41. Renshaw AA, Nappi D, Sugarbaker DJ, Swanson S. Effusion cytology of esophageal carcinoma. Cancer. 1997;81:365–72.

42. Gamez RG, Jessurun J, Berger MJ, Pambuccian SE. Cytology of metastatic cervical squamous cell carcinoma in pleural fluid: report of a case confirmed by human papillomavirus typing. Diagn Cytopathol. 2009;37:381–7.

43. Semczuk A, Skomra D, Rybojad P, Jeczeń R, Rechberger T. Endometrial carcinoma with pleural metastasis: a case report. Acta Cytol. 2006;50:697–700.

44. Kogan J, Golzman B, Turkot S, Ben-Dor D, Charkowsky T, Oren S. Malignant pericardial effusion and cardiac tamponade as a late complication of endometrial carcinoma. Eur J Intern Med. 2004;15:318–20.

45. Jamshed A, Khafaga Y, El-Husseiny G, Gray AJ, Manji M. Pericardial metastasis in carcinoma of the uterine cervix. Gynecol Oncol. 1996;61:451–3.

46. Santala M, Puistola U, Kauppila A. Endometrial adenocarcinoma complicated by malignant pericardial effusion. Gynecol Oncol. 1995;56:444–5.

47. Rieke JW, Kapp DS. Successful management of malignant pericardial effusion in metastatic squamous cell carcinoma of the uterine cervix. Gynecol Oncol. 1988;31:338–51.

48. Hayashi Y, Iwasaka T, Hachisuga T, Kishikawa T, Ikeda N, Sugimori H. Malignant pericardial effusion in endometrial adenocarcinoma. Gynecol Oncol. 1988;29:234–9.

49. Arville B, Al Diffalha S, Mehrotra S. Cervical squamous cell carcinoma metastatic to pericardial fluid--large cell balls masquerade as adenocarcinoma. Diagn Cytopathol. 2015;43:912–5.

50. Ikoma S, Nicolas M, Jagirdar J, Policarpio-Nicolas ML. Chondrosarcoma-like metastasis from a poorly differentiated uterine cervical squamous cellcarcinoma. A unique morphology and diagnostic pitfall in cytology. Diagn Cytopathol. 2017;45:750–3.

51. Huang CC, Michael CW. Cytomorphological features of metastatic squamous cell carcinoma in serous effusions. Cytopathology. 2014;25:112–9.

52. Silver SA, Devouassoux-Shisheboran M, Mezzetti TP, Tavassoli FA. Mesonephric adenocarcinomas of the uterine cervix: a study of 11 cases with immunohistochemical findings. Am J Surg Pathol. 2001;25:379–87.

53. Khunamornpong S, Siriaunkgul S, Suprasert P. Cytology of small-cell carcinoma of the uterine cervix in serous effusion: a report on two cases. Diagn Cytopathol. 2001;24:253–5.

54. Atahan S, Ekinci C, Içli F, Erdoğan N. Cytology of clear cell carcinoma of the female genital tract in fine needle aspirates and ascites. Acta Cytol. 2000;44:1005–9.

55. Zhou C, Gilks CB, Hayes M, Clement PB. Papillary serous carcinoma of the uterine cervix: a clinicopathologic study of 17 cases. Am J Surg Pathol. 1998;22:113–20.

56. Johnston WW. The malignant pleural effusion. A review of cytopathologic diagnoses of 584 specimens from 472 consecutive patients. Cancer. 1985;56:905–9.

57. McGrath SM, Rana DN, Lynch M, Desai M. Metastatic transitional cell carcinoma causing a unilateral pleural effusion: a case report. Acta Cytol. 2008;52:351–3.

58. Renshaw AA, Madge R, Granter SR. Intracytoplasmic eosinophilic inclusions (Melamed-Wolinska bodies). Association with metastatic transitional cell carcinoma in pleural fluid. Acta Cytol. 1997;41:995–8.

59. Fabozzi SJ, Newton JR Jr, Moriarty RP, Schellhammer PF. Malignant pericardial effusion as initial solitary site of metastasis from transitional cell carcinoma of the bladder. Urology. 1995;45:320–2.

60. Xiao GQ. Cytomorphology of urothelial carcinomatous peritoneal effusion. Cytopathology. 2008;19:131–3.

61. Kim SS, Choi YD, Nam JH, Kwon DD, Juhng SW, Choi C. Cytologic features of primary signet ring cell carcinoma of the bladder: a case report. Acta Cytol. 2009;53:309–12.

62. Cimino-Mathews A, Ali SZ. Metastatic urothelial carcinoma with signet ring features: Cytomorphologic findings in abdominal paracentesis. Diagn Cytopathol. 2011;39:132–4.

63. Islam N, Ahmedani MY. Renal carcinoma presenting as cardiac tamponade: a case report and review of literature. Int J Cardiol. 1998;64:207–11.

64. Peck JR, Hitchcock CL, Maguire S, Dickerson J, Bush C. Isolated cardiac metastasis from plasmacytoid urothelial carcinoma of the bladder. Exp Hematol Oncol. 2012;1:16.

65. Katsuya Y, Fukusumi M, Morita S, Ibe T, Wakuda K, Mouri A, Hamamoto Y, Yamada K, Kamimura M. Pseudomesotheliomatous carcinoma due to pleural metastasis from renal pelvic cancer. Intern Med. 2014;53:871–4.

66. Huang CC, Attele A, Michael CW. Cytomorphologic features of metastatic urothelial carcinoma in serous effusions. Diagn Cytopathol. 2013;41:569–74.

67. Mai KT, Roustan Delatour NL, Assiri A, Al-Maghrabi H. Secondary prostatic adenocarcinoma: a cytopathological study of 50 cases. Diagn Cytopathol. 2007;35:91–5.

68. Renshaw AA, Nappi D, Cibas ES. Cytology of metastatic adenocarcinoma of the prostate in pleural effusions. Diagn Cytopathol. 1996;15:103–7.

69. Saif MW, Figg WD, Hewitt S, Brosky K, Reed E, Dahut W. Malignant ascites as only manifestation of metastatic prostate cancer. Prostate Cancer Prostatic Dis. 1999;2:290–3.

70. Saif MW. Malignant ascites associated with carcinoma of the prostate. J Appl Res. 2005;5:305–11.

71. Catton PA, Hartwick RW, Srigley JR. Prostate cancer presenting with malignant ascites: signet-ring cell variant of prostatic adenocarcinoma. Urology. 1992;39:495–7.

72. Brimo F, Epstein JI. Immunohistochemical pitfalls in prostate pathology. Hum Pathol. 2012;43:313–24.

73. Sears D, Hajdu SI. The cytologic diagnosis of malignant neoplasms in pleural and peritoneal effusions. Acta Cytol. 1987;31:85–97.

74. Renshaw AA, Comiter CV, Nappi D, Granter SR. Effusion cytology of renal cell carcinoma. Cancer. 1998;84:148–52.

75. Gupta R, Mathur SR, Iyer VK, Kumar AS, Seth A. Cytomorphologic consideration in malignant ascites with renal cell carcinoma: a report of two cases. Cytojournal. 2010;7:4.

76. Teresa P, Maria Grazia Z, Doriana M, Irene P, Michele S. Malignant effusion of chromophobe renal-cell carcinoma: cytological and immunohistochemical findings. Diagn Cytopathol. 2012;40:56–61.

77. Davion S, Rohan S, Nayar R, Kulesza P. Metastatic chromophobe renal cell carcinoma in pleural fluid cytology: review of literature and report of a case. Diagn Cytopathol. 2012 Sep;40(9):826–9.

78. Ellis CL, Burroughs F, Michael CW, Li QK. Cytology of metastatic renal medullary carcinoma in pleural effusion: a study of two cases. Diagn Cytopathol. 2009;37:843–8.

79. Caraway NP, Wojcik EM, Katz RL, Ro JY, Ordóñez NG. Cytologic findings of collecting duct carcinoma of the kidney. Diagn Cytopathol. 1995;13:304–9.

80. Drut R. Malignant rhabdoid tumor of the kidney diagnosed by fine-needle aspiration cytology. Diagn Cytopathol. 1990;6:124–6.

81. Chute DJ, Kong CS, Stelow EB. Immunohistochemistry for the detection of renal cell carcinoma in effusion cytology. Diagn Cytopathol. 2011;39:118–23.

82. Knoepp SM, Kunju LP, Roh MH. Utility of PAX8 and PAX2 immunohistochemistry in the identification of renal cell carcinoma in diagnostic cytology. Diagn Cytopathol. 2012;40:667–72.

83. Waters L, Crumley S, Truong L, Mody D, Coffey D. PAX2 and PAX8: useful markers for metastatic effusions. Acta Cytol. 2014;58:60–6.

84. Wiseman W, Michael CW, Roh MH. Diagnostic utility of PAX8 and PAX2 immunohistochemistry in the identification of metastatic Müllerian carcinoma in effusions. Diagn Cytopathol. 2011;39:651–6.

85. Tong GX, Devaraj K, Hamele-Bena D, Yu WM, Turk A, Chen X, Wright JD, Greenebaum E. Pax8: a marker for carcinoma of Müllerian origin in serous effusions. Diagn Cytopathol. 2011;39:567–74.

86. Hajdu SI, Nolan MA. Exfoliative cytology of malignant germ cell tumors. Acta Cytol. 1975;19:255–60.

87. Geisinger KR, Hajdu SI, Helson L. Exfoliative cytology of nonlymphoreticular neoplasms in children. Acta Cytol. 1984;28:16–28.

88. Wong JW, Pitlik D, Abdul-Karim FW. Cytology of pleural, peritoneal and pericardial fluids in children. A 40-year summary. Acta Cytol. 1997;41:467–73.

89. Kashimura M, Tsukamoto N, Matsuyama T, Kashimura Y, Sugimori H, Taki I. Cytologic findings of ascites from patients with ovarian dysgerminoma. Acta Cytol. 1983;27:59–62.

90. Roncalli M, Gribaudi G, Simoncelli D, Servida E. Cytology of yolk-sac tumor of the ovary in ascitic fluid. Report of a case. Acta Cytol. 1988;32:113–6.

91. Selvaggi SM. Cytologic features of malignant ovarian monodermal teratoma with an ependymal component in peritoneal washings. Int J Gynecol Pathol. 1992;11:299–303.

92. Valente PT, Schantz HD, Edmonds PR, Hanjani P. Peritoneal cytology of uncommon ovarian tumors. Diagn Cytopathol. 1992;8:98–106.

93. Selvaggi SM, Guidos BJ. Immature teratoma of the ovary on fluid cytology. Diagn Cytopathol. 2001;25:411–4.

94. Abe T, Shinohara N, Harabayashi T, Tsuchiya K, Suzuki S, Itoh T, Seki T, Togashi M, Nonomura K, Koyanagi T. Peritoneal carcinomatosis in refractory seminoma. Int J Urol. 2004;11:184–6.

95. Ikeda K, Tate G, Suzuki T, Mitsuya T. Cytomorphologic features of immature ovarian teratoma in peritoneal effusion: a case report. Diagn Cytopathol. 2005;33:39–42.

96. Murugan P, Siddaraju N, Sridhar E, Soundararaghavan J, Habeebullah S. Unusual ovarian malignancies in ascitic fluid: a report of 2 cases. Acta Cytol. 2010;54:611–7.

97. Izban KF, Candel AG, Hsi ED, Selvaggi SM. Metastatic melanoma of the vulva identified by peritoneal fluid cytology. Diagn Cytopathol. 1999;20:152–5.

98. Baniak N, Podberezin M, Kanthan SC, Kanthan R. Primary pulmonary/pleural melanoma in a 13 year-old presenting as pleural effusion. Pathol Res Pract. 2017;213:161–4.

99. Longatto Filho A, de Carvalho LV, Santos Gda C, Oyafuso MS, Lombardo V, Bortolan J, Neves JI. Cytologic diagnosis of melanoma in serous effusions. A morphologic and immunocytochemical study. Acta Cytol. 1995;39:481–4.

100. Beaty MW, Fetsch P, Wilder AM, Marincola F, Abati A. Effusion cytology of malignant melanoma. A morphologic and immunocytochemical analysis including application of the MART-1 antibody. Cancer. 1997;81:57–63.

101. Ikeda K, Tate G, Iezumi K, Suzuki T, Kitamura T, Mitsuya T. Effusion cytomorphology and immunocytochemistry of malignant melanoma: five cases of melanotic melanoma and one case of amelanotic melanoma. Diagn Cytopathol. 2009;37: 516–21.

102. Niemann TH, Thomas PA. Melanoma with signet-ring cells in a peritoneal effusion. Diagn Cytopathol. 1995;12:241–4.

103. Pinto MM. An immunoperoxidase study of S-100 protein in neoplastic cells in serous effusions. Use as a marker for melanoma. Acta Cytol. 1986;30:240–4.

104. Conner JR, Cibas ES, Hornick JL, Qian X. Wilms tumor 1/cytokeratin dual-color immunostaining reveals distinctive staining patterns in metastatic melanoma, metastatic carcinoma, and mesothelial cells in pleural fluids: an effective first-line test for the workup of malignant effusions. Cancer Cytopathol. 2014;122:586–95.

105. Watson CW, Friedman KJ. Cytology of metastatic neuroendocrine (Merkel-cell) carcinoma in pleural fluid. A case report. Acta Cytol. 1985;29:397–402.

106. Payne MM, Rader AE, McCarthy DM, Rodgers WH. Merkel cell carcinoma in a malignant pleural effusion: case report. Cytojournal. 2004;1:5.

107. Policarpio-Nicolas ML, Avery DL, Hartley T. Merkel cell carcinoma presenting as malignant ascites: A case report and review of literature. Cytojournal. 2015;12:19.

108. Cohen I, Loberant N, King E, Herskovits M, Sweed Y, Jerushalmi J. Rhabdomyosarcoma in a child with massive pleural effusion: cytological diagnosis from pleural fluid. Diagn Cytopathol. 1999;21:125–8.

109. Abadi MA, Zakowski MF. Cytologic features of sarcomas in fluids. Cancer. 1998;84:71–6.

110. Longatto-Filho A, Bisi H, Bortolan J, Granja NV, Lombardo V. Cytologic diagnosis of metastatic sarcoma in effusions. Acta Cytol. 2003;47:317–8.

111. Ikeda K, Tsuta K. Effusion cytomorphology of small round cell tumors. J Cytol. 2016;33:85–92.

112. Ahmed AA, Andraws N, Almutairi AM, Saied HM, Elbagir-Mohamed AM. Cytologic and immunophenotypic features of malignant cells in pediatric body fluids. Acta Cytol. 2015;59:332–8.

113. Allsbrook WC Jr, Stead NW, Pantazis CG, Houston JH, Crosby JH. Embryonal rhabdomyosarcoma in ascitic fluid. Immunocytochemical and DNA flow cytometric study. Arch Pathol Lab Med. 1986;110:847–9.

114. Thompson KS, Jensen JD, Bhoopalam N, Reyes CV. Pleural effusion cytology of embryonal rhabdomyosarcoma. Diagn Cytopathol. 1997;16:270–3.

115. Cribbs RK, Shehata BM, Ricketts RR. Primary ovarian rhabdomyosarcoma in children. Pediatr Surg Int. 2008;24:593–5.

116. Yao JC, Wang WC, Tseng HH, Hwang WS. Primary rhabdomyosarcoma of the prostate. Diagnosis by needle biopsy and immunocytochemistry. Acta Cytol. 1988;32:509–12.

117. Ohi S. Characterization, anticancer drug susceptibility and atRA-induced growth inhibition of a novel cell line (HUMEMS) established from pleural effusion of alveolar rhabdomyosarcoma of breast tissue. Hum Cell. 2007;20:39–51.

118. Kaw YT, Cramer HM. Cytologic diagnosis of rhabdomyosarcoma in a patient with germ cell tumor. A case report. Acta Cytol. 1995;39:249–51.

119. Alderman MA, Thomas DG, Roh MH. Diagnostic evaluation of metastatic rhabdomyosarcoma in effusion specimens. Diagn Cytopathol. 2013;41:955–9.

120. Bhattacharya B, Sariya D, Reddy VB, Kluskens L, Gould VE, Gattuso P. Application of adjunct techniques in cytologic material in the diagnosis of rhabdomyosarcoma: case report and review of the literature. Diagn Cytopathol. 2002;26:384–6.

121. Thiryayi SA, Rana DN, Roulson J, Crosbie P, Woodhead M, Eyden BP, Hasleton PS. Diagnosis of alveolar rhabdomyosarcoma in effusion cytology: a diagnostic pitfall. Cytopathology. 2010;21:273–5.

122. Theunissen P, Cremers M, van der Meer S, Bot F, Bras J. Cytologic diagnosis of rhabdomyosarcoma in a child with a pleural effusion. A case report. Acta Cytol. 2004;48:249–53.

123. Yuregir OO, Sahin FI, Avci Z, Yilmaz Z, Celasun B, Sarialioglu F. Multiple chromosome abnormalities in the pleural fluid of a patient with recurrent Ewing sarcoma. Pediatr Hematol Oncol. 2009;26:267–72.

124. Schiavo R, Tullio C, La Grotteria M, Andreotti IC, Scarpati B, Romiti L, Bozzi F, Pedrazzoli P, Establishment SS. characterization of a new Ewing's sarcoma cell line from a malignant pleural effusion. Anticancer Res. 2007;27:3273–8.

125. Nishio J, Iwasaki H, Ishiguro M, Ohjimi Y, Fujita C, Yanai F, Nibu K, Mitsudome A, Kaneko Y, Kikuchi M. Establishment and characterization of a novel human desmoplastic small round cell tumor cell line, JN-DSRCT-1. Lab Investig. 2002;82:1175–82.

126. Hallman JR, Geisinger KR. Cytology of fluids from pleural, peritoneal and pericardial cavities in children. A comprehensive survey. Acta Cytol. 1994;38:209–17.

127. Hattori Y, Yoshida A, Sasaki N, Shibuki Y, Tamura K, Tsuta K. Desmoplastic small round cell tumor with sphere-like clusters mimicking adenocarcinoma. Diagn Cytopathol. 2015;43:214–7.

128. Zhu H, McMeekin EM, Sturgis CD. Desmoplastic small round cell tumor, a "Floating Island" pattern in pleural fluid cytology: a case report and review of the literature. Case Rep Pathol. 2015;2015:676894.

129. Berry GJ, Anderson CJ, Pitts WC, Neitzel GF, Weiss LM. Cytology of angiosarcoma in effusions. Acta Cytol. 1991;35:538–42.

130. Boucher LD, Swanson PE, Stanley MW, Silverman JF, Raab SS, Geisinger KR. Cytology of angiosarcoma. Findings in fourteen fine-needle aspiration biopsy specimens and one pleural fluid specimen. Am J Clin Pathol. 2000;114:210–9.

131. Davidson B, Abeler VM. Primary ovarian angiosarcoma presenting as malignant cells in ascites: case report and review of the literature. Diagn Cytopathol. 2005;32:307–9.

132. Shin OR, Cho U, Chang E, Seo KJ. Metastatic pleural angiosarcoma: a diagnostic pitfall might be overcome by morphologic clues and clinical correlation. Diagn Cytopathol. 2015;43:669–72.

133. Antic T, Staerkel G. Mediastinal epithelioid hemangioendothelioma metastatic to lymph nodes and pleural fluid: report of a case. Diagn Cytopathol. 2010;38:113–6.

134. Buggage RR, Soudi N, Olson JL, Busseniers AE. Epithelioid hemangioendothelioma of the lung: pleural effusion cytology, ultrastructure, and brief literature review. Diagn Cytopathol. 1995;13:54–60.

135. Enbom ET, Abasolo PA, Dixon JR, Nikolaenko LM, French SW, Duane GB. Cytomorphological features of epithelioid hemangioendothelioma in ascitic fluid with radiological, clinical and histopathological correlations. Acta Cytol. 2014;58:211–6.

136. Sayah M, VandenBussche C, Maleki Z. Epithelioid hemangioendothelioma in pleural effusion. Diagn Cytopathol. 2015;43: 751–5.

137. Wengerkievicz AC, Corá AP, de Almeida LP, Duarte NJ, Siqueira SA, Antonangelo L. Neoplastic ascites in osteosarcoma: a case report. Acta Cytol. 2010;54:845–8.

138. Geisinger KR, Naylor B, Beals TF, Cytopathology NPM. including transmission and scanning electron microscopy, of pleomorphic liposarcomas in pleural fluids. Acta Cytol. 1980;24:435–41.

139. Dagli AF, Pehlivan S, Ozercan MR. Pleural liposarcoma mimicking carcinoma in pleural effusion cytology: a case report. Acta Cytol. 2010;54:601–4.

140. Kudo N, Ogose A, Hotta T, Kawashima H, Gu W, Umezu H, Toyama T, Endo N. Establishment of novel human dedifferentiated chondrosarcoma cell line with osteoblastic differentiation. Virchows Arch. 2007;451:691–9.

141. Ikemoto S, Sugimura K, Yoshida N, Nakatani T. Chondrosarcoma of the urinary bladder and establishment of a human chondrosarcoma cell line (OCUU-6). Hum Cell. 2004;17:93–6.

142. Chen KT. Effusion cytology of metastatic extraskeletal myxoid chondrosarcoma. Diagn Cytopathol. 2003;28:222–3.

143. Tsuchido K, Yamada M, Satou T, Otsuki Y, Shimizu S, Kobayashi H. Cytology of sclerosing epithelioid fibrosarcoma in pleural effusion. Diagn Cytopathol. 2010;38:748–53.

144. Hagiwara Y, Nakamura K, Taguchi M, Ashiwa A, Nishioka C, Kono T, Matsuzaki N, Yuba Y. Myxofibrosarcoma of the heart: a case report with positive pleural effusion cytology. Diagn Cytopathol. 2016;44:1112–6.

145. Nguyen GK, Jeannot A. Cytology of synovial sarcoma metastases in pleural fluid. Acta Cytol. 1982;26:517–20.

146. Sonobe H, Manabe Y, Furihata M, Iwata J, Oka T, Ohtsuki Y, Mizobuchi H, Yamamoto H, Kumano O, Abe S. Establishment and characterization of a new human synovial sarcoma cell line, HS-SY-II. Lab Investig. 1992;67:498–505.

147. Ng WK, Lui PC, Ma L. Peritoneal washing cytology findings of disseminated myxoid leiomyosarcoma of uterus: report of a case with emphasis on possible differential diagnosis. Diagn Cytopathol. 2002;27:47–52.

148. Awasthi A, Gupta N, Srinivasan R, Nijhawan R, Rajwanshi A. Cytopathological spectrum of unusual malignant pleural effusions at a tertiary care centre in north India. Cytopathology. 2007;18:28–32.

149. Knapik J, Yachnis AT, Ripley D, Biegel JA, Rathor S, Hardt NS, Talerman A, Wilkinson EJ. Aggressive uterine sarcoma with rhabdoid features: diagnosis by peritoneal fluid cytology and absence of INI1 gene mutation. Hum Pathol. 2001;32:884–6.

150. Hirakawa E, Kobayashi S, Miki H, Haba R, Saoo K, Yamakawa K, Ohkura I, Kira Y. Ascitic fluid cytology of adenosarcoma of the ovary: a case report. Diagn Cytopathol. 2001;24:343–6.

151. Keller JM, Listrom MB, Hart JB, Olson NJ, Jordan SW. Cytologic detection of penile malignant melanoma of soft parts in pleural effusion using monoclonal antibody HMB-45. Acta Cytol. 1990;34:393–6.

152. Jaffer S, Woodruff JM. Cytology of melanotic schwannoma in a fine needle aspirate and pleural fluid. A case report. Acta Cytol. 2000;44:1095–100.

153. Lee JC, Wu JM, Liau JY, Huang HY, Lo CY, Jan IS, Hornick JL, Qian X. Cytopathologic features of epithelioid inflammatory myofibroblastic sarcoma with correlation of histopathology, immunohistochemistry, and molecular cytogenetic analysis. Cancer Cytopathol. 2015;123:495–504.

154. Motoyama T, Watanabe H. Ascitic fluid cytologic features of a malignant mixed mesodermal tumor of the ovary. Acta Cytol. 1987;31:63–7.

155. Farr GH, Hajdu SI. Exfoliative cytology of metastatic neuroblastoma. Acta Cytol. 1972;16:203–6.

156. Baliga M, Holmquist N, Warrier RP. Alteration of Wilms' tumor staging by cytologic detection of malignant cells in chylous ascites. Diagn Cytopathol. 1995;12:357–9.

157. Vernon AN, Sheeler LR, Biscotti CV, Stoller JK. Pleural effusion resulting from metastatic papillary carcinoma of the thyroid. Chest. 1992;101:1448–50.

158. Vassilopoulou-Sellin R, Sneige N. Pleural effusion in patients with differentiated papillary thyroid cancer. South Med J. 1994;87:1111–6.

159. Hyman MP. Papillary and undifferentiated thyroid carcinoma presenting as a metastatic papillary serous effusion. A case report. Acta Cytol. 1979;23:483–6.

160. Siddaraju N, Viswanathan VK, Saka VK, Basu D, Shanmugham C. Fine needle aspiration of follicular variant of papillary thyroid carcinoma presenting with pleural effusion: a case report. Acta Cytol. 2007;51:911–5.

161. Hsu KF, Hsieh CB, Duh QY, Chien CF, Li HS, Shih ML. Hürthle cell carcinoma of the thyroid with contralateral malignant pleural effusion. Onkologie. 2009;32:47–9.

162. Rosa M. Cytological features of medullary thyroid carcinoma in ascitic effusion. Diagn Cytopathol. 2017;45:1030–2.

163. Geisinger KR, Steffee CH, McGee RS, Woodruff RD, Buss DH. The cytomorphologic features of sclerosing mucoepidermoid carcinoma of the thyroid gland with eosinophilia. Am J Clin Pathol. 1998;109:294–301.

164. Olson MT, Nuransoy A, Ali SZ. Malignant pleural effusion resulting from metastasis of thyroid primaries: a cytomorphological analysis. Acta Cytol. 2013;57:177–83.

165. Lew M, Pang JC, Roh MH, Jing X. Cytologic Features and Immunocytochemical Profiles of Malignant Effusions with Metastatic Papillary Thyroid Carcinoma: A Case Series from a Single Institution. Acta Cytol. 2015;59:412–7.

166. Vyas M, Harigopal M. Metastatic thyroid carcinoma presenting as malignant pleural effusion: a cytologic review of 5 cases. Diagn Cytopathol. 2016;44:1085–9.

167. Seok JY, Lee KG. Cytologic features of metastatic lymphoepithelial carcinoma in pleural fluid: a case report. Acta Cytol. 2009;53:215–8.

168. Florentine BD, Fink T, Avidan S, Braslavsky D, Raza A, Cobb CJ. Extra-salivary gland presentations of adenoid cystic carcinoma: a report of three cases. Diagn Cytopathol. 2006;34:491–4.

169. Benchetritt M, Butori C, Long E, Ilie M, Ferrari E, Hofman P. Pericardial effusion as primary manifestation of metastatic cutaneous adenoid cystic carcinoma: diagnostic cytopathology from an exfoliative sample. Diagn Cytopathol. 2008;36:351–4.

Part II

# Biology, Therapy, and Prognosis

# Lung Cancer

8

## Katalin Dobra and Anders Hjerpe

## Introduction

Lung cancer is worldwide the leading cause of cancer-related death [1–3]. Over 75% of the newly detected lung cancer patients have at the time of the diagnosis already distal or regional metastases [4]. Malignant pleural effusions represent advanced metastatic disease. Such metastatic involvement of the serosal cavities occurs in 15–26% of the cases [5, 6], often being the first clinical manifestation of a malignant process. With appropriate adjuvant analyses, the serous effusions can provide the necessary diagnostic information for choice of therapy. This is in particular true also for predictive analyses of tumor genetics, the unfixed effusions, in fact, being more suitable for analyses of nucleic acids than formalin-fixed paraffin-embedded tissue.

Although most lung cancers supposedly develop from the same epithelium lining the bronchial or bronchiolar-alveolar walls, the histological appearances of these tumor tissues vary considerably. Non-small-cell lung cancer (NSCLC) accounts for about 80% of all lung cancer cases, whereas the remaining 20% corresponds to small-cell lung carcinoma (SCLC). Traditionally, NSCLCs are further categorized into tree main groups: squamous cell carcinoma (SCC), adenocarcinoma (AC), and large-cell carcinoma (LCC). The WHO subdivides each of these further into subgroups, and together with some less common tumor types, such as tumors from mucosal glands and sarcomas, the classification describes some 50 different histological growth patterns of malignant lung tumors [7]. When a malignant condition is diagnosed in a serous cavity, however, molecular characterization is clinically more important, and the histogenetic classification is often limited to the main tumor phenotypes. Although therapy often has profound effects on the subgroup of patients with targetable mutations, only limited improvements have been achieved in

the overall 5-year survival of lung cancer when treated with chemotherapy, which remains stably around 15% [8]. This might at least partly be attributed to late detection, morphological and biological heterogeneity, and frequent occurrence of primary or secondary resistance to chemotherapy.

## Histogenetic Classification of Lung Cancers

Lung AC shows the largest variability within the tumor group. By light microscopy these glandular tumors sometimes form mucins that can be demonstrated by histochemistry and immunohistochemistry. Correspondingly various types of secretory granules can be seen by electron microscopy (Fig. 8.1a). Glandular differentiation of lung cancer is often associated with the expression of cytokeratins (CKs) 7 and 18 and mucin type 1 (MUC1). Napsin A and TTF-1 are also typically expressed in most lung ACs [9]. These epitopes are, however, not too infrequently expressed also in the other types of bronchogenic carcinoma and serve better to distinguish primary lung cancers from metastases. Particular forms of lung ACs are those originating from the peripheral parts of the bronchial tree. Based on the latest WHO classification [7], however, the term bronchioloalveolar carcinoma (BAC) should be restricted to an in situ condition with lepidic spread along pre-existing alveolar walls, respecting the basement membrane. Ultrastructurally, tumors with pneumocytic phenotype contain typical surfactant multilamellar bodies. These structures can also be seen in tumors with unequivocal infiltrative growth (Fig. 8.2), and surfactant can be recognized immunohistochemically. Still, invasive cancers with bronchioloalveolar cell phenotype are just classified as ACs. Following the WHO classification, lung ACs can be categorized into altogether 14 subgroups.

SCCs constitute a similarly large group. The cells are often keratinized and form intercellular bridges—the result of desmosome junctions becoming visible because of shrinkage during preparation. Ultrastructurally these cells show abundant desmosomes with tonofilaments formed by coarse

K. Dobra, M.D., Ph.D. (✉) · A. Hjerpe, M.D., Ph.D.
Division of Pathology, Department of Laboratory Medicine,
Karolinska Institute, Stockholm, Sweden
e-mail: katalin.dobra@ki.se

© Springer International Publishing AG, part of Springer Nature 2018
B. Davidson et al. (eds.), *Serous Effusions*, https://doi.org/10.1007/978-3-319-76478-8_8

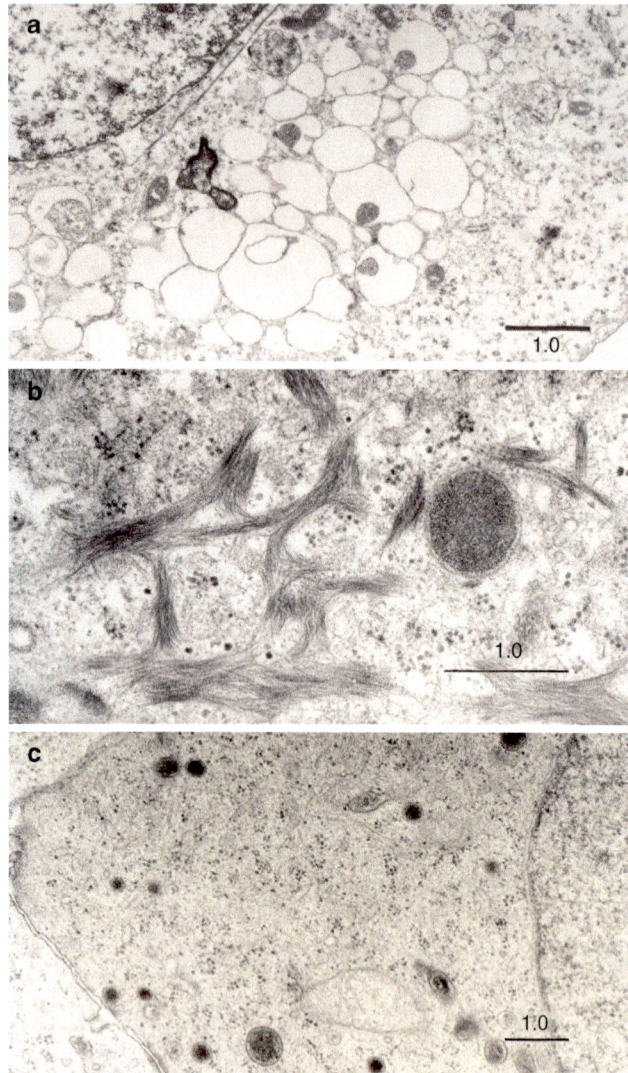

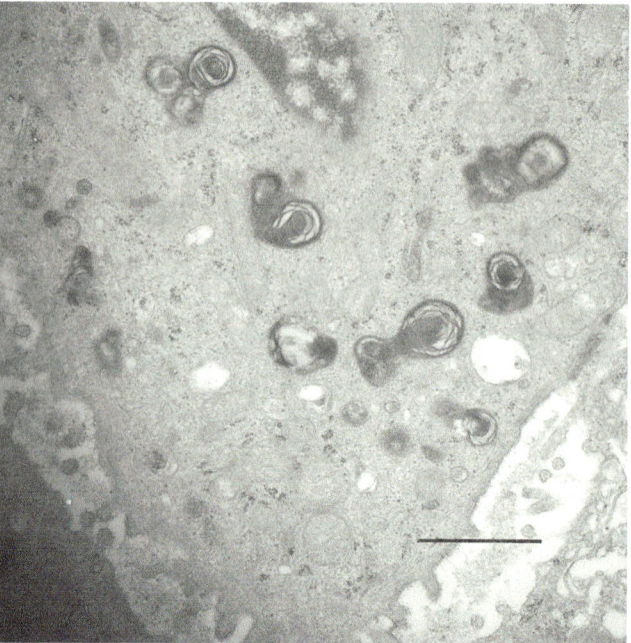

**Fig. 8.2** Electron microscopy of adenocarcinoma cells in a pleural effusion. The multilamellated bodies indicate the differentiation into a pneumocyte phenotype. Bar 5 μm

**Fig. 8.1** Three pleural effusions with carcinoma cells, showing small-cell morphology in light microscopy. The presence of secretory granules, shown by electron microscopy (**a**) reveals, however, that this tumor in fact is an adenocarcinoma, while the abundant tonofilaments (**b**) demonstrates the epidermoid phenotype of a squamous cell carcinoma. Cells from the third tumor (**c**) contain numerous neurosecretory granules verifying the true neuroendocrine phenotype of a small-cell lung carcinoma. Bar 1 μm

be characterized by showing immunoreactivity to epitopes like CD56, chromogranin, and synaptophysin. Biologically, these tumors differ from other forms of invasive lung cancer, and the main divider in classification of lung cancers is the neuroendocrine SCLC vs. NSCLC.

A number of different terms have previously been used for this biologically separate category of small-cell lung cancers: small-cell anaplastic carcinoma, oat-cell carcinoma, lymphocyte-like carcinoma, and recently also neuroendocrine carcinoma grade 3. To be categorized into this group, the neuroendocrine nature should be established. This can be done by immunocytochemistry (ICC) and/or by electron microscopy. Similar neuroendocrine differentiation is also seen in carcinoids, which can be distinguished based on their rate of proliferation, using the MIB1/Ki-67 antibody. The biology, and perhaps also the presumed histogenesis, of SCLC is, however, quite different from that of the carcinoids, and the term SCLC is preferred for these cancers instead of neuroendocrine cancer grade 3.

LCC constitutes a group of non-small-cell carcinomas that are too poorly differentiated to allow the distinction between epidermoid or glandular differentiation. The proportion of cases referred to this group varies from one material to another, and with the adjunct of ICC, many of these cases will be referred to one of the other three groups, large-cell undifferentiated carcinoma becoming in this way rare. A particular form of LCC displays neuroendocrine differentiation (large-cell neuroendocrine cancers, LCNEC). The neu-

bundles of CKs (Fig. 8.1b). Immunohistochemically, they can be recognized by expression of CKs 5 and 17 together with p63. According to the WHO classification, five different patterns of squamous differentiation can be recognized.

SCLC constitutes the third common form of lung cancer. Lung cancers with small-cell morphology are heterogeneous and show variable ultrastructure and immunophenotype, some cases merely being poorly differentiated SCCs and others ACs. The tumor cells of the particular SCLC group contain neurosecretory granules (Fig. 8.1c), which also can

roendocrine phenotype is established by ICC and distinguished from SCLC by the nuclear size and structure.

Tumors considered to develop from other structures than the epithelium lining the airway surfaces are less frequent. Most common of these are the carcinoids and atypical carcinoids. They belong to the group of neuroendocrine tumors (neuroendocrine cancer grades 1 and 2, respectively) with immunophenotypes similar to the SCLCs. Less commonly carcinomas may also develop from submucosal glands. The tumors formed are identical to those seen in salivary glands, i.e., mucoepidermoid carcinoma, adenoid cystic carcinoma, and epithelial-myoepithelial carcinoma.

The importance of classifying lung cancers is to provide guidance in the choice of therapy and prognosis, i.e., to deduce biological information of clinical importance from the morphology. The number of diagnostically relevant groups is then, however, small. As emphasized earlier, the main divider is the distinction of SCLC from NSCLC. These two groups show major differences in aggressiveness, chemosensitivity, and prognosis, while the different subgroups of NSCLC show only limited variability of these parameters.

One must in this context be aware of the poor correlation between light microscopy, electron microscopy, and ICC, when it comes to subclassification of NSCLCs. Thus in the light microscope, a mixed adenosquamous phenotype is considered to be rare [7]. Electron microscopy, however, reveals that a majority of non-small-cell carcinomas simultaneously exhibit both secretory granules and abundant tonofilaments, in fact indicating that adenosquamous differentiation is the most common phenotype [10].

The use of ICC for classifying lung cancers indicates a spectrum more similar to that obtained with electron microscopy and different from that obtained with routine histology. It therefore seems as if light microscopy has a limited ability to classify the tumors according to their biological behavior, this capacity probably being improved by the adjunct of ICC. Still, for practical reasons, therapy is often based on diagnoses from light microscopy. With increased understanding of factors necessary for drug effects and the development of targeted therapies, a classification based on molecular characteristics will be increasingly important, probably replacing much of the histology.

## Etiology and Pathogenesis

### Carcinogenesis

Exposure to tobacco smoke, radon, asbestos, arsenic, and other forms of air pollution is the main etiological factor connected to lung cancer. Although smoking is the leading cause of lung cancer in about 80–90% of cases, approximately 10% of patients have never smoked [11]. Environmental factors and genetic susceptibility together are thought to contribute to cancer development. These factors are orchestrated, and they trigger oncogene activation, tumor suppressor gene silencing, and widespread loss of heterozygosity.

Among the 55 carcinogens identified in cigarette smoke, 20 are involved in pulmonary carcinogenesis. Of these, polycyclic aromatic hydrocarbons and tobacco-specific N-nitrosamines, especially nitrosamine 4-(methylnitrosamino)-1-1(3-pyridyl)-1-butanone (NNK), seem to play major roles. The carcinogens start a metabolic activation process, leading to formation of DNA adducts. If the DNA adducts escape cellular clearance and repair mechanisms and persist, they lead to permanent DNA damage, which may hit critical oncogenes such as KRAS, MYC, and tumor suppressor genes including p53, p16, pRB, and FHIT; for review see [11].

Differences in the susceptibility to lung cancer among individuals are likely to occur, and genetic polymorphisms have been identified in proteins associated with carcinogen metabolism. Several novel lung cancer susceptibility genes, located on chromosomes 5p15.33, 6p21, and 15q24-25.1, have been identified by large-scale genome-wide association studies [12]. The 15q25 region contains three nicotine acetylcholine receptor (nAChR) genes [13], and their polymorphisms have also been reported to be associated with nicotine dependence. The 6q23-25 and 13q31.3 regions were also identified as being associated with risk for lung cancer, particularly in never-smokers [12].

## Chromosomal Aberrations in Lung Cancer

One of the most frequent and early changes in lung cancer pathogenesis relates to chromosome 3. Amplifications are commonly involving the chromosome arm 3q, and allele losses occur at multiple losses of heterozygosity (LOH) sites on chromosome arm 3p [14]. Frequent regions with amplifications (14q13.3, 12q15, 12p12.1, 8q24.21, 7p11.2, and 8q21.13) and deletions (9p21.3, 9p23, 10q23.31) of lung AC specimens have been identified, residing known oncogenes such as MYC, EGFR, KRAS, and tumor suppressor genes such as CDKN2A/CDKN2B [15] and the thyroid transcription factor (TTF-1) located on chromosome 14q13.3 [16, 17].

A well-known cofactor for lung carcinogenesis is asbestos, a mineral fiber that is known to cause chromosomal aberrations. Lung cancers in patients exposed to asbestos often show a number of additional aberrations (2p21-p16.3, 5q35.3, 9q33.3-q34.11, 9q34.13-q34.3, 11p15.5, 14q11.2, and 19p13.1-p13.3) [18–20].

## The Role of Microenvironment in the Survival of Metastatic Cancer Cells in Serosal Effusions

Mesothelial cells play a key role in maintaining the homeostasis of the serosal cavities and possess mechanisms that prevent tumor spread and metastasis [21, 22]. Lung cancer cells, however, show a high predilection to metastasize to the pleural space, where they adopt an anchorage-independent growth in effusion, survive, and proliferate despite the unfavorable condition provided by the serous surface. The molecular basis of this predilection is not fully understood but is most likely based on reciprocal tumor-microenvironment interactions [23–27]. Metastatic tumor cells that disseminate to the serosal cavities possess a strong autonomous proliferative drive, and the presence of malignant cells in the pleural space indicates that the malignant cell has overcome the pleural defense mechanisms [28, 29].

One such potential defense mechanism of the mesothelium against invading malignant cells is endostatin, which inhibits angiogenesis and endothelial cell migration, induces cell cycle arrest and apoptosis, and thereby reduces tumor growth [30]. Polyanionic compounds such as glycosaminoglycans [31] and sialomucins [32] present on the mesothelial surface are other factors having a capacity to counteract tumor attachment and growth. Interestingly, a mechanism by which malignant cells present themselves as innocuous to the mesothelial cellular environment is the expression of the hyaluronan-binding proteoglycan CD44 [33], which acts as a receptor for surfaces carrying hyaluronan.

Cells obtained from malignant pleural effusion show aberrant glucose metabolism [34]. Malignant cells also acquire growth advantage by autocrine and paracrine growth stimulation and developing resistance to apoptosis. They actively modulate the microenvironment in the pleural fluid by inducing a pro-angiogenic shift, by secreting growth factors such as vascular endothelial growth factor (VEGF), basic FGF (bFGF), and transforming growth factor beta (TGF-β) [35–37]) and by inducing benign mesothelial cells to release growth factors [38]. In this way metastatic malignant cells contribute to convert the repressive micromilieu of the pleural space to a permissive one, further facilitating tumor growth. Indeed, the level of VEGF from pleural effusions of lung cancer patients is up to 25-fold higher compared to patients with active infectious diseases [39–43]. Platelet-derived growth factor (PDGF) levels are also selectively higher in lung AC, compared to SCLC and nonmalignant pleural effusions [44]. Various cytokines, interleukins, and interferons, including IL-2, IL-4, TNF-α, and INF-γ, are widespread in malignant effusions, and their relative abundance correlates with each other, suggesting cross talk between them [45, 46].

Recent advances in cancer biology point to a role for inflammatory signaling in cancer. Lung cancer patients with malignant pleural effusion seem to have weaker immune defense than those with TB pleurisy, both locally and systemically [47]. Inflammatory markers were significantly expressed in pleural effusions, and values in pleura-invading tumor-associated effusions in lung cancer patients were typically higher than those of other tumors. IL-8 and VEGF correlated negatively with survival, reflecting to some extent also the tumor origin [48].

## The Molecular Biology of Lung Cancer

The molecular signature of lung cancer has been subject of extensive research activity, and NSCLCs, particularly adenocarcinomas, are today very well characterized with regard to their molecular changes. At the same time, emerging data show distinctive molecular signatures also for squamous carcinomas and SCLC; these latter two are, however, not yet included in the clinical routine workflow as no targeted therapeutic options are available. In this chapter the most frequent actionable mutations and molecular changes will be described. These changes carry therapeutic consequences and are already integrated in molecular diagnostics and clinical management as a part of personalized cancer medicine approach. Many laboratories have already integrated ICC- and next-generation sequencing (NGS)-based screening approaches in their workflow, following specific algorithms that allow molecular subtyping, treatment prediction, and selection of patients for targeted therapeutic options.

### The Molecular Signature of Lung Adenocarcinoma

Both genetic and epigenetic changes are known to be common events in lung cancer. Driver mutations are responsible for both the initiation and maintenance of the malignancy. To date, *EGFR*, *KRAS*, *BRAF*, *PIK3CA*, and *ERBB2* gene mutations, *EML4-ALK*, *ROS-1*, and *RET-1* fusion genes and *MET* amplifications are the most widely recognized alterations involved in both the biology and the clinical management of NSCLC [49, 50].

### *EGFR* Mutation

The epidermal growth factor receptor (EGFR) family of receptor tyrosine kinases (RTKs) is deregulated in a subset of NSCLC by activating mutations, increased copy number, or protein overexpression. *EGFR* is mutated in up to 7–10%

of Caucasian and about 32% of East-Asian patients with NSCLC [51]. Approximately 50% of *EGFR*-mutated cases also show increased *EGFR* copy number [52]. *EGFR* over-expression is present in >60% of metastatic NSCLC and it correlates with poor prognosis [53]. Upon ligand binding, homo- or heterodimerization of EGFR leads to autophos-phorylation of the intracellular domain and subsequent activation of the Ras/mitogen-activated protein kinase (MAPK) and PI3K/Akt pathways, resulting in increased cell survival, proliferation, invasion, and metastasis. Activating mutations in exons 18–21 of the *EGFR* gene [54] render tumor cells independent of ligand activation of the TK. Deletions in exon 19 and point mutations of L8555R constitute about 90% of all *EGFR*-activating muta-tions (for review, see [55]).

Patients with malignant pleural effusions related to lung AC have a higher rate of *EGFR* mutations than patients with primary tumors [56, 57], and this constitutes the most fre-quent molecular change in pulmonary AC presenting with malignant effusion at the time of the first diagnosis [58]. *EGFR* status predicts tumor responsiveness to treatment and clinical outcome [59–62]. *EGFR* gene mutations were found in the tumor tissue from 25% of NSCLC patients and in 23% of plasma samples [62]. Mutations are most frequently pres-ent in females, never-smokers, and ACs with bronchioloal-veolar features.

## *KRAS, BRAF, PIK3CA,* and *ERBB2* Mutations

Recent studies showed that activating *EGFR, KRAS, BRAF,* and *ERBB2* mutations exhibit mutually exclusive patterns in lung AC, suggesting that they represent inde-pendent ways of oncogenic pathways [52, 63, 64], and they differ in terms of epidemiological, morphological, biological, and clinical aspects. EGFR and ERBB2 are two signaling receptors upstream of the other three. It is there-fore sufficient for the stimulation of MAPK and mTOR in tumor cells if only one of them has a mutation that results in autonomous signaling. This is probably the explanation why they so often are mutually exclusive and indicates that this signaling pathway is important for the development of a lung carcinoma. Still another common situation when mTOR is activated is when there is a loss of the phospha-tase and tensin homolog (PTEN) activity. This tumor sup-pressor gene (TSG) negatively regulates the PI3K activity, and mutations and deletions of *PTEN* then result in increased cell proliferation and reduced apoptosis [15, 65–77].

*KRAS* mutants show often morphological features of mucinous AC and occur preferentially in males, smokers, and Caucasians [78]. Depending on the screening method used, up to 25% of patients are carrying *KRAS* mutations, whereas mutation of *BRAF* and class-1a phosphoinositide-(3,4,5)-kinase (*PIK3CA*) are less frequent and occur only in <5% of lung cancers [49]. Molecular profiling of metastatic NSCLC derived from malignant effusions shows higher fre-quency of genetic abnormalities, mainly corresponding to *EGFR* and *KRAS* mutations, together occurring in 59% of the cases [79]. In a clinical mutational profiling of 1006 lung cancers by NGS, the well-known V600E *BRAF* mutation accounted, however, for only 24% of all *BRAF* mutations, whereas kinase-impaired mutations affecting codons 466 and 594 were seen in 25%, highlighting the diversity of BRAF mutations in this setting.

Even though most driver mutations are mutually exclu-sive, accumulating evidence suggest more complex altera-tions particularly in advanced cases, involving clonality. A large prospective molecular characterization revealed fre-quent co-occurring targetable mutations of which some showed at least three concurrent alterations [80], often affecting *EGFR* and *PIK3CA*. Moreover, detailed study of variant allele frequencies together with knowledge of previ-ous EGFR-TKI therapy uncovered the presence of coexist-ing mutations, one being a dominant, the other a sub-clonal population. In the light of this complexity, a comprehensive broad molecular screening will help us better understand the evolution of individual tumors. Based on this it will be pos-sible to tailor our future therapies, considering also simulta-neous targeting of different actionable alterations. At the same time this might pose serious future challenge in defin-ing the best choice of therapy among many possible options. Ex vivo sensitivity testing together with molecular character-ization might serve as a useful tool in combining different therapeutic options.

## *EML4-ALK* Rearrangements

The fusion of echinoderm microtubule-associated protein-like 4 (*EML4*) and anaplastic lymphoma kinase (*ALK*) results in constitutive tyrosine kinase activity and activation of the downstream MAP kinase pathway. The *EML4-ALK* fusion gene is formed by a small inversion within chromosome 2p, resulting in the fusion of these genes [81]. It occurs in 3–13 % of NSCLC, and apart from rare exceptions, *EML4-ALK* and *EGFR* mutations are mutually exclusive, but patients share many clinical characteristics [82–85].

*EML-ALK* rearrangements can be detected by ICC, fluo-rescent in situ hybridization (FISH), and molecular tests comprising RT-PCR or NGS from cytological specimens obtained from malignant pleural effusions. Sensitive anti-bodies are now available such as the rabbit monoclonal anti-body D5F3 (Ventana Medical Systems, Inc., Switzerland), described to yield 100% sensitivity and specificity [86]. Recent comparative studies revealed that ICC shows reliable results also when compared to break-apart FISH, often considered the gold standard with high sensitivity, specificity, and positive predictive values [87–89]. Thus, ICC is an excellent tool for screening [90], virtually covering all rearrangements. Discrepancies may, however, occur between various analyses, and the FISH analysis can yield both false-positive and false-negative results. ICC-positive but FISH-negative cases most likely correspond to false-negative FISH results and reflect the limited ability of the FISH analysis to cover all different fusion variants.

NGS offers multiplexed analysis comprising the targetable *ALK*, *ROS1*, and *RET*, among others [91]. By NGS, apart from the *EML4-ALK*, previously unreported fusion partners were identified [92].

## *ROS1* and *RET* Rearrangements

The ROS proto-oncogene is a RTK with structural similarities to ALK. The precise physiological function of this protein is not known, although it has been associated with cell growth and differentiation. In 1–2% of NSCLC, its gene, *ROS1*, may act as a driver following rearrangement with *CD74*, *EZR*, *SLC24A2*, and *FIG* genes [93]. This translocation is mutually exclusive from *EGFR* mutations and *ALK* rearrangements. The *ROS1* translocation, to which targeted therapies now are available, can be demonstrated by FISH using break-apart probes and by ICC demonstrating the overexpressed protein. Detection of ROS1 with the D4D6 monoclonal antibody (Cell Signaling Technology) may yield false-positive results, and only moderate to strong reactivity should be considered staining >50% of tumor cells [94]. Patients with *ROS1* fusions respond initially to crizotinib, similarly to *ALK* rearrangements, but resistance mechanisms are already known that necessitate new therapeutic strategies to overcome treatment failure [95].

*RET* rearrangements occur in 1–2% of NSCLC, and the *KIF5B-RET* is the most common fusion gene [96], yielding partial response to cabozantinib in a subset of patients (28%) [97].

## Other Mutations

Among other oncogenes, MYC and cyclin D1 are amplified or overexpressed in 5–10% of lung cancer cases [98], whereas the anti-apoptotic Bcl-2 is overexpressed in about 25% of cases [99]. These alterations, however, are not targeted in clinical settings.

*MET* exon 14 skipping mutations and high-level amplification in the *MET* gene also occur relatively to a high extent,

ranging from 3 to 17%, respectively, in various types of lung cancer and indicating poor prognosis [100, 101]. They also open up for new therapeutic options and can serve as useful biomarkers [102, 103].

## Small-Cell Lung Cancer (SCLC)

The molecular biology of SCLC differs greatly or in many aspects from NSCLC [104].

Dominant oncogenes of the *MYC* family are frequently overexpressed in both SCLC and NSCLC, while the *KRAS* oncogene is never mutated in SCLC but is mutated in 30% of NSCLCs.

The most frequent genetic abnormalities involve TSGs. SCLC and NSCLC differ significantly also in the TSGs that are inactivated during the pathogenesis of lung cancer. There were 22 different "hot spots" for loss of heterozygosity, 13 of them with a preference for SCLC, 7 for NSCLC, and 2 affecting both. Alterations of both p53 and retinoblastoma suppressor protein (pRB) are central for the carcinogenesis of SCLC. The *TP53* gene, coding for the TSG p53, is mutated in more than 90% of SCLCs and more than 50% of NSCLCs, while pRB is inactivated in over 90% of SCLC but only 15% of NSCLCs. Consequently, p16, which regulates pRB, is almost never mutated in SCLC, while this is found in more than 50% of NSCLCs [105].

## MicroRNAs in Lung Cancer

MicroRNAs (miRNAs) are small, noncoding, endogenous, single-stranded RNA fragments consisting of approximately 22–23 nucleotides [106, 107]. They play important regulatory roles in a wide variety of developmental and oncogenic pathways [108–112]. Interestingly, genetic dissection of hot spots for chromosomal abnormalities revealed that about half of the miRNAs are located within or near chromosomal fragile sites, common breakpoints, or minimal regions with amplification or loss of heterozygosity [113–115]. The combination of nonrandom chromosomal abnormalities and other genetic alterations or epigenetic events contributes to downregulation or overexpression of miRNAs.

The specific miRNA expression pattern, which characterizes lung cancers, may be useful in the future as a biomarker [116]. A unique miRNA molecular profile, consisting of miR-17-3p, miR-21, miR-106a, miR-146, miR-155, miR-191, miR-192, miR-203, miR-205, miR-210, miR-212, and miR-214, was claimed to be diagnostic of NSCLC [117]. Furthermore, circulating exosomal miRNA signatures mirror those of the primary lung cancer and may discriminate cancer patients from controls.

Detection of miRNA might thus be suitable for screening and early detection of lung cancer [118, 119]. This gives hope also of using them not only as biomarkers but also as therapeutic targets [120].

## Gene Expression Profiling

A molecular diagnostic test for distinguishing lung AC from other malignant tumors in pleural effusions has been established [121]. Certain patterns of gene expression have been associated with the different phenotypes of lung cancer and with their prognosis. Thus, deregulation of the Ras oncogenic pathway was found in most lung ACs as opposed to SCCs. Patients with high Ras activity had lower levels of MYC, E2F3, β-catenin, and Src activity, and this pattern could be associated with a less favorable prognosis [122].

Genomic amplification at 3q26.33 has been shown in many cases of lung SCCs. This region contains the transcription factor SOX2, which is necessary for squamous differentiation. Furthermore, SOX2 expression is required for proliferation and anchorage-independent growth of lung cancer cell lines, and SOX2-driven tumors show expression of markers of both squamous differentiation and pluripotency [66].

Activation of the WNT pathway was identified as a determinant of metastasis to the brain and bone during lung AC progression. Data are, however, lacking regarding the involvement of this pathway in metastatic spread to the pleura [123].

## Epigenetic Alterations

Epigenetic alterations are considered to play important roles in lung cancer. Hypermethylation of the promoter region of key genes is one of the most common mechanisms that tumors use to inactivate the function of tumor suppressor and other genes. Epigenetic analysis of pleural fluid improves the diagnostic yield and accuracy of the current cytologic examination [124]. Hypermethylation [125] or homozygous deletion of p16 [126] is frequently detected in malignant pleural fluids. Significant differences were also detected in the methylation profiles between the two major types of NSCLC, whereas SCLC clustered together with carcinoids [127]. Patients with methylation of *p16INK4a*, RAS association domain family 1A (*RASSF1A*), or retinoic acid receptor *β* (*RARβ*) were 5.68 times more likely to have malignant effusions than patients without methylation. Furthermore, methylations per patient were more numerous for lung cancer patients than for nonmalignant pulmonary conditions [128]. Differences in the frequency of *RARβ*

methylation pattern correspond to 70% for SCLC and 40% for NSCLCs [105].

Interestingly, *KRAS* mutations were significantly higher in *p16* (*INK4A*)-methylated cases than in unmethylated cases, and the methylation index was higher in *KRAS*-mutant cases than in wild-type cases [129].

A comparison of mutation and methylation demonstrated that *EGFR* mutation had an inverse correlation with methylation of *SPARC* (secreted protein acidic and rich in cysteine), an extracellular $Ca^{2+}$-binding glycoprotein associated with the regulation of cell adhesion and growth, and the *p16INK4A* gene [130].

## Integrative Approach to Molecular Profiling

The integrative approach to analyze parallel dimensions enables the identification of genes that are disrupted by multiple mechanisms and/or pathways that are disrupted at multiple components at low frequency. The MUC1 glycoprotein interacts with EGFR, ERBB2, and c-Src in a way that activates cell proliferation. EGFR here seems to regulate the binding of MUC1 to c-Src [131, 132]. The MUC1 gene shows such a concerted disruption, displaying concurrent copy number increase, hypomethylation, and overexpression [133].

## Proteomics

Expression patterns obtained with genomic analyses are preferably paralleled with corresponding wide screening for the pattern of proteins formed. The techniques for such analyses develop rapidly, and thousands of proteins can now be identified using a tumor volume of $0.01$ mm$^3$ [99]. Studies have indicated that the protein patterns can be used for establishing the presence of a lung cancer and to further indicate the histological type of tumor [99, 111]. It has also been possible to correlate the obtained protein patterns with prognosis and even to indicate possible therapeutic targets [99, 111–113]. These studies have mainly analyzed proteins obtained from the tumor tissue, but similar results can also be obtained by analyzing effusion supernatants and serum [134–136]. This possibility for a wide proteomics screen is highly promising. The analysis can reveal novel biomarkers and specific expression patterns as a diagnostic tool that extends far beyond the determination of only a few biomarkers. The analyses still await standardization for use in clinical routines. Once this is done, the clinical utility of effusion analyses may increase greatly. Integrative approaches, adding also RNA sequencing to DNA and proteomic data, will improve this molecular characterization of tumors.

## Ancillary Methods in Diagnostic Effusion Cytology

One cause of an effusion is the establishment of a malignant condition in the serous cavity. When the fluid is taken for diagnostic examination by clinical cytology, the primary question is always whether there is a malignant condition or not. There are, however, conditions when the mesothelium is stimulated to proliferate for other reasons. This stimulation will change the morphology of the mesothelial cells, which will be polymorphic with distinct and sometimes multiple nucleoli, and the cells will pile up to form papillary structures. This proliferative process, also called "mesotheliosis," is perhaps the most difficult pitfall in effusion cytology. Therefore, a correct malignant diagnosis often requires the help of adjuvant analyses, either ICC [137, 138] or molecular biology techniques [139, 140], as described elsewhere in this book.

The most common primary for a malignant involvement of the pleura is a lung cancer. The tumors usually shed both dissociated cells and cell groups into the fluid. The basic morphology of these cells does not differ significantly in cytological preparations from the primary tumor. Among the NSCLCs, however, the adenomatous differentiation is by far the most common. It may be that peripheral lung carcinomas, more often being ACs, will spread to the serous cavity earlier than centrally growing tumors. This is, however, not the entire explanation. Other factors must also contribute, and reciprocal tumor-microenvironment interactions are most likely to be involved. The diagnostic features for these tumors and a substantial amount of possible ICC adjuncts are described elsewhere in this book. It may be wise to routinely include a minimal battery of these ICC reactions whenever diagnosing a malignant effusion: thyroid transcription factor-1 (TTF-1) to support lung origin, CK5 and p63 to show squamous differentiation, CK7 for adenomatous cells, and in case of small-cell morphology also CD56, synaptophysin, and chromogranin.

## Electron Microscopy

Electron microscopy of effusion cell pellets can be an adjunct, although its role in diagnostic effusion cytology is limited. This analysis of an effusion cell pellet is most often employed to establish the diagnosis of a malignant mesothelioma, but it can sometimes also define the phenotype in metastatic lung carcinomas. The ultrastructural presentation of the adenomatous and epidermoid phenotypes is well known, but will classify the tumor cells different from light microscopy, sometimes with tonofilaments and secretory vacuoles simultaneously present in the same cell [10]. In par-

ticular, there are two tumor types that can be recognized at the ultrastructural level. The first of these is AC cell with the pneumocyte type 2 phenotype that contains the typical multilaminated bodies associated with the production of surfactant (Fig. 8.2). The second main type of lung cancer that can be recognized by electron microscopy of an effusion cell pellet is the SCLC. Cells of this phenotype contain electron-dense neurosecretory granules, supporting a diagnosis of neuroendocrine cancer. This diagnosis is, however, often better achieved with ICC.

## Analysis of Aneuploidy by FISH

Malignant cells in effusions are readily demonstrated with the UroVysion kit (Abbott Molecular Inc., Des Plaines, IL), labeling the 9p21 locus (p16 region) and the centromeric regions of chromosomes 3, 7, and 17 [139]. Similar accurate definition of malignancy can be obtained with a set of probes labeling 5p15.2, 6p11.1-q11, 7p12 (*EGFR*), and 8q24.12–24.13 (*CMYC*) [141]. The probes were formerly offered as a kit ("LaVysion," Abbott Molecular Inc.), particularly aiming for the detection of lung cancer in cytologic specimen, and they are now available as isolated reagents. While these reagents reveal the presence of a malignant condition, there are so far no established and routinely used techniques that provide information regarding tumor origin or tumor type.

## NGS

NGS is already incorporated in the clinical workflow of many laboratories. Actionable mutations can be detected by specifically tailored lung cancer-related gene panels comprising a limited number of genes. Regardless of the method used, multiplexed molecular profiling of pleural effusions includes typically *EGFR, KRAS, BRAF, PIK3CA, NRAS, MEK1, AKT1, PTEN, HER2, MET, FGFR1, FGFR2* and *ALK, ROS1,* and *RET* fusions [142]. However, considerable challenges are posed by the bioinformatics, as lung cancer panels are gradually expanded to whole exome sequencing (WES) and whole genome sequencing (WGS) [143]. This analytical challenge might limit the broad clinical applicability of NGS for genotype-tailored treatments [144].

## Treatment Options

A malignant effusion corresponds to a disseminated tumor beyond possibilities to cure. Thus, chemotherapy with a palliative purpose or best supportive care is the main therapeutic alternative. Severe dyspnea occurs in 60–80% of the patients with malignant pleural effusion; therefore its management is primarily aimed to reduce symptoms by repeated pleurocentesis or pleurodesis. Pleurodesis involves insufflation of a sclerosing agent, most often talc, into the pleural space, causing an acute inflammatory response, followed by an extensive fibrosis, thus preventing the recurrence of malignant pleural effusions [145]. Talc insufflation alters the angiogenic balance in the pleural space from a biologically active and angiogenic environment to a more angiostatic milieu [146], and a large surface area covered with normal mesothelial cells is a prerequisite for a successful pleurodesis.

Multiple trials have established the benefit of chemotherapy for palliation and disease control of patients with malignant effusion, compared to best supportive care [147–149]. The response to therapy, however, differs between the tumor phenotypes, the largest difference being between SCLC and NSCLC. For optimal therapy it is therefore important not only to establish the malignant condition but also to obtain a more detailed diagnosis of tumor phenotype.

## Chemotherapy Regimens Based on Clinical Trials and Empirical Data

### NSCLC

Chemotherapy prolongs the survival of patients with advanced NSCLC when compared to best supportive care alone. Platinum-based combination chemotherapy seems to be the most effective according to meta-analyses [149, 150]. Among the two most frequently used platinum-based drugs, carboplatin has a more favorable toxicity profile and similar efficacy compared to cisplatin, which is highly nephrotoxic [151]. Gemcitabine and paclitaxel are anticancer agents with significant single-agent activity against advanced NSCLC. They have different mechanisms of action and their toxicities are nonoverlapping [152], which also makes them attractive in combination treatment. Indeed, adding carboplatin to either gemcitabine or paclitaxel resulted in better response and survival rates [153, 154]. Drugs that may be combined with platinum include the third-generation cytotoxic drugs docetaxel, gemcitabine, irinotecan, paclitaxel, pemetrexed, and vinorelbine [155].

### SCLC

SCLC is considered a chemotherapy-responsive disease, and etoposide-platinum is the standard first-line treatment. Despite initial response rates of more than 60% of the patients and complete response rates of 20–30%, the median survival time and efficacy of systemic chemotherapy have not been significantly improved in the past decades [156]. Taxanes, topoisomerase inhibitors, and antimetabolites such as pemetrexed and gemcitabine have been demonstrated to be efficient both as single drugs and in combination with platinum-based drugs [157, 158].

## Targeted Therapy

With the identification of driver mutations in patients with defined clinical and morphological characteristics, a new arsenal of therapeutic options is available for the treatment of patients with lung cancer [159, 160]. A recent prospective study revealed that a high proportion of patients harboring sensitizing EGFR mutations or ALK and ROS1 fusions received matched targeted therapy and also showed clinical benefit in most cases [80], highlighting the impact of molecular predictive testing for improved clinical outcome.

### Targeting Epidermal Growth Factor Receptor (EGFR)

The most widely studied targeted therapy is related to the epidermal growth factor (EGF) pathway [161]. Patients with advanced NSCLC harboring EGFR mutations have a significantly better response rate when treated with RTK inhibitors than patients with wild-type EGFR.

EGFR signaling can be disrupted at numerous points. The most common is the blockade of the cell surface receptor by monoclonal antibodies and inhibition of the activity of the tyrosine kinase domain by tyrosine kinase inhibitors. Only a small proportion of patients will have significant response to EGFR inhibitors in unselected patient material, but the presence of activating mutations in the kinase domain of EGFR increases the response rate to 75–90% [159, 161–164].

Patients with pleural effusion showing activating EGFR mutations have a significantly better response rate to EGFR tyrosine kinase inhibitors compared to patients with wild-type EGFR. Their median progression-free survival corresponded to 11.2 vs. 2.7 months, and overall survival was 21.8 vs. 5.8 months, compared to patients with wild-type EGFR [62]. Thus, the presence of EGFR mutations highly predicts the efficacy of EGFR tyrosine kinase inhibitors (TKIs) also in advanced NSCLC, giving a significant survival advantage.

Most patients will, however, acquire resistance against TKIs. Major resistance mechanisms comprise a secondary threonine-790 to methionine point mutation (T790M) in the EGFR gene and amplification of the MET proto-oncogene [165]. The T790M mutation causes steric hindrance and impairs the binding of TKIs. Interference on multiple levels with the EGFR signaling pathway or development of irreversible inhibitors of EGFR may help to overcome this problem. Other frequent mechanisms conferring resistance to TKIs comprise HER2 and MET amplifications and PIK3CA mutation [166]. In a recent study, many T790M-negative patients showed activation of *ERBB2*, *MET*, *FGFR1*, and *ALK* or the RAS/MEK/ERK and PI3K/AKT/mTOR pathways [166]. Furthermore, new resistance-related molecular alterations, such as *TET2* mutation and *SOX2* amplification, were detected.

### Targeting EML4-ALK and ROS1

Therapies targeted against ALK are currently under development, and they are already included in clinical trials for NSCLC patients harboring the *ALK4-EML* fusion [81]. Crizotinib, an orally administered dual inhibitor of the c-Met and ALK pathways, has recently been evaluated and showed dramatic clinical benefit for patients with advanced NSCLC. Activation of the analogue *ROS1* gene shows similarly positive results following treatment with crizotinib. However, relapse and acquired resistance mechanisms have also been registered [167].

### Targeting the PD-1/PD-L1 Axis

A novel approach to treat NSCLC involves interference with processes that makes it possible for tumor cells to evade recognition of immune cells. In particular the inhibition of the PD-1/PD-L1 axis is now an established and successful therapeutic option [168]. The programmed death-1 receptor (PD-1) is present on activated T cells, and when bound to a PD-L1 ligand on the tumor cells, this has an immunosuppressive effect on the T cell. Tumors that express PD-L1 can be identified by ICC. Attempts to block PD-1 or PD-L1 by antibody-based treatment have efficiently improved the response rates for treatment. In addition to PD-L1 expression, high neo-antigen and non-synonymous mutational burden, DNA repair pathway defects with microsatellite instability, mismatch-repair deficiency, and presence of activating T cells are all related to treatment efficacy and improved patient survival [169–171].

### Targeting Angiogenesis

Inhibition of VEGF impairs angiogenesis and disrupts metastatic tumor spread. Bevacizumab is a monoclonal antibody that binds to VEGF and blocks interaction with its cell surface receptor. Clinical trials have demonstrated that disruption of these signaling pathways can improve survival in advanced lung cancer. The addition of bevacizumab to paclitaxel and carboplatin improves survival compared with chemotherapy alone in patients with previously untreated metastatic non-squamous NSCLC [172].

### Other Agents and Experimental Approaches

Folate antimetabolites (pemetrexed), proteasome inhibitors (bortezomib), modified glutathione analogues, and other agents are currently being evaluated in patients with lung cancer [173]. Experimental evidence suggests that bortezo-mib is able to specifically target and counteract the effusion-inducing phenotype of lung AC [174]. Bortezomib is a proteasome inhibitor, which targets the ubiquitin-proteasome pathway, with subsequent inhibition of the degradation of proteins involved in cell cycle regulation and cancer cell survival [175]. Recent clinical trials further demonstrate the importance of histology in governing individualized treatment, based on both safety and efficacy considerations. For example, bevacizumab and pemetrexed are currently restricted to patients with non-squamous NSCLC. Bevacizumab causes severe pulmonary hemorrhages in patients with squamous cell histology, whereas pemetrexed seems to be more efficient in patients with non-squamous cell morphology [176].

### Assay-Directed Chemotherapy

Systematic reviews of chemotherapy sensitivity and resistance assays performed during the last decades reveal higher response rates for patients receiving assay-guided therapy compared to patients treated with empiric chemotherapy [177, 178]. Of particular interest is optimization of ex vivo assay-based methods selecting treatment regimens with the greatest chance of inducing a response in patients with malignant effusions, since the functional status and short median survival of these patients usually do not allow repeated chemotherapy regimens [179, 180]. These assays have only been applied in a few centers and are not yet integrated into general routine oncology. Reasons for this may be due to problems with performing tumor cell-specific measurements and the lack of larger randomized trials. The possibility to personalize treatment also including tests of drugs outside standardized first- and second-line regimens is, however, most challenging.

## Molecular Biomarkers for Lung Cancer

### Diagnostic Tumor Markers

Tumor tissue that has established a metastatic growth in a serous cavity may shed or secrete various cell components into the fluid. These compounds are delivered either as secretory products or as a consequence of tumor cell decay. The demonstration of such biochemical compounds can have diagnostic importance, particularly if the biomarker is unique to the tumor tissue or is associated with drug sensitivity or prognosis. One marker indicating deterioration of cell integrity is cholesterol, and together with the simultaneous determination of more specific tumor markers such as CEA, it is possible to indicate presence of a malignant condition [181–184]. Attempts to define malignant involvement of the serous cavities by biomarker analyses specifically directed toward malignancy-associated epitopes included also Her-2/neu

[185], CYFRA 21-1 [186, 187], CA-19.9 [188], CA 125 [189, 190] CA15-3, VEGF [191], and HGF/SF [192]. Similarly, the measurement of TTF-1 and napsin A can be used to define the presence of a bronchogenic carcinoma.

## Predictive Markers for Optimal Treatment Response

The goal in the management of lung cancer is to achieve optimal treatment response for each patient. However, only a minority of patients benefit from a given cancer treatment. This has led to interest in the identification of gene expression-based predictive signatures. Given the high biological heterogeneity of lung cancer, molecular biomarkers are required for optimal decision-making and to predict the likelihood of success or failure of a given therapy. A well-validated genotyping can give a good basis for personalized treatment.

## Prediction of EGFR Tyrosine Kinase Inhibitors

The observation that only a minority of patients responds to EGFR-targeted therapies, in combination with their toxicity and high costs, has driven the search for validating molecular markers which can predict treatment response [193]. Screening for *EGFR* mutation status is to date the most relevant approach for selecting lung cancer patients for treatment [52, 194]. Apart from the malignant cells, the cell-free pleural fluid may also be a feasible clinical specimen for *EGFR* mutation detection in advanced NSCLC, if proper and sensitive detection methods are employed [195]. As direct sequencing can miss a significant portion of mutations in these heterogeneous specimens, more sensitive methods, such as mutant-enriched PCR and gene scan, may provide more reliable mutational information [196–198].

*EGFR* amplifications are less informative from a clinical point of view, since *EGFR* mutations relate best to treatment response to EGFR tyrosine kinase inhibitors. Patients with tumors lacking *EGFR* mutations and with *EGFR* amplification have dramatically lower response rates, corresponding to approximately 8% [199] compared to 70–90% for those with *EGFR* mutations. In addition to molecular methods, EGFR can be demonstrated by ICC, and antibodies specifically directed toward the mutated *EGFR* epitopes are available. This provides an alternative way to predict response to EGFR inhibitors. This is particularly useful on effusions with insufficient cells for molecular testing [200].

## Markers Indicating Primary or Acquired Resistance to EGFR Inhibitors

Primary resistance to EGFR TKIs is seen in association with activating mutations of downstream compounds. Thus lung ACs, harboring activating mutations in the downstream *KRAS*, are associated with a lack of sensitivity to gefitinib (Iressa) and erlotinib (Tarceva), suggesting that treatment decisions regarding use of these kinase inhibitors might be improved by determining the mutational status not only of *EGFR* but also *KRAS* [64], although the two often are mutually exclusive. Activating mutations on codons 12, 13, and 61 of *KRAS* are predictors of resistance to EGFR inhibitors and of poor prognosis. Mutations in the *KRAS* oncogene constitute a negative predictive marker in this clinical setting, and their presence can be used to predict which patients are unlikely to benefit from treatment with EGFR-directed therapy [52, 201]. Similarly, patients with EML4-ALK fusions do not benefit from EGFR tyrosine kinase-based therapy [84].

Acquired resistance to EGFR inhibitors is often connected to amplification of the gene encoding for the MET receptor or a second gatekeeper threonine-790 to methionine point mutation (T790M) [202–204]. Activating mutations of the main downstream effectors of *KRAS*, i.e., *BRAF* (V600E), also signal treatment failure with EGFR inhibitors [205]. Other parameters indicating acquired resistance to EGFR inhibitors are EGFR polysomy, mutations in codons 9 and 20 of the lipid kinase *PIK3CA*, expression of PTEN, which causes the inhibition of *PIK3CA*. Homozygous loss of *PTEN* contributes to erlotinib resistance in *EGFR*-mutant lung cancer by activation of Akt and EGFR [70].

## Predictive Markers for Treatment Response

Thymidylate synthase (TS) catalyzes reductive methylation of deoxyuridine monophosphate (dUMP) to deoxythymidinemonophosphate (dTMP), providing the only de novo source of thymidylate required for DNA replication and DNA repair [206]. This enzyme is the primary target of pemetrexed (Alimta), and high expression levels counteract the effects of this drug, making the tumor resistant [206–208].

Advanced NSCLC expresses excision repair cross-complementing group 1 gene (ERCC1) and ribonucleotide reductase subunit M1 (RRM1) in 35% and 40% of patients, respectively. This expression, whether determined by ICC or RT-PCR, predicts resistance to platinum-based drugs and an unfavorable outcome after platinum-based treatment [209–212].

Drugs like vinorelbine, taxane, and paclitaxel are antimitotic agents, with preferential action directed against tubulin. In NSCLCs the expression of IIIβ tubulin is reported to indicate resistance to such microtubule inhibition [213–215].

## Predictive Biomarkers in Clinical Trials

Lung cancer clinical trials account for 14% of ongoing oncology trials worldwide [216]. Although biomarker analysis was included in 38% of the ongoing NSCLC clinical trials registered in the ClinicalTrials.gov website, only 8% of the trials used actual biomarkers for patient selection. EGFR expression or mutation status was the most common biomarker, used to select patients in 44% of clinical trials, followed by *KRAS* mutation status in 13% of the trials [217]. Molecular tests including *EGFR, KRAS, ERCC1, RRM1,* VEGF, and serum tumor markers are not routinely used yet, but they might have clinical relevance in the near future [155].

## Prognostic Biomarkers

Lung AC is one of the most frequent metastatic tumors occurring in the serosal cavities [218, 219]. It often causes a malignant effusion corresponding to a disseminated disease beyond possibilities to cure [220]. Patients with malignant effusion have a limited life expectancy, with median survival times ranging from 4 to 13 months in different studies [221, 222]. A number of biomarkers have been suggested to distinguish patients with better prognosis. A meta-analysis based on 53 published studies identified *KRAS* mutation as a negative prognostic factor [223], while *EGFR* mutations were associated with a better prognosis [224]. Gene expression-based prognostic signatures for NSCLC have, however, not yet been standardized for clinical application [225].

Attempts have also been done to find prognostic markers by genome-wide screening and ICC. Using a tissue microarray from NSCLC specimens, it could be shown that syndecan-1 and EGFR expression was associated with a 30% reduction in the risk of death, independent of histology and other confounders. It can be hypothesized that loss of expression of these receptors reflects a less differentiated tumor with a more pronounced biologic aggressiveness, explaining the worse outcome for patients with such tumors [226].

On the other hand many markers detected in pleural fluids are negatively correlated to patient survival such as survivin [227, 228], IL-8, VEGF [48, 229], lactate dehydrogenase [230], and weak telomerase activity [231].

## Concluding Remarks

Lung carcinoma cells exfoliated into an effusion can often provide a diagnostic basis sufficient for clinical management. The development of new analytical techniques and the increased understanding of tumors will gradually shift the focus of tumor characterization toward biological parameters defined by molecular biology, epigenetics, and protein expression. This means that the analysis of isolated cells will be increasingly important for the choice of therapy and the diagnostic information can be made available earlier in the diagnostic process.

Tumor cells from an effusion can routinely be obtained without previous aldehyde fixation and will therefore provide a better material for the analysis of their DNA or protein contents, as compared to paraffin embedded tissues. Furthermore, the spread of a lung cancer to a serous cavity implies a more advanced stage of the disease. It can therefore be recommended in these cases that the search for therapy targets preferably should be performed using cells from the effusion rather than from the primary tumor tissue. Such a development toward increased use of cytological material requires attention to the handling of samples, perhaps including the development of routines for tumor cell enrichment and cell culturing.

## References

1. Jemal A, Thun MJ, Ries LA, Howe HL, Weir HK, Center MM, Ward E, Wu XC, Eheman C, Anderson R, et al. Annual report to the nation on the status of cancer, 1975-2005, featuring trends in lung cancer, tobacco use, and tobacco control. J Natl Cancer Inst. 2008;100(23):1672–94.
2. Jemal A, Siegel R, Ward E, Hao Y, Xu J, Murray T, Thun MJ. Cancer statistics, 2008. CA Cancer J Clin. 2008;58(2):71–96.
3. Jemal A, Siegel R, Xu J, Ward E. Cancer statistics, 2010. CA Cancer J Clin. 2010;60(5):277–300.
4. Jemal A, Siegel R, Ward E, Murray T, Xu J, Smigal C, Thun MJ. Cancer statistics, 2006. CA Cancer J Clin. 2006;56(2):106–30.
5. Porcel JM, Esquerda A, Vives M, Bielsa S. Etiology of pleural effusions: analysis of more than 3,000 consecutive thoracenteses. Arch Bronconeumol. 2014;50(5):161–5.
6. Porcel JM, Gasol A, Bielsa S, Civit C, Light RW, Salud A. Clinical features and survival of lung cancer patients with pleural effusions. Respirology. 2015;20(4):654–9.
7. Travis WDBE, Müller-Hermelink HK, Harris CC. Pathology and genetics of tumours of the lung, pleura, thymus and heart. Lyon: IARC Press; 2004.
8. Goldstraw P, Crowley J, Chansky K, Giroux DJ, Groome PA, Rami-Porta R, Postmus PE, Rusch V, Sobin L. The IASLC Lung Cancer Staging Project: proposals for the revision of the TNM stage groupings in the forthcoming (seventh) edition of the TNM Classification of malignant tumours. J Thorac Oncol. 2007;2(8):706–14.
9. Mukhopadhyay S, Katzenstein AL. Subclassification of non-small cell lung carcinomas lacking morphologic differentiation on biopsy specimens: Utility of an immunohistochemical panel containing TTF-1, napsin A, p63, and CK5/6. Am J Surg Pathol. 2011;35(1):15–25.
10. McDowell EM, McLaughlin JS, Merenyl DK, Kieffer RF, Harris CC, Trump BF. The respiratory epithelium. V. Histogenesis of lung carcinomas in the human. J Natl Cancer Inst. 1978;61(2):587–606.
11. Hecht SS. Tobacco smoke carcinogens and lung cancer. J Natl Cancer Inst. 1999;91(14):1194–210.
12. Yokota J, Shiraishi K, Kohno T. Genetic basis for susceptibility to lung cancer recent progress and future directions. Adv Cancer Res. 2010;109:51–72.
13. Hung RJ, McKay JD, Gaborieau V, Boffetta P, Hashibe M, Zaridze D, Mukeria A, Szeszenia-Dabrowska N, Lissowska J, Rudnai P, et al. A susceptibility locus for lung cancer maps to nicotinic acetylcholine receptor subunit genes on 15q25. Nature. 2008;452(7187):633–7.
14. Wistuba II, Behrens C, Virmani AK, Mele G, Milchgrub S, Girard L, Fondon JW III, Garner HR, McKay B, Latif F, et al. High resolution chromosome 3p allelotyping of human lung cancer and preneoplastic/preinvasive bronchial epithelium reveals multiple,

discontinuous sites of 3p allele loss and three regions of frequent breakpoints. Cancer Res. 2000;60(7):1949–60.

15. Weir BA, Woo MS, Getz G, Perner S, Ding L, Beroukhim R, Lin WM, Province MA, Kraja A, Johnson LA, et al. Characterizing the cancer genome in lung adenocarcinoma. Nature. 2007;450(7171):893–8.

16. Kendall J, Liu Q, Bakleh A, Krasnitz A, Nguyen KC, Lakshmi B, Gerald WL, Powers S, Mu D. Oncogenic cooperation and coamplification of developmental transcription factor genes in lung cancer. Proc Natl Acad Sci U S A. 2007;104(42):16663–8.

17. Tanaka H, Yanagisawa K, Shinjo K, Taguchi A, Maeno K, Tomida S, Shimada Y, Osada H, Kosaka T, Matsubara H, et al. Lineage-specific dependency of lung adenocarcinomas on the lung development regulator TTF-1. Cancer Res. 2007;67(13):6007–11.

18. Nymark P, Wikman H, Ruosaari S, Hollmen J, Vanhala E, Karjalainen A, Anttila S, Knuutila S. Identification of specific gene copy number changes in asbestos-related lung cancer. Cancer Res. 2006;66(11):5737–43.

19. Kettunen E, Aavikko M, Nymark P, Ruosaari S, Wikman H, Vanhala E, Salmenkivi K, Pirinen R, Karjalainen A, Kuosma E, et al. DNA copy number loss and allelic imbalance at 2p16 in lung cancer associated with asbestos exposure. Br J Cancer. 2009;100(8):1336–42.

20. Nymark P, Kettunen E, Aavikko M, Ruosaari S, Kuosma E, Vanhala E, Salmenkivi K, Pirinen R, Karjalainen A, Knuutila S, et al. Molecular alterations at 9q33.1 and polyploidy in asbestos-related lung cancer. Clin Cancer Res. 2009;15(2):468–75.

21. Mutsaers SE. The mesothelial cell. Int J Biochem Cell Biol. 2004;36(1):9–16.

22. Mutsaers SE, Wilkosz S. Structure and function of mesothelial cells. Cancer Treat Res. 2007;134:1–19.

23. Graves EE, Vilalta M, Cecic IK, Erler JT, Tran PT, Felsher D, Sayles L, Sweet-Cordero A, Le QT, Giaccia AJ. Hypoxia in models of lung cancer: implications for targeted therapeutics. Clin Cancer Res. 2010;16(19):4843–52.

24. Graves EE, Maity A, Le QT. The tumor microenvironment in non-small-cell lung cancer. Semin Radiat Oncol. 2010;20(3):156–63.

25. Kassis J, Klominek J, Kohn EC. Tumor microenvironment: what can effusions teach us? Diagn Cytopathol. 2005;33(5):316–9.

26. Kohn EC, Travers LA, Kassis J, Broome U, Klominek J. Malignant effusions are sources of fibronectin and other promigratory and proinvasive components. Diagn Cytopathol. 2005;33(5):300–8.

27. Quaranta V, Giannelli G. Cancer invasion: watch your neighbourhood. Tumori. 2003;89(4):343–8.

28. Jantz MA, Antony VB. Pathophysiology of the pleura. Respiration. 2008;75(2):121–33.

29. Lynch CC, Matrisian LM. Matrix metalloproteinases in tumor-host cell communication. Differentiation. 2002;70(9 10):561 73.

30. O'Reilly MS, Boehm T, Shing Y, Fukai N, Vasios G, Lane WS, Flynn E, Birkhead JR, Olsen BR, Folkman J. Endostatin: an endogenous inhibitor of angiogenesis and tumor growth. Cell. 1997;88(2):277–85.

31. Gulyas M, Dobra K, Hjerpe A. Expression of genes coding for proteoglycans and Wilms' tumour susceptibility gene 1 (WT1) by variously differentiated benign human mesothelial cells. Differentiation. 1999;65(2):89–96.

32. Sharma RK, Mohammed KA, Nasreen N, Hardwick J, Van Horn RD, Ramirez-Icaza C, Antony VB. Defensive role of pleural mesothelial cell sialomucins in tumor metastasis. Chest. 2003;124(2):682–7.

33. Ponta H, Wainwright D, Herrlich P. The CD44 protein family. Int J Biochem Cell Biol. 1998;30(3):299–305.

34. Lin CC, Chen LC, Tseng VS, Yan JJ, Lai WW, Su WP, Lin CH, Huang CY, Su WC. Malignant pleural effusion cells show

aberrant glucose metabolism gene expression. Eur Respir J. 2011;37(6):1453–65.

35. Grove CS, Lee YC. Vascular endothelial growth factor: the key mediator in pleural effusion formation. Curr Opin Pulm Med. 2002;8(4):294–301.

36. Cheng D, Lee YC, Rogers JT, Perkett EA, Moyers JP, Rodriguez RM, Light RW. Vascular endothelial growth factor level correlates with transforming growth factor-beta isoform levels in pleural effusions. Chest. 2000;118(6):1747–53.

37. Lee YC, Lane KB. The many faces of transforming growth factor-beta in pleural diseases. Curr Opin Pulm Med. 2001;7(4):173–9.

38. Gary Lee YC, Melkerneker D, Thompson PJ, Light RW, Lane KB. Transforming growth factor beta induces vascular endothelial growth factor elaboration from pleural mesothelial cells in vivo and in vitro. Am J Respir Crit Care Med. 2002;165(1):88–94.

39. Kishiro I, Kato S, Fuse D, Yoshida T, Machida S, Kaneko N. Clinical significance of vascular endothelial growth factor in patients with primary lung cancer. Respirology. 2002;7(2):93–8.

40. Yanagawa H, Takeuchi E, Suzuki Y, Ohmoto Y, Bando H, Sone S. Vascular endothelial growth factor in malignant pleural effusion associated with lung cancer. Cancer Immunol Immunother. 1999;48(7):396–400.

41. Thickett DR, Armstrong L, Millar AB. Vascular endothelial growth factor (VEGF) in inflammatory and malignant pleural effusions. Thorax. 1999;54(8):707–10.

42. Ishimoto O, Saijo Y, Narumi K, Kimura Y, Ebina M, Matsubara N, Asou N, Nakai Y, Nukiwa T. High level of vascular endothelial growth factor in hemorrhagic pleural effusion of cancer. Oncology. 2002;63(1):70–5.

43. Tomimoto H, Yano S, Muguruma H, Kakiuchi S, Sone S. Levels of soluble vascular endothelial growth factor receptor 1 are elevated in the exudative pleural effusions. J Med Invest. 2007;54(1-2):146–53.

44. Safi A, Sadmi M, Martinet N, Menard O, Vaillant P, Gallati H, Hosang M, Martinet Y. Presence of elevated levels of platelet-derived growth factor (PDGF) in lung adenocarcinoma pleural effusions. Chest. 1992;102(1):204–7.

45. Xirouchaki N, Tzanakis N, Bouros D, Kyriakou D, Karkavitsas N, Alexandrakis M, Siafakas NM. Diagnostic value of interleukin-1alpha, interleukin-6, and tumor necrosis factor in pleural effusions. Chest. 2002;121(3):815–20.

46. Aoe K, Hiraki A, Murakami T, Murakami K, Makihata K, Takao K, Eda R, Maeda T, Sugi K, Darzynkiewicz Z, et al. Relative abundance and patterns of correlation among six cytokines in pleural fluid measured by cytometric bead array. Int J Mol Med. 2003;12(2):193–8.

47. Chen YM, Yang WK, Whang-Peng J, Tsai CM, Perng RP. An analysis of cytokine status in the serum and effusions of patients with tuberculous and lung cancer. Lung Cancer. 2001;31(1):25–30.

48. Kotyza J, Havel D, Vrzalova J, Kulda V, Pesek M. Diagnostic and prognostic significance of inflammatory markers in lung cancer-associated pleural effusions. Int J Biol Markers. 2010;25(1):12–20.

49. Pao W, Iafrate AJ, Su Z. Genetically informed lung cancer medicine. J Pathol. 2011;223(2):230–40.

50. Bronte G, Rizzo S, La Paglia L, Adamo V, Siragusa S, Ficorella C, Santini D, Bazan V, Colucci G, Gebbia N, et al. Driver mutations and differential sensitivity to targeted therapies: a new approach to the treatment of lung adenocarcinoma. Cancer Treat Rev. 2010;36(Suppl 3):S21–9.

51. Mitsudomi T, Yatabe Y. Mutations of the epidermal growth factor receptor gene and related genes as determinants of epidermal growth factor receptor tyrosine kinase inhibitors sensitivity in lung cancer. Cancer Sci. 2007;98(12):1817–24.

52. Ladanyi M, Pao W. Lung adenocarcinoma: guiding EGFR-targeted therapy and beyond. Mod Pathol. 2008;21(Suppl 2):S16–22.

53. Sharma SV, Bell DW, Settleman J, Haber DA. Epidermal growth factor receptor mutations in lung cancer. Nat Rev Cancer. 2007;7(3):169–81.

54. Shigematsu H, Gazdar AF. Somatic mutations of epidermal growth factor receptor signaling pathway in lung cancers. Int J Cancer. 2006;118(2):257–62.

55. Kumar A, Petri ET, Halmos B, Boggon TJ. Structure and clinical relevance of the epidermal growth factor receptor in human cancer. J Clin Oncol. 2008;26(10):1742–51.

56. Wu SG, Gow CH, Yu CJ, Chang YL, Yang CH, Hsu YC, Shih JY, Lee YC, Yang PC. Frequent epidermal growth factor receptor gene mutations in malignant pleural effusion of lung adenocarcinoma. Eur Respir J. 2008;32(4):924–30.

57. Zou J, Bella AE, Chen Z, Han X, Su C, Lei Y, Luo H. Frequency of EGFR mutations in lung adenocarcinoma with malignant pleural effusion: Implication of cancer biological behaviour regulated by EGFR mutation. J Int Med Res. 2014;42(5):1110–7.

58. Rodriguez EF, Shabihkhani M, Carter J, Maleki Z. Molecular alterations in patients with pulmonary adenocarcinoma presenting with malignant pleural effusion at the first diagnosis. Acta Cytol. 2017;61(3):214–22.

59. Hung MS, Lin CK, Leu SW, Wu MY, Tsai YH, Yang CT. Epidermal growth factor receptor mutations in cells from non-small cell lung cancer malignant pleural effusions. Chang Gung Med J. 2006;29(4):373–9.

60. Soh J, Toyooka S, Aoe K, Asano H, Ichihara S, Katayama H, Hiraki A, Kiura K, Aoe M, Sano Y, et al. Usefulness of EGFR mutation screening in pleural fluid to predict the clinical outcome of gefitinib treated patients with lung cancer. Int J Cancer. 2006;119(10):2353–8.

61. Soh J, Toyooka S, Ichihara S, Suehisa H, Kobayashi N, Ito S, Yamane M, Aoe M, Sano Y, Kiura K, et al. EGFR mutation status in pleural fluid predicts tumor responsiveness and resistance to gefitinib. Lung Cancer. 2007;56(3):445–8.

62. Jian G, Songwen Z, Ling Z, Qinfang D, Jie Z, Liang T, Caicun Z. Prediction of epidermal growth factor receptor mutations in the plasma/pleural effusion to efficacy of gefitinib treatment in advanced non-small cell lung cancer. J Cancer Res Clin Oncol. 2010;136(9):1341–7.

63. Soung YH, Lee JW, Kim SY, Seo SH, Park WS, Nam SW, Song SY, Han JH, Park CK, Lee JY, et al. Mutational analysis of EGFR and K-RAS genes in lung adenocarcinomas. Virchows Arch. 2005;446(5):483–8.

64. Pao W, Wang TY, Riely GJ, Miller VA, Pan Q, Ladanyi M, Zakowski MF, Heelan RT, Kris MG, Varmus HE. KRAS mutations and primary resistance of lung adenocarcinomas to gefitinib or erlotinib. PLoS Med. 2005;2(1):e17.

65. Zhu CQ, Ding K, Strumpf D, Weir BA, Meyerson M, Pennell N, Thomas RK, Naoki K, Ladd-Acosta C, Liu N, et al. Prognostic and predictive gene signature for adjuvant chemotherapy in resected non-small-cell lung cancer. J Clin Oncol. 2010;28(29):4417–24.

66. Bass AJ, Watanabe H, Mermel CH, Yu S, Perner S, Verhaak RG, Kim SY, Wardwell L, Tamayo P, Gat-Viks I, et al. SOX2 is an amplified lineage-survival oncogene in lung and esophageal squamous cell carcinomas. Nat Genet. 2009;41(11):1238–42.

67. Wagner PL, Perner S, Rickman DS, LaFargue CJ, Kitabayashi N, Johnstone SF, Weir BA, Meyerson M, Altorki NK, Rubin MA. In situ evidence of KRAS amplification and association with increased p21 levels in non-small cell lung carcinoma. Am J Clin Pathol. 2009;132(4):500–5.

68. Ramos AH, Dutt A, Mermel C, Perner S, Cho J, Lafargue CJ, Johnson LA, Stiedl AC, Tanaka KE, Bass AJ, et al. Amplification of chromosomal segment 4q12 in non-small cell lung cancer. Cancer Biol Ther. 2009;8(21):2042–50.

69. Sos ML, Michel K, Zander T, Weiss J, Frommolt P, Peifer M, Li D, Ullrich R, Koker M, Fischer F, et al. Predicting drug suscep-

tibility of non-small cell lung cancers based on genetic lesions. J Clin Invest. 2009;119(6):1727–40.

70. Sos ML, Koker M, Weir BA, Heynck S, Rabinovsky R, Zander T, Seeger JM, Weiss J, Fischer F, Frommolt P, et al. PTEN loss contributes to erlotinib resistance in EGFR-mutant lung cancer by activation of Akt and EGFR. Cancer Res. 2009;69(8):3256–61.

71. Barletta JA, Perner S, Iafrate AJ, Yeap BY, Weir BA, Johnson LA, Johnson BE, Meyerson M, Rubin MA, Travis WD, et al. Clinical significance of TTF-1 protein expression and TTF-1 gene amplification in lung adenocarcinoma. J Cell Mol Med. 2009;13(8B):1977–86.

72. Ding L, Getz G, Wheeler DA, Mardis ER, McLellan MD, Cibulskis K, Sougnez C, Greulich H, Muzny DM, Morgan MB, et al. Somatic mutations affect key pathways in lung adenocarcinoma. Nature. 2008;455(7216):1069–75.

73. Perner S, Wagner PL, Soltermann A, LaFargue C, Tischler V, Weir BA, Weder W, Meyerson M, Giordano TJ, Moch H, et al. TTF1 expression in non-small cell lung carcinoma: association with TTF1 gene amplification and improved survival. J Pathol. 2009;217(1):65–72.

74. Shedden K, Taylor JM, Enkemann SA, Tsao MS, Yeatman TJ, Gerald WL, Eschrich S, Jurisica I, Giordano TJ, Misek DE, et al. Gene expression-based survival prediction in lung adenocarcinoma: a multi-site, blinded validation study. Nat Med. 2008;14(8):822–7.

75. Minami Y, Shimamura T, Shah K, LaFramboise T, Glatt KA, Liniker E, Borgman CL, Haringsma HJ, Feng W, Weir BA, et al. The major lung cancer-derived mutants of ERBB2 are oncogenic and are associated with sensitivity to the irreversible EGFR/ ERBB2 inhibitor HKI-272. Oncogene. 2007;26(34):5023–7.

76. Thomas RK, Weir B, Meyerson M. Genomic approaches to lung cancer. Clin Cancer Res. 2006;12(14 Pt 2):4384s–91s.

77. Zhao X, Weir BA, LaFramboise T, Lin M, Beroukhim R, Garraway L, Beheshti J, Lee JC, Naoki K, Richards WG, et al. Homozygous deletions and chromosome amplifications in human lung carcinomas revealed by single nucleotide polymorphism array analysis. Cancer Res. 2005;65(13):5561–70.

78. Suda K, Tomizawa K, Mitsudomi T. Biological and clinical significance of KRAS mutations in lung cancer: an oncogenic driver that contrasts with EGFR mutation. Cancer Metastasis Rev. 2010;29(1):49–60.

79. Carter J, Miller JA, Feller-Kopman D, Ettinger D, Sidransky D, Maleki Z. Molecular profiling of malignant pleural effusion in metastatic non-small-cell lung carcinoma. The effect of preanalytical factors. Ann Am Thorac Soc. 2017;14(7):1169–76.

80. Jordan EJ, Kim HR, Arcila ME, Barron D, Chakravarty D, Gao J, Chang MT, Ni A, Kundra R, Jonsson P, et al. Prospective comprehensive molecular characterization of lung adenocarcinomas for efficient patient matching to approved and emerging therapies. Cancer Discov. 2017;7(6):596–609.

81. Soda M, Choi YL, Enomoto M, Takada S, Yamashita Y, Ishikawa S, Fujiwara S, Watanabe H, Kurashina K, Hatanaka H, et al. Identification of the transforming EML4-ALK fusion gene in non-small-cell lung cancer. Nature. 2007;448(7153):561–6.

82. Inamura K, Takeuchi K, Togashi Y, Nomura K, Ninomiya H, Okui M, Satoh Y, Okumura S, Nakagawa K, Soda M, et al. EML4-ALK fusion is linked to histological characteristics in a subset of lung cancers. J Thorac Oncol. 2008;3(1):13–7.

83. Sasaki T, Rodig SJ, Chirieac LR, Janne PA. The biology and treatment of EML4-ALK non-small cell lung cancer. Eur J Cancer. 2010;46(10):1773–80.

84. Shaw AT, Yeap BY, Mino-Kenudson M, Digumarthy SR, Costa DB, Heist RS, Solomon B, Stubbs H, Admane S, McDermott U, et al. Clinical features and outcome of patients with non-small-cell lung cancer who harbor EML4-ALK. J Clin Oncol. 2009;27(26):4247–53.

85. Zhang X, Zhang S, Yang X, Yang J, Zhou Q, Yin L, An S, Lin J, Chen S, Xie Z, et al. Fusion of EML4 and ALK is associated with development of lung adenocarcinomas lacking EGFR and KRAS mutations and is correlated with ALK expression. Mol Cancer. 2010;9:188.

86. Zhong J, Li X, Bai H, Zhao J, Wang Z, Duan J, An T, Wu M, Wang Y, Wang S, et al. Malignant pleural effusion cell blocks are substitutes for tissue in EML4-ALK rearrangement detection in patients with advanced non-small-cell lung cancer. Cytopathology. 2016;27(6):433–43.

87. Zhou J, Yao H, Zhao J, Zhang S, You Q, Sun K, Zou Y, Zhou C. Cell block samples from malignant pleural effusion might be valid alternative samples for anaplastic lymphoma kinase detection in patients with advanced non-small-cell lung cancer. Histopathology. 2015;66(7):949–54.

88. Wang W, Tang Y, Li J, Jiang L, Jiang Y, Su X. Detection of ALK rearrangements in malignant pleural effusion cell blocks from patients with advanced non-small cell lung cancer: a comparison of Ventana immunohistochemistry and fluorescence in situ hybridization. Cancer Cytopathol. 2015;123(2):117–22.

89. Savic S, Bode B, Diebold J, Tosoni I, Barascud A, Baschiera B, Grilli B, Herzog M, Obermann E, Bubendorf L. Detection of ALK-positive non-small-cell lung cancers on cytological specimens: high accuracy of immunocytochemistry with the 5A4 clone. J Thorac Oncol. 2013;8(8):1004–11.

90. Liu L, Zhan P, Zhou X, Song Y, Yu L, Wang J. Detection of EML4-ALK in lung adenocarcinoma using pleural effusion with FISH, IHC, and RT-PCR methods. PLoS One. 2015;10(3):e0117032.

91. Yamamoto G, Kikuchi M, Kobayashi S, Arai Y, Fujiyoshi K, Wakatsuki T, Kakuta M, Yamane Y, Iijima Y, Mizutani H, et al. Routine genetic testing of lung cancer specimens derived from surgery, bronchoscopy and fluid aspiration by next generation sequencing. Int J Oncol. 2017;50(5):1579–89.

92. Ali SM, Hensing T, Schrock AB, Allen J, Sanford E, Gowen K, Kulkarni A, He J, Suh JH, Lipson D, et al. Comprehensive genomic profiling identifies a subset of Crizotinib-responsive ALK-rearranged non-small cell lung cancer not detected by fluorescence in situ hybridization. Oncologist. 2016;21(6):762–70.

93. Bergethon K, Shaw AT, Ou SH, Katayama R, Lovly CM, McDonald NT, Massion PP, Siwak-Tapp C, Gonzalez A, Fang R, et al. ROS1 rearrangements define a unique molecular class of lung cancers. J Clin Oncol. 2012;30(8):863–70.

94. Rossi G, Ragazzi M, Tamagnini I, Mengoli MC, Vincenzi G, Barbieri F, Piccioli S, Bisagni A, Vavala T, Righi L, et al. Does immunohistochemistry represent a robust alternative technique in determining drugable predictive gene alterations in non-small cell lung cancer? Curr Drug Targets. 2017;18(1):13–26.

95. Drilon A, Somwar R, Wagner JP, Vellore NA, Eide CA, Zabriskie MS, Arcila ME, Hechtman JF, Wang L, Smith RS, et al. A novel Crizotinib-resistant solvent-front mutation responsive to Cabozantinib therapy in a patient with ROS1-rearranged lung cancer. Clin Cancer Res. 2016;22(10):2351–8.

96. Wang R, Hu H, Pan Y, Li Y, Ye T, Li C, Luo X, Wang L, Li H, Zhang Y, et al. RET fusions define a unique molecular and clinicopathologic subtype of non-small-cell lung cancer. J Clin Oncol. 2012;30(35):4352–9.

97. Drilon A, Rekhtman N, Arcila M, Wang L, Ni A, Albano M, Van Voorthuysen M, Somwar R, Smith RS, Montecalvo J, et al. Cabozantinib in patients with advanced RET-rearranged non-small-cell lung cancer: an open-label, single-centre, phase 2, single-arm trial. Lancet Oncol. 2016;17(12):1653–60.

98. Sekido Y, Fong KM, Minna JD. Progress in understanding the molecular pathogenesis of human lung cancer. Biochim Biophys Acta. 1998;1378(1):F21–59.

99. Salgia R, Skarin AT. Molecular abnormalities in lung cancer. J Clin Oncol. 1998;16(3):1207–17.

100. Tong JH, Yeung SF, Chan AW, Chung LY, Chau SL, Lung RW, Tong CY, Chow C, Tin EK, Yu YH, et al. MET amplification and Exon 14 splice site mutation define unique molecular subgroups of non-small cell lung carcinoma with poor prognosis. Clin Cancer Res. 2016;22(12):3048–56.

101. Cassidy RJ, Zhang X, Patel PR, Shelton JW, Escott CE, Sica GL, Rossi MR, Hill CE, Steuer CE, Pillai RN, et al. Next-generation sequencing and clinical outcomes of patients with lung adenocarcinoma treated with stereotactic body radiotherapy. Cancer. 2017;123(19):3681–90.

102. Paik PK, Drilon A, Fan PD, Yu H, Rekhtman N, Ginsberg MS, Borsu L, Schultz N, Berger MF, Rudin CM, et al. Response to MET inhibitors in patients with stage IV lung adenocarcinomas harboring MET mutations causing exon 14 skipping. Cancer Discov. 2015;5(8):842–9.

103. Cortot AB, Kherrouche Z, Descarpentries C, Wislez M, Baldacci S, Furlan A, Tulasne D. Exon 14 deleted MET receptor as a new biomarker and target in cancers. J Natl Cancer Inst. 2017;109(5).

104. Kitamura H, Yazawa T, Sato H, Okudela K, Shimoyamada H. Small cell lung cancer: significance of RB alterations and TTF-1 expression in its carcinogenesis, phenotype, and biology. Endocr Pathol. 2009;20(2):101–7.

105. Wistuba II, Gazdar AF, Minna JD. Molecular genetics of small cell lung carcinoma. Semin Oncol. 2001;28(2 Suppl 4):3–13.

106. Bartel DP. MicroRNAs: genomics, biogenesis, mechanism, and function. Cell. 2004;116(2):281–97.

107. Bartel DP. MicroRNAs: target recognition and regulatory functions. Cell. 2009;136(2):215–33.

108. He X, He L, Hannon GJ. The guardian's little helper: microRNAs in the p53 tumor suppressor network. Cancer Res. 2007;67(23):11099–101.

109. He L, He X, Lowe SW, Hannon GJ. microRNAs join the p53 network--another piece in the tumour-suppression puzzle. Nat Rev Cancer. 2007;7(11):819–22.

110. He L, He X, Lim LP, de Stanchina E, Xuan Z, Liang Y, Xue W, Zender L, Magnus J, Ridzon D, et al. A microRNA component of the p53 tumour suppressor network. Nature. 2007;447(7148):1130–4.

111. Johnson SM, Grosshans H, Shingara J, Byrom M, Jarvis R, Cheng A, Labourier E, Reinert KL, Brown D, Slack FJ. RAS is regulated by the let-7 microRNA family. Cell. 2005;120(5):635–47.

112. Lu J, Getz G, Miska EA, Alvarez-Saavedra E, Lamb J, Peck D, Sweet-Cordero A, Ebert BL, Mak RH, Ferrando AA, et al. MicroRNA expression profiles classify human cancers. Nature. 2005;435(7043):834–8.

113. Calin GA, Sevignani C, Dumitru CD, Hyslop T, Noch E, Yendamuri S, Shimizu M, Rattan S, Bullrich F, Negrini M, et al. Human microRNA genes are frequently located at fragile sites and genomic regions involved in cancers. Proc Natl Acad Sci U S A. 2004;101(9):2999–3004.

114. Calin GA, Croce CM. MicroRNAs and chromosomal abnormalities in cancer cells. Oncogene. 2006;25(46):6202–10.

115. Calin GA, Croce CM. MicroRNA signatures in human cancers. Nat Rev Cancer. 2006;6(11):857–66.

116. Chen X, Ba Y, Ma L, Cai X, Yin Y, Wang K, Guo J, Zhang Y, Chen J, Guo X, et al. Characterization of microRNAs in serum: a novel class of biomarkers for diagnosis of cancer and other diseases. Cell Res. 2008;18(10):997–1006.

117. Yanaihara N, Caplen N, Bowman E, Seike M, Kumamoto K, Yi M, Stephens RM, Okamoto A, Yokota J, Tanaka T, et al. Unique microRNA molecular profiles in lung cancer diagnosis and prognosis. Cancer Cell. 2006;9(3):189–98.

118. Rabinowits G, Gercel-Taylor C, Day JM, Taylor DD, Kloecker GH. Exosomal microRNA: a diagnostic marker for lung cancer. Clin Lung Cancer. 2009;10(1):42–6.

119. Lin PY, Yu SL, Yang PC. MicroRNA in lung cancer. Br J Cancer. 2010;103(8):1144–8.

120. Heneghan HM, Miller N, Kerin MJ. MiRNAs as biomarkers and therapeutic targets in cancer. Curr Opin Pharmacol. 2010;10(5):543–50.

121. Holloway AJ, Diyagama DS, Opeskin K, Creaney J, Robinson BW, Lake RA, Bowtell DD. A molecular diagnostic test for distinguishing lung adenocarcinoma from malignant mesothelioma using cells collected from pleural effusions. Clin Cancer Res. 2006;12(17):5129–35.

122. Bild AH, Yao G, Chang JT, Wang Q, Potti A, Chasse D, Joshi MB, Harpole D, Lancaster JM, Berchuck A, et al. Oncogenic pathway signatures in human cancers as a guide to targeted therapies. Nature. 2006;439(7074):353–7.

123. Nguyen DX, Chiang AC, Zhang XH, Kim JY, Kris MG, Ladanyi M, Gerald WL, Massague J. WNT/TCF signaling through LEF1 and HOXB9 mediates lung adenocarcinoma metastasis. Cell. 2009;138(1):51–62.

124. Brock MV, Hooker CM, Yung R, Guo M, Han Y, Ames SE, Chang D, Yang SC, Mason D, Sussman M, et al. Can we improve the cytologic examination of malignant pleural effusions using molecular analysis? Ann Thorac Surg. 2005;80(4):1241–7.

125. Ng CS, Zhang J, Wan S, Lee TW, Arifi AA, Mok T, Lo DY, Yim AP. Tumor p16M is a possible marker of advanced stage in non-small cell lung cancer. J Surg Oncol. 2002;79(2):101–6.

126. Gui S, Liu H, Zhang L, Zuo L, Zhou Q, Fei G, Wang Y. Clinical significance of the detection of the homozygous deletion of P16 gene in malignant pleural effusion. Intern Med. 2007;46(15):1161–6.

127. Toyooka S, Toyooka KO, Maruyama R, Virmani AK, Girard L, Miyajima K, Harada K, Ariyoshi Y, Takahashi T, Sugio K, et al. DNA methylation profiles of lung tumors. Mol Cancer Ther. 2001;1(1):61–7.

128. Katayama H, Hiraki A, Aoe K, Fujiwara K, Matsuo K, Maeda T, Murakami T, Toyooka S, Sugi K, Ueoka H, et al. Aberrant promoter methylation in pleural fluid DNA for diagnosis of malignant pleural effusion. Int J Cancer. 2007;120(10):2191–5.

129. Toyooka S, Tokumo M, Shigematsu H, Matsuo K, Asano H, Tomii K, Ichihara S, Suzuki M, Aoe M, Date H, et al. Mutational and epigenetic evidence for independent pathways for lung adenocarcinomas arising in smokers and never smokers. Cancer Res. 2006;66(3):1371–5.

130. Suzuki M, Shigematsu H, Iizasa T, Hiroshima K, Nakatani Y, Minna JD, Gazdar AF, Fujisawa T. Exclusive mutation in epidermal growth factor receptor gene, HER-2, and KRAS, and synchronous methylation of nonsmall cell lung cancer. Cancer. 2006;106(10):2200–7.

131. Schroeder JA, Thompson MC, Gardner MM, Gendler SJ. Transgenic MUC1 interacts with epidermal growth factor receptor and correlates with mitogen-activated protein kinase activation in the mouse mammary gland. J Biol Chem. 2001;276(16):13057–64.

132. Li Y, Ren J, Yu W, Li Q, Kuwahara H, Yin L, Carraway KL III, Kufe D. The epidermal growth factor receptor regulates interaction of the human DF3/MUC1 carcinoma antigen with c-Src and beta-catenin. J Biol Chem. 2001;276(38):35239–42.

133. Pao W, Kris MG, Iafrate AJ, Ladanyi M, Janne PA, Wistuba II, Miake-Lye R, Herbst RS, Carbone DP, Johnson BE, et al. Integration of molecular profiling into the lung cancer clinic. Clin Cancer Res. 2009;15(17):5317–22.

134. Jacot W, Lhermitte L, Dossat N, Pujol JL, Molinari N, Daures JP, Maudelonde T, Mange A, Solassol J. Serum proteomic profiling of lung cancer in high-risk groups and determination of clinical outcomes. J Thorac Oncol. 2008;3(8):840–50.

135. Tyan YC, Wu HY, Lai WW, Su WC, Liao PC. Proteomic profiling of human pleural effusion using two-dimensional nano liquid chromatography tandem mass spectrometry. J Proteome Res. 2005;4(4):1274–86.

136. Tyan YC, Wu HY, Su WC, Chen PW, Liao PC. Proteomic analysis of human pleural effusion. Proteomics. 2005;5(4):1062–74.

137. Kim JH, Choi YD, Lee JS, Lee JH, Nam JH, Choi C. Utility of thyroid transcription factor-1 and CDX-2 in determining the primary site of metastatic adenocarcinomas in serous effusions. Acta Cytol. 2010;54(3):277–82.

138. Dejmek A, Naucler P, Smedjeback A, Kato H, Maeda M, Yashima K, Maeda J, Hirano T. Napsin A (TA02) is a useful alternative to thyroid transcription factor-1 (TTF-1) for the identification of pulmonary adenocarcinoma cells in pleural effusions. Diagn Cytopathol. 2007;35(8):493–7.

139. Flores-Staino C, Darai-Ramqvist E, Dobra K, Hjerpe A. Adaptation of a commercial fluorescent in situ hybridization test to the diagnosis of malignant cells in effusions. Lung Cancer. 2010;68(1):39–43.

140. Fiegl M, Massoner A, Haun M, Sturm W, Kaufmann H, Hack R, Krugmann J, Fritzer-Szekeres M, Grunewald K, Gastl G. Sensitive detection of tumour cells in effusions by combining cytology and fluorescence in situ hybridisation (FISH). Br J Cancer. 2004;91(3):558–63.

141. Voss JS, Kipp BR, Halling KC, Henry MR, Jett JR, Clayton AC, Rickman OB. Fluorescence in situ hybridization testing algorithm improves lung cancer detection in bronchial brushing specimens. Am J Respir Crit Care Med. 2010;181(5):478–85.

142. Akamatsu H, Koh Y, Kenmotsu H, Naito T, Serizawa M, Kimura M, Mori K, Imai H, Ono A, Shukuya T, et al. Multiplexed molecular profiling of lung cancer using pleural effusion. J Thorac Oncol. 2014;9(7):1048–52.

143. Kruglyak KM, Lin E, Ong FS. Next-generation sequencing and applications to the diagnosis and treatment of lung cancer. Adv Exp Med Biol. 2016;890:123–36.

144. Zugazagoitia J, Rueda D, Carrizo N, Enguita AB, Gomez-Sanchez D, Diaz-Serrano A, Jimenez E, Merida A, Calero R, Lujan R et al. Prospective clinical integration of an amplicon-based next-generation sequencing method to select advanced non-small-cell lung cancer patients for genotype-tailored treatments. Clin Lung Cancer. 2017.

145. Antony VB. Pathogenesis of malignant pleural effusions and talc pleurodesis. Pneumologie. 1999;53(10):493–8.

146. Nasreen N, Mohammed KA, Brown S, Su Y, Sriram PS, Moudgil B, Loddenkemper R, Antony VB. Talc mediates angiostasis in malignant pleural effusions via endostatin induction. Eur Respir J. 2007;29(4):761–9.

147. Grilli R, Oxman AD, Julian JA. Chemotherapy for advanced non-small-cell lung cancer: how much benefit is enough? J Clin Oncol. 1993;11(10):1866–72.

148. Souquet PJ, Chauvin F, Boissel JP, Cellerino R, Cormier Y, Ganz PA, Kaasa S, Pater JL, Quoix E, Rapp E, et al. Polychemotherapy in advanced non small cell lung cancer: a meta-analysis. Lancet. 1993;342(8862):19–21.

149. Carbone DP, Minna JD. Chemotherapy for non-small cell lung cancer. BMJ. 1995;311(7010):889–90.

150. D'Addario G, Pintilie M, Leighl NB, Feld R, Cerny T, Shepherd FA. Platinum-based versus non-platinum-based chemotherapy in advanced non-small-cell lung cancer: a meta-analysis of the published literature. J Clin Oncol. 2005;23(13):2926–36.

151. Klastersky J, Sculier JP, Lacroix H, Dabouis G, Bureau G, Libert P, Richez M, Ravez P, Vandermoten G, Thiriaux J, et al. A randomized study comparing cisplatin or carboplatin with etoposide in patients with advanced non-small-cell lung cancer: European Organization for Research and Treatment of Cancer Protocol 07861. J Clin Oncol. 1990;8(9):1556–62.

152. Kroep JR, Giaccone G, Voorn DA, Smit EF, Beijnen JH, Rosing H, van Moorsel CJ, van Groeningen CJ, Postmus PE, Pinedo HM, et al. Gemcitabine and paclitaxel: pharmacokinetic and pharmaco-

dynamic interactions in patients with non-small-cell lung cancer. J Clin Oncol. 1999;17(7):2190–7.

153. Mori K, Kobayashi H, Kamiyama Y, Kano Y, Kodama T. A phase II trial of weekly chemotherapy with paclitaxel plus gemcitabine as a first-line treatment in advanced non-small-cell lung cancer. Cancer Chemother Pharmacol. 2009;64(1):73–8.

154. Li C, Sun Y, Pan Y, Wang Q, Yang S, Chen H. Gemcitabine plus paclitaxel versus carboplatin plus either gemcitabine or paclitaxel in advanced non-small-cell lung cancer: a literature-based meta-analysis. Lung. 2010;188(5):359–64.

155. Azzoli CG, Giaccone G, Temin S. American Society of Clinical Oncology Clinical Practice Guideline Update on chemotherapy for Stage IV non-small-cell lung cancer. J Oncol Pract. 2010;6(1):39–43.

156. Davies AM, Lara PN, Lau DH, Gandara DR. Treatment of extensive small cell lung cancer. Hematol Oncol Clin North Am. 2004;18(2):373–85.

157. Socinski MA, Weissman C, Hart LL, Beck JT, Choksi JK, Hanson JP, Prager D, Monberg MJ, Ye Z, Obasaju CK. Randomized phase II trial of pemetrexed combined with either cisplatin or carboplatin in untreated extensive-stage small-cell lung cancer. J Clin Oncol. 2006;24(30):4840–7.

158. Chiappori AA, Rocha-Lima CM. New agents in the treatment of small-cell lung cancer: focus on gemcitabine. Clin Lung Cancer. 2003;4(Suppl 2):S56–63.

159. McDermott U, Settleman J. Personalized cancer therapy with selective kinase inhibitors: an emerging paradigm in medical oncology. J Clin Oncol. 2009;27(33):5650–9.

160. Besse B, Ropert S, Soria JC. Targeted therapies in lung cancer. Ann Oncol. 2007;18(Suppl 9):ix135–42.

161. Lynch TJ, Bell DW, Sordella R, Gurubhagavatula S, Okimoto RA, Brannigan BW, Harris PL, Haserlat SM, Supko JG, Haluska FG, et al. Activating mutations in the epidermal growth factor receptor underlying responsiveness of non-small-cell lung cancer to gefitinib. N Engl J Med. 2004;350(21):2129–39.

162. Paez JG, Janne PA, Lee JC, Tracy S, Greulich H, Gabriel S, Herman P, Kaye FJ, Lindeman N, Boggon TJ, et al. EGFR mutations in lung cancer: correlation with clinical response to gefitinib therapy. Science. 2004;304(5676):1497–500.

163. Pao W, Miller V, Zakowski M, Doherty J, Politi K, Sarkaria I, Singh B, Heelan R, Rusch V, Fulton L, et al. EGF receptor gene mutations are common in lung cancers from "never smokers" and are associated with sensitivity of tumors to gefitinib and erlotinib. Proc Natl Acad Sci U S A. 2004;101(36):13306–11.

164. Pao W, Miller VA, Kris MG. 'Targeting' the epidermal growth factor receptor tyrosine kinase with gefitinib (Iressa) in non-small cell lung cancer (NSCLC). Semin Cancer Biol. 2004;14(1):33–40.

165. Janne PA. Challenges of detecting EGFR T790M in gefitinib/erlotinib-resistant tumours. Lung Cancer. 2008;60(Suppl 2):S3–9.

166. Jin Y, Shao Y, Shi X, Lou G, Zhang Y, Wu X, Tong X, Yu X. Mutational profiling of non-small-cell lung cancer patients resistant to first-generation EGFR tyrosine kinase inhibitors using next generation sequencing. Oncotarget. 2016;7(38):61755–63.

167. Gerber DE, Minna JD. ALK inhibition for non-small cell lung cancer: from discovery to therapy in record time. Cancer Cell. 2010;18(6):548–51.

168. Gandini S, Massi D, Mandala M. PD-L1 expression in cancer patients receiving anti PD-1/PD-L1 antibodies: a systematic review and meta-analysis. Crit Rev Oncol/Hematol. 2016;100:88–98.

169. Rizvi NA, Hellmann MD, Snyder A, Kvistborg P, Makarov V, Havel JJ, Lee W, Yuan J, Wong P, Ho TS, et al. Cancer immunology. Mutational landscape determines sensitivity to PD-1 blockade in non-small cell lung cancer. Science. 2015;348(6230):124–8.

170. Le DT, Uram JN, Wang H, Bartlett BR, Kemberling H, Eyring AD, Skora AD, Luber BS, Azad NS, Laheru D, et al. PD-1 blockade in tumors with mismatch-repair deficiency. N Engl J Med. 2015;372(26):2509–20.

171. Grigg C, Rizvi NA. PD-L1 biomarker testing for non-small cell lung cancer: truth or fiction? J Immunother Cancer. 2016;4:48.

172. Subramanian J, Morgensztern D, Govindan R. Vascular endothelial growth factor receptor tyrosine kinase inhibitors in non-small-cell lung cancer. Clin Lung Cancer. 2010;11(5):311–9.

173. Kennedy B, Gargoum F, Bystricky B, Curran DR, O'Connor TM. Novel agents in the management of lung cancer. Curr Med Chem. 2010;17(35):4291–325.

174. Psallidas I, Karabela SP, Moschos C, Sherrill TP, Kollintza A, Magkouta S, Theodoropoulou P, Roussos C, Blackwell TS, Kalomenidis I, et al. Specific effects of bortezomib against experimental malignant pleural effusion: a preclinical study. Mol Cancer. 2010;9:56.

175. Russo A, Bronte G, Fulfaro F, Cicero G, Adamo V, Gebbia N, Rizzo S. Bortezomib: a new pro-apoptotic agent in cancer treatment. Curr Cancer Drug Targets. 2010;10(1):55–67.

176. Langer CJ, Besse B, Gualberto A, Brambilla E, Soria JC. The evolving role of histology in the management of advanced non-small-cell lung cancer. J Clin Oncol. 2010;28(36):5311–20.

177. Schrag D, Garewal HS, Burstein HJ, Samson DJ, Von Hoff DD, Somerfield MR. American Society of Clinical Oncology Technology Assessment: chemotherapy sensitivity and resistance assays. J Clin Oncol. 2004;22(17):3631–8.

178. Samson DJ, Seidenfeld J, Ziegler K, Aronson N. Chemotherapy sensitivity and resistance assays: a systematic review. J Clin Oncol. 2004;22(17):3618–30.

179. Roscilli G, De Vitis C, Ferrara FF, Noto A, Cherubini E, Ricci A, Mariotta S, Giarnieri E, Giovagnoli MR, Torrisi MR, et al. Human lung adenocarcinoma cell cultures derived from malignant pleural effusions as model system to predict patients chemosensitivity. J Transl Med. 2016;14:61.

180. Otvos R, Szulkin A, Hillerdal CO, Celep A, Yousef-Fadhel E, Skribek H, Hjerpe A, Szekely L, Dobra K. Drug sensitivity profiling and molecular characteristics of cells from pleural effusions of patients with lung adenocarcinoma. Genes Cancer. 2015;6(3-4):119–28.

181. Gulyas M, Kaposi AD, Elek G, Szollar LG, Hjerpe A. Value of carcinoembryonic antigen (CEA) and cholesterol assays of ascitic fluid in cases of inconclusive cytology. J Clin Pathol. 2001;54(11):831–5.

182. Radjenovic-Petkovic T, Pejcic T, Nastasijevic-Borovac D, Rancic M, Radojkovic D, Radojkovic M, Djordjevic I. Diagnostic value of CEA in pleural fluid for differential diagnosis of benign and malign pleural effusion. Med Arh. 2009;63(3):141–2.

183. Huang WW, Tsao SM, Lai CL, Su CC, Tseng CE. Diagnostic value of Her-2/neu, Cyfra 21-1, and carcinoembryonic antigen levels in malignant pleural effusions of lung adenocarcinoma. Pathology. 2010;42(3):224–8.

184. Toda K, Takahashi J, Tabuchi Y, Koizumi T, Nishimura R, Nishio W, Tsubota N, Matsuoka H. Clinical usefulness of CEA-mRNA determination in minor effusion. J Exp Clin Cancer Res. 2005;24(3):423–9.

185. Hung TL, Chen FF, Liu JM, Lai WW, Hsiao AL, Huang WT, Chen HH. Su WC: Clinical evaluation of HER-2/neu protein in malignant pleural effusion-associated lung adenocarcinoma and as a tumor marker in pleural effusion diagnosis. Clin Cancer Res. 2003;9(7):2605–12.

186. Szturmowicz M, Tomkowski W, Fijalkowska A, Kupis W, Cieslik A, Demkow U, Langfort R, Wiechecka A, Orlowski T, Torbicki A. Diagnostic utility of CYFRA 21-1 and CEA assays in pericardial fluid for the recognition of neoplastic pericarditis. Int J Biol Markers. 2005;20(1):43–9.

187. Li CS, Cheng BC, Ge W, Gao JF. Clinical value of CYFRA21-1, NSE, CA15-3, CA19-9 and CA125 assay in the elderly patients with pleural effusions. Int J Clin Pract. 2007;61(3):444–8.

188. Hackbarth JS, Murata K, Reilly WM, Algeciras-Schimnich A. Performance of CEA and CA19-9 in identifying pleural effusions caused by specific malignancies. Clin Biochem. 2010;43(13-14):1051–5.

189. Kuralay F, Tokgoz Z, Comlekci A. Diagnostic usefulness of tumour marker levels in pleural effusions of malignant and benign origin. Clin Chim Acta. 2000;300(1-2):43–55.

190. Bielsa S, Esquerda A, Salud A, Montes A, Arellano E, Rodriguez-Panadero F, Porcel JM. High levels of tumor markers in pleural fluid correlate with poor survival in patients with adenocarcinomatous or squamous malignant effusions. Eur J Intern Med. 2009;20(4):383–6.

191. Fiorelli A, Vicidomini G, Di Domenico M, Napolitano F, Messina G, Morgillo F, Ciardiello F, Santini M. Vascular endothelial growth factor in pleural fluid for differential diagnosis of benign and malignant origin and its clinical applications. Interact Cardiovasc Thorac Surg. 2011;12(3):420–4.

192. Eagles G, Warn A, Ball RY, Baillie-Johnson H, Arakaki N, Daikuhara Y, Warn RM. Hepatocyte growth factor/scatter factor is present in most pleural effusion fluids from cancer patients. Br J Cancer. 1996;73(3):377–81.

193. Richman SD, Hutchins GG, Seymour MT, Quirke P. What can the molecular pathologist offer for optimal decision making? Ann Oncol. 2010;21(Suppl 7):vii123–9.

194. Pao W, Chmielecki J. Rational, biologically based treatment of EGFR-mutant non-small-cell lung cancer. Nat Rev Cancer. 2010;10(11):760–74.

195. Zhang X, Zhao Y, Wang M, Yap WS, Chang AY. Detection and comparison of epidermal growth factor receptor mutations in cells and fluid of malignant pleural effusion in non-small cell lung cancer. Lung Cancer. 2008;60(2):175–82.

196. Pan Q, Pao W, Ladanyi M. Rapid polymerase chain reaction-based detection of epidermal growth factor receptor gene mutations in lung adenocarcinomas. J Mol Diagn. 2005;7(3):396–403.

197. Asano H, Toyooka S, Tokumo M, Ichimura K, Aoe K, Ito S, Tsukuda K, Ouchida M, Aoe M, Katayama H, et al. Detection of EGFR gene mutation in lung cancer by mutant-enriched polymerase chain reaction assay. Clin Cancer Res. 2006;12(1):43–8.

198. Molina-Vila MA, Bertran-Alamillo J, Reguart N, Taron M, Castella E, Llatjos M, Costa C, Mayo C, Pradas A, Queralt C, et al. A sensitive method for detecting EGFR mutations in non-small cell lung cancer samples with few tumor cells. J Thorac Oncol. 2008;3(11):1224–35.

199. Miller VA, Riely GJ, Zakowski MF, Li AR, Patel JD, Heelan RT, Kris MG, Sandler AB, Carbone DP, Tsao A, et al. Molecular characteristics of bronchioloalveolar carcinoma and adenocarcinoma, bronchioloalveolar carcinoma subtype, predict response to erlotinib. J Clin Oncol. 2008;26(9):1472–8.

200. Brevet M, Arcila M, Ladanyi M. Assessment of EGFR mutation status in lung adenocarcinoma by immunohistochemistry using antibodies specific to the two major forms of mutant EGFR. J Mol Diagn. 2010;12(2):169–76.

201. Garcia J, Riely GJ, Nafa K, Ladanyi M. KRAS mutational testing in the selection of patients for EGFR-targeted therapies. Semin Diagn Pathol. 2008;25(4):288–94.

202. Pao W, Miller VA, Politi KA, Riely GJ, Somwar R, Zakowski MF, Kris MG, Varmus H. Acquired resistance of lung adenocarcinomas to gefitinib or erlotinib is associated with a second mutation in the EGFR kinase domain. PLoS Med. 2005;2(3):e73.

203. Yun CH, Mengwasser KE, Toms AV, Woo MS, Greulich H, Wong KK, Meyerson M, Eck MJ. The T790M mutation in EGFR kinase causes drug resistance by increasing the affinity for ATP. Proc Natl Acad Sci U S A. 2008;105(6):2070–5.

204. Suda K, Onozato R, Yatabe Y, Mitsudomi T. EGFR T790M mutation: a double role in lung cancer cell survival? J Thorac Oncol. 2009;4(1):1–4.

205. Vakiani E, Solit DB. KRAS and BRAF: drug targets and predictive biomarkers. J Pathol. 2011;223(2):219–29.

206. Ceppi P, Monica V, Righi L, Papotti M, Scagliotti GV. Emerging role of thymidylate synthase for the pharmacogenomic selection of patients with thoracic cancer. Int J Clin Pharmacol Ther. 2010;48(7):481–2.

207. Bepler G, Sommers KE, Cantor A, Li X, Sharma A, Williams C, Chiappori A, Haura E, Antonia S, Tanvetyanon T, et al. Clinical efficacy and predictive molecular markers of neoadjuvant gemcitabine and pemetrexed in resectable non-small cell lung cancer. J Thorac Oncol. 2008;3(10):1112–8.

208. Kamoshida S, Suzuki M, Shimomura R, Sakurai Y, Komori Y, Uyama I, Tsutsumi Y. Immunostaining of thymidylate synthase and p53 for predicting chemoresistance to S-1/cisplatin in gastric cancer. Br J Cancer. 2007;96(2):277–83.

209. Wang X, Zhao J, Yang L, Mao L, An T, Bai H, Wang S, Liu X, Feng G, Wang J. Positive expression of ERCC1 predicts a poorer platinum-based treatment outcome in Chinese patients with advanced non-small-cell lung cancer. Med Oncol. 2010;27(2):484–90.

210. Ikeda S, Takabe K, Suzuki K. Expression of ERCC1 and class IIIbeta tubulin for predicting effect of carboplatin/paclitaxel in patients with advanced inoperable non-small cell lung cancer. Pathol Int. 2009;59(12):863–7.

211. Cobo M, Isla D, Massuti B, Montes A, Sanchez JM, Provencio M, Vinolas N, Paz-Ares L, Lopez-Vivanco G, Munoz MA, et al. Customizing cisplatin based on quantitative excision repair cross-complementing 1 mRNA expression: a phase III trial in non-small-cell lung cancer. J Clin Oncol. 2007;25(19):2747–54.

212. Azuma K, Sasada T, Kawahara A, Hattori S, Kinoshita T, Takamori S, Ichiki M, Imamura Y, Ikeda J, Kage M, et al. Expression of ERCC1 and class III beta-tubulin in non-small cell lung cancer patients treated with a combination of cisplatin/docetaxel and concurrent thoracic irradiation. Cancer Chemother Pharmacol. 2009;64(3):565–73.

213. Seve P, Mackey J, Isaac S, Tredan O, Souquet PJ, Perol M, Lai R, Voloch A, Dumontet C. Class III beta-tubulin expression in tumor cells predicts response and outcome in patients with non-small cell lung cancer receiving paclitaxel. Mol Cancer Ther. 2005;4(12):2001–7.

214. Seve P, Isaac S, Tredan O, Souquet PJ, Pacheco Y, Perol M, Lafanechere L, Penet A, Peiller EL, Dumontet C. Expression of class III {beta}-tubulin is predictive of patient outcome in patients with non-small cell lung cancer receiving vinorelbine-based chemotherapy. Clin Cancer Res. 2005;11(15):5481–6.

215. Dumontet C, Isaac S, Souquet PJ, Bejui-Thivolet F, Pacheco Y, Peloux N, Frankfurter A, Luduena R, Perol M. Expression of class III beta tubulin in non-small cell lung cancer is correlated with resistance to taxane chemotherapy. Bull Cancer. 2005;92(2):E25–30.

216. Seruga B, Hertz PC, Le LW, Tannock IF. Global drug development in cancer: a cross-sectional study of clinical trial registries. Ann Oncol. 2010;21(4):895–900.

217. Subramanian J, Madadi AR, Dandona M, Williams K, Morgensztern D, Govindan R. Review of ongoing clinical trials in non-small cell lung cancer: a status report for 2009 from the ClinicalTrials.gov website. J Thorac Oncol. 2010;5(8):1116–9.

218. Bedrossian CW. Diagnostic problems in serous effusions. Diagn Cytopathol. 1998;19(2):131–7.

219. Lynch TJ Jr. Management of malignant pleural effusions. Chest. 1993;103(4 Suppl):385S–9S.

220. van den Toorn LM, Schaap E, Surmont VF, Pouw EM, van der Rijt KC, van Klaveren RJ. Management of recurrent malignant pleural

effusions with a chronic indwelling pleural catheter. Lung Cancer. 2005;50(1):123–7.

221. Antunes G, Neville E, Duffy J, Ali N. BTS guidelines for the management of malignant pleural effusions. Thorax. 2003;58(Suppl 2):ii29–38.

222. Grossi F, Pennucci MC, Tixi L, Cafferata MA, Ardizzoni A. Management of malignant pleural effusions. Drugs. 1998;55(1):47–58.

223. Mascaux C, Iannino N, Martin B, Paesmans M, Berghmans T, Dusart M, Haller A, Lothaire P, Meert AP, Noel S, et al. The role of RAS oncogene in survival of patients with lung cancer: a systematic review of the literature with meta-analysis. Br J Cancer. 2005;92(1):131–9.

224. Kosaka T, Yatabe Y, Onozato R, Kuwano H, Mitsudomi T. Prognostic implication of EGFR, KRAS, and TP53 gene mutations in a large cohort of Japanese patients with surgically treated lung adenocarcinoma. J Thorac Oncol. 2009;4(1):22–9.

225. Subramanian J, Simon R. Gene expression-based prognostic signatures in lung cancer: ready for clinical use? J Natl Cancer Inst. 2010;102(7):464–74.

226. Shah L, Walter KL, Borczuk AC, Kawut SM, Sonett JR, Gorenstein LA, Ginsburg ME, Steinglass KM, Powell CA. Expression of syndecan-1 and expression of epidermal growth factor receptor are associated with survival in patients with nonsmall cell lung carcinoma. Cancer. 2004;101(7):1632–8.

227. Lan CC, Wu YK, Lee CH, Huang YC, Huang CY, Tsai YH, Huang SF, Tsao TC. Increased survivin mRNA in malignant pleural effusion is significantly correlated with survival. Jpn J Clin Oncol. 2010;40(3):234–40.

228. Wu YK, Chen KT, Kuo YB, Huang YS, Chan EC. Quantitative detection of survivin in malignant pleural effusion for the diagnosis and prognosis of lung cancer. Cancer Lett. 2009;273(2): 331–5.

229. Hsu IL, Su WC, Yan JJ, Chang JM, Lai WW. Angiogenetic biomarkers in non-small cell lung cancer with malignant pleural effusion: correlations with patient survival and pleural effusion control. Lung Cancer. 2009;65(3):371–6.

230. Bielsa S, Salud A, Martinez M, Esquerda A, Martin A, Rodriguez-Panadero F, Porcel JM. Prognostic significance of pleural fluid data in patients with malignant effusion. Eur J Intern Med. 2008;19(5):334–9.

231. Zendehrokh N, Franzen L, Dejmek A. Weak telomerase activity in malignant cells in metastatic serous effusions correlation to short survival time. Acta Cytol. 2007;51(3):412–6.

# Ovarian Cancer

9

Ben Davidson

## Introduction

The epidemiology, clinical presentation, and treatment of ovarian carcinoma (OC), as well as the morphology and differential diagnosis of this cancer, are discussed in Chap. 3. In the years that passed since the publication of the first edition of this book, a large body of literature has been published regarding the genomic landscape of OC, particularly high-grade serous carcinoma (HGSC), many applying next-generation sequencing (NGS). The most comprehensive genomic analysis of OC was the Cancer Genome Atlas (TCGA) analysis of HGSC [1]. Much focus has additionally been directed at determining the origin of the various histotypes of OC, with the fallopian tube currently recognized to be the origin of the majority of HGSC. While these studies are beyond the scope of this chapter, those that have included effusion specimens will be discussed below. Tumors originating from the ovary, the fallopian tube, or the peritoneum are collectively referred to as OC for the sake of simplicity.

The presence of metastatic disease dramatically worsens the outcome of patients with cancer, including those with OC [2]. The main anatomic site involved by OC metastasis is the abdominal cavity [3]. In view of the central role of metastasis within the serosal cavities in OC progression, especially in serous carcinoma, it is not surprising that the scientific literature focusing on OC effusions is far more extensive than that related to any other cancer form. Two additional issues that have received growing attention in recent years are the involvement of tumor cells in effusions and of the ascites fluid itself in chemoresistance (reviewed in [4, 5]) and the feasibility of culturing cells from ascites for assessment of standard and experimental therapeutics (see below).

B. Davidson, M.D., Ph.D.
Department of Pathology, The Norwegian Radium Hospital, Oslo University Hospital, Oslo, Norway

Faculty of Medicine, Institute of Clinical Medicine, University of Oslo, Oslo, Norway
e-mail: bend@medisin.uio.no; bdd@ous-hf.no

Papers dealing with the biology of OC in effusions may generally be divided into three categories:
1. Studies of clinical specimens
2. Studies in which ascites supernatants have been applied to tumor cells (OC or other) in vitro
3. Animal models in which the OC model of intraperitoneal dissemination has been reproduced in vivo

Naturally, these three research approaches are closely linked, and some studies have accordingly utilized more than one of them. Nevertheless, as this book has cytopathologists as its primary target audience, the focus of this chapter will be on scientific work related to clinical specimens. Research performed on effusion specimens will be discussed separately for different aspects of tumor biology and the tumor-host interaction, including adhesion, invasion and metastasis, growth factors, proliferation and apoptosis, interaction with the immune response, intracellular signaling and transcription, spheroid- and cancer stem cell (CSC)-related studies, and analyses of various molecules that cannot be classified into one of the above groups. Discussion of studies using high-throughput methodology, including NGS, and ex vivo culturing will constitute the final part of this chapter.

## Adhesion, Invasion, and Metastasis

The processes of invasion and metastasis involve extensive changes in the expression of adhesion molecules, proteases, and angiogenic molecules, as well as in intracellular signaling networks and transcription factors regulating the expression of these molecules, in cancer cells compared to their normal counterparts. Adhesion or other surface molecules that have been shown to be expressed in OC include cadherins, integrins, immunoglobulin superfamily members, proteoglycans, and mucins, whereas the main proteases that mediate invasion and metastasis in this tumor, as well as in many others, are the matrix metalloproteinase (MMP) family and the urinary-type plasminogen activator (uPA) pathway. This section will focus on these molecules.

© Springer International Publishing AG, part of Springer Nature 2018
B. Davidson et al. (eds.), *Serous Effusions*, https://doi.org/10.1007/978-3-319-76478-8_9

## Cadherins and Their Regulators

Cadherins, a family of Ca²⁺-dependent integral membrane glycoproteins, are located at the cell-cell adherens junctions, where they mediate homophilic contact with neighboring cells [6]. Cadherins are connected via their carboxy-terminal intracytoplasmic domain to p120 catenin, β-catenin, and γ-catenin, which in turn bind α-catenin, forming a link to actin in the cytoskeleton [7]. Cadherins have a central role in differentiation and tissue organization during embryogenesis and participate in maintaining tissue structure in the mature organism. E-cadherin, the major epithelial cadherin, inhibits invasion and is regarded as a tumor suppressor molecule [8]. Its loss through inactivation or downregulation occurs through genetic (mutations) and epigenetic (CpG promoter hypermethylation, transcriptional regulation, and posttranslational modification) mechanisms and has been shown to be associated with tumor progression in various tumors [9–11]. Loss of E-cadherin may be accompanied by expression of pro-invasive mesenchymal markers, including N-cadherin, vimentin, and collagens, a process termed epithelial-to-mesenchymal transition (EMT), occurring in cancer cells as a pathological version of a process normally occurring during embryogenesis [12]. Epigenetic silencing of the E-cadherin promoter by transcription factors is a central mechanism in EMT, and the main negative transcriptional regulators of E-cadherin in human cancer are Snail and Slug, members of the Snail superfamily, as well as Twist, Zeb, and Smad-interacting protein 1 (SIP1), members of the crystallin enhancer binding factor 1 family [13, 14].

Mutations in the *CDH1* gene, encoding E-cadherin, are rare in OC, and those in the *CTNNB1* gene, encoding β-catenin, are largely limited to endometrioid carcinomas [15, 16]. However, the E-cadherin complex is differentially expressed along tumor progression in OC, suggesting epigenetic regulation, with EMT regulators having a central role in the biology of this cancer (reviewed in [17]).

E-cadherin protein was found to be overexpressed in OC effusions compared to patient-matched primary carcinomas [18], and E-cadherin was subsequently reported to be co-expressed with the EMT-associated N-cadherin, as well as with P-cadherin, in OC cells in effusions [19] (Fig. 9.1a–c).

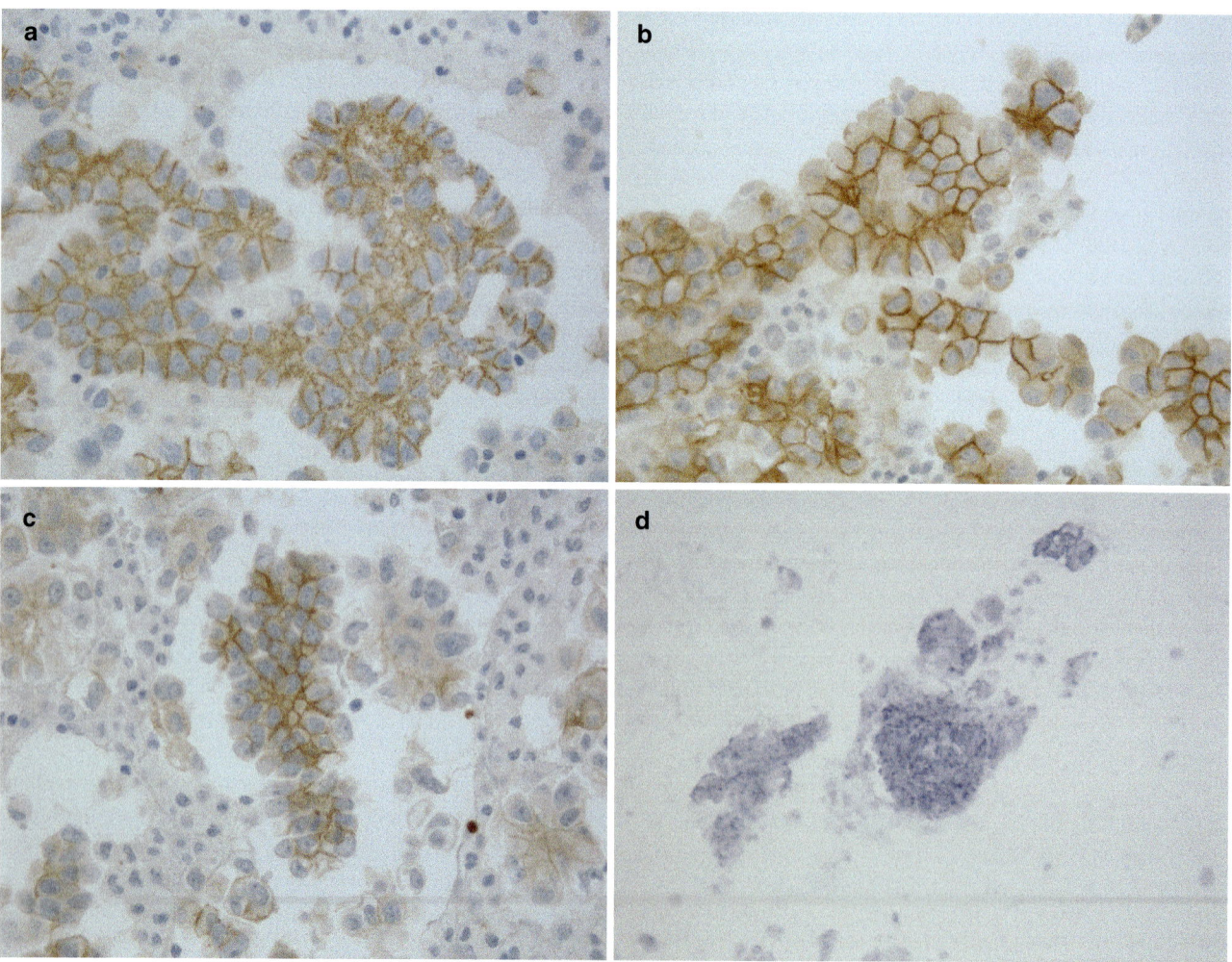

**Fig. 9.1** Cadherins and their transcriptional regulators in ovarian carcinoma. (**a–c**) Immunostaining for E-cadherin (**a**), N-cadherin (**b**), and P-cadherin (**c**); (**d**) mRNA in situ hybridization for *Snail* (NBT-BCIP as chromogen)

Lower E-cadherin mRNA levels in OC effusions were associated with shorter progression-free survival (PFS) [20]. However, a more recent analysis of 100 HGSC effusions by immunohistochemistry (IHC) did not show a prognostic role for E-cadherin, N-cadherin, or P-cadherin protein expression [21]. Conversely, proteomics analysis of 51 OC effusions identified the 4-protein signature of E-cadherin, N-cadherin, AKT, and phospho-paxillin (p-paxillin) as marker of significantly improved PFS [22].

Snail, Slug, and SIP1 mRNA was expressed in the majority of OC effusions (Fig. 9.1d), and higher SIP1/E-cadherin mRNA ratio was associated with poor overall survival (OS) [20]. However, Snail and Slug protein expression is significantly lower in effusions compared to primary tumors, suggesting a mechanism for the E-cadherin upregulation in effusions [23]. In addition, Snail protein localizes to the cytoplasm rather than the nucleus in uncultured OC cells from effusions, suggesting that it is not functional in these cells [23]. Recently, the mRNA levels of three additional EMT markers, Twist1, Zeb1, and Vimentin, were found to be significantly higher in solid OC metastases compared to primary carcinomas and effusions [24]. Vimentin and Zeb1 protein expression by IHC was significantly related to poor chemotherapy response at diagnosis in the abovementioned study of 100 OC effusions [21]. These data suggest that OC does not fully follow the classical model of EMT and that OC cells in effusions probably undergo at least partially the reverse process of mesenchymal-to-epithelial transition (MET).

## Integrins

Integrins are a family of heterodimeric glycoproteins composed of α- and β-subunits that are involved in invasion, metastasis, angiogenesis, proliferation, and apoptosis. At least 18α and 8β subunits forming 24 heterodimers have been identified to date. Intracellular signaling via integrin receptors is initiated in response to cues originating from other cells (e.g., stromal myofibroblasts) or different extracellular matrix (ECM) proteins, including laminin, fibronectin, collagen, vitronectin, entactin, tenascin, and fibrinogen, and mediates synthesis of many cancer-associated molecules. Altered expression of integrins (down- or upregulation) has been detected in the majority of malignant tumors but varies considerably according to the origin of the neoplasm [25–27]. In vitro studies have demonstrated that integrins are crucial for the interaction of OC cells with ECM molecules and that attachment to the peritoneal mesothelium involves the β1 integrin subunit and CD44, an adhesion molecule of the immunoglobulin superfamily [28–30].

Decreased expression of the α6 and β4 integrin subunits was found in 6 ascites specimens compared to 24 patient-matched solid primary and metastatic lesions, whereas expression of the α2, α3 and β1 integrin subunits was compa-

rable [31]. In another study, protein expression of the α2, α3, α5, α6, αv, and β1 integrin subunits was found in nine tissue and ascites specimens [32]. Comparative analysis of 121 OC effusions and 30 solid primary and metastatic tumors showed frequent expression of the αv integrin subunit at all anatomic sites but higher expression of the β1 subunit in effusions compared to solid lesions (Fig. 9.2a, b). Tumor cell synthesis of the two subunits was shown using mRNA in situ hybridization (ISH) [33]. Expression of the two integrin subunits in effusions showed no relationship with survival. However, analysis of solid OC specimens from two groups of patients with long-term and short-term survival and follow-up of up to 20 years demonstrated correlation between αv integrin subunit mRNA expression by ISH and poor survival [34].

Laminin levels are increased in effusions from patients with serous OC compared to normal peritoneal fluid [35]. In an additional study, expression of laminin receptors, including the 67-kD non-integrin laminin receptor (67-kD LR) and the α6 integrin subunit, was analyzed in 88 OC effusions and 116 corresponding solid tumors. The α6 subunit mRNA expression was higher in effusions compared to corresponding solid tumors, and its protein product was localized to carcinoma cells in 17/27 effusions using flow cytometry (FCM; Fig. 9.2c) [36]. The 67-kDa receptor was frequently expressed in both effusions and solid lesions at both the mRNA and protein level. Of note, application of ascites to OC cell lines in vitro results in upregulation of α6 integrin, without affecting the levels of the αv, β1, and β4 subunits [37].

The expression of several of the ECM ligands of integrins has been investigated in effusion specimens. Type IV collagen expression was shown to be significantly reduced in OC effusions compared to primary carcinomas [38]. In contrast, the levels of procollagen types I and III have been shown to be markedly increased in OC effusions compared to normal peritoneal fluid and benign cysts using immunoassay [39, 40]. In the study by Cracchiolo et al., higher levels of procollagen type III were associated with poor disease-free interval and OS, being a stronger prognosticator than residual disease volume [39].

Kohn et al. identified the ECM protein fibronectin in malignant ascites, predominantly from OC patients, as a promigratory factor for melanoma cells in vitro [41]. Fibronectin was additionally shown to be immunosuppressive, based on its ability to inhibit proliferation of lectin-stimulated lymphocytes [42]. In another study, both fibronectin and oncofetal fibronectin, a protein involved in trophoblast adhesion and expressed in different cancers, were detected at higher levels in OC ascites specimens compared to benign effusions [43].

The dynamic expression of ECM receptors in OC and the presence of ECM proteins in OC effusions in a tumor-specific manner suggest that these molecular interactions are central in the biology of this cancer within the serosal cavities.

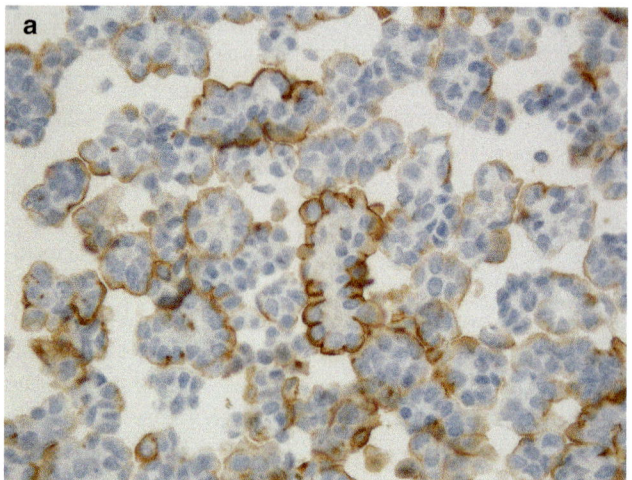

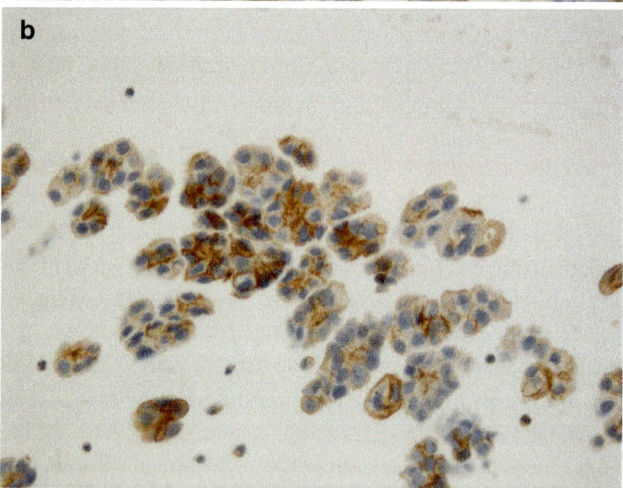

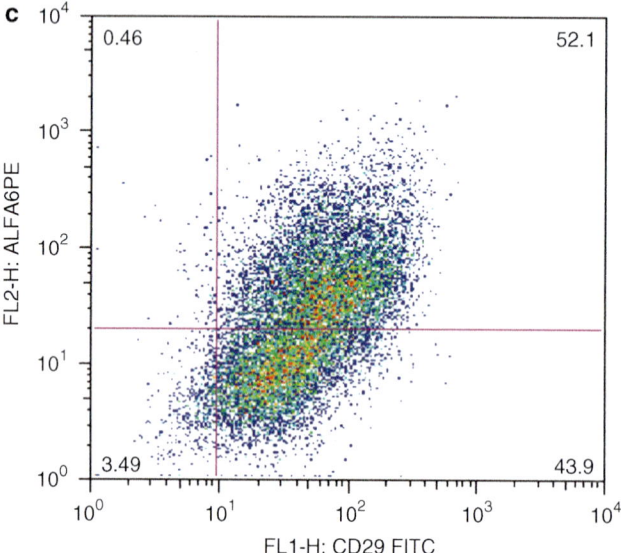

**Fig. 9.2** Integrins. (**a**, **b**) Immunostaining for the αv (**a**) and β1 (**b**) subunits. (**c**) Flow cytometry analysis for the α6 and β1 subunits showing co-expression in 52% of tumor cells

## Claudins

Claudins are a family of tight junction-specific integral membrane proteins, currently including 24 members. Tight junctions are located in the apical aspect of epithelial or endothelial cells, where they maintain cell polarity and regulate the paracellular transport of solutes and the diffusion of proteins and lipids. Claudins form homo- or heterodimeric contacts between neighboring cells. Claudin-3 and claudin-4 contain a binding site for *Clostridium perfringens* enterotoxin. Claudin expression is deregulated in multiple cancer types, making them potential targets for targeted therapy [44].

Claudin-7 was found to be expressed in OC cells in ascites and was absent from leukocytes and reactive mesothelial cells [45]. A similar cancer-specific expression pattern was shown for claudin-4 in two studies [46, 47]. Comparative gene expression array analysis of OC and diffuse malignant peritoneal mesothelioma (DMPM) effusions showed significantly higher expression of the genes coding for claudin-3, claudin-4, and claudin-6 in OC/PPC compared to DMPM, a finding that was validated for claudin-3 and claudin-4 using quantitative RT-PCR (qRT-PCR) and IHC [48]. A subsequent analysis of the diagnostic role of claudin-1, claudin-3, and claudin-7 in 325 effusions showed higher expression of claudins in OC compared to adenocarcinomas of other origin, malignant mesotheliomas (MM) and benign reactive mesothelial cells (RMC) [49]. Analysis of the anatomic site-related expression and prognostic role of claudins in OC included effusions (*n* = 218), primary OC (*n* = 81), and solid metastases (*n* = 164) immunostained for claudin-1, claudin-3, claudin-4, and caludin-7 [50]. All four claudins were expressed in the majority of tumors at all anatomic sites (Fig. 9.3a–d). However, the percentage of immunostained cells was significantly higher in effusions compared to primary carcinomas and solid metastases for claudin-1, claudin-3, and claudin-7. Higher claudin-3 and caludin-7 expression in effusions was associated with shorter survival in univariate and multivariate analysis.

These studies demonstrate that claudins are widely expressed in OC, with significant overexpression of some family members in effusions. Claudin expression in OC effusions has both diagnostic and prognostic value, and their cancer-specific expression suggests that they may be a therapeutic target in this disease.

## CD44

The immunoglobulin superfamily member CD44, the principal receptor for hyaluronic acid, has received much atten-

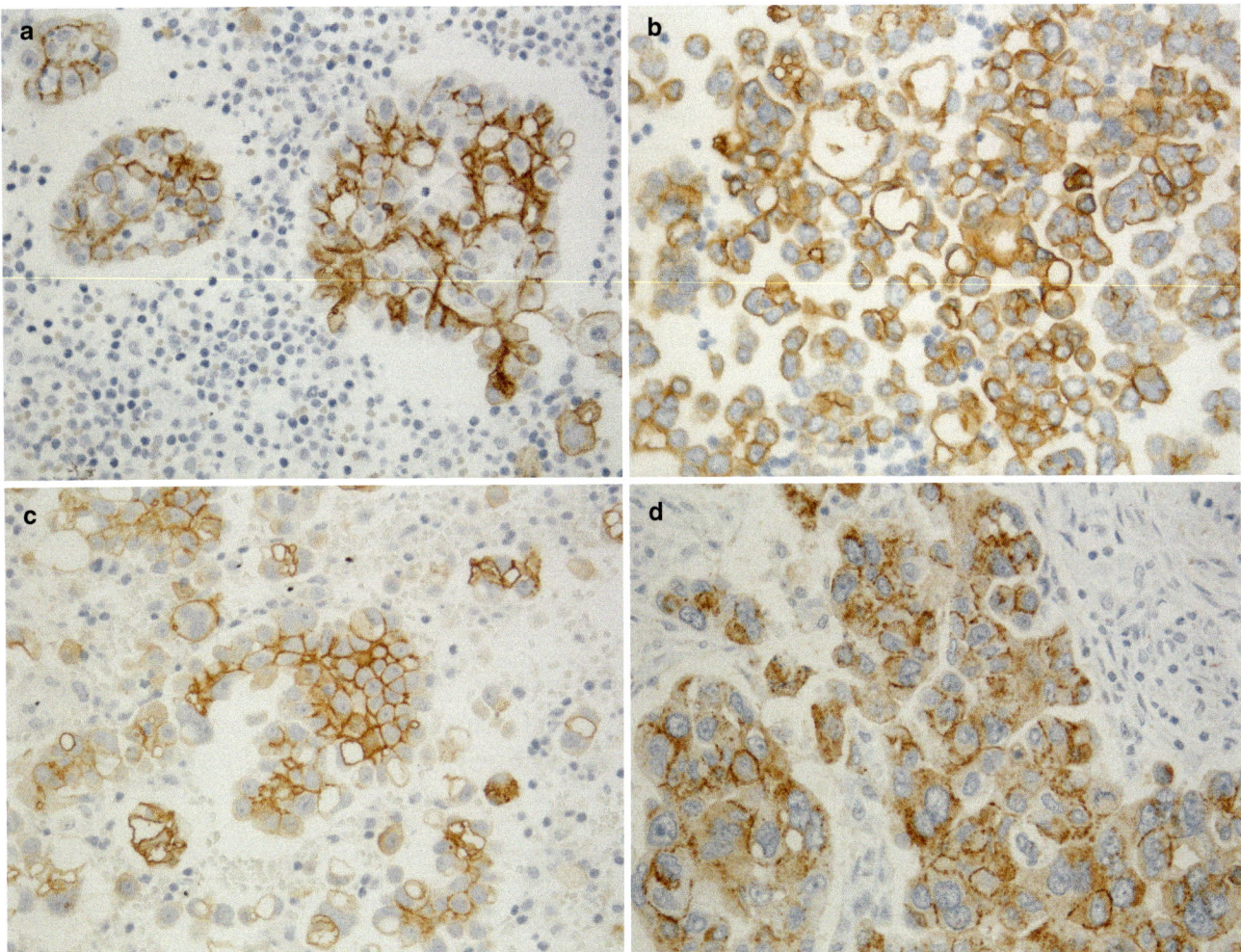

**Fig. 9.3** Claudins. (**a–c**) Immunostaining in effusions, showing expression of claudin-1 (**a**), claudin-4 (**b**), and claudin-7 (**c**). (**d**) Claudin-3 expression in primary ovarian carcinoma

tion as both molecular partner of integrins and as an ECM receptor by itself. It additionally interacts with osteopontin and MMPs. CD44 is a transmembrane glycoprotein which is widely expressed in hematopoietic and mesodermal cells. The CD44 gene is composed of 20 exons, of which ten are constitutively expressed in almost all cell types, coding for a heavily glycosylated ~85-kDa molecule called the standard form (CD44s). The remaining exons can be alternatively spliced in various combinations, producing different CD44 isoforms. CD44 is involved in lymphocyte homing, hematopoiesis, differentiation, inflammation, wound healing, embryonic development, and apoptosis, as well as in tumor cell invasion and metastasis [51–53]. In recent years, CD44 has been receiving attention for its potential role as a cancer stem cell marker, including in OC [53, 54].

CD44 was shown to be involved in attachment of OC cells to mesothelial cells in vitro, and analysis of 16 solid OC lesions and 8 effusions showed reduced CD44 expression in tumor cells in effusions, postulated to facilitate the release of tumor cells into the peritoneal cavity [55]. It was shown to be upregulated in OC cells exposed to ascites from patients with ovarian tumors in vitro [56, 57].

Analysis of 59 malignant and benign effusions, of which the former were predominantly from OC patients, nevertheless showed more frequent CD44s expression in reactive mesothelial cells (RMC), with the opposite finding with respect to CD44v3-10 [58]. Furthermore, CD44s was more highly expressed in OC cells in effusions compared to solid primary and metastatic tumors [59]. Expression of both CD44s and CD44v3-10 was unrelated to survival [59]. Bar and co-workers found comparable CD44v6 expression in

OC cells in effusions and solid tumors, as well as in benign tumors [38], whereas soluble CD44v6 was reported to differentiate between benign and malignant effusions, the latter including 8 OC [60]. In agreement with the latter report, Taylor et al. found high levels of the v4/5 and v6 CD44 isoforms in analysis of ascites and sera from OC patients [61].

## MUC4

Mucins are a family of glycoproteins that constitute part of the mucous layer protecting epithelial cells lining the respiratory, genitourinary, and digestive tract from physical, chemical, and microbial damage. Mucins are coded by 20 genes (*MUC1-20*) and are divided into secreted gel-forming, soluble, and transmembrane mucins. They are heavily glycosylated, with a carbohydrate moiety that may contribute 50–90% of their molecular weight. Expression of mucins is altered in a large number of cancers compared to their normal tissue counterparts. Furthermore, mucins are thought to mediate a variety of tumor-promoting effects, including loss of adhesion, prevention of apoptosis, metastasis, and prosurvival signal transduction [62–64].

MUC4 is a transmembrane mucin involved in receptor tyrosine kinase (RTK)-related signal transduction, metastasis, and suppression of apoptosis based on in vitro studies. In clinical material, MUC4 is expressed in carcinomas of different origin and has been shown to have a prognostic role in lung, pancreatic, and bile duct carcinoma [63, 65]. It is considered to be a candidate therapeutic target in pancreatic carcinoma [66].

Validation analysis in our array paper showed MUC4 expression using IHC in 117/122 (96%) OC specimens, the majority of which were solid tumors, compared to 1/30 (3%) DMPM [48]. In a subsequent study, MUC4 expression was found in 141/142 (99%) OC effusions (Fig. 9.4), while RMC were uniformly negative [67]. These data suggest that MUC4 is a good marker for differentiating OC from benign or malignant mesothelial cells.

## EMMPRIN

EMMPRIN (extracellular matrix metalloproteinase inducer, CD147), member of the immunoglobulin superfamily, is a membrane glycoprotein that mediates signaling events leading to MMP synthesis. EMMPRIN has multiple partner proteins, including key signaling membrane proteins such as caveolin-1 and integrins, as well as protein chaperones of the cyclophilin family [68]. EMMPRIN has been shown to be involved in tissue repair and in lymphocyte migration and activation, as well as in several pathological processes, including ischemic disease, Alzheimer's disease, and cancer [68]. A recent meta-analysis showed association between EMMPRIN and chemoresistance and poor outcome in different cancers [69].

EMMPRIN mRNA and protein are widely expressed on OC cells in effusions and solid tumors, and its presence is associated with MMP and integrin subunit expression and with activation of the mitogen-activated protein kinase (MAPK) signaling pathway [70, 71] (Fig. 9.5). However, whereas EMMPRIN expression on peritumoral stromal and endothelial cells in solid OC correlated with poor survival, no such relationship was demonstrated for tumor cell expression in effusions [70]. Parenthetically, caveolin-1, the major constituent of caveolae, flask-shaped invaginations of cell membranes that are involved in molecule transport, adhesion, and signal transduction, is frequently expressed in OC effusions, although its expression is unrelated to clinicopathologic parameters [72].

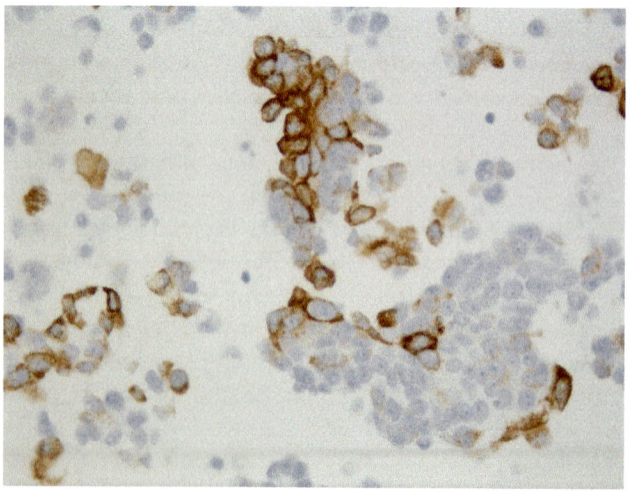

**Fig. 9.4** MUC4 immunostaining in effusion

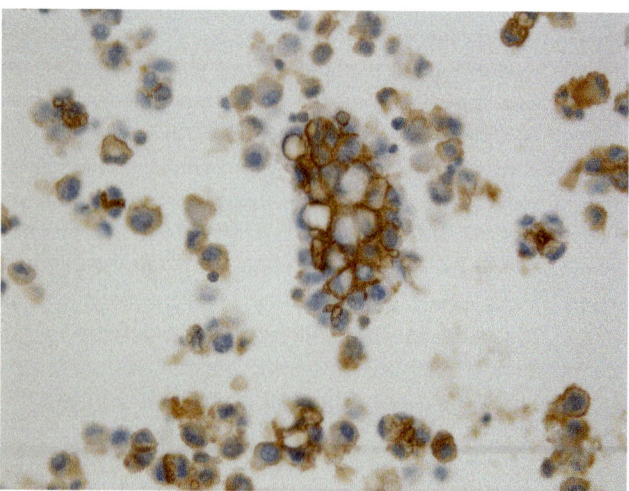

**Fig. 9.5** EMMPRIN immunostaining in effusion

## Nerve Growth Factor (NGF) Receptors

Neurotrophins are a family of growth factors, consisting in mammals of nerve growth factor (NGF), brain-derived neurotrophic factor (BDNF), NT-3, and NT-4/5. Neurotrophins bind in a specific manner to the tyrosine kinase receptors TrkA, TrkB, and TrkC, leading to receptor autophosphorylation and activation of intracellular signaling via ras, MAPK, phosphoinositol-3-kinase (PI3K)/AKT, and phospholipase-γ (PLC-γ), with resulting survival and proliferation. p75, an additional neutrophin receptor, belongs to the tumor necrosis receptor (TNF) superfamily, has a different structure, lacks intrinsic catalytic activity, and is able to bind all neurotrophins. p75 is able to activate both pro-survival and pro-apoptotic signaling pathways [73, 74]. Trk family members have been shown to be expressed in a variety of neural and non-neural tumors, the latter consisting primarily of carcinomas [75]. In contrast, p75 was shown to be expressed in some neural and soft tissue tumors, with little expression in carcinomas [76].

Fusions in *NTRK1*, *NTRK2*, and *NTRK3*, encoding TrkA, TrkB, and TrkC, respectively, have been found in different cancers, including carcinomas, sarcomas, brain tumors, and hematological cancers, suggesting that targeting these receptors may have clinical benefit [77, 78].

Total Trk and p-TrkA expression was shown to be higher in primary OC and solid metastases compared to effusions, while the opposite was true for p75. NGF was frequently expressed in OC cells [79, 80] (Fig. 9.6a–d). In solid lesions, p-TrkA was additionally expressed in endothelial cells, supporting its postulated role as an angiogenic factor, and its expression in tumor cells was associated with poor survival [80]. High expression of TrkB and BDNF was recently reported in OC, with particularly high levels in omental metastases and in OC cells in ascites [81].

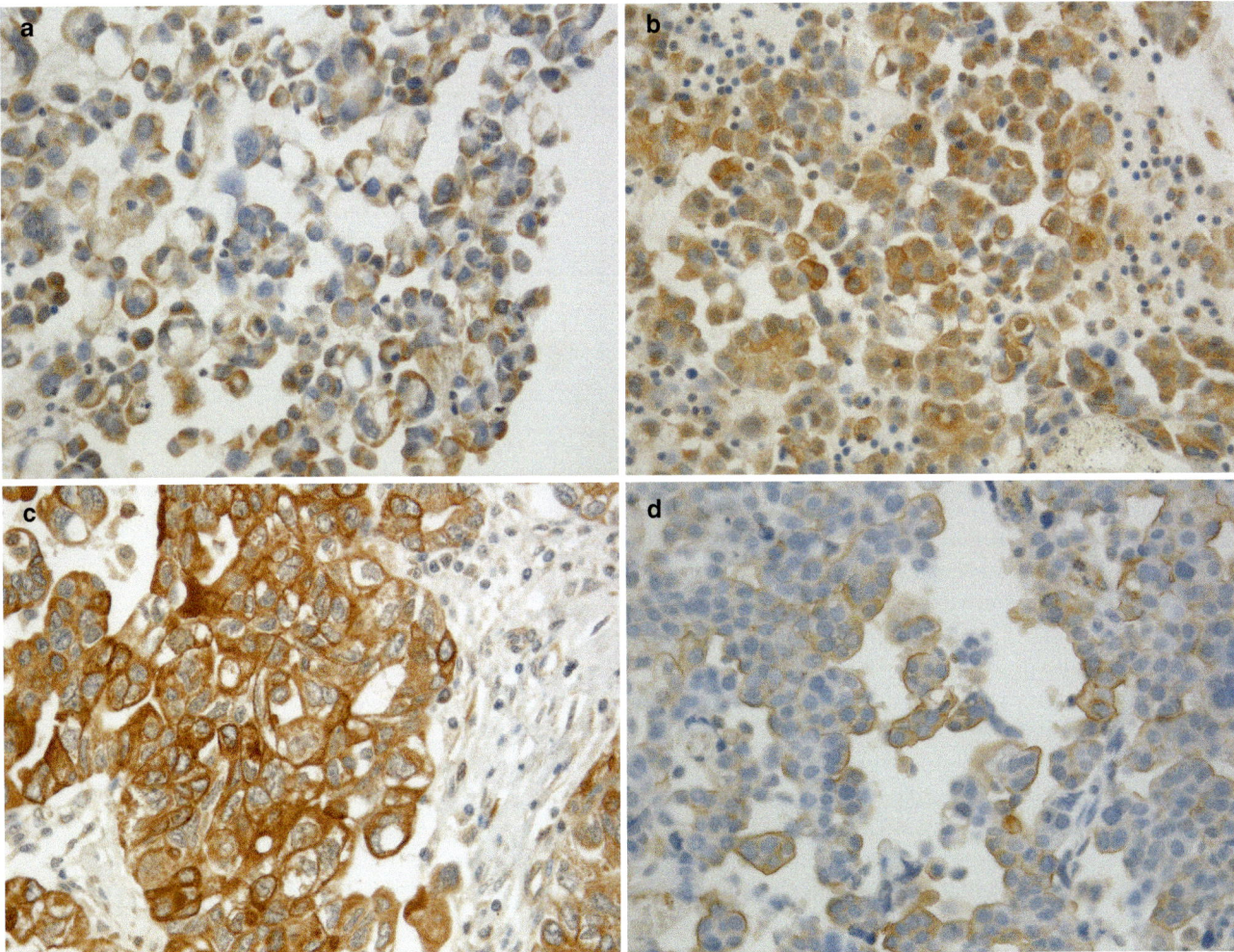

**Fig. 9.6** Nerve growth factor (NGF) and its receptor TrkA. (**a**, **b**) Effusions. NGF and total (pan-)TrkA immunostaining. (**c**, **d**) Primary carcinoma. Pan-TrkA and phospho-(p-)TrkA immunostaining in **c**, **d**, respectively

These data support a role for the neurotrophin autocrine pathway in OC tumor progression and suggest that Trk receptors may be an attractive target for molecular therapy in this cancer.

## Proteases

The ability to invade adjacent tissues and metastasize to distant organs is one of the central characteristics of cancer cells. The two main families involved in this process in OC are the MMP family and the uPA pathway, and members of both families have been shown to be expressed in OC effusions.

### MMP

MMPs are zinc- and calcium-dependent enzymes that degrade a large variety of basement membrane and ECM components. Twenty-three MMPs have been identified in humans, with no functional redundancy among them. MMP-2 (gelatinase A, 72-kD type IV collagenase) and MMP-9 (gelatinase B, 92-kD type IV collagenase), the only enzymes with a gelatin-binding domain, are crucial for tumor metastasis due to their ability to degrade collagen type IV, a component of all basement membranes. Additional MMP substrates include other MMP members, proteinases of different families (e.g., plasminogen), growth factors (transforming growth factor, TGF), tyrosine kinase receptors (Her2/neu, FGFR1), adhesion molecules (CD44, E-cadherin, αv integrin), and other molecules. MMP activity is negatively regulated in a reversible manner by specific inhibitors, TIMP1-4, through the formation of a 1:1 stoichiometric binding, as well as by α2 macroglobulins, thrombospondins, and the membrane-bound RECK protein. However, TIMP-2 also participates in cell surface-mediated activation of MMP-2 with membrane type I MMP (MT1-MMP, MMP-14). MMP synthesis is positively regulated by different ECM proteins, growth factors, and cytokines (e.g., via integrins) and is regulated at the transcriptional level by Ets family members, AP-1 and AP-2, and additional factors [82, 83].

MMPs have been shown to have an important role in normal tissue homeostasis, as well as in a range of pathological conditions, including cancer. Their role in invasion, metastasis, and angiogenesis is now supplemented by data documenting their participation in other processes, such as regulation of cytokines and chemokines, intracellular signaling, and transcriptional regulation. Although attempts to target MMPs therapeutically have been disappointing to date, efforts in this direction are still being made [84, 85].

Both MMP-2 and MMP-9 were identified in ascites fluid from advanced-stage OC patients using zymography [86], and both enzymes were secreted by OC cells of different anatomic locations, including ascites, in short-term cultures [87], although MMP-2 was the main gelatinolytic MMP secreted and activated [88]. MMP-2, MMP-9, and TIMP-2 were identi-

fied in malignant effusions, predominantly from OC patients, by Kohn et al. [41]. In an additional study, MMP-2 and MMP-9 activity was shown to be higher in malignant ascites, including that of 6 OC, compared to ascites from patients with cirrhosis or tuberculosis using zymography [89].

MMP-1, MMP-2, MMP-9, and TIMP-2 were shown to be expressed in OC effusions and solid lesions at the mRNA and/or protein levels by ISH and IHC, respectively (Fig. 9.7a). Comparative analysis of OC at different anatomic sites showed significantly higher expression of MMP-2 and lower expression of TIMP-2 in effusions compared to primary tumors [90]. In contrast to data for solid lesions, MMP and TIMP expression in effusions did not correlate with survival, suggesting that the clinical role of these molecules may be limited to the former specimens. In another study, MT1-MMP, which activates MMP-2 at the cell surface, was detected in OC effusions and solid lesions using ISH (Fig. 9.7b). MT1-MMP and MT2-MMP mRNA was detected in OC effusions using RT-PCR, with no expression of MT3-MMP [91].

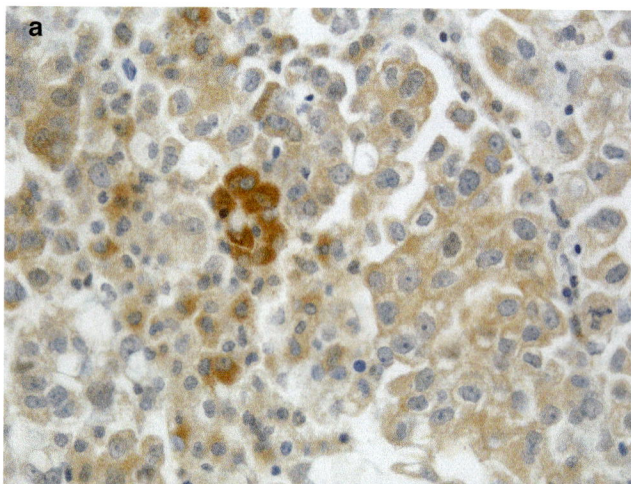

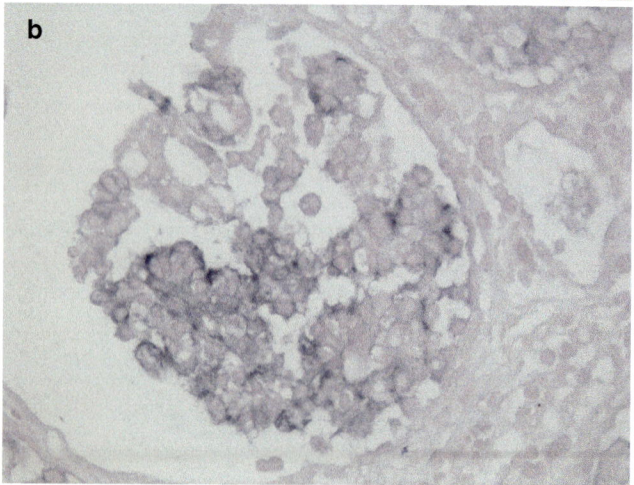

**Fig. 9.7** Matrix metalloproteinases (MMP) in effusions. (**a**) Immunostaining for MMP-1; (**b**) mRNA in situ hybridization for *MMP14* (NBT-BCIP as chromogen)

## uPA

The urokinase-type plasminogen activator (uPA) is a serine protease that is synthesized as a latent proenzyme. uPA activation is achieved by the formation of a two-chain enzyme and is mediated by several proteases, including plasmin, trypsin, cathepsins B and L, and kallikreins. uPA and its homologue tissue-type PA (tPA) cleave plasminogen to plasmin, thereby activating the degradation of fibrin and other ECM proteins and the activation of several MMPs, including MMP-9, and growth factors that are known to play a role in OC, such as basic fibroblast growth factor (bFGF), insulin growth factor (IGF), and TGFβ. This system is negatively regulated by the plasminogen activator inhibitors PAI-1 and PAI-2 and the plasmin inhibitor α2 antiplasmin. The uPA receptor uPAR is a glycosylphosphatidylinositol (GPI)-anchored protein that is additionally able to bind the ECM protein vitronectin and interacts with different integrins (primarily with the α3β1 and α5β1 fibronectin receptors), G-coupled proteins, and caveolin. This leads to the activation of major intracellular signaling via the MAPK and PI3K pathways. uPAR is cleaved to yield a soluble form (suPAR). The uPA system is involved in various cancer-related processes, including proliferation, adhesion, invasion, migration, and regulation of apoptosis, making it an attractive cancer therapy target [92–94].

Fishman et al. found only low uPA production in primary cultures of OC cells, but ascites-derived cells had higher uPA levels compared to those from primary carcinomas and solid metastases [87]. High uPA levels were found in 15/19 OC ascites specimens using zymography [95]. uPA lacking the GPI anchor was isolated from OC ascites [96], and a subsequent study showed that both uPAR and the D2D3 fragment of suPAR are present at this anatomic site [97]. The application of ascites to OC cell lines in vitro was shown to mediate expression of uPA and uPAR and increase invasiveness [37]. Higher PAI-2 levels in ascites were associated with poor disease-free survival for patients with stage III disease, a finding that was hypothesized to be related to the presence of macrophage colony-stimulating factor-1 (CSF-1) in these cases [98]. Higher ascites CSF-1 levels were associated with longer OS in analysis of 44 cases [99]. A urinary trypsin inhibitor that inhibits trypsin and plasmin activities was identified in the ascites fluid in analysis of 22 specimens [100].

## Kallikreins

Human tissue kallikreins are a family of serine proteases, currently consisting of 15 different members, all encoded by a single gene cluster located at chromosome region 19q13.4. Their biological roles include regulation of blood pressure, seminal fluid liquefaction, skin desquamation, and synaptic neuronal plasticity. Kallikreins have been shown to be deregulated in several cancers [101].

The levels of several KLK members, including KLK5–8, 10, 11, 13, and 14, were shown to be significantly higher in OC effusion supernatants compared to benign effusions, and KLK6, 7, 8, and 10 additionally distinguished OC from other cancers by ELISA [102]. In agreement with this report, KLK6–8 were overexpressed in OC/PPC compared to DMPM at the gene level using gene arrays [48]. KLK4 was detected in the majority of OC specimens, including both effusions and solid lesions [103]. KLK7 was recently shown to be more highly expressed in OC effusions compared to patient-matched primary tumors in a limited series of six cases [104].

These data document that multiple protease classes and protease inhibitors are present in OC effusions. Some of these undoubtedly have their origin in the serum, while the majority is locally produced. Proteases may be important for our understanding of OC metastasis, as diagnostic markers, and potentially as therapeutic targets, although the latter is clearly limited by their ubiquitous distribution and central role in processes beneficial for the host, such as wound healing.

## Lysyl oxidase (LOX)

The LOX family consists of 5 copper-binding secreted enzymes, LOX and LOX-like (LOXL)1–4. LOX is required in the synthesis of elastin and collagen. Expression of LOX family members has been reported in multiple cancers [105].

Analysis of the expression of LOXL2, LOXL3, and LOXL4 in solid specimens and effusions from patients with OC, breast carcinoma, and MM using RT-PCR detected 2 new alternative splice variants of LOXL4. The spliced segments were exon 9 (splice variant 1) or both exons 8 and 9 (splice variant 2). In OC, splice variant 1 was significantly elevated in effusions compared to solid lesions, whereas splice variant 2 appeared only in effusions. LOXL2 and LOXL3 expression was comparable in solid specimens and effusions [106]. A follow-up study using a mouse model showed that the LOXL4 splice variants promote metastasis and tumor progression in ES2 OC cells [107].

## Growth Factors

Cancer cells in effusions are dependent on growth factors for proliferation and survival, possibly even more than their counterparts in solid lesions, as they have no direct access to the vasculature, and the microenvironment of effusions is rich in such proteins [108]. Growth factor signaling occurs predominantly, though not uniquely, via tyrosine kinase receptors that are often overexpressed on tumor cells. Current data regarding growth factors in OC effusions are discussed in this section. Angiogenic molecules are additionally discussed, as many of them are growth factors. Cytokines are discussed in the section dealing with the immune response, as many of these proteins have their origin in leukocytes and/or affect their function.

## The Insulin-Like Growth Factor (IGF) System

The IGF system consists of the peptide hormones insulin, IGF-I, and IGF-II; the cell surface receptors insulin receptor (IR), IGF-1R, and IGF-2R and hybrid IGF-1R/IR receptors, of which all except IGF-2R possess tyrosine kinase activity; and a family of circulating IGF-binding proteins (IGFBP). Activation of IGF receptors leads to phosphorylation of adaptor proteins of the IRS family or SHC, with subsequent activation of the MAPK family member ERK and the PI3K signaling pathway, resulting in cell proliferation and survival, differentiation, metabolism, and EMT, the latter affecting adhesion, migration, invasion, and metastasis [109].

The six IGFBP members are present in the serum extracellularly, and in the circulation positively or negatively regulate the biological activity of IGF-I and IGF-II. They additionally interact with the ECM proteins fibronectin, collagen I, osteopontin, and vitronectin and with cellular proteins, including integrins and caveolin. IGF is released by proteolysis of IGFBP which is mediated by multiple proteases, including plasmin, thrombin, and members of the MMP family, or by the binding of IGFBP to the ECM [110, 111].

The IGF system is under investigation for its possible role as a target for molecular therapy in cancer, though results to date have not been encouraging [109].

The *IGFBP3* and *IGF-II* genes were overexpressed in OC compared to DMPM effusions by gene expression arrays [48] and were subsequently shown to be more highly expressed at the protein level in carcinomas of various origins, including OC, compared to MM (Fig. 9.8a, b). IGFBP3 was found in the effusion supernatant of all OC, as well as in breast carcinomas and 16 mesotheliomas using ELISA. High IGFBP3 expression in pre-chemotherapy and high IGF-II expression in post-chemotherapy OC effusions correlated with poor OS, and IGF-II expression in post-chemotherapy effusions was an independent prognostic factor in Cox multivariate analysis [112].

## Angiogenic Factors

The ability of solid tumors to grow locally, and subsequently disseminate to distant organs, is dependent upon the formation of new blood vessels (angiogenesis), the presence of which increases nutrient supply and facilitates vascular invasion by tumor cells. This process involves a large number of angiogenic factors, including vascular endothelial growth factor (VEGF), bFGF and acidic FGF (aFGF), TGFα and

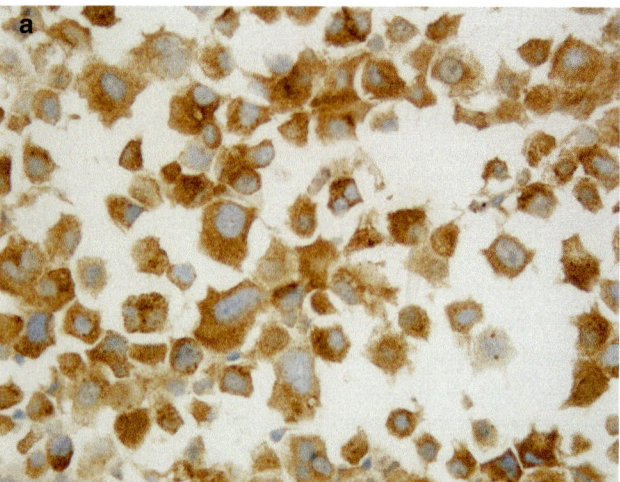
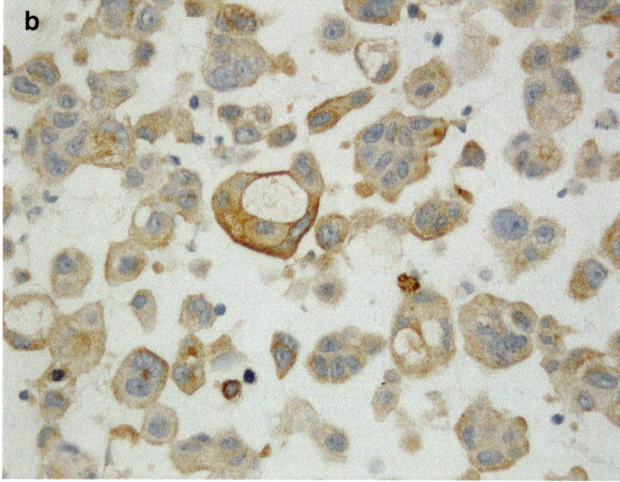

**Fig. 9.8** The insulin growth factor pathway. (**a**, **b**) IGFBP3 and IGF-2 immunostaining in effusions

TGFβ, platelet-derived growth factor (PDGF), interleukin-8 (IL-8), and heparanase [113, 114].

The VEGF family currently consists of seven members, VEGF-A to VEGF-F and placental growth factor (PlGF), that mediate their effects through the tyrosine kinase receptors VEGFR1-3. VEGF-A has 6 isoforms consisting of 121–206 amino acid residues, as a result of alternative splicing. It induces proliferation, sprouting, migration, and tube formation in endothelial cells and is a key molecule in tumor angiogenesis [115]. As discussed in Chap. 3, VEGF (previously also termed vascular permeability factor) increases vessel permeability, thereby contributing to the accumulation of effusions. Bevacizumab (Avastin), a monoclonal antibody against VEGF, is now included in the treatment of patients with advanced-stage OC in combination with standard chemotherapy in Europe [116].

bFGF (FGF-2), a 146-amino-acid polypeptide, is part of a family that at present consists of 22 members in vertebrates, the majority of which are secreted. FGF signaling involves various receptors, including FGFR, which are RTK, integrins, and heparan sulfate proteoglycans, and induces, in addition to angiogenesis, inflammation, tumor growth, and chemoresistance. *FGFR* genes are amplified in many cancers. FGF signaling is under assessment for potential relevance in the context of targeted therapy [117, 118].

IL-8 (CXCL8) is a member of the chemokine family, small molecules that regulate the immune response and mediate several cancer-related events, including angiogenesis. IL-8 also promotes survival of tumor stem cells and attracts myeloid cells mediating suppression of the immune response. It is primarily produced by tumor cells and its serum levels therefore are a good indicator of tumor burden [119].

Different VEGF isoforms were detected in OC ascites and shown to be produced by tumor cells [120]. OC cells in ascites and OC cell lines were shown to express VEGF and its receptors KDR and flt at the mRNA level, supporting the presence of an autocrine VEGF pathway in this tumor [121]. Barton et al. analyzed 36 ascites specimens from patients with advanced-stage OC for angiogenin, VEGF, and bFGF levels using ELISA. Wide variation was seen across samples, and angiogenic marker expression was not interrelated in a given specimen, although VEGF and bFGF levels in the whole group were higher than in the patient-matched serum samples. No association was seen between serum or ascites levels of the measured factors and tumor vascularity [122]. VEGF levels were reported to effectively differentiate between benign and malignant effusions, including 8 OC, in the study by Dong and co-workers [60], and were found to be high in an additional analysis of 6 OC effusions [123]. These results are in agreement with an additional report, in which VEGF levels in malignant effusions, including 35 OC, were higher than matched serum levels and were higher than ascites levels in specimens from patients with liver cirrhosis [124]. OC cells in primary OC and OC cell lines were shown to express FGFR 2-IIIb and its ligands FGF-1 and FGF-7, and the latter two proteins were found in ascites fluid from OC patients [125].

OC cells in peritoneal and pleural effusions expressed *IL-8*, *VEGF*, and *bFGF* mRNA, evidence that these cells produce angiogenic factors, as well as their protein products (Fig. 9.9a, b). However, OC cells in effusions had significantly lower *VEGF* mRNA expression compared to primary OC and solid metastases, as well as lower *IL-8* mRNA expression compared to solid metastases. Angiogenic gene expression in effusions was unrelated to clinicopathologic parameters or patient survival [126].

Heparanase is an endoglycosidase that degrades heparan sulfate, component of proteoglycans on the membranes of eukaryotic cells (syndecans and glypicans) or in the ECM (perlecans). Heparan sulfate chains bind a large variety of molecules, such as ECM structural proteins, growth factors, chemokines, and enzymes, thereby affecting adhesion, proliferation, survival, and differentiation. This diversity of interactions is reflected in the role of heparan sulfate interactions in embryogenesis, inflammation, tissue repair, angiogenesis, and tumorigenesis. Heparanase mediates angiogenesis through the release of HS-bound angiogenic factors, including VEGF and bFGF, from the ECM and basement membrane and the release of HS degradation fragments that stimulate the binding of bFGF to its receptor [127, 128]. Recently described roles for heparanase include regulation of exosome biogenesis and function and increase of chemoresistance via enhanced autophagy [128]. Exosomes are discussed below.

Heparanase was expressed in the majority of OC effusions (Fig. 9.9c) and was found in effusion supernatants. Its expression at the tumor cell membrane was associated with significantly shorter OS for patients with post-chemotherapy disease recurrence effusions [129].

## Other Growth Factors

GEP (progranulin/PC cell-derived growth factor) is a 68-kDa secreted protein with multiple glycosylated variants, the most common of which is 88kDa in size. GEP is also cleaved into granulins (epithelins), small proteins of 6kDa in size that have inhibitory function, opposing that of GEP. GEP has a role in physiological processes, such as embryogenesis and wound repair, as well as in tumorigenesis [130]. GEP synthesis is regulated by endothelin-1 (ET-1) and lysophosphatidic acid (LPA), two additional growth factors for OC cells, and by cyclic AMP (cAMP) in vitro [131].

GEP was shown to be frequently expressed in OC at all anatomic sites (Fig. 9.9d). However, staining was higher in primary carcinomas and solid metastases compared to effusions. Its expression in OC cells was unrelated to survival, although expression in the peritumoral stroma correlated with worse overall survival [132].

The TGFβ family regulates tissue homeostasis, proliferation, differentiation, apoptosis, adhesion, motility, migration, and invasion and consequently has an important role in cancer progression. The effects of TGFβ are mediated by the ligand isoforms TGFβ1, TGFβ2, and TGFβ3 through TGFβ type I and II receptors, which have serine/threonine kinase activity. TGFβRI propagates signaling by recruitment and phosphorylation of Smad2 and Smad3, which then translocate to the nucleus and modulate gene expression. This pathway is often referred to as the canonical signaling pathway. Noncanonical TGFβ involves the mitogen-activated protein kinase (MAPK) pathway, the phosphoinositol-3-kinase (PI3K)/AKT signaling pathway, and Rho-like GTPases, regulating many processes, including EMT and apoptosis [133–136].

The levels of TGFα, member of the EGF family, were found to be lower in OC ascites compared to controls [137].

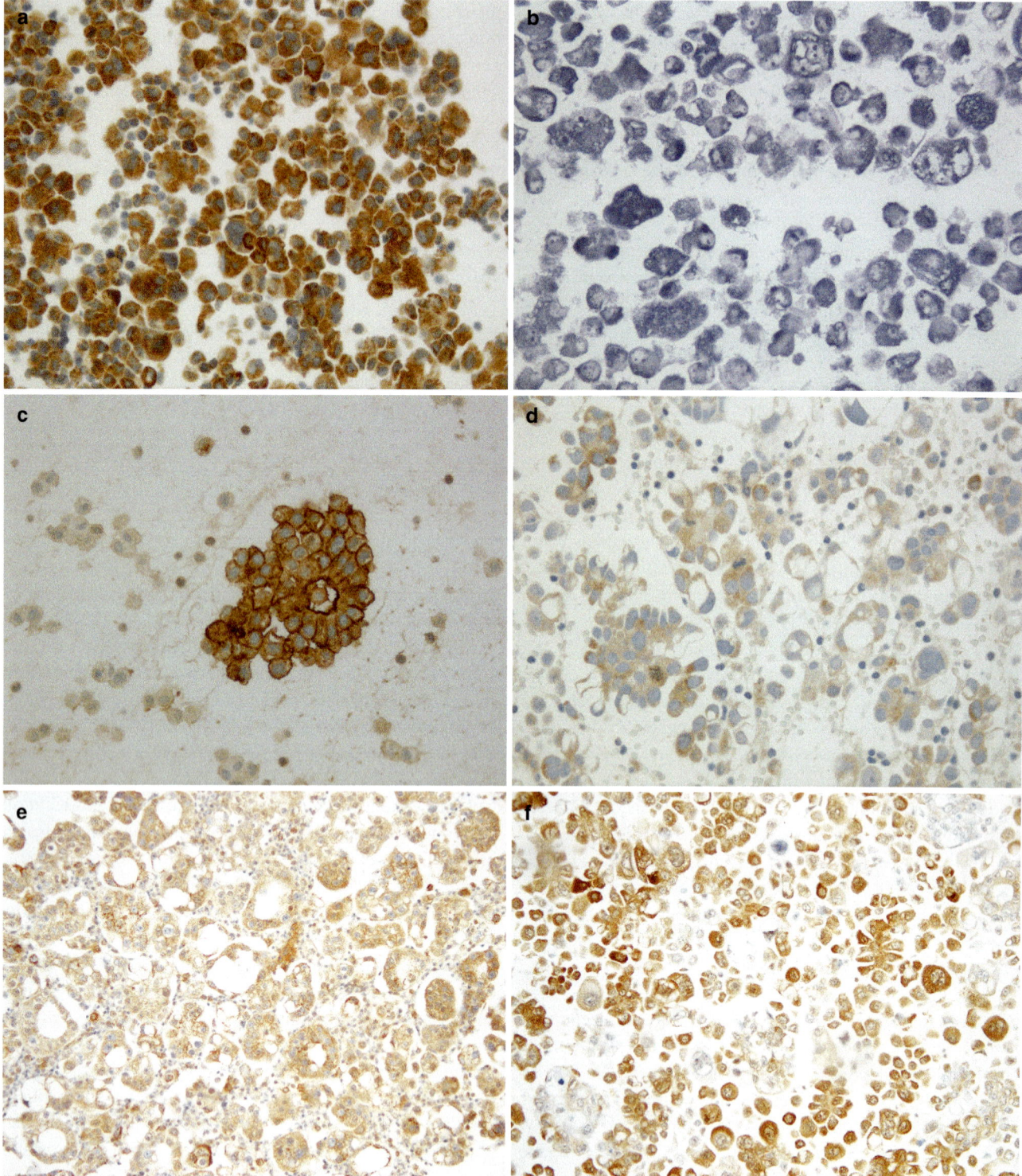

**Fig. 9.9** Growth factor expression in effusions. (**a**) VEGF protein, (**b**) *FGF2* in situ hybridization (NBT-BCIP as chromogen), (**c**) heparanase protein, (**d**) Granulin-Epithelin Precursor (GEP) protein, (**e**) TGFβ3, (**f**) p-Smad2, (**g**) p-Smad3

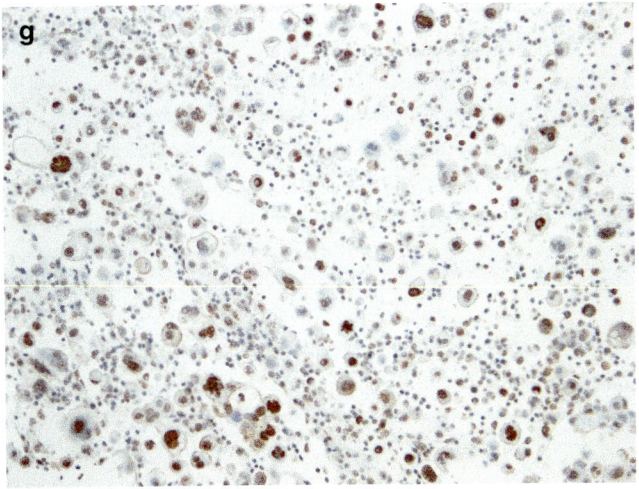

**Fig. 9.9** (continued)

In a recent study, *TGFβRI* and *TGFβRII* mRNA by qPCR was overexpressed in HGSC effusions and solid metastases compared to the ovarian tumors, whereas Smad2, p-Smad2, and p-Smad3 were overexpressed in solid specimens compared to effusions. In univariate survival analysis, higher *TGFβ2* variant 1 and *TGFβRIII* mRNA levels were associated with a trend for shorter OS in patients with post-chemotherapy effusions, and the latter finding was an independent prognostic marker in Cox multivariate analysis. Smad3 protein expression was associated with a trend for shorter OS in univariate survival analysis (Fig. 9.9e–g) [138].

In another study, the concentration of soluble growth differentiation factor-15 (GDF-15), member of the TGFβ family, was measured in 195 effusion supernatants from 162 OC patients by an immunoradiometric assay. Tumor cell GDF-15 expression by IHC was analyzed in 114 effusions. GDF-15 was detected in all effusion supernatants, with overexpression in post-chemotherapy effusions, and IHC showed expression in OC cells in 111/114 (97%) specimens. High GDF-15 effusion concentration was associated with poor response to chemotherapy at first disease recurrence and poor OS in univariate and Cox multivariate analysis. High tumor cell GDF-15 expression in pre-chemotherapy specimens was associated with poor PFS [139].

Endoglin (CD105) is a transmembrane glycoprotein composed of two 95-kDa subunits that form a homodimeric 180-kDa protein and is an auxiliary receptor for several TGFβ family proteins. There are two splice isoforms of the protein, termed short (S)-endoglin and long (L)-endoglin based on differences in its cytoplasmic part. In addition, a soluble form of the protein (sEng) is probably formed by proteolytic shedding. Endoglin is primarily expressed on endothelial cells but has been detected in mesenchymal and hematopoietic cells, as well as in different cancers. TGFβ binding results in activin-like kinase (ALK) recruitment and signaling propagation to the nucleus via Smad proteins that act as transcription repressors or activators. Mutations in endoglin or ALK-1 are the molecular cause for hereditary hemorrhagic telangiectasia (Osler-Weber-Rendu disease), a condition that is characterized by vascular malformations and severe bleeding episodes [140, 141]. Its involvement in multiple pathologic conditions related to altered angiogenesis led to its identification as a potential therapeutic target of a range of diseases, including cancer [142].

Endoglin expression by IHC was found in OC cells and RMC in 95/211 (45%) and 133/211 (63%) effusions, respectively. Tumor cell expression was significantly associated with younger patient age and post-chemotherapy status. No association was found between cellular endoglin expression and its soluble effusion concentration by ELISA, measured in 95 patient-matched effusions. Endoglin expression was significantly higher in solid metastases compared to effusions in analysis of 34 patient-matched specimens. Endoglin expression was unrelated to survival [143].

The two PDGF isoforms A and B were found in ascites from OC patients, and their levels were higher than those measured in nonmalignant effusions [144]. Finally, the presence of anti-angiogenic factors was observed in malignant effusions, including specimens from OC patients, in vitro using the chick chorioallantoic membrane model [145]. These factors were subsequently shown to be fibrin degradation products, as detailed above [100].

## Proliferation and Apoptosis

The ability to divide without limit and resistance to cell death are two major characteristics of tumor biology that greatly limit our ability to cure cancer once tumor cells have spread beyond the organ of origin. OC cells in effusions have high degree of proliferation, which may exceed that of the primary tumor, and little apoptosis (Fig. 9.10a, b) [146]. As in other areas, data regarding expression of molecules related to proliferation and apoptosis in effusions are limited, although some information has been gathered, as detailed below.

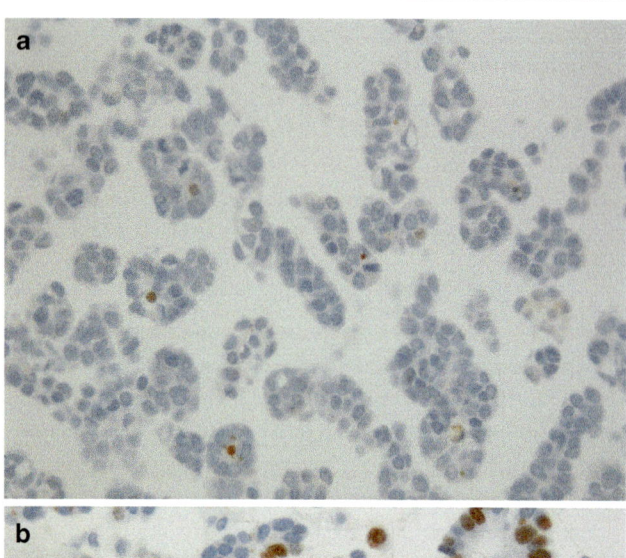

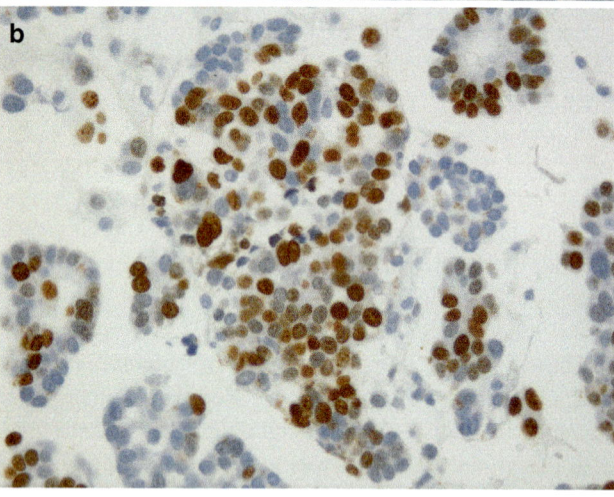

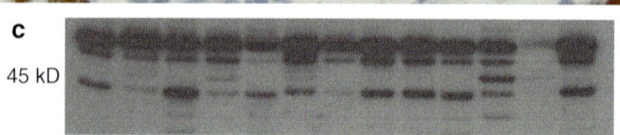

45 kD

**Fig. 9.10** Proliferation and apoptosis in effusions. (**a**) p85 PARP fragment immunostaining. Nuclear expression is limited to a few cells, denoting low degree of apoptosis; (**b**) Ki-67 immunostaining, showing high proliferation; (**c**) Western blotting for cyclin E in ovarian carcinoma effusions, showing the presence of low molecular weight fragments in the majority of effusions

## Cell Cycle Markers

The exit of cells from the quiescent state and progression along the cell cycle is regulated at several checkpoints—the G0→G1, G1→S, and G2→M transition. These events are mediated by members of the cyclin and cyclin-dependent kinase (Cdk) families. Cyclins, the regulatory unit, bind Cdk, the catalytic component, in a specific manner. These complexes exert a regulatory role by phosphorylation of key proteins, such as the retinoblastoma gene product (pRB), which together with p53 is a major regulator of the cell cycle. Cdk-cyclin complexes are negatively regulated by p15[INK4b], p16[INK4a], p21[WAF1/CIP1], and p27[kip1] [147–149].

Deletion of the area encompassing the *CDKN2A* and *CDKN2B* genes, encoding for p16[INK4a] and p15 [INK4b], respectively, at chromosome 9p21 was found in OC ascites [150]. Higher p16[INK4a] protein expression in OC cells in ascites was related to better response to first-line chemotherapy and longer survival in analysis of 37 effusions [151]. p27[kip1] protein expression was frequently observed in OC cells in effusions using IHC and Western blotting (WB). Staining was higher in pre- compared to post-chemotherapy, but was unrelated to clinicopathologic parameters or survival [152]. p21[WAF1/CIP1] was only infrequently and focally expressed in another study using the same methods [80].

Cyclin A is expressed from late G1 phase to mitosis. It forms a complex with Cdk2, resulting in kinase activity detected in S phase, which is crucial for the entry into mitosis. Cyclin A is frequently detected in OC cells in effusions and is significantly expressed with the proliferation marker Ki-67. However, its expression is associated with longer OS [152].

The cyclin E-Cdk2 complex mediates the G1→S transition through phosphorylation and thereby inactivates pRb by releasing the E2F transcription factor. The *CCNE1* gene encoding for cyclin E is overexpressed in OC/PPC compared to DMPM [48]. The presence of low molecular weight (LMW) cyclin E forms, reported to have higher biological activity than the full cyclin E molecule, by WB similarly differentiated OC from MM and RMC and was associated with shorter OS and PFS (Fig. 9.10c) [153]. Measurement of cyclin E DNA fragments by quantitative real-time PCR effectively differentiated between benign ($n = 70$) and malignant ($n = 198$) effusions, the latter including 88 OC [154].

Discordance in the *TP53* mutation status between primary OC and patient-matched ascites was reported in two studies [155, 156]. The presence of p53 autoantibodies in OC ascites was reported in 18 and 19% of specimens in two independent studies [157, 158]. Their presence coincided with absent p53 expression in one of these reports [157], suggesting that their presence may interfere with p53 detection. However, in a third study, in which sera, cyst fluid, and/or ascites specimens were analyzed, p53 autoantibodies were infrequently found in both p53-overexpressing and p53-non-overexpressing cases [159]. In the study by Abendstein et al., the presence of p53 autoantibodies was a marker of poor OS and PFS, with the finding for PFS shown to be independent in multivariate analysis [158].

## The Death Receptor Family

Death receptors (DRs) are members of the TNFR superfamily that are able to induce the extrinsic apoptosis signaling pathway upon ligand binding. In addition to exhibiting the cysteine-rich extracellular domain typical of the TNFR family, DRs are characterized by a conserved cytoplasmic domain of approximately 80 amino acids, the death domain (DD), which is essential for transduction of the apoptotic signal. The best characterized DR members, Fas (CD95/Apo-1), TNFR1, TRAILR1 (DR4), and TRAILR2 (DR5), have as respective ligands FasL (CD95L/Apo-1L), TNF, and TRAIL, the latter binding both DR4 and DR5. Three other receptors, TRAILR3 (DcR1), TRAILR4 (DcR2), and the soluble receptor osteoprotegerin, lack functional cytoplasmic domains and do not transmit the apoptotic signal following binding to TRAIL [160, 161]. DR activation as a modality for cancer treatment has been extensively investigated in recent years, with generally disappointing results [162]. This may be related to absence of these receptors on tumor cells, but, not less significantly, to the fact that Fas, DR4, and DR5 mediate non-apoptotic effects as well, including promoting cell survival and proliferation, inducing inflammation, and mediating tumorigenesis and tumor progression [163, 164].

Malignant ascites from OC patients was shown to protect OC cells in vitro from TRAIL-induced apoptosis through Akt activation in an αvβ5 integrin-dependent process [165]. The $IC_{50}$ of TRAIL increased in vitro in the presence of clinical ascites specimens, and higher $IC_{50}$ was associated with shorter disease-free survival for 35 OC patients from whom the ascites specimens were tapped [166].

In agreement with these data, OC ascites was recently shown to inhibit FasL-mediated apoptosis. Ascites specimens contained the decoy receptor DcR3, and higher levels of this protein by ELISA were associated with stage IV disease and platinum resistance [167].

As opposed to normal ovarian surface epithelial cells, OC cells obtained from ascites did not express FasL on their surface, but secreted the full FasL protein, as well as a heavily glycosylated variant of this protein. Both secreted forms mediated apoptosis in vitro, from which the authors hypothesized a role for this protein in the killing of immune cells by tumor cells and thereby evasion of the immune response [168].

High Fas expression was previously found in OC ascites compared to primary and recurrent solid specimens [169]. Quantitative analysis of DR4, DR5, Fas, TNFR1, and TNFR2 status in OC effusions using FCM showed frequent DR4, DR5, and Fas expression on tumor cells in the majority of effusions, with less frequent expression of TNFR1 and TNFR2 (Fig. 9.11a–c) [170]. DR4 and TNFR2 expression was higher in FIGO stage IV compared to stage III tumors. Effusions from patients who responded poorly to chemotherapy at first disease recurrence had significantly higher DR4, DR5, and Fas expression. Higher DR4 expression correlated with poor OS and PFS in univariate survival analysis, as well as in multivariate Cox analysis.

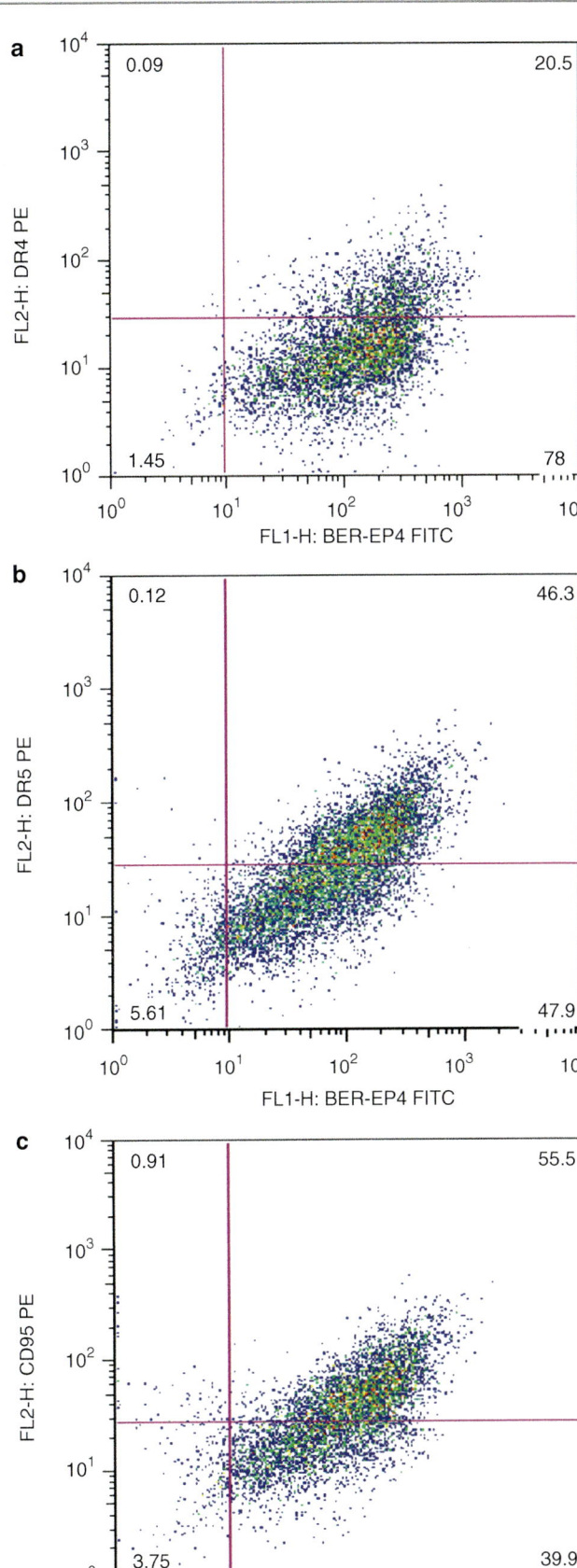

**Fig. 9.11** Death receptors. Flow cytometry analysis showing expression of DR4 (**a**), DR5 (**b**), and Fas (**c**) in carcinoma cells in effusion (co-labeled by Ber-EP4)

## Caspases and Their Inhibitors

Apoptosis, or programmed cell death, is a process regulating cell death following irreparable DNA damage and is additionally important for controlling cell number during normal development. Apoptosis is mediated by caspases, a family of cysteinyl aspartate-specific proteases. Caspases are activated by two major pathways, which have considerable crosstalk. The extrinsic pathway is initiated by ligation of DR members, including Fas/CD95, TNFR, and TRAILR, to activate membrane-proximal caspases (caspase-8 and caspase-10), which in turn cleave and activate caspase-3, caspase-6, and caspase-7 or B-cell chronic lymphocytic leukemia/lymphoma 2 (Bcl-2) proteins, depending on cell type. The intrinsic pathway is activated by different stimuli, including chemotherapy, kinase inhibitors, hypoxia, growth factor withdrawal, and radiation. It involves disruption of the mitochondrial membrane; release of mitochondrial proteins that regulate apoptosis, including cytochrome $c$, into the cytoplasm; and the formation of complex between cytochrome $c$, adaptor protein apoptotic protease-activating factor 1 (APAF1), and pro-caspase-9, in which pro-caspase-9 is activated. Caspase-9 downstream activates effector caspases, most notably caspase-3, resulting in apoptosis [171, 172].

The levels of cleaved (activated) caspases, as well as the degree of dUTP incorporation, another method of measuring apoptosis, can be quantitatively measured in OC effusions using FCM [173]. Analysis of 76 OC effusions showed caspase-3 and caspase-8 cleavage and dUTP incorporation in <10% of tumor cells in the majority of effusions (Fig. 9.12a, b), with comparable levels in pre- and post-chemotherapy effusions. Higher-than-median cleaved caspase-3 levels correlated with longer OS and PFS [174].

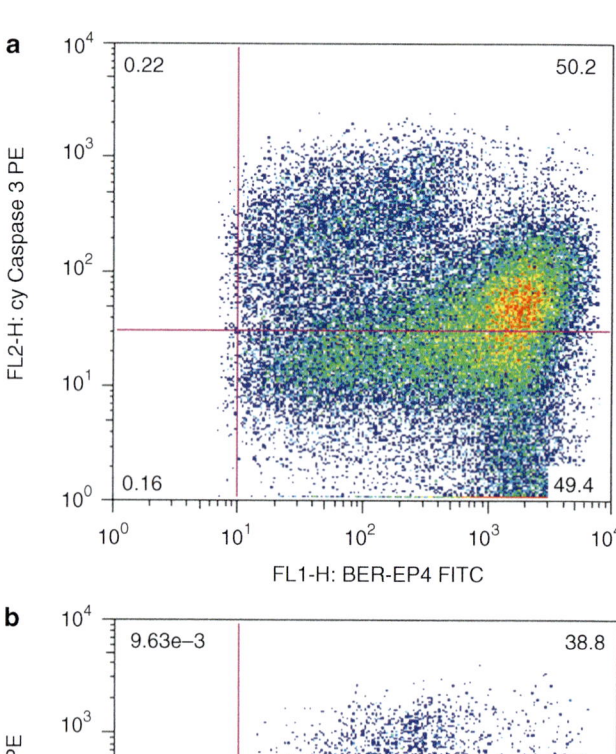

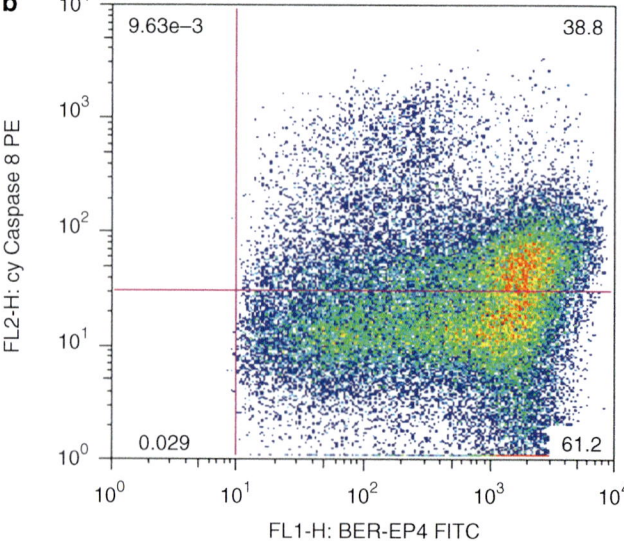

**Fig. 9.12** Caspases. Flow cytometry analysis showing expression of cleaved caspase-3 (**a**) and cleaved caspase-8 (**b**) in carcinoma cells in effusion (labeled by Ber-EP4). This specimen had an unusually high degree of apoptosis, whereas the majority of specimens expressed caspases in <10% of cells

The widely used Annexin-V assay measures phosphatidylserine cell surface exposure as marker of apoptosis but in fact labels also cells in stress that are not apoptotic. FCM analysis of Annexin-V expression in 76 OC effusions showed more frequent labeling compared to cleaved caspase levels and dUTP incorporation. Higher percentage of Annexin-V-expressing cells in post-chemotherapy effusions was associated with poor OS and PFS. The higher Annexin-V expression compared to more reliable apoptosis markers and its association with poor survival were concluded to support a role in cell survival rather than apoptosis in effusions [175].

FCM analysis measuring the expression of the anti-apoptotic protein c-FLIP in serous effusions was established by the author's group, and c-FLIP expression was assessed for clinical relevance in a series of 69 OC effusions. c-FLIP expression was detected in tumor cells in all specimens (expression range 21–100%, median 80%), with no association to clinicopathologic parameters, chemoresponse at diagnosis, or survival [176].

Inhibitors of apoptosis (IAPs) are a family of 8 cytoplasmic proteins that prevent apoptosis by specifically inhibiting caspase-3, caspase-7, and caspase-9, consisting of neuronal AIP (NAIP), cellular IAP1 (cIAP1), cellular IAP2 (cIAP2), X chromosome-linked IAP (XIAP), survivin, baculovirus IAP repeat (BIR)-containing ubiquitin-conjugating enzyme (BRUCE/Apollon), melanoma IAP (ML-IAP, previously called Livin), and IAP-like protein 2 (ILP-2). IAPs contain one or more repeats of a highly conserved 70–80-amino-acid zinc-binding domain, termed the baculovirus IAP repeat (BIR), which mediates the binding of caspases. Certain IAPs additionally interact with the MAPK, TGFβ, and nuclear factor-kB (NF-kB) signal transduction pathways, and survivin is additionally expressed at the mitotic apparatus in the nucleus in the G2/M phase, where it is thought to facilitate cell division. As with several of the above-discussed proteins, efforts to target IAP family members, and survivin in particular, in cancer have generally been unsuccessful, although new approaches, e.g., small molecules that mimic the binding domain of the endogenous IAP antagonist second mitochondrial activator of caspases (Smac) to IAP proteins, are under evaluation [177, 178].

XIAP expression was detected in tumor cells in 54/81 malignant effusions, including 13/13 OC, compared to 2/35 benign effusions, suggesting a diagnostic role for this protein [179].

XIAP and Survivin expression was found in >90% of effusions in analysis of 106 specimens studied using Western blotting, whereas Livin was absent. XIAP expression by IHC was significantly higher in effusions compared to solid primary and metastatic lesions (Fig. 9.13a, b). Nuclear Survivin was significantly positively related to Ki-67 score, and its presence was associated with longer PFS and OS in univariate analysis. For PFS, this was reproduced in Cox multivariate analysis [180].

Bcl-2 and Bcl-$X_L$ are closely linked anti-apoptotic cytoplasmic proteins containing Bcl-2 homology (BH) domains mediating binding and inactivation of pro-apoptotic family members [181]. Several drugs targeting Bcl-2 proteins are under clinical investigation, and the highly selective BCL-2 inhibitor venetoclax was recently approved in the USA for the treatment of patients with chronic lymphocytic leukemia with 17p deletion who have received at least one prior therapy [182].

Data is limited regarding the clinical role of Bcl-2 and Bcl-$X_L$ in OC effusions. Bcl-$X_L$ was shown to be expressed in 7/7 OC effusions in one study [183]. In a larger series of 188 effusions and 124 patient-matched primary carcinomas and 81 solid metastases, Bcl-2 expression was significantly higher in primary carcinomas and solid metastases compared to effusions, whereas Bcl-$X_L$ expression was highest in effusions (Fig. 9.13c). Bcl-$X_L$ expression was additionally associated with poor response to chemotherapy at diagnosis [184].

Heat shock proteins (HSP), divided into groups based on molecular weight, are chaperones of cellular proteins, involved in assembly, folding, and maturation of multiple proteins, thereby affecting critical cellular functions, such as differentiation, proliferation, and apoptosis. HSP27 and HSP70 family members independently regulate apoptosis upstream of the mitochondria by inhibiting stress-inducing signals, at the mitochondrial level by preventing membrane permeability and release of cytochrome $c$, and downstream of the mitochondria by suppressing caspase activation. They regulate apoptosis by binding multiple proteins involved in cell death and survival, including caspases, apoptosis-inducing factor (AIF), the intracellular signaling proteins AKT and JNK-1, and the transcription factor Stat3 [185–188]. HSP family members have been shown to be expressed in multiple cancer types, where they mediate tumor-related processes, including migration, invasion, metastasis, and EMT, and have been associated with adverse outcome in many of these malignancies. They are consequently under investigation as therapeutic targets, with particular effort directed at inhibiting HSP90 [188, 189].

In the abovementioned study of Bcl-2 proteins [184], HSP27 was expressed exclusively in the cytoplasm, while HSP70 was expressed in both the cytoplasm and the nucleus (Fig. 9.13d). HSP27 expression was more frequent in high-grade tumors. Nuclear and cytoplasmic HSP70 expression was significantly higher in primary carcinomas and solid metastases compared to effusions. However, increased cytoplasmic HSP70 staining in effusions correlated with poor OS in univariate analysis.

In a follow-up study, HSP90 expression by IHC was analyzed in 265 effusions from patients with advanced-stage OC. HSP90 was expressed in the cytoplasm and nucleus of tumor cells in 97% and 18% of specimens, respectively.

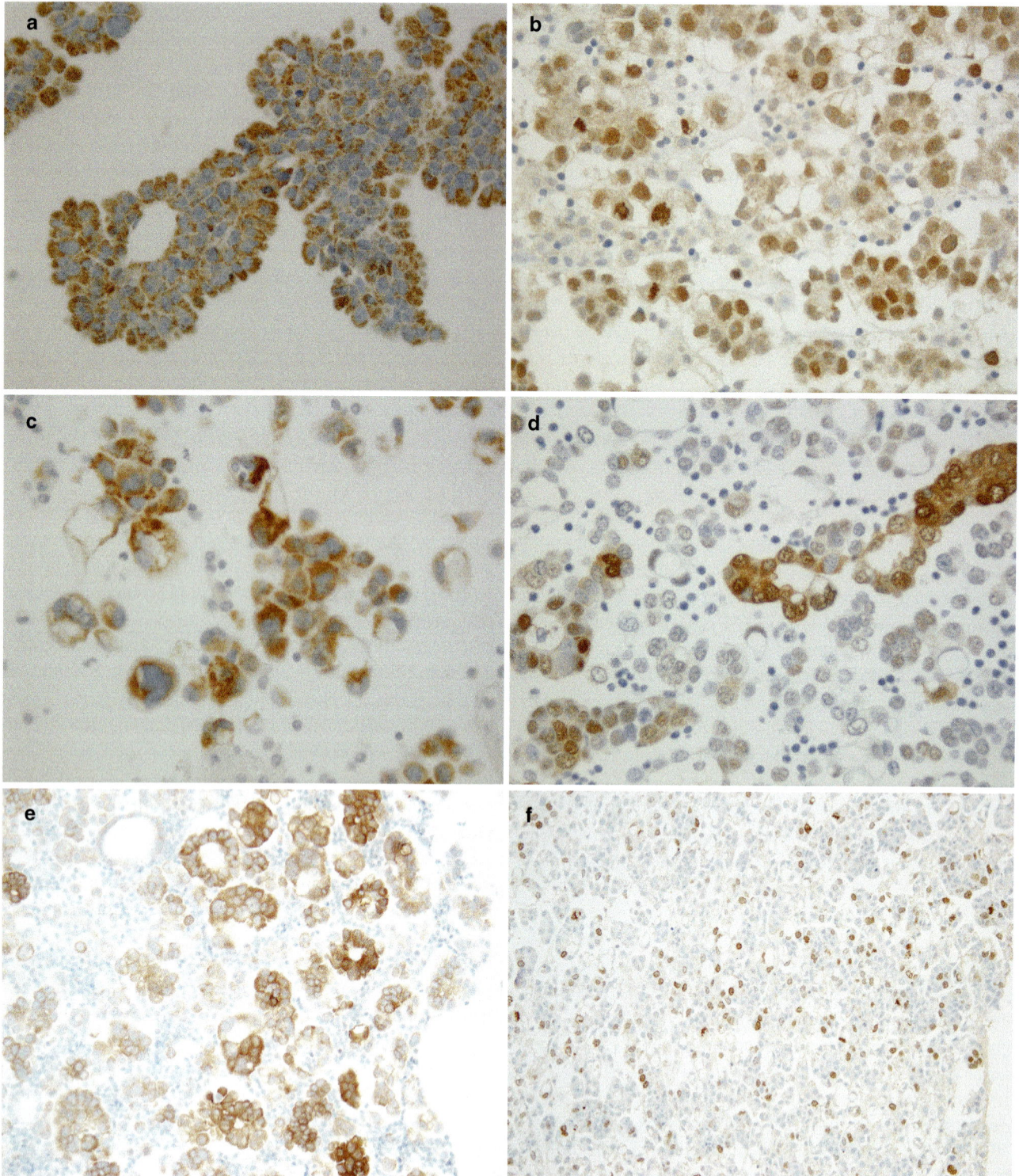

**Fig. 9.13** Apoptosis inhibitors. Immunostaining for XIAP (**a**), Survivin (**b**), Bcl-XL (**c**), HSP-70 (**d**), HSP-90 (**e**), Aurora-B (**f**), and Wee1 (**g**) in effusions

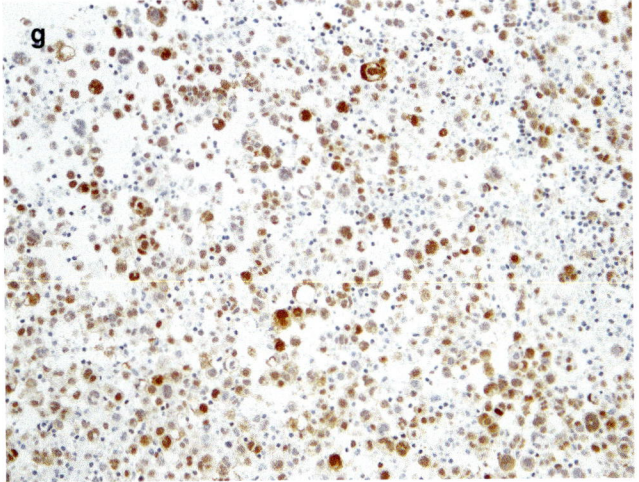

**Fig. 9.13** (continued)

Nuclear HSP90 expression was significantly higher in post-compared to pre-chemotherapy effusions, but no association was observed with chemoresponse or survival (Fig. 9.13e) [190].

A third family of proteins analyzed in this study was the Bag family. Bag proteins bind HSP70, thereby regulating its activity in protein degradation. They additionally interact with Bcl-2, enhancing its anti-apoptotic effect. In addition, Bag-4, also known as silencer of death domain (SODD), binds to TNFR1, suppressing pro-apoptotic signal transduction [191]. As was true for HSP and Bcl-2 proteins, Bag-1 and Bag-4/SODD expression in effusions differed from that in solid lesions, with higher Bag-1 in primary carcinomas and solid metastases and higher Bag-4 expression in effusions [184].

## Regulation of Mitosis

Mitosis is a highly regulated stepwise process, including centrosome maturation, bipolar spindle assembly, microtubule attachments, and cytokinesis. Failure of the mitotic process, including deregulation of kinases involved in this process, results in genome instability and cancer development [192].

Aurora kinases are key regulators of mitosis and have received considerable attention as therapeutic targets in cancer [193]. Aurora-A is a serine/threonine kinase involved in centrosome function and bipolar spindle assembly [194]. Aurora-B is member of the chromosomal passenger complex

mediating chromosome-microtubule interactions, chromosome condensation, sister chromatid cohesion, the spindle assembly checkpoint (SAC), and cytokinesis [195].

Analysis of the expression and clinical role of Aurora-A and Aurora-B in serous OC using qPCR and IHC was recently performed. *AURKA* and *AURKB* mRNA and their protein product were demonstrated in all primary carcinomas ($n = 38$), solid metastases ($n = 52$), and effusions ($n = 88$) (Fig. 9.13f), with higher expression of *AURKA* mRNA and Aurora-A protein in effusions compared to solid specimens. Low Aurora-B protein expression was associated with primary chemotherapy resistance and poor treatment response in pre-chemotherapy effusions. No significant association was found between Aurora-A kinase expression at the mRNA or protein level and PFS or OS [196].

Analysis of the mRNA and protein expression of Bub1, another mitosis-related protein, using qPCR and WB was performed as follow-up study in the same material. *BUB1* mRNA levels in both effusions and solid lesions were significantly related to the mRNA levels of *AURKA* and *AURKB*. *BUB1* mRNA expression was additionally significantly higher in chemo-naïve solid lesions compared to specimens obtained after neoadjuvant chemotherapy. However, no association with chemotherapy exposure was found in effusions, nor was any relationship with survival found at any of the anatomic sites [197].

DNA damage during cell cycle progression may result in cell cycle arrest/delay at three major DNA-damage checkpoints, i.e., G1/S, intra-S, and G2/M. Since p53, which controls the G1/S checkpoint, is often inactivated in cancer, tumor cells rely on the S and G2/M checkpoints for repairing DNA damage. The Wee1-like kinase (Wee1) is a tyrosine kinase negatively regulating G2/M transition by phosphorylating and thereby inhibiting cyclin-dependent kinase-1 (CDK1), also known as CDC2. It additionally stabilizes DNA during S-phase, thereby preventing unscheduled replication initiation. Based on these functions, Wee1 is regarded as a tumor-promoting molecule and is therapeutically targeted in cancer [198].

Wee1 protein expression analysis in 287 serous OC effusions showed nuclear expression in 265/287 (92%) specimens (Fig. 9.13g), and this was validated using WB, showing expression in 45/45 analyzed effusions. Wee1 expression by IHC was significantly higher in post- compared to pre-chemotherapy effusions and was significantly related to poor OS in the former group, a finding which remained significant in Cox multivariate analysis [199].

## The Immune System

Efforts to harness the immune response to combat OC have started several decades ago. Regrettably, they have to date not been successful in curing patients with this cancer, and improvements at prolonging PFS or OS have been modest at best. The reason for this disappointing outcome owes, as in many other tumors, to the ability of OC cells to evade destruction by immune effectors, which combines both changes in their antigenic profile and the ability to inhibit the immune system or modify it to have tumor-promoting action. A new effort is likely to be directed at modulating the immune response in gynecological cancer in general and OC in particular given the recent introduction of such therapy in other cancers [200–202]. Overview of the literature in this area in studies of OC effusions is detailed below.

The ability of ascites to suppress DNA synthesis in lymphocytes was reported more than 30 years ago [203]. High levels of HSP10, a protein which suppresses CD3-zeta expression on T lymphocytes, and thereby their activation via TcR, were found in OC ascites and serum, while sera from controls had undetectable levels of this protein [204]. Membrane vesicles, or exosomes, secreted by OC cells, suppressed the expression of the lymphocyte signaling proteins CD3-zeta and JAK3, resulting in apoptosis [205]. Monocytes/macrophages from blood and ascites of OC patients have reduced antibody-dependent cell-mediated cytotoxicity and phagocytic activity compared to cells from normal donor blood [206]. Tumor-associated T lymphocytes and natural killer (NK) cells from OC ascites have reduced CD3 and CD16 expression, respectively, as well as reduced activity of the tyrosine kinase p56$^{lck}$. Both cell classes have reduced proliferation compared to peripheral blood lymphocytes from normal controls [207]. IL-10-producing monocytes were detected in OC ascites and shown to inhibit T-cell proliferation and cytokine production [208]. Macrophages from OC ascites stimulate proliferation of OC cells in vitro, and this effect was postulated to be mediated via Stat3 activation by IL-6 and IL-10 [209]. OC ascites inhibits NK cell activation in response to lipid presented by CD1-expressing cells [210].

HLA-G, together with HLA-E, is a nonclassical major histocompatibility complex (MHC) class I antigen that is thought to bind to the CD8 T-cell receptor and is involved in interaction with NK cells. HLA-G is present as a membrane-bound or a soluble form, and its expression in normal tissues is limited to trophoblastic cells, where it is postulated to mediate immune tolerance during pregnancy. However, it is widely expressed in cancer cells, in which it has been hypothesized to play a role in evasion of immunosurveillance by host T lymphocytes and NK cells [211, 212].

Measurement of HLA-G in 42 malignant ascites specimens, including 25 OC, and 18 reactive effusions by ELISA showed significantly higher HLA-G levels in malignant effusions compared to their benign counterparts [213]. HLA-G protein expression was found in 49/148 (33%) OC effusions using IHC and was significantly lower in post- compared to pre-chemotherapy effusions. Surprisingly, HLA-G tumor expression in pre-chemotherapy effusions correlated with better OS in univariate analysis [214].

Several other aspects related to the role of the immune system in OC biology are presented below.

Cytokines have been extensively investigated for their presence and role in OC. TNF mRNA was localized to tumor and/or inflammatory cells in analysis of seven ascites specimens. The same study showed the presence of the p55 and p75 TNF receptors on tumor cells in solid lesions, suggesting the presence of an autocrine/paracrine pathway [215]. TNF-α and IL-1β stimulated VEGF production in mesothelial cells and OC cell lines in vitro, and the levels of IL-1β and VEGF were significantly related to both inflammatory and OC effusions [216]. Elevated levels of soluble IL-2Rα were found in 86/86 (100%) ascites specimens and 67/85 (79%) serum samples from OC patients, compared to 12/25 (48%) benign ascites specimens and 1/88 (1%) serum samples from controls [217]. In agreement with this observation, soluble IL-2Rα ascites levels by ELISA were higher in OC than in normal females and were additionally elevated compared to patient-matched serum samples for the 23 OC patients [218].

The clinical role of IL-6 and other cytokines in OC has been the subject of several studies. Analysis of the clinical role of *IL-6* polymorphisms at position 174 showed significant association between the presence of the GG genotype and longer OS. However, the presence of this genotype was unrelated to IL-6 ascites or serum levels [219]. Higher levels of IL-6 were measured in sera and ascites specimens from patients with stage III–IV compared to stage I–II OC [220]. OC IL-6 and TNF-α ascites levels were significantly higher than in control specimens [221]. In analysis of 70 patients, IL-6 levels in ascites correlated significantly with ascites volume and marginally with primary tumor size but were unrelated to clinical parameters, including survival [222].

IL-13 and IL-15 levels by ELISA were reported to be higher in OC effusions compared to benign specimens [223]. Zeimet et al. analyzed the expression of multiple cytokines in serum and ascites from 76 OC patients. IL-10 and IL-12 were found in all ascites specimens, whereas IL-4 was detected in 43%. The majority of cytokines were more highly expressed in ascites than in serum samples, and high levels of neopterin, TNF-α, and IL-12 were associated with shorter disease-free and overall survival, a finding that retained its significance for IL-12 in multivariate analysis [224]. In another study, lower ascitic levels of IL-1 RA, an anti-inflammatory cytokine that competes with IL-1α and IL-1β on binding IL-1 receptor, but has no intrinsic activity, were associated with better PFS and OS, including in multivariate analysis [225]. Higher levels of osteoprotegerin, IL-10, and leptin in OC ascites were associated with shorter PFS in analysis of ten specimens [226]. In a study of 70 patients, higher IL-6 and TNF-α levels in ascites were significantly related to shorter PFS [227]. Ascites from OC patients was shown to increase the release of IL-6, IL-1β, and the chemokines CCL2 and CXCL8 (see below) in peripheral blood mononuclear cells from healthy volunteers. It additionally increased the release of the anti-inflammatory cytokine IL-10 and inhibited the production of interferon-γ and IL-12 [228].

Chemokines are a family of small secreted proteins that regulate the immune response and are produced by multiple cell classes in the tumor microenvironment, including cancer and stromal cells, endothelial cells, macrophages, and neutrophils. They are divided into four classes, C-C, C-X-C, C, and C-X₃-C, depending on the location of the first two cysteines in their sequence. Chemokines exert their biological role through 18 G-protein-coupled chemokine receptors expressed on tumor cells, creating an autocrine loop that mediates proliferation, regulates angiogenesis and cancer stemlike cell properties, and promotes invasion and metastasis [229, 230].

OC cells in ascites expressed the chemokine receptor CXCR4 using FCM and its ligand CXCL12 was found in the ascites fluid [231]. OC cells isolated from ascites produced TNF-α in response to CXCL12 [232]. In an additional study, several CC chemokines were found in ascites fluid in analysis of 66 OC effusions using ELISA, and cells expressing chemokine protein and mRNA were detected in these specimens using FCM and RT-PCR, respectively. The chemokine receptors CCR1, CCR2, and CCR5 were detected on macrophages in the majority of specimens, whereas lymphocyte expression was more variable and differed between CD4+ and CD8+ cells. Cellular chemokine expression was not significantly related to the secreted levels of these proteins [233].

Analysis of 73 OC effusions using FCM showed expression of CXCR4 and CCR7 on lymphocytes in all specimens, with less frequent expression of CXCR1, CCR2, and CCR5. Monocytes were frequently positive for CXCR1, CXCR4, CCR2, and CCR5, with only rare expression of CCR7. Carcinoma cells only rarely expressed chemokine receptors, with one to three specimens positive for each of the five receptors (Fig. 9.14a–c) [234].

In an additional study, CCL2, CCL3, CCL18, and CXCL8 were found in OC effusions, with lower levels of CCL7 and CCL20. CCL18 and CXCL8 levels were higher in OC effusions compared to specimens obtained from patients with other malignancies or with benign conditions [235].

The nature of the leukocyte cell classes in OC effusions and their clinical relevance have been the focus of several studies. The presence of CD4+/CD25+ regulatory cells, CD3+/CD56+ NK cells, and HLA-DR-expressing T cells was higher in OC effusions compared to blood from OC patients or effusions from patients with cirrhosis, and changes in the blood-to-ascites ratio in the former two parameters were related to histological grade and platinum resistance [236]. Another study by the same group showed inverse correlation between the presence of CD4+/CD25+ regulatory and CD3+/CD56+ NK cells and levels of TNF-α and VEGF, respectively. Lower VEGF and higher TNF-α levels were associated with platinum sensitivity and improved survival [237]. Intraperitoneal tumor-infiltrating CD3+ lymphocytes were shown to express the co-stimulatory molecules CD80 and CD86, as well as their receptors CD28 and CTLA-4, in OC ascites, and the numbers of these cells were higher than in the peripheral blood [238].

Comparative analysis of patient-matched blood and ascites specimens from 17 patients, the majority with HGSC, showed accumulation of CD8+ cytotoxic T cells and regulatory T cells (Tregs) in ascites compared to peripheral blood, with a skewing toward the CD45RA-effector/memory cells. Regulatory T cells in ascites were more activated and proliferated more than their counterparts in the blood, and their number was positively related to that of the tumor cells [239].

B cells were previously reported to be absent from the peritoneal cavity, based on analysis of peritoneal specimens from ten OC patients and eight controls, where the presence of occasional cells was attributed to contamination with peripheral blood [240]. However, the author's group observed consistent presence of these cells in analysis of 73 specimens. Furthermore, the presence of B cells and NK cells in OC effusions was associated with poor survival [234].

Macrophages have been receiving growing attention as tumor-promoting cells in recent years [241, 242] and are present in large numbers in effusions, often underappreciated due to confusion with RMC [243]. It was recently reported that monocytes/macrophages stimulated by coagulation factor XII upregulate several transcription factors, including AP-1 and Stat family members, and that OC cells have increased invasive capability in their presence [244].

Analysis of macrophage populations and cytokine profiles in OC ascites showed association between alternatively activated (M2) macrophages expressing CD163, measured in 20 patients, and IL-6 and IL-10 levels, and these parameters were significantly related to shorter relapse-free survival [245]. This population was shown to be characterized by interferon signaling in a subsequent study [246].

**Fig. 9.14** Chemokine receptors. Flow cytometry analysis showing expression of CXCR4 in lymphocytes (**a**), CCR5 in macrophages (**b**), and CXCR4 in carcinoma cells (**c**), co-labeled for CD45, CD14, and Ber-EP4, respectively

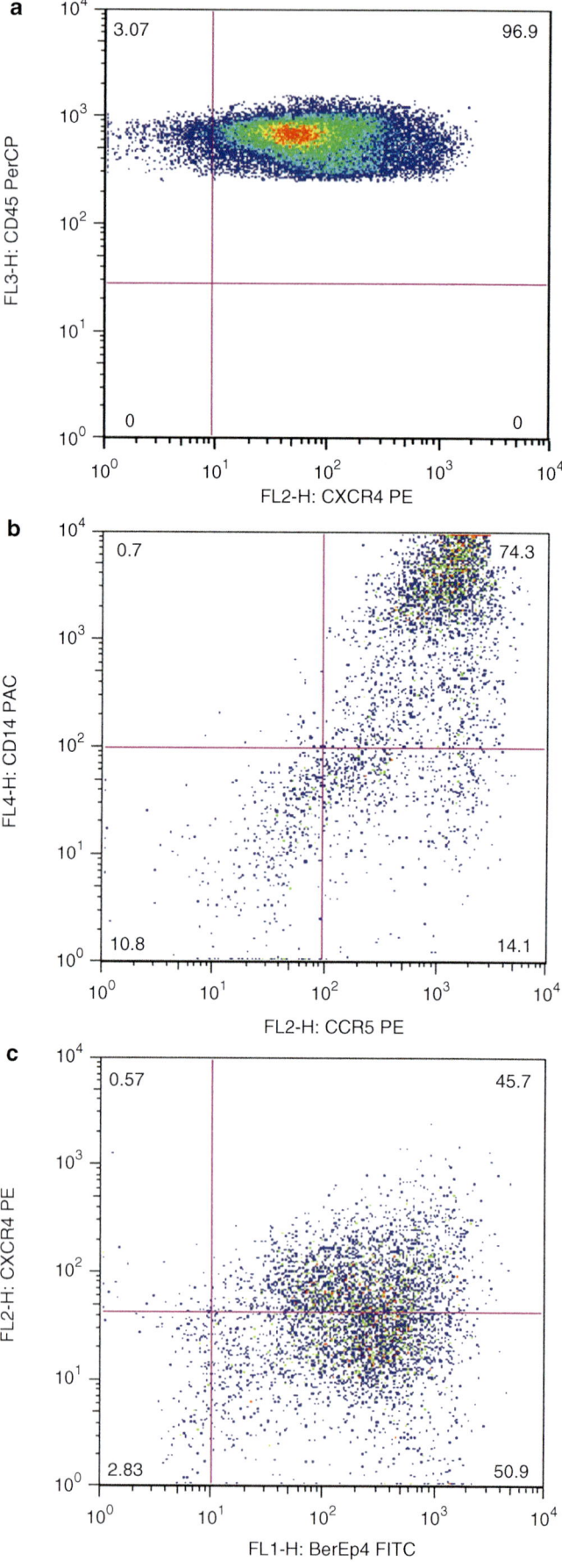

## Intracellular Signaling and Transcriptional Regulation

As discussed above, many of the molecules that were already presented in this chapter mediate cell signaling, affecting transcription and synthesis of cancer-associated molecules and through it major aspects of tumor cell biology, such as cell survival, apoptosis, proliferation, invasion, and metastasis. This section deals in more detail with the intracellular part of these signaling pathways.

## The MAPK Signaling Pathway

The MAPK pathway is a four-level cascade, in which each kinase activates the following kinase substrate through a complex network, enabling the cell to maintain diversity and specificity while responding to various extracellular cues. MAPK double phosphorylation at tyrosine and threonine residues at the final level of the cascade occurs in an enzyme-specific manner by the MEK family of MAPK kinases. Two MAPK family members, c-jun amino-terminal kinase (JNK) and the high osmolarity glycerol response kinase (p38), are activated by stress-related stimuli, whereas the extracellular-regulated kinase (ERK) is largely activated by growth factor signals. MAPK activation leads to phosphorylation of a variety of cytosolic substrates, and to their own translocation to the nucleus, where they activate a large number of transcription factors, including AP-1 and Ets-1. p38 and JNK activation may result in apoptosis or cell survival, depending on the nature of the signal, as well as in proliferation, differentiation, and inflammation, while ERK promotes differentiation, proliferation, and migration. MAPK activity is negatively regulated by dual-specificity phosphatases (DUSP) that deactivate the enzymes [247, 248]. Activation of the RAS/RAF/MEK/ERK cascade is involved in chemoresistance [249].

WB analysis of 64 fresh-frozen OC effusions showed frequent expression and activation of ERK, JNK, and p38 (Fig. 9.15) [250]. Surprisingly, expression of all three family members was associated with clinicopathologic parameters related to less aggressive clinical course and/or longer survival. Higher levels of p-p38 and total (pan-)JNK were significantly associated with younger age and lower histological grade, respectively, and higher level of pan-ERK, p-ERK, and pan-JNK correlated with longer OS. The finding for pan-ERK and pan-JNK retained its prognostic role in Cox multivariate analysis.

In agreement with this finding, higher mRNA expression of PAC1, member of the DUSP family, in OC effusions was associated with poor survival [251].

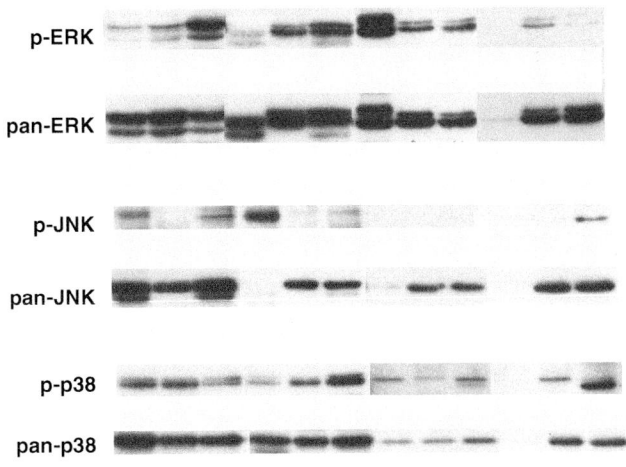

**Fig. 9.15** Western blotting for the MAPK members ERK, JNK, and p38, showing total expression (pan) and activation (p-MAPK) in effusions

In an additional study using proteomics, significantly higher p-ERK levels were found in OC effusions compared to benign effusions [252]. Notably, in this study, higher p38 and p-JNK levels were related to poor survival in separate analyses of pre- and post-chemotherapy specimens, respectively.

The Ras oncogene is part of the ERK signaling pathway. Frequent mutations in *KRAS* were found in analysis of 47 peritoneal effusions and washings from OC patients using PCR restriction fragment length polymorphism (RFLP) analysis, whereas *NRAS* and *HRAS* mutations were infrequent [253].

## The PI3K/AKT/mTOR Signaling Pathway

Dysregulation of the PI3K/AKT/mTOR signaling pathway is a central event in cancer. Following activation by receptor tyrosine kinases, PI3K converts phosphatidylinositol (4,5) bisphosphate (PIP$_2$) to phosphatidylinositol (3,4,5) triphosphate (PIP$_3$) which then acts as a second messenger activating downstream pathways involving AKT, mTOR, and other proteins. The tumor suppressor phosphatase and tensin homology (PTEN) negatively regulates PI3K activity and is mutated or deleted in multiple cancer types. The serine/threonine kinase AKT comprises three homologous family members (AKT1, AKT2, and AKT3) and is activated by double phosphorylation at Thr308 and Ser473. PI3K signaling promotes cell growth, protein translation, and cell survival, antagonizes cell cycle arrest, impacts metabolism, modulates the immune response, and regulates angiogenesis and invasion. A major target in the downstream cascade of AKT activity is mTOR, a protein residing in two functionally distinct complexes, mTORC1 and mTORC2. mTORC1 phosphory-lates 4E-BP1 (eukaryotic initiation factor 4E-binding protein 1) and p70S6K (ribosomal p70S6 kinase), both regulators of mRNA translation and cell growth, as well as the PI3K/AKT pathway itself. Research directed at identifying PI3K/AKT/mTOR signaling pathway inhibitors has received much focus in recent years [254, 255].

Proteomics analysis showed significantly higher AKT levels in OC effusions compared to benign effusions, as well as a trend for shorter survival for patients with disease recurrence post-chemotherapy effusions with high AKT activation level [252], though the latter association was not reproduced in a subsequent study using the same methodology [22].

In another study [256], the expression of PTEN and its inhibitor DJ-1, an oncogene overexpressed in different cancers [257], was analyzed. DJ-1 mRNA was frequently expressed in OC and was positively associated with that of its transcriptional regulators Sp1 and Sp3. DJ-1 expression was significantly higher in post- compared to pre-chemotherapy effusions and predicted shorter PFS in univariate analysis for patients with post-chemotherapy effusions. PTEN protein expression by IHC was low and was unrelated to DJ-1 levels or patient survival.

In a follow-up study, protein expression of AKT, mTOR, and DJ-1 in OC was studied (Fig. 9.16a, b) [258]. p-AKT expression in effusions by IHC was highest in high-grade tumors, and high p-mTOR protein expression in effusions was associated with poor PFS for patients with post-chemotherapy effusions in univariate and multivariate analysis. FCM analysis showed significant co-expression of AKT, mTOR, and DJ-1 in effusions. Higher p-AKT Thr308/pan-AKT ratio by WB was associated with more advanced FIGO stage and a trend for poor response to chemotherapy at first disease recurrence.

## NF-κB

The NF-κB family consists of five proteins, named RelA (p65), RelB, c-Rel, p50/p105 (NF-κB1), and p52/p100 (NF-κB2), that form homodimers or heterodimers. NF-κB is localized in the cytoplasm in complex with inhibitors of NF-κB (IκBs). Cell stimulation results in IκB phosphorylation in a site-specific manner by activated IκB kinase (IKK) complexes, of which the most common contain IKKα, IKKβ, and a regulatory IKKγ subunit.

The "canonical" NF-κB pathway is activated by TNF-α, IL-1, and other stimuli and involves IκBα phosphorylation at ser32 and ser36 predominantly by IKKβ. IκBα is subsequently ubiquitinated and degraded in the 26S proteasome, thereby releasing the NF-κB p65/p50 heterodimer to translo-

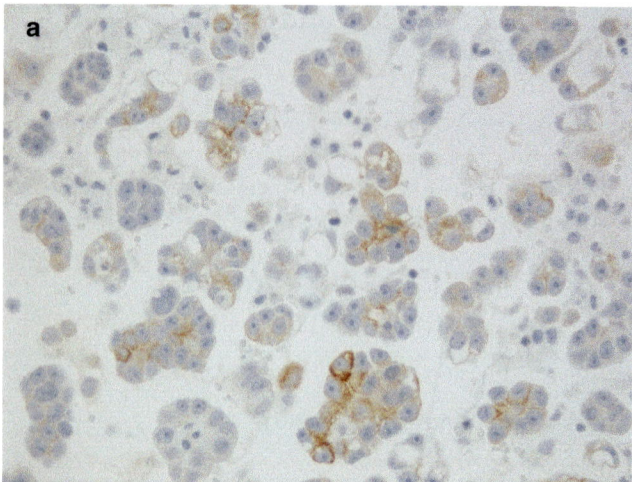
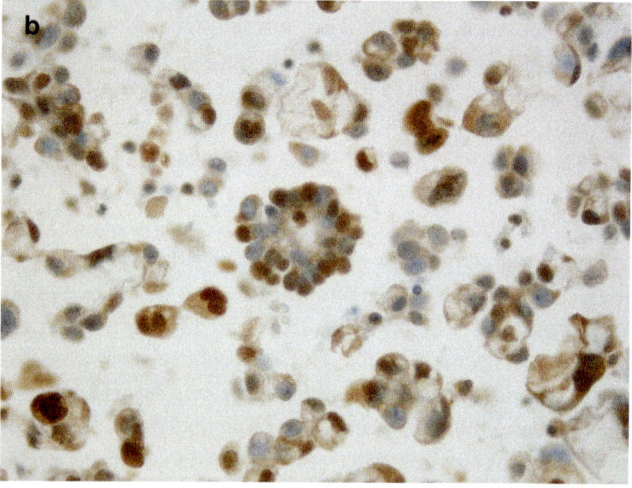

**Fig. 9.16** PI3K pathway. Immunostaining for p-mTOR (**a**) and p-AKT (**b**) in effusions

cate into the nucleus. Other NF-κB activation pathways have been described. In the nucleus, NF-κB may induce or repress the expression of numerous genes, affecting cell proliferation and survival, inflammation, the immune response, and apoptosis [259–261].

NF-κB p65 and IκBα protein expression was recently studied in OC effusions, primary carcinomas, and solid metastases [174]. A significantly higher percentage of cells expressed both proteins in solid lesions compared to effusions, although nuclear NF-κB p65 expression, indicating NF-κB activation, was observed in the majority of tumors irrespective of anatomic site (Fig. 9.17a). NF-κB p65 phosphorylation at Ser536 was found in 94% of 75 OC effusions using WB (Fig. 9.17b). In effusions, nuclear NF-κB p65 expression was significantly associated with larger volume of residual disease and poor response to chemotherapy at disease recurrence, as well as with poor PFS in univariate and Cox multivariate analysis.

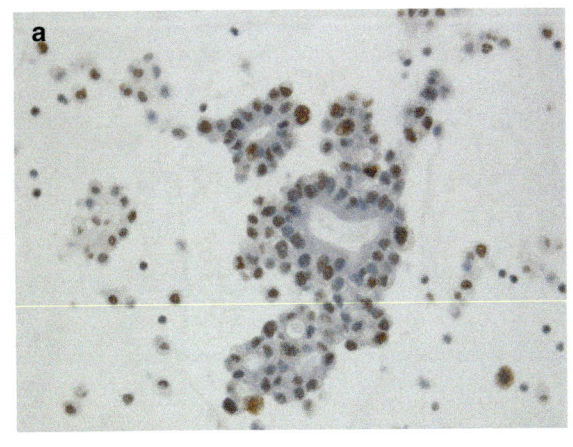

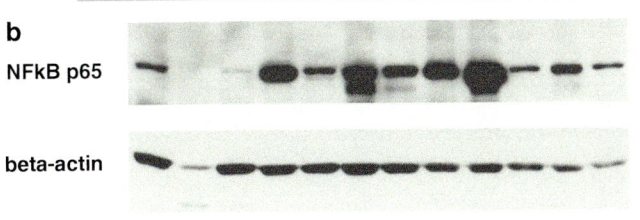

**Fig. 9.17** NF-κB. (**a**) Immunostaining for NF-κB p65, (**b**) Western blotting for the activated form, NF-κB p-p65 (Ser536)

## Ets Transcription Factors

The Ets family of transcriptional factors consists of 28 members in humans and is highly conserved across different species. All family members contain an 85-amino-acid DNA-binding domain (the Ets domain) that confers the ability to bind to DNA sequences having the core motif GGAA/T (Ets-binding site, EBS). Another conserved area that is present in 11 members is the pointed (PNT) domain, which mediates protein-protein interactions and oligomerization. Ets factors have 200 known target genes, including proteases (MMP-1, MMP-3, and MMP-9, cathepsin) and their inhibitors (TIMP-1), cell cycle molecules (cyclin D1, p21), apoptosis promoters and inhibitors (Fas, PARP, Bcl-2, Bcl-XL), adhesion molecules (E-cadherin, integrins), immune response mediators (interleukins, immunoglobulins), and angiogenesis mediators (the VEGF receptors Flt-1 and flk-1, Tie-1 and Tie-2). In these multiple target genes, ETS factors can mediate transcriptional activation or repression according to the binding factor and the DNA sequence involved [262–264]. Ets members are aberrantly expressed in a range of solid tumors through gene amplification, overexpression of gene products, or creation of fusion genes with multiple partners [265].

Four members of the Ets family – Ets-1, Ets-2, Erg, and PEA3 – have been shown to be expressed in OC effusions at the mRNA levels using ISH, and the presence of Ets-1 and PEA3, studied in a large number of specimens, was associated with poor survival. Ets members were significantly co-expressed with their target genes or regulators, including integrins, MMP, and angiogenic molecules [266, 267].

mRNA expression, a fifth member of this family, *EHF*, previously found to be overexpressed in OC compared to DMPM by gene expression array analysis [48], was studied using qPCR. *EHF* levels were significantly higher in OC effusions and primary carcinomas compared to MM effusions, and higher levels in pre-chemotherapy effusions were associated with poor PFS in univariate and multivariate analysis [268].

## The Peroxisome Proliferator-Activated Receptor (PPAR) Family and Lipid Signaling

PPARs, consisting of PPAR-α, PPAR-β/δ, and PPAR-γ, are transcription factors belonging to the nuclear hormone receptor (NHR) superfamily, together with the steroid, thyroid hormone, vitamin D, and retinoid receptors. PPAR-α and PPAR-β/δ are widely expressed in normal tissues, whereas PPAR-γ has more limited distribution, mainly in adipose tissue. PPARs function as heterodimers bound to the retinoid receptor (RXR) and are activated by polyunsaturated fatty acids (e.g., arachidonic and linoleic acid) and their derivatives, generated through the action of the lipoxygenase and cyclooxygenase (COX) pathways. PPAR-α activation has an anti-inflammatory effect, whereas all PPARs have been shown to have tumor-inhibitory effects, probably through suppression of proliferation and induction of differentiation and apoptosis. PPAR-γ is highly expressed in multiple cancer types but has been most often associated with improved survival [269, 270].

PPAR-α, PPAR-β, and PPAR-γ mRNA was frequently expressed in OC using RT-PCR, with significantly higher PPAR-α and PPAR-β levels in effusions compared to primary carcinomas and solid metastases. PPAR-γ mRNA and protein were detected in carcinoma cells using ISH and IHC, respectively (Fig. 9.18a). Higher effusion mRNA levels of all PPARs were associated with less favorable response to chemotherapy at diagnosis, as well as poor PFS and OS in univariate, though not in multivariate survival analysis [271].

In a related study, expression of members of the phospholipase A₂ family, which hydrolyze arachidonic acid from phospholipids at the cell membrane, in OC effusions was found to be related to patient survival [272]. Other investigators found higher levels of prostaglandin E2, which is synthesized by COX enzymes, in ascites from OC patients compared to specimens from patients with other cancers or cirrhosis [273].

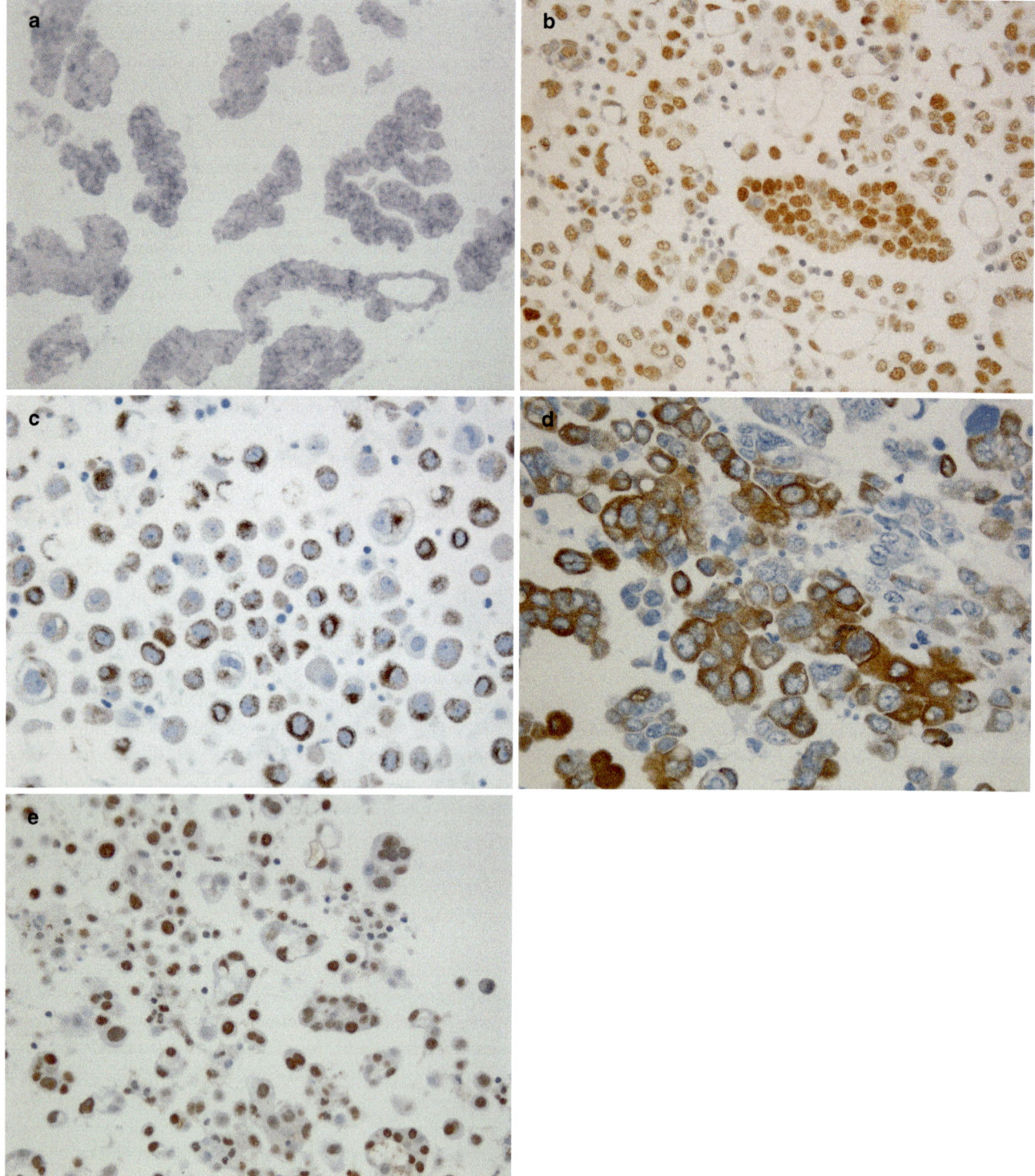

**Fig. 9.18** Stem cell and transcription-related markers. (**a**) mRNA in situ hybridization for *PPAR-γ* (NBT-BCIP as chromogen). (**b–e**) Immunostaining for Rsf-1 (**b**), Nestin (**c**), class III β-tubulin (**d**), and XPA (**e**)

In the context of lipid-mediated signaling in OC, it is essential to mention lysophosphatidic acid (LPA), a phospholipid with growth factor properties. LPA was detected in the effusion fluid in analysis of 62 malignant specimens from patients with various cancers, and levels were highest in the 13 OC effusions in this series [274]. Lysophospholipids, including LPA, were similarly shown to be present at higher levels in OC effusions compared to benign effusions by mass spectrometry [275]. Recently, OC ascites was shown to be a stronger mediator of migration of adipose tissue-derived stem cells in vitro, an effect mediated by LPA [276].

Recently, mRNA expression of the phospholipase D (PLD) isoforms PLD1 and PLD2 by qPCR was studied in 125 HGSC specimens (73 effusions, 28 ovarian tumors, 24 solid metastases). PLD1 and PLD2 isoforms were found in most specimens at all anatomic sites, but PLD2 mRNA levels were significantly higher in effusions compared with both carcinomas in the ovary and solid metastases. Higher levels of both isoforms were associated with higher CA 125 levels at diagnosis, and higher PLD2 mRNA levels in effusions were associated with unfavorable response to chemotherapy, though not to survival [277].

## Activating Protein 2γ (AP-2γ)

AP-2γ, member of a family of DNA-binding transcription factors, is encoded by the *TFAP2C* gene located on chromosome 20q13.2 in humans. AP-2 family members are required for normal growth and morphogenesis during mammalian development but regulate at the transcriptional level molecules known to be dysregulated in cancer, including those involved in proliferation (HER-2/*neu*), cell cycle regulation (p21$^{WAF1/CIP1}$), hormonal regulation (ER), inhibition of apoptosis (c-kit, Bcl-2), adhesion (MCAM/MUC18 and E-cadherin), and invasion/angiogenesis (MMP-2 and MMP-9, PAI-1, VEGF, and the thrombin receptor PAR-1) [278, 279].

Nuclear AP-2γ expression by IHC was detected in tumor cells in 28/75 (37%) borderline tumors, 13/22 (59%) FIGO stage I OC, and 255/306 (83%) advanced-stage OC, the latter including 202 effusions, a difference that was statistically significant. WB showed AP-2γ expression in 59/61 effusions. AP-2γ expression did not correlate with clinicopathologic parameters or survival [280].

## Rsf-1

Genetic material in human cells is stored in the form of chromatin, which consists of nucleoprotein complexes containing DNA and protein. DNA is wrapped around an octamer core of histones whose position and density are regulated through chromatin remodeling complexes, consisting in eukaryotes of the SWI/SNF2, ISWI, CHD, and INO80 families. Among these families, mSWI/SNF2, consisting of BAF (BRG1- or BRM-associated factors) and PBAF (polybromo-associated BAF), is the most commonly associated with disease, and 20% of cancers harbor mutations in genes belonging to this family [281].

RSF is a chromatin-remodeling complex that is composed of two subunits, hSNF2H and p325 (Rsf-1), and is involved in the formation of RNA polymerase II complexes. A truncated form of RSF-p325 encodes for the hepatitis B virus transcription repressor HBXAP. Amplification at the 11q13.5 chromosome region and overexpression of Rsf-1 were found in HGSC using digital karyotyping. Analysis of Rsf-1 amplification using FISH in primary tumors and of Rsf-1 mRNA levels in effusions using quantitative real-time PCR showed that its amplification and overexpression are associated with poor survival in two OC cohorts [282].

Tumor cell Rsf-1 protein expression by IHC was found in 157/168 (93%) OC effusions (Fig. 9.18b) and was significantly associated with more advanced disease (FIGO stage IV). Rsf-1 expression level was significantly lower in primary OC and in solid metastases. Higher Rsf-1 staining in effusions from patients tapped at disease recurrence was significantly associated with shorter OS in univariate and Cox multivariate survival analysis [283].

## NAC1

The BTB/POZ (bric-a-brac tramtrack broad complex/poxvirus and zinc domain) family consists of a large number of genes that are conserved among species from yeast to human and encode for zinc finger family transcription factors or actin-binding proteins. BTB/POZ proteins participate in a variety of cellular events that affect transcriptional regulation, protein ubiquitination and degradation, cytoskeletal regulation, and ion channel function [284, 285].

The BTB/POZ family member NAC1 was first discovered in the nucleus accumbens in the brain of rats, where it was shown to be upregulated following chronic cocaine administration [286]. Serial analysis of gene expression (SAGE) analysis showed overexpression of the *NAC1* gene in OC compared to benign ovarian epithelium, and NAC1 protein was shown to be sufficient for induction of the oncogenic phenotype and essential for tumor cell growth and survival in an experimental model [287].

Analysis of 176 OC effusions and 197 patient-matched primary tumors and solid metastases using IHC showed NAC1 expression in >90% of tumors, with significantly higher staining intensity and extent in effusions compared to solid tumors. NAC1 expression intensity was additionally significantly higher in specimens obtained after the administration of chemotherapy and correlated with shorter PFS for patients with post-chemotherapy effusions in univariate survival analysis [288].

Comparative proteomics analysis of SKOV-3 OC cells with and without a dominant negative NAC1 construct showed negative association between NAC1 silencing and levels of the *FASN* gene, encoding for FAS, a protein involved in fatty acid synthesis. In agreement with this, FAS and NAC1 were significantly co-expressed in OC effusions [289].

## Notch3

Notch proteins are evolutionarily conserved membrane receptors involved in embryogenesis and tissue homeostasis, affecting cellular differentiation, proliferation, survival, and apoptosis. The canonical Notch signaling pathway includes DSL ligands, having a *D*elta, *S*errate, and *L*ag2 domain, Notch receptors, and nuclear effectors. In mammals, these constitute four receptors, Notch1–4, and five ligands, including Jagged1–2 and Delta-like 1, 3, and 4. Interaction between a ligand and the N-terminal EGF-repeat region of the Notch extracellular domain (ECD) initiates a conformational change in the receptor, triggering two sequential proteolytic cleavages by the ADAM family of metalloproteases and γ-secretase. The end result of the protease cleavages is the release of the Notch intracellular domain (NICD), which is then translocated into the nucleus where it cooperates with the DNA-binding protein CSL and its co-activator Mastermind (Mam) to activate transcription of Notch downstream effectors [290, 291]. Notch signaling is dysregulated in different cancers [292] and is under active investigation for its role in cancer stem cell biology and as a therapeutic target [293]. However, the Notch pathway also has tumor suppressor activities [294].

*Notch3* gene amplification at chromosome 19p13.12 was found in 19.5% of HGSC using digital karyotyping and SNP array analysis, and *Notch3* DNA copy number was positively associated with Notch3 protein expression based on parallel IHC and FISH analysis of solid specimens and effusions. Functional inactivation of Notch3 resulted in suppression of cell proliferation and induction of apoptosis in cell lines overexpressing this molecule [295].

In a subsequent study, Jagged-1 was shown to be expressed on peritoneal mesothelial cells, and Jagged-1 knockdown resulted in reduced adhesion and proliferation in OC cells [296]. High *Notch3* in post-chemotherapy disease recurrence OC effusions by qPCR was recently shown to be associated with poor OS and PFS. Ectopic expression of *Notch3* resulted in upregulation of several stem cell markers, including Nanog, OCT4, Rex1, RIF1, and SALL4 [297].

## Spheroid and CSC-Related Studies

Though not directly related to signaling and transcription, these aspects of OC biology may certainly be briefly discussed here, as the natural continuation of the above paragraph dealing with Notch3 signaling. Both the spheroid and stem cell aspects of OC biology have been under research in recent years, not least due to their postulated role in mediating chemoresistance.

Tumor cell spheroids from ascites of patients with advanced-stage OC were shown to adhere to the ECM proteins fibronectin and type I collagen, as well as to hyaluronan

and to mesothelial cells, in part via β1 integrin, supporting that they mediate dissemination of OC cells within the peritoneal cavity. Invasion of the mesothelial layer was seen in some tumors [298, 299].

The above-discussed adhesion molecule CD44 is a postulated stem cell marker expressed in OC. Comparison of CD44-positive and CD44-negative cells isolated from primary and metastatic OC, including ascites, showed expression of β-catenin and co-expression of Toll-like receptor 4 (TLR4) and myeloid differentiation factor 88, which activate NF-κB signaling in CD44-positive tumors. These cells had constitutive NF-κB activation, were chemoresistant, and formed spheroids [300]. CD24, a membrane-linked glycoprotein expressed in multiple cancer types and another stem cell marker, was found in OC exosomes in ascites specimens [301] and was recently reported to be frequently overexpressed in OC cells in effusions compared to solid lesions [302].

A CD44+/CD24- fraction >25% was associated with higher risk of recurrence and significantly shorter PFS in a study of 19 serous OC ascites specimens [303], and the presence of a higher (>15%) fraction of ALDH-positive cells was related to shorter PFS in analysis of 15 ascites specimens [304].

Serous OC cells isolated from effusions from patients with chemoresistant tumors have higher mRNA expression of E-cadherin, EpCAM, and the CSC markers Oct4 and Stat3 compared to specimens from chemosensitive tumors [305]. Activation of JAK2 and Stat3 was observed in serous OC cells isolated from ascites following treatment with paclitaxel [306].

OC ascites was shown to contain CSC-like side populations (SP) that express the ABC transporter *ABCB1* (encoding P-glycoprotein) and the histone methyltransferase *EZH2*, and this cell population increased after chemotherapy in patient-matched sequential specimens [307].

Nestin is an intermediate filament expressed in proliferating cells during developmental stages in a variety of embryonic and fetal tissues and shown to be a CSC marker in several cancers, including OC [308, 309]. Analysis of nestin protein expression in 217 OC effusions using IHC documented its expression in tumor cells in 95.6% of specimens (Fig. 9.18c). However, no association was found between the percentage of cells expressing this protein and clinicopathologic parameters, including chemotherapy response and survival [310].

## Other Molecules

A myriad of other molecules have been investigated with respect to their expression, biological role, and clinical relevance in OC effusions. Many of these are directly or indirectly related to the above-described cancer-related cellular pathways. They are nevertheless discussed separately, as they do not belong to these pathways.

Folate (vitamin B9) is involved in one-carbon transfer reactions that are essential for RNA and DNA synthesis. Folate is also involved in the remethylation of homocysteine to methionine, an important step in the biosynthesis of S-adenosylmethionine, which provides methyl groups for methylation of DNA, RNA, proteins, and phospholipids. Cellular folate uptake is mediated by several molecules, including the folate receptor (FR) family, which consists of four family members, termed FR-α, FR-β, FR-γ, and FR-δ. The genes coding for FR, *FOLR1-4*, are located on the long arm of chromosome 11 and have about 70% sequence homology. *FOLR1* and *FOLR2* encode for membrane-bound glycoproteins, whereas *FOLR3* encodes for a secreted protein, FR-γ or FR-γ', the latter of which is a mutated form. The protein product of *FOLR4* has not been identified to date.

FR members are differentially expressed in normal and tumor tissues. FR-α, the most extensively studied family member, is expressed in urogenital organs, the female genital tract, salivary and bronchial glands, the choroid plexus, retinal pigment cells, and the placenta. High FR-α levels have been detected in genital and non-genital carcinomas. FR-β is expressed by hematopoietic cells and the placenta, as well as by leukemia and lymphoma cells. FR-γ has been detected in normal and malignant hematopoietic cells, as well as in genital carcinomas [311, 312].

FR-α has been investigated for its potential role as a target for molecular therapy, as modulator of the immune system, and as a diagnostic marker in imaging [311]. Therapeutic approaches for blocking FR-α in cancer include the use of antibodies or folic acid conjugates and vaccines targeting this protein. Many of these approaches are applied in clinical studies of OC [313].

FR-α was detected in 60% of OC ascites using an immunoradiometric assay with the MOv18/MOv19 antibodies [314]. Reduced intracellular folate availability was hypothesized to induce folate receptor expression in OC, and this parameter was therefore compared between OC ascites/cyst fluid and ascites from patients with other malignancies or benign conditions by measuring extracellular homocysteine levels. Normal folate levels were found in OC specimens. However, higher homocysteine levels in ascites/cyst fluid compared to patient-matched serum were observed in OC, postulated to result from impaired remethylation of homocysteine to methionine [315]. Forster et al. established an FCM assay for measuring FR-α in OC effusions, applying Ber-EP4 and CD45 as epithelial and leukocyte markers, respectively, in which tumor cells in all 25 studied ascites specimens expressed FR-α [316].

*FOLR1* and *FOLR3* were identified as genes that are overexpressed in OC/PPC compared to DMPM effusions [48]. In a validation study, *FOLR1*and *FOLR3* gene expression and FR-α protein expression were analyzed in a large effusion series using qPCR and FCM, respectively. *FOLR1* and

*FOLR3* mRNA and FR-α protein levels were significantly higher in OC compared to MM and breast carcinoma effusions. *FOLR1* and *FOLR3* levels were directly interrelated in OC effusions. However, *FOLR1* and *FOLR3* mRNA and FR-α protein expression in OC effusions was unrelated to clinical parameters or survival [317].

Microtubules are involved in a diverse range of cellular functions, including mitosis. Paclitaxel, a chemotherapeutic agent used in first-line chemotherapy in OC, blocks cell division by inhibition of the mitotic spindle, causing cell death. Resistance toward paclitaxel is thought to be multifactorial and involves regulation by tubulin isotypes, as well as overexpression of the multidrug transporter P-glycoprotein (P-gp), altered metabolism of the drug, decreased sensitivity to death-inducing stimuli, altered microtubule dynamics, and altered binding of paclitaxel to the microtubule [318, 319].

OC cells in four ascites specimens had significantly higher levels of class I, III, and IVa β-tubulin compared to seven untreated primary carcinomas [320]. Class III β-tubulin was found in 98.6% of 217 OC effusions using IHC in another study (Fig. 9.18d), with comparable staining extent in pre- and post-chemotherapy effusions. High class III beta-tubulin expression in pre-chemotherapy effusions was significantly associated with primary chemoresistance and with poor OS in univariate survival analysis, though not in Cox multivariate analysis [310].

P-gp, product of the *MDR1* gene, was found in 7/10 malignant effusions from OC and breast cancer patients [321]. P-gp protein and *MDR1* mRNA were found in only 14 and 19 of 75 studied OC effusions, respectively, in another study [72]. Higher expression of lung resistance-related protein (LRP) and higher degree of resistance to carboplatin in serous OC ascites compared to patient-matched omental metastases were found in analysis of 25 cases, and LRP expression predicted recurrence at 1 year. P-glycoprotein and canalicular multispecific organic anion transporter (MRP2) were absent at both anatomic sites in this study [322]. Eleven differentially expressed proteins were found in comparative analysis of ascites specimens from 12 chemosensitive and 7 intrinsically resistant serous OC using two-dimensional gel electrophoresis and mass spectrometry. Ceruloplasmin was shown to be differentially expressed using ELISA in a validation series [323].

Glutathione S-transferase-π, another protein related to chemoresistance, was expressed in 63% of 87 surgical OC specimens, including 25/28 (89%) of tumors that were resistant to cisplatin. Expression in OC cells in effusions (*n* = 24) was similar to that in the surgical specimen in the majority of cases [324].

Cellular response to DNA damage is a complex and rapidly expanding area of research, and alterations in expression and structure of molecules related to these pathways impacts on the response to radiotherapy and chemotherapy. Targeting of molecules involved in DNA repair is currently in clinical use or under clinical investigation in many cancers [325].

Hypermethylation of at least some of six analyzed genes, including the DNA repair gene *BRCA1*, mutated in hereditary OC, was found in tumor specimens, serum, and peritoneal fluids from OC patients [326].

Comparative analysis of the expression of hMSH2 and C-terminal-binding protein (CTBP) in 11 OC effusions and 9 solid tumors showed higher expression of the former in solid lesions, with comparable CTBP expression. hMSH2 expression was directly associated with better response to chemotherapy [327].

The nucleotide excision repair protein XPA was detected in OC cells in 136/142 (96%) analyzed effusions (Fig. 9.18e), and expression was significantly higher in specimens from patients who had complete response to chemotherapy compared to those with partial or no response. XPA expression in >25% of tumor cells in post-chemotherapy disease recurrence effusions was associated with longer PFS and OS in univariate analysis, and XPA was an independent predictor of PFS in multivariate analysis [328].

Several additional molecules which do not distinctly belong in one of the abovementioned pathways have been studied in OC effusions. Telomerase, the enzyme that synthesizes telomeric DNA and contributes to the ability of cancer cells to avoid aging and replicate endlessly, was shown to be expressed in OC cells in ascites and was absent in the non-tumor fraction from these specimens [329]. In another study, the presence of telomerase, as measured by the telomeric repeat amplification protocol (TRAP), was found in 27/27 peritoneal washing specimens containing OC cells, compared to 2/20 benign specimens, performing slightly better than morphology in diagnosing these specimens [330]. In analysis of 19 ascites and peritoneal washing specimens from patients with gynecological malignancies, including 10 OC, using the TRAP assay, telomerase activity was found in 5 of 6 specimens with positive cytology, 1 of 4 samples with suspicious cytology, and 1 of 9 samples with negative cytology [331].

α1-Acid glycoprotein, a 42–44-kD serum protein synthesized in the liver, was isolated from OC ascites and shown to negatively modulate the immune response in vitro [332]. The same group analyzed the association between the levels of haptoglobin, an acute-phase protein, in 21 ascites specimens and the presence of tumor at second-look laparotomy. No association was found between these two parameters. However, the group with negative findings consisted of only four patients [333].

Transthyretin, previously called prealbumin, is part of a family of proteins involved in thyroid hormone transport and additionally participates in vitamin A metabolism. Its levels are reduced in the serum of OC patients compared to controls and, although found in its full and truncated form in ascites, does not appear to originate from OC cells [334]. In

a related study, the levels of carotenoids, α-tocopherol, and retinol were found to be lower in plasma from OC patients compared to controls, and these micronutrients were detected in ascites from these OC patients at levels comparable to their plasma levels [335].

Periostin, an ECM protein shown to be produced by osteoclasts and mediate adhesion and binding to heparin in these cells, is synthesized by OC cells, was shown to be present in 20/21 OC ascites specimens by WB, and promoted integrin-mediated adhesion of OC cells [336].

Expression of mRNA of the so-called tumor rejection proteins *MAGE*, *BAGE*, and *GAGE* was found in 7–63% of 27 OC peritoneal specimens (ascites or washings), most frequently for *BAGE*. With the exception of one *BAGE*-positive specimen, 17 benign effusions were negative for these molecules [337].

Glycodelin A, a glycoprotein produced by endometrial and decidual cells, was shown to be expressed by OC cells in solid lesions and was isolated from five OC ascites specimens. It was further shown to inhibit proliferation of blood mononuclear leukocytes in vitro [338].

Analysis of the expression of cell surface aminopeptidases, involved in small peptide degradation, showed dipeptidyl peptidase IV levels in benign mesothelial cells to be the highest among four family members studied. Enzyme activity was increased following exposure to OC, but not benign ascites [339].

OC cells in ascites bound Müllerian-inhibiting substance (MIS) in 15/27 specimens analyzed and mRNA of its type II receptor was detected in 8/9 tested specimens. Inhibition of colony formation was observed in 9/11 cases in which MIS-responsive OC cells grew on soft agarose [340].

The membrane protein B7-H4 was found to be overexpressed at the gene level in OC and breast carcinoma compared to normal tissues, and its protein product was subsequently shown to be more highly expressed in OC specimens, including ascites, compared to normal tissue using WB and ELISA. Serum levels by ELISA were higher in OC patients compared to controls or patients with benign gynecological disease, and the combination of B7-H4 with CA 125 resulted in increased sensitivity in detecting OC compared to CA 125 alone [341].

Nitric oxide (NO) synthesis by NO synthase (NOS) was found in 14/38 (37%) ovarian tumors, including both solid lesions and ascites specimens, of which the majority were carcinomas. Analysis of ten patient-matched cases with both solid lesion and ascites showed similar NOS activity, evidenced by conversion of L-arginine to citrulline, measured radioactively [342].

The presence of incompletely degraded soluble products of fibrin that possess anti-angiogenic activity was recently demonstrated in ascites specimens [343]. The levels of thrombomodulin, a cell surface receptor for the serine protease thrombin, were shown to be higher in asci-tes from advanced-stage OC patients compared to benign exudates [344].

Apolipoprotein E (ApoE), a molecule involved in lipid transport and identified as overexpressed in OC by SAGE analysis [345], was studied in OC cell lines and clinical specimens. ApoE mediated cell proliferation and survival in vitro, and its expression in OC cell nuclei in primary diagnosis effusions (Fig. 9.19a) was associated with longer OS [346].

Membralin, a gene localized to chromosome 19p13.3, was shown to be highly expressed in serous OC, with tumor cells in effusions having higher expression levels than their counterparts in solid lesions [347].

Homozygous deletion of the *MKK4* gene, encoding for the tumor suppressor MAPK kinase-4, was found in high-grade serous OC, and qPCR showed reduced level of *MKK4* mRNA in OC compared to benign ovarian tissue [348].

Endothelin-converting enzyme-1 (ECE-1) , an enzyme mediating the cleavage of endothelin-1, an OC growth factor, into its active form, is significantly more highly expressed in solid OC lesions (primary and metastatic) compared to effusions, and its silencing in OC cells in vitro results in reduced signaling via the MAPK ERK1/2, reduced invasiveness, and increased E-cadherin expression and adhesion to the basement membrane proteins laminin-1 and collagen type IV [349].

S100A4, a small acidic Ca$^{2+}$-binding protein that has been shown to promote metastasis, was widely expressed in advanced-stage OC (Fig. 9.19b), and significantly higher expression was found in tumor cell nuclei in primary OC and solid metastases compared to effusions. The presence of S100A4 in primary carcinomas was associated with poor OS [350].

Osteopontin (OPN), a soluble protein present in all body fluids, is involved in signaling pathways related to adhesion and extracellular matrix interactions, affecting multiple cellular functions, including inflammation, angiogenesis, and

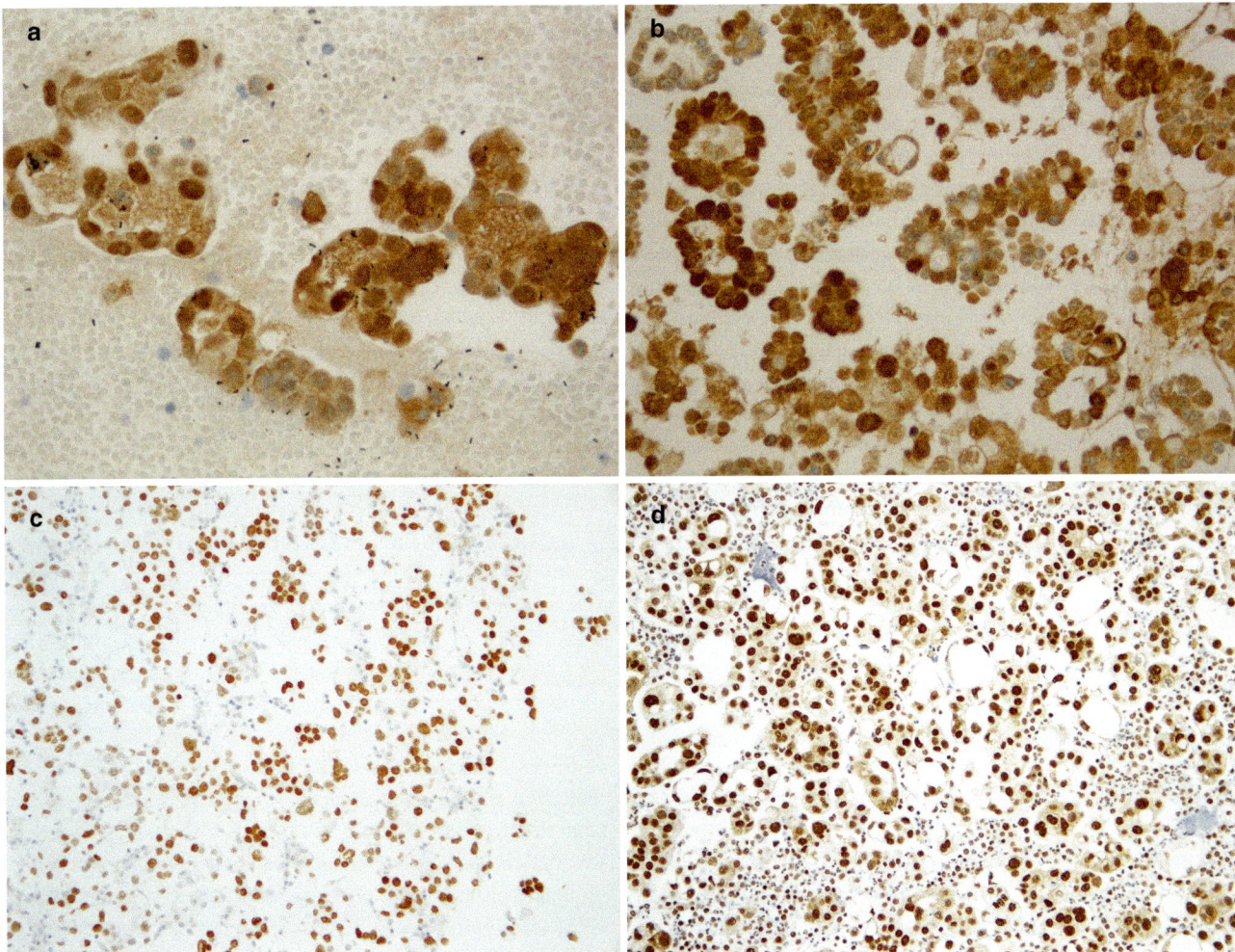

**Fig. 9.19** Various cancer-associated markers. Immunostaining for APO-E (**a**), S100A4 (**b**), HMGA2 (**c**), and HuR (**d**) in ovarian serous carcinoma effusions

tumor metastasis. OPN was detected in 126/170 (74%) OC effusions, but unexpectedly, its expression in primary diagnosis specimens was associated with longer PFS in univariate analysis [351].

Expression of members of the protein of regenerating liver (PRL) phosphatase family was analyzed in 186 OC specimens, including primary carcinomas, effusions, and solid metastases. *PRL1-3* mRNA was expressed in the majority of tumors, but *PRL-1* mRNA levels were highest in effusions. Higher *PRL-1* and *PRL-2* mRNA expression in effusions was associated with longer OS, whereas *PRL-3* mRNA and PRL-3 protein expression was unrelated to disease outcome [352].

Pregnancy-associated plasma protein A (PAPP-A), which promotes the IGF pathway, was reported to be highly expressed in OC ascites specimens ($n = 33$). Combination of chemotherapy with a neutralizing monoclonal PAPP-A antibody in a mouse model sensitized OC cells to platinum and reduced ascites formation [353].

Equilibrative and concentrative nucleoside transporters (ENTs and CNTs) mediate the cellular uptake of nucleosides used in anticancer therapy. The expression of 4 of these proteins—ENT1, ENT2, ENT4, and CNT3—was quantitatively studied in 66 OC effusions using FCM. Expression of all four molecules was detected in practically all specimens, but was unrelated to chemotherapy response or survival [354].

Calreticulin is a multifunctional $Ca^{2+}$-binding chaperone of the endoplasmic reticulum mediating cell adhesion, transcriptional regulation of steroid and other receptors, and nuclear export of glucocorticoid receptors. Calreticulin has been shown to be involved in embryogenesis, wound healing, Alzheimer's disease, and cancer. Analysis of calreticulin mRNA and protein expression in HGSC, as well as measurement of its levels in HGSC effusions supernatants, showed anatomic site-related differences between effusions, solid metastases, and primary carcinomas, with overexpression in solid lesions, as well as between peritoneal and pleural effusions. Higher protein expression in effusions was associated with better response to chemotherapy at diagnosis, but not to survival [355].

Microsomal glutathione transferase 1 (MGST1), member of the MAPEG (membrane-associated proteins in eicosanoid and glutathione metabolism) family, is a membrane protein of the endoplasmic reticulum and the outer mitochondrial membrane that protects cells from oxidative stress. As calreticulin, MGST1 mRNA was shown to be overexpressed in solid OC specimens compared to effusions. No association with clinicopathologic parameters or survival was found [356].

HMGA2, a high-mobility group AT hook (HMGA) protein, is a nonhistone nuclear protein involved in chromatin remodeling and gene transcription, which is involved in embryogenesis and cancer, mediating EMT in tumor cells. Analysis of HMGA2 protein expression by IHC in 199 effu-

sions and in 50 patient-matched primary tumors and solid metastases showed frequent expression of this molecule (Fig. 9.19c) but failed to show significant association with anatomic site or disease outcome [357].

Expression of the RNA-binding protein Hu antigen R (HuR), aka ELAV (embryonic lethal, abnormal vision, *Drosophila*)-like protein 1 (ELAVL1), member of the ELAV/Hu family, was recently studied in HGSC. Higher HuR mRNA expression in effusions (Fig. 9.19d) was significantly related to poor OS in both the entire cohort and in patients with prechemotherapy effusions tapped at diagnosis, a finding that was reproduced in Cox multivariate survival analysis [358].

Ezrin and p130Cas are cytoplasmic structural proteins modulating signaling pathways affecting the cytoskeleton and regulating cell motility and proliferation. Ezrin overexpression was found in OC cells cultured in vitro as spheroids mimicking effusion morphology compared to cells cultured on alginate scaffold and in clinical effusion specimens compared to solid tumors. Expression of neither of the two proteins was not associated with survival [359].

## Genetics and High-Throughput Analyses

Studies focusing on a single molecule, a family of molecules, or one signaling pathway may yield invaluable data that promotes our understanding of the biologically and clinically relevant events in OC effusions. Nevertheless, the possibility to obtain a larger volume of data applying high-throughput technology is an attractive approach that has been extensively utilized in studies of all cancers, including OC, in recent years. In the context of OC effusions, such studies may be informative in several respects:

1. Expanding our knowledge regarding molecular differences between various cancers affecting the serosal cavities or between tumor cells and benign cells
2. Analyses of anatomic site-related expression profiles, by comparing effusions to solid specimens
3. Analyses of OC effusions with the aim of identifying genes or proteins related to tumor biology, treatment response, and/or patient survival

Several studies based on high-throughput technology, including SAGE, digital karyotyping, and proteomics, have been described in previous sections of this chapter. This section details data regarding additional studies in this field.

Ioakim-Liossi and co-workers applied cytogenetics to short-term cultures of OC effusions, breast carcinoma effusions, and benign effusions from patients with different conditions. No genetic aberrations were found in benign effusions, whereas OC and breast carcinoma cells were frequently aneuploid and displayed an array of numerical and structural chromosomal anomalies, most frequently affecting chromosomes 1, 3, 6, 7, 8, 9, 11, 12, and 17 [360]. Frequent aneuploidy was additionally observed in a comparative study of primary serous OC and patient-matched OC effusions (Fig. 9.20) [146].

Chang et al. compared the allelic status of 20 malignant effusions, the majority from OC patients, and 20 benign effusions using digital single nucleotide polymorphism (SNP) analysis. Allelic imbalance in at least 1 of 7 studied markers was observed in 19/20 malignant effusions compared to 1/20 benign specimens [361]. In another study, loss of heterozygosity at chromosome 3p was investigated at 16 loci in a large series of OC, borderline tumors, and benign tumors, the former including 19 ascites specimens. LOH for at least 1 of the markers was observed in 21/58 malignant specimens [362].

Nagel et al. applied comparative genomic hybridization to 15 malignant cytological specimens, of which 11 were effusions and 8 were OC, and found 14 of them to be informative. Gains of genetic material were generally more frequently observed than losses, and OC specimens had most frequently gain of part or the entire long arm of chromosomes 8, 20, and 3. High amplification sites were found at 8q, at 20q, or in both 17q and 20p [363]. Although the latter study did not address the diagnostic relevance of CGH applied to effusions, it did demonstrate that these specimens are optimal for high-throughput analyses.

The ability of gene expression array analysis to differentiate cancers affecting the serosal cavities was investigated in two studies. The first one, in which serous OC specimens were compared to DMPM, has already been referred to in this chapter [48], and some of the follow-up studies validating molecules that are overexpressed in OC/PPC have been discussed earlier in this chapter [49, 50, 67, 112, 153, 268, 302, 317]. mRNA and protein expression of

PRAME (preferentially expressed antigen of melanoma), repressor of retinoic acid receptor signaling, were similarly confirmed to be higher in OC compared to MM, using qPCR and WB, respectively [364]. Rab25, an epithelial-specific member of the Rab family of small GTPases, was similarly confirmed to be overexpressed in OC compared to MM at the mRNA and protein level using qPCR and IHC, respectively [365]. MMP-7, the protein product of another gene shown to be overexpressed in OC in the gene expression analysis, was recently shown to effectively differentiate OC from MM and RMC [366]. In two additional studies, the *TNXB* and *PINCH2* genes, encoding for the ECM protein Tenascin-X and the adhesion molecule PINCH-2, were shown to be overexpressed in MM compared to OC, a finding that was also observed at the protein level for Tenascin-X [367, 368].

In a subsequent study using the same platform, the gene expression profiles of serous OC and breast carcinoma of the infiltrating ductal type (currently termed infiltrating carcinoma of no special type, NST) were compared, and 288 unique probes were found to be significantly differentially expressed in the two cancers [369]. Four validation studies of these findings were performed [370–373], of which three focused on genes overexpressed in serous OC.

mRNA levels by qPCR of scavenger receptor class A, member 3 (*SCARA3*), a molecule protecting cells by scavenging reactive oxygen species, were significantly higher in OC compared to both MM and breast carcinoma. In OC, *SCARA3* mRNA levels were significantly higher in post-compared to pre-chemotherapy effusions, but no association with survival was found [370].

*GPX3*, encoding the antioxidant enzyme glutathione peroxidase 3, and *APO1A*, encoding apolipoprotein A–I, component of high-density lipoprotein (HDL), which also has anti-inflammatory and antioxidant properties, are two addi-

**Fig. 9.20** Ploidy analysis of an aneuploid serous carcinoma with high S-phase in effusion

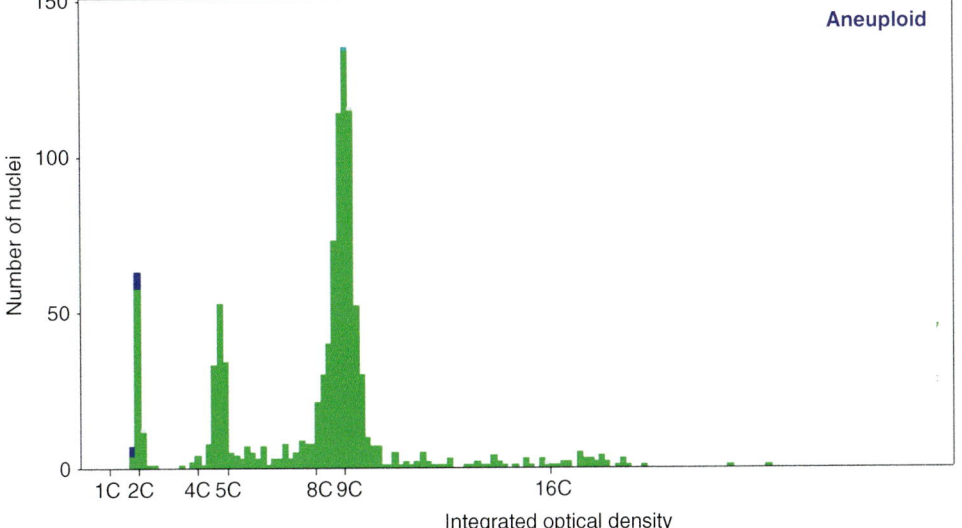

tional genes validated as overexpressed in OC compared to breast carcinoma. Additionally, higher *APOA1* mRNA levels in primary diagnosis pre-chemotherapy effusions were significantly related to longer OS in both univariate and Cox multivariate survival analysis [371].

*HOXB5* and *HOXB8*, members of the homeobox transcription factor family, are two additional genes found to be overexpressed in OC compared to breast carcinoma effusions. Analysis of HOXB5 and HOXB8 protein expression by IHC in 286 serous OC effusions and 76 patient-matched solid lesions (27 primary carcinomas, 49 metastases) showed anatomic site-related differences in the expression of both proteins. HOXB5 expression was significantly higher in post-chemotherapy compared to pre-chemotherapy effusions. In univariate survival analysis of the effusion cohort, cytoplasmic HOXB8 expression was associated with significantly shorter PFS, whereas nuclear HOXB8 expression was associated with significantly shorter OS in patients with post-chemotherapy effusions [372].

Gene expression array analysis was also used for comparing OC cells in effusions and the ovarian tumors. Analysis of 38 effusions (28 peritoneal, 10 pleural) and 8 patient-matched primary OC revealed 112 unique genes of known function that were differentially expressed between effusions (all specimens) and primary carcinomas. Genes overexpressed in effusions included *CLD7*, *KRT7*, and *KRT19*, whereas *IGFBP7*, *SPARC*, and *APOD* were among the genes overexpressed in primary OC. Peritoneal and pleural effusions were remarkably similar, with only 19 genes that were significantly differentially expressed at these 2 anatomic sites [374].

MicroRNAs (miRNAs), small noncoding RNAs that exert a regulatory effect posttranscriptionally by binding target mRNAs and inhibiting gene translation, are deregulated in cancer. Analysis of 13 OC effusions and 8 primary carcinomas using miRNA array platforms identified 3 sets of miRNAs—overexpressed in primary carcinomas, overexpressed in effusions, and highly expressed in both groups. qPCR was applied in analysis of a validation series consisting of 30 effusions and 15 primary OC. Reduced miR-145 and miR-214 and elevated let-7f, miR-182, miR-210, miR-200c, miR-222, and miR-23a levels were found in effusions in both sets. In silico target prediction programs identified potential target genes for some of the differentially expressed miRNAs. Expression of ZEB1 and c-Myc, targets of miR-200c, as well as of PAK1 and PTEN, predicted targets of miR-222, was analyzed. Inverse correlations between expression levels of the indicated miRNAs and of the predicted target genes were found. In addition, higher expression of the miRNA-processing molecules Ago1, Ago2, and Dicer was observed in effusions compared to primary carcinomas [375].

Expanded analysis of the mRNA expression of the latter 3 molecules, as well as Drosha, another miRNA-processing molecule, was subsequently performed in 144 specimens, including effusions, primary tumors, and solid metastases. Dicer, Ago1, and Ago2 protein levels were analyzed by WB. Ago1, Ago2, and Drosha mRNA levels were highest in effusions, whereas Ago1 protein expression was highest in solid metastases. Higher Ago2 protein levels in pre-chemotherapy effusions were related to shorter PFS in univariate and multivariate survival analysis [376].

Recently, the clinical role of 9 miRNAs found to be overexpressed in effusions in the abovementioned study [375] was analyzed in a series of 148 HGSC effusions. miR-29a levels were inversely related to protein expression by WB of its target DNA methyltransferase 3A (DNMT3A). Higher miR-29a levels were significantly associated with longer OS, whereas higher DNMT3A expression was significantly related to poor OS in univariate and Cox multivariate survival analysis [377].

Exosomes, 30–100 nm lipoprotein vesicles that are secreted from cells and present in most body fluids, contain proteins, mRNAs, and miRNAs. Exosomes have been gaining increasing attention as carriers of tumor messages promoting angiogenesis, tumor growth, drug resistance, and metastasis and have relevance within the biological, diagnostic, and prognostic aspects of liquid biopsies [378–380].

miRNA profiling identified 99 highly expressed miRNAs in exosomes isolated from serous OC effusion supernatants. High levels of miRNA-21, miRNA-23b, and miRNA-29a were associated with poor PFS, whereas high expression of miRNA-21 was significantly related with poor OS, the latter also in Cox multivariate analysis. LP9 mesothelial cells and ES2 OC cells exposed to effusion-derived exosomes had reduced tumor spheroid expansion and reduced mesothelial clearance area. SCID mice treated with OC exosomes had larger OC tumor load, more infiltrative tumors, and shorter survival [381].

Cappellesso and co-workers assessed the association between the tumor suppressor programmed cell death 4 (PDCD4) and its regulator miR-21 in normal ovaries, serous cystadenomas, ovarian serous OC, and cells and exosomes from benign and OC effusions using IHC, ISH, and qPCR. Gradual loss of PDCD4 and gain of miR-21 were observed from normal ovaries to OC. This inverse relationship between PDCD4 and miR-21 was also observed in cells and exosomes from effusion specimens, where benign specimens had high expression of PDCD4 and low miR-21 levels, whereas the opposite was true for OC specimens [382].

Recently, the expression and clinical role of molecules involved in exosome synthesis and secretion, including ARF6, nSMase2, TSAP6, Rab27a, and Rab27b, were analyzed in HGSC effusions and solid specimens by qPCR and WB. Secreted ARF6, nSMase2, and Rab27a protein levels in exosomes from effusion supernatants were additionally studied. nSMase2 and TSAP6 mRNA was overexpressed in effusions compared to solid specimens, whereas the opposite was true for ARF6, nSMase2, TSAP6, and Rab27a protein levels. Exosomes from effusion supernatants contained ARF6, nSMase2, and Rab27a. Higher TSAP6 protein levels in HGSC cells in effusions were associated with shorter OS, whereas higher levels of exosomal Rab27a protein were significantly related to longer OS [383].

As OC cells in effusions are chemoresistant and have CSC characteristics, there is a clear rationale in identifying molecules involved in chemoresistance in this cancer. Analysis of 32 serous OC effusions for a 380 MDR-linked gene signature using TaqMan-based qRT-PCR assay identified gene signatures predicting OS and PFS [384]. A subsequent qPCR validation analysis including 150 advanced-stage serous OC effusions focused on 14 genes shown to be associated with chemotherapy response and/or PFS in the TaqMan-based qRT-PCR assay, including *AKR1C1*, *ABCA4*, *ABCA13*, *ABCB10*, *BIRC6*, *CASP9*, *CIAPIN1*, *FAS*, *MGMT*, *MUTYH*, *POLH*, *SRC*, *TBRKB*, and *XPA*. Higher *ABCA4* and *POLH* mRNA expression was significantly related to better (complete) chemotherapy response at diagnosis. Higher mRNA expression of the anti-apoptotic molecule *CIAPIN1* was significantly related to shorter OS and PFS in univariate survival analysis for patients with pre-chemotherapy effusions, whereas *ABCA13* mRNA expression was significantly related to shorter OS. The findings for *CIAPIN1* remained an independent marker in Cox multivariate analysis of OS [385].

Several analyses of the OC effusion proteome have been performed, in addition to the analyses previously described in this chapter [22, 252].

Gortzak-Uzan et al. combined proteomics and web-based microarray data to analysis of ascites specimens with the aim of identifying robustly expressed OC-specific proteins. Eighty candidate biomarkers were identified, including proteins present in urine and plasma in addition to ascites, proteins present only in ascites, and proteins involved in protein-protein interactions, providing a basis for further research into the role of these molecules [386].

In an additional study, autoantibody signatures of OC cells were studied using high-density protein arrays. Comparative analysis of 30 OC effusions and 30 benign effusions identified 15 tumor-associated antigens, of which nine had a known cellular function [387].

Puiffe and co-workers applied ascites from 54 patients to OV-90 OC cells and observed inhibitory or stimulatory effects on different cellular parameters, including invasion, proliferation, and spheroid formation. The gene expression profiles of OV-90 cells exposed to invasion-inhibitory and invasion-stimulatory ascites were compared, revealing 243 probe sets that were significantly differentially expressed [388].

Differences in the proteomes of patient-matched primary diagnosis pre-chemotherapy and disease recurrence post-chemotherapy serous OC effusions were recently studied using liquid chromatography coupled with mass spectrometry. Analysis of nine paired specimens showed upregulation of several proteins, including CP, FN1, SYK, CD97, AIF1, WNK1, SERPINA3, APOD, URP2, STAT5B, and RELA (NF-κB p65), and data were validated by quantitative RT-PCR. In vitro analysis of OC cells using different assays showed association between RELA and STAT5B expression and reduced response to carboplatin [389].

Another STAT family member, STAT3, was recently shown to be constitutively activated in OC cells in ascites specimens. pSTAT3 expression was associated with large primary tumor and widespread peritoneal metastases in a mouse model. Treatment with the STAT3 inhibitor HO-3867 suppressed tumor growth, angiogenesis, and metastasis in vivo and had cytotoxic activity in ex vivo cultures of human OC, including in chemoresistant tumors [390].

Metabolomics is another method that has been applied to OC effusion research. Analysis of 115 effusion supernatants by high-resolution magnetic resonance (MR) spectroscopy showed that OC specimens ($n = 95$) had elevated levels of ketones and lactate compared to MM ($n = 10$) and breast carcinomas ($n = 10$), whereas the latter had higher levels of glucose, alanine, and pyruvate. Analysis of eight pairs of patient-matched pre- and post-chemotherapy OC effusions showed a significant increase in glucose and lipid levels in the latter [391].

A recent MR analysis of 48 benign and 44 malignant effusions, the latter including five OC, identified increased signals related to lipids, branched amino acids, and lactate in the malignant specimens [392].

## Future Perspectives

OC remains a highly lethal disease due to late detection and primary or acquired chemoresistance. The key to improving the dismal outcome of patients with this cancer is early detection. However, as this approach is yet to be proven cost-effective, efforts must be made in parallel to improve the treatment of OC patients, especially through the addition of targeted therapy to aggressive surgery and optimized chemotherapy.

The body of data presented in this chapter provides evidence regarding the complexity of protein and gene expression patterns in OC cells in effusions. While this complexity characterizes all cancers, it is fairly safe to state that the common predilection of OC, especially of the serous type, to the unique microenvironment of the serosal cavities, is responsible for biological patterns that are shared by no other malignancy. As evident from many of the studies presented in this chapter, cancer-associated molecules are additionally often differentially expressed in primary OC, effusions, and solid metastases. Furthermore, pre- and post-chemotherapy effusions have different expression patterns, and a given molecule may have a different predictive and prognostic role at diagnosis vs. disease recurrence.

Designing new therapeutic strategies against cancer requires understanding of the biological mechanisms which sustain and promote tumor cell proliferation and survival. In particular, our understanding of the cellular mechanisms mediating resistance to chemotherapy is crucial for overcoming this major obstacle in treating cancer patients. While precious knowledge has been and is currently gained through in vitro and animal studies, studies of patient material from large and well-characterized cohorts are the ultimate test of relevance and are the ones to decide the clinical role of new molecules considered as possible candidates for targeted therapy. In OC, such studies must include effusion specimens, both at diagnosis and at each disease recurrence, as these are present in the majority of patients with advanced disease, and contribute significantly to the morbidity and mortality from this disease. Indeed, this fact has been gaining the attention of many research groups in recent years. Culturing of OC cells from effusions in the objective of testing current or novel therapeutics can yield important information directing therapy [393]. The use of cutting-edge genomic approaches, including NGS, in analysis of disease heterogeneity and progression, either in analyses focused on effusions or in analyses of multiple anatomic sites in which some effusion specimens have been included, has been increasingly evident [394–398]. It is to be hoped that these technological advances will result in better understanding and treatment of this cancer.

# References

1. Cancer Genome Atlas Research Network. Integrated genomic analyses of ovarian carcinoma. Nature. 2011;474:609–15.
2. Steeg PS. Targeting metastasis. Nat Rev Cancer. 2016;16:201–18.
3. Thibault B, Castells M, Delord JP, Couderc B. Ovarian cancer microenvironment: implications for cancer dissemination and chemoresistance acquisition. Cancer Metastasis Rev. 2014;33:17–39.
4. Ahmed N, Stenvers KL. Getting to know ovarian cancer ascites: opportunities for targeted therapy-based translational research. Front Oncol. 2013;3:256.
5. Davidson B. Recently identified drug resistance biomarkers in ovarian cancer. Expert Rev Mol Diagn. 2016;16:569–78.
6. Shirayoshi Y, Hatta K, Hosoda M, Tsunasawa S, Sakiyama F, Takeichi M. Cadherin cell adhesion molecules with distinct binding specificities share a common structure. EMBO J. 1986;5:2485–8.
7. Behrens J. Cadherins and catenins: role in signal transduction and tumor progression. Cancer Metastasis Rev. 1999;18:15–30.
8. Vleminckx K, Vakaet L Jr, Mareel M, Fiers W, van Roy F. Genetic manipulation of E-cadherin expression by epithelial tumor cells reveals an invasion suppressor role. Cell. 1991;66:107–19.
9. Hajra KM, Fearon ER. Cadherin and catenin alterations in human cancer. Genes Chromosomes Cancer. 2002;34:255–68.
10. Bruner HC, Derksen PWB. Loss of E-Cadherin-dependent cell-cell adhesion and the development and progression of cancer. Cold Spring Harb Perspect Biol. 2018;10(3):pii: a029330.
11. Kourtidis A, Lu R, Pence LJ, Anastasiadis PZ. A central role for cadherin signaling in cancer. Exp Cell Res. 2017;358:78–85.
12. Zeisberg M, Neilson EG. Biomarkers for epithelial-mesenchymal transitions. J Clin Invest. 2009;119:1429–37.
13. Peinado H, Olmeda D, Cano A. Snail, Zeb and bHLH factors in tumour progression: an alliance against the epithelial phenotype? Nat Rev Cancer. 2007;7:415–28.
14. Kalluri R, Weinberg RA. The basics of epithelial-mesenchymal transition. J Clin Invest. 2009;119:1420–8.
15. Risinger JI, Berchuck A, Kohler MF, Boyd J. Mutations of the E-cadherin gene in human gynecologic cancers. Nat Genet. 1994;7:98–102.
16. Palacios J, Gamallo C. Mutations in the beta-catenin gene (CTNNB1) in endometrioid ovarian carcinomas. Cancer Res. 1998;58:1344–7.
17. Davidson B, Tropé CG, Reich R. Epithelial-mesenchymal transition in ovarian carcinoma. Front Oncol. 2012;2:33.
18. Davidson B, Berner A, Nesland JM, Risberg B, Berner HS, Tropé CG, Kristensen GM, Bryne M, Flørenes VA. E-cadherin and α-, β- and γ-catenin protein expression is up-regulated in ovarian carcinoma cells in serous effusions. J Pathol. 2000;192:460–9.
19. Sivertsen S, Berner A, Michael C, Bedrossian B, Davidson B. Ovarian carcinoma and malignant mesothelioma cells in effusions have comparable cadherin expression. Acta Cytol. 2006;50:603–7.
20. Elloul S, Bukholt Elstrand M, Nesland JM, Tropé CG, Kvalheim G, Goldberg I, Reich R, Davidson B. Snail, Slug, and Smad-interacting protein 1 as novel parameters of disease aggressiveness in metastatic ovarian and breast carcinoma. Cancer. 2005;103:1631–43.
21. Davidson B, Holth A, Hellesylt E, Tan TZ, Huang RYJ, Tropé CG, Nesland JM, Thiery JP. The clinical role of epithelial-mesenchymal transition and stem cell markers in advanced-stage serous ovarian carcinoma effusions. Hum Pathol. 2015;46:1–8.
22. Kim G, Davidson B, Henning R, Wang J, Yu M, Annunziata C, Hetland T, Kohn EC. Adhesion molecule protein signature in ovarian cancer effusions is prognostic of patient outcome. Cancer. 2012;118:1543–53.
23. Elloul S, Silins I, Tropé CG, Benshushan A, Davidson B, Sitedependent RR. expression of E-cadherin transcriptional regulators in ovarian carcinoma. Virchows Arch. 2006;449:520–8.
24. Elloul S, Vaksman O, Tuft Stavnes H, Tropé CG, Davidson B, Reich R. Mesenchymal-to-epithelial transition determinants as characteristics of ovarian carcinoma effusions. Clin Exp Metastasis. 2010;27:161–72.
25. Hood JD, Cheresh DA. Role of integrins in cell invasion and migration. Nat Rev Cancer. 2002;2:91–100.
26. Sanders RJ, Mainiero F, Giancotti FP. The role of integrins in tumorigenesis and metastasis. Cancer Invest. 1998;16:329–44.
27. Seguin L, Desgrosellier JS, Weis SM, Cheresh DA. Integrins and cancer: regulators of cancer stemness, metastasis, and drug resistance. Trends Cell Biol. 2015;25:234–40.
28. Moser TL, Pizzo SV, Bafetti LM, Fishman DA, Stack MS. Evidence for preferential adhesion of ovarian epithelial carcinoma cells to type I collagen mediated by the α2β1 integrin. Int J Cancer. 1996;67:695–701.
29. Strobel T, Cannistra SA. β1-integrins partly mediate binding of ovarian cancer cells to peritoneal mesothelium in vitro. Gynecol Oncol. 1999;73:362–7.
30. Lessan K, Aguiar DJ, Oegema T, Siebenson L, Skubitz AP. CD44 and β1 integrin mediate ovarian carcinoma cell adhesion to peritoneal mesothelial cells. Am J Pathol. 1999;154:1525–37.

31. Skubitz APN, Bast RC Jr, Wayner EA, Letourneau PC, Wilke MS. Expression of α6 and β4 integrins in serous ovarian carcinoma correlates with expression of the basement membrane protein laminin. Am J Pathol. 1996;148:1445–61.

32. Cannistra SA, Ottensmeier C, Niloff J, Orta B, DiCarlo J. Expression and function of β1 and αvβ3 integrins in ovarian cancer. Gynecol Oncol. 1995;58:216–25.

33. Davidson B, Goldberg I, Reich R, Tell L, Dong HP, Tropé CG, Risberg B, Kopolovic J. αv and β1 integrin subunits are commonly expressed in malignant effusions from ovarian carcinoma patients. Gynecol Oncol. 2003;90:248–57.

34. Goldberg I, Davidson B, Reich R, Gotlieb WH, Ben-Baruch G, Bryne M, Berner A, Nesland JM, Kopolovic J. αV integrin is a novel marker of poor prognosis in advanced-stage ovarian carcinoma. Clin Cancer Res. 2001;7:4073–9.

35. Byers LJ, Osborne JL, Carson LF, Carter JR, Haney AF, Weinberg JB, Ramakrishnan S. Increased levels of laminin in ascitic fluid of patients with ovarian cancer. Cancer Lett. 1995;88:67–72.

36. Givant-Horwitz V, Davidson B, van de Putte G, Dong HP, Goldberg I, Amir S, Kristensen GB, Reich R. Expression of the 67kDa laminin receptor and the α6 integrin subunit in serous ovarian carcinoma. Clin Exp Metastasis. 2003;20:599–609.

37. Ahmed N, Riley C, Oliva K, Rice G, Quinn M. Ascites induces modulation of alpha6beta1 integrin and urokinase plasminogen activator receptor expression and associated functions in ovarian carcinoma. Br J Cancer. 2005;92:1475–85.

38. Bar JK, Grelewski P, Popiela A, Noga L, Rabczyñski J. Type IV collagen and CD44v6 expression in benign, malignant primary and metastatic ovarian tumors: correlation with Ki-67 and p53 immunoreactivity. Gynecol Oncol. 2004;95:23–31.

39. Cracchiolo BM, Hanauske-Abel HM, Schwartz PE, Chambers JT, Holland B, Chambers SK. Procollagen-derived biomarkers in malignant ascites of ovarian cancer. Independent prognosticators for progression-free interval and survival. Gynecol Oncol. 2002;87:24–33.

40. Zhu GG, Risteli J, Puistola U, Kauppila A, Risteli L. Progressive ovarian carcinoma induces synthesis of type I and type III procollagens in the tumor tissue and peritoneal cavity. Cancer Res. 1993;53:5028–32.

41. Kohn EC, Travers LA, Kassis J, Broome U, Klominek J. Malignant effusions are sources of fibronectin and other promigratory and proinvasive components. Diagn Cytopathol. 2005;33:300–8.

42. Olt G, Berchuck A, Soisson AP, Boyer CM, Bast RC Jr. Fibronectin is an immunosuppressive substance associated with epithelial ovarian cancer. Cancer. 1992;70:2137–42.

43. Menzin AW, Loret de Mola JR, Bilker WB, Wheeler JE, Rubin SC, Feinberg RF. Identification of oncofetal fibronectin in patients with advanced epithelial ovarian cancer: detection in ascitic fluid and localization to primary sites and metastatic implants. Cancer. 1998;82:152–8.

44. Tabariès S, Siegel PM. The role of claudins in cancer metastasis. Oncogene. 2017;36:1176–90.

45. Tassi RA, Bignotti E, Falchetti M, Ravanini M, Calza S, Ravaggi A, Bandiera E, Facchetti F, Pecorelli S, Santin AD. Claudin-7 expression in human epithelial ovarian cancer. Int J Gynecol Cancer. 2008;18:1262–71.

46. Lonardi S, Manera C, Marucci R, Santoro A, Lorenzi L, Facchetti F. Usefulness of Claudin 4 in the cytological diagnosis of serosal effusions. Diagn Cytopathol. 2011;39:313–7.

47. Jo VY, Cibas ES, Pinkus GS. Claudin-4 immunohistochemistry is highly effective in distinguishing adenocarcinoma from malignant mesothelioma in effusion cytology. Cancer Cytopathol. 2014;122:299–306.

48. Davidson B, Zhang Z, Kleinberg L, Li M, Flørenes VA, Wang TL, IeM S. Gene expression signatures differentiate ovarian/peritoneal serous carcinoma from diffuse malignant peritoneal mesothelioma. Clin Cancer Res. 2006;12:5944–50.

49. Kleinberg L, Holth A, Fridman E, Schwartz I, Shih IM, Davidson B. The diagnostic role of claudins in serous effusions. Am J Clin Pathol. 2007;127:928–37.

50. Kleinberg L, Holth A, Tropé CG, Reich R, Davidson B. Claudin upregulation in ovarian carcinoma effusions is associated with poor survival. Hum Pathol. 2008;39:747–57.

51. Underhill C. CD44: the hyaluronan receptor. J Cell Sci. 1992;103:293–8.

52. Orian-Rousseau V. CD44, a therapeutic target for metastasising tumours. Eur J Cancer. 2010;46:1271–7.

53. Senbanjo LT, Chellaiah MA. CD44: a multifunctional cell surface adhesion receptor is a regulator of progression and metastasis of cancer cells. Front Cell Dev Biol. 2017;5:18.

54. Muinao T, Deka Boruah HP, Pal M. Diagnostic and prognostic biomarkers in ovarian cancer and the potential roles of cancer stem cells—an updated review. Exp Cell Res. 2018;362(1):1–10.

55. Cannistra SA, Kansas GS, Niloff J, DeFranzo B, Kim Y, Ottensmeier C. Binding of ovarian cancer cells to peritoneal mesothelium in vitro is partly mediated by CD44H. Cancer Res. 1993;53:3830–8.

56. Meunier L, Puiffe ML, Le Page C, Filali-Mouhim A, Chevrette M, Tonin PN, Provencher DM, Mes-Masson AM. Effect of ovarian cancer ascites on cell migration and gene expression in an epithelial ovarian cancer in vitro model. Transl Oncol. 2010;3:230–8.

57. Yang W, Toffa SE, Lohn JW, Seifalian AM, Winslet MC. Malignant ascites increases the antioxidant ability of human ovarian (SKOV-3) and gastric adenocarcinoma (KATO-III) cells. Gynecol Oncol. 2005;96:430–8.

58. Berner HS, Davidson B, Berner A, Risberg B, Nesland JM. Differential expression of CD44s and CD44v3-10 in adenocarcinoma cells and reactive mesothelial cells in effusions. Virchows Arch. 2000;436:330–5.

59. Berner HS, Davidson B, Berner A, Risberg B, Kristensen GB, Tropé CG, Van de Putte G, Nesland JM. Expression of CD44 in effusions of patients diagnosed with serous ovarian carcinoma—diagnostic and prognostic implications. Clin Exp Metastasis. 2000;18:197–202.

60. Dong WG, Sun XM, Yu BP, Luo HS, Yu JP. Role of VEGF and CD44v6 in differentiating benign from malignant ascites. World J Gastroenterol. 2003;9:2596–600.

61. Taylor DD, Gercel-Taylor C, Gall SA. Expression and shedding of CD44 variant isoforms in patients with gynecologic malignancies. J Soc Gynecol Investig. 1996;3:289–94.

62. Byrd JC, Bresalier RS. Mucins and mucin binding proteins in colorectal cancer. Cancer Metastasis Rev. 2004;23:77–99.

63. Carraway KL 3rd, Funes M, Workman HC, Sweeney C. Contribution of membrane mucins to tumor progression through modulation of cellular growth signaling pathways. Curr Top Dev Biol. 2007;78:1–22.

64. van Putten JPM, Strijbis K. Transmembrane mucins: signaling receptors at the intersection of inflammation and cancer. J Innate Immun. 2017;9:281–99.

65. Singh AP, Chaturvedi P, Batra SK. Emerging roles of MUC4 in cancer: a novel target for diagnosis and therapy. Cancer Res. 2007;67:433–6.

66. Gautam SK, Kumar S, Cannon A, Hall B, Bhatia R, Nasser MW, Mahapatra S, Batra SK, Jain M. MUC4 mucin- a therapeutic target for pancreatic ductal adenocarcinoma. Expert Opin Ther Targets. 2017;21:657–69.

67. Davidson B, Baekelandt M, Shih IM. MUC4 is upregulated in ovarian carcinoma effusions and differentiates carcinoma cells from mesothelial cells. Diagn Cytopathol. 2007;35:756–60.

68. Iacono KT, Brown AL, Greene MI, Saouaf SJ. CD147 immuno-globulin superfamily receptor function and role in pathology. Exp Mol Pathol. 2007;83:283–95.

69. Xin X, Zeng X, Gu H, Li M, Tan H, Jin Z, Hua T, Shi R, Wang H. CD147/EMMPRIN overexpression and prognosis in cancer: A systematic review and meta-analysis. Sci Rep. 2016;6:32804.

70. Davidson B, Goldberg I, Berner A, Kristensen GB, Reich R. EMMPRIN (extracellular matrix metalloproteinase inducer) is a novel marker of poor outcome in serous ovarian carcinoma. Clin Exp Metastasis. 2003;20:161–9.

71. Davidson B, Givant-Horwitz V, Lazarovici P, Risberg B, Nesland JM, Tropé CG, Schaefer E, Reich R. Matrix metalloproteinases (MMP), EMMPRIN (extracellular matrix metalloproteinase inducer) and mitogen-activated protein kinases (MAPK): co-expression in metastatic serous ovarian carcinoma. Clin Exp Metastasis. 2003;20:621–31.

72. Davidson B, Goldberg I, Givant-Horwitz V, Nesland JM, Berner A, Bryne M, Risberg B, Kopolovic J, Kristensen GB, Tropé CG, van de Putte G, Reich R. Caveolin-1 expression in ovarian carcinoma is MDR1 independent. Am J Clin Pathol. 2002;117:225–34.

73. Patapoutian A, Reichardt LF. Trk receptors: mediators of neurotrophin action. Curr Opin Neurobiol. 2001;11:272–80.

74. Teng KK, Hempstead BL. Neurotrophins and their receptors: signaling trios in complex biological systems. Cell Mol Life Sci. 2004;61:35–48.

75. Nakagawara A. Trk receptor tyrosine kinases: A bridge between cancer and neural development. Cancer Lett. 2001;169:107–14.

76. Fanburg-Smith JC, Miettinen M. Low-affinity nerve growth factor receptor (p75) in dermatofibrosarcoma protuberans and other nonneuronal tumors: a study of 1,150 tumors and fetal and adult normal tissues. Hum Pathol. 2001;32:976–83.

77. Vaishnavi A, Le AT, Doebele RC. TRKing down an old oncogene in a new era of targeted therapy. Cancer Discov. 2015;5:25–34.

78. Khotskaya YB, Holla VR, Farago AF, Mills Shaw KR, Meric-Bernstam F, Hong DS. Targeting TRK family proteins in cancer. Pharmacol Ther. 2017;173:58–66.

79. Davidson B, Lazarovici P, Ezersky A, Nesland JM, Berner A, Risberg B, Tropé CG, Kristensen GB, Goscinski M, van de Putte G, Reich R. Expression levels of the NGF receptors TrkA and p75 in effusions and solid tumors of serous ovarian carcinoma patients. Clin Cancer Res. 2001;7:3457–64.

80. Davidson B, Reich R, Lazarovici P, Nesland JM, Risberg B, Tropé CG, Flørenes VA. Expression and activation of the nerve growth factor receptor TrkA in serous ovarian carcinoma. Clin Cancer Res. 2003;9:2248–59.

81. Yu X, Liu L, Cai B, He Y, Wan X. Suppression of anoikis by the neurotrophic receptor TrkB in human ovarian cancer. Cancer Sci. 2008;99:543–52.

82. Egeblad M, Werb Z. New functions for the matrix metalloproteinases in cancer progression. Nat Rev Cancer. 2002;2:161–74.

83. Bjorklund M, Koivunen E. Gelatinase-mediated migration and invasion of cancer cells. Biochim Biophys Acta. 2005;1755:37–69.

84. Levin M, Udi Y, Solomonov I, Sagi I. Next generation matrix metalloproteinase inhibitors—novel strategies bring new prospects. Biochim Biophys Acta. 2017;1864:1927–39.

85. Jobin PG, Butler GS, Overall CM. New intracellular activities of matrix metalloproteinases shine in the moonlight. Biochim Biophys Acta. 2017;1864:2043–55.

86. Young TN, Rodriguez GC, Rinehart AR, Bast RCJ, Pizzo SV, Stack MS. Characterization of gelatinases linked to extracellular matrix invasion in ovarian adenocarcinoma: purification of matrix metalloproteinase 2. Gynecol Oncol. 1996;62:89–99.

87. Fishman DA, Bafetti LM, Banionis S, Kearns AS, Chilukuri K, Stack MS. Production of extracellular matrix-degrading proteinases by primary cultures of human epithelial ovarian carcinoma cells. Cancer. 1997;80:1457–63.

88. Fishman DA, Bafetti LM, Stack MS. Membrane-type matrix metalloproteinase expression and matrix metalloproteinase-2 activation in primary human ovarian epithelial carcinoma cells. Invasion Metastasis. 1996;16:150–9.

89. Sun XM, Dong WG, Yu BP, Luo HS, Yu JP. Detection of type IV collagenase activity in malignant ascites. World J Gastroenterol. 2003;9:2592–5.

90. Davidson B, Reich R, Berner A, Givant-Horwitz V, Goldberg I, Risberg B, Kristensen GB, Tropé CG, Bryne M, Kopolovic J, Nesland JM. Ovarian carcinoma cells in serous effusions show altered MMP-2 and TIMP-2 mRNA levels. Eur J Cancer. 2001;37:2040–9.

91. Davidson B, Goldberg I, Berner A, Nesland JM, Givant-Horwitz V, Bryne M, Risberg B, Kristensen GB, Tropé CG, Kopolovic J, Reich R. Expression of membrane-type 1,2 and 3 matrix metalloproteinases messenger RNA in ovarian carcinoma cells in serous effusions. Am J Clin Pathol. 2001;115:517–24.

92. Duffy MJ, Duggan C. The urokinase plasminogen activator system: a rich source of tumour markers for the individualized management of patients with cancer. Clin Biochem. 2004;37:541–8.

93. Blasi F, Carmeliet P. uPAR: a versatile signalling orchestrator. Nat Rev Mol Cell Biol. 2002;3:932–42.

94. Su SC, Lin CW, Yang WE, Fan WL, Yang SF. The urokinase-type plasminogen activator (uPA) system as a biomarker and therapeutic target in human malignancies. Expert Opin Ther Targets. 2016;20:551–66.

95. Young TN, Rodriguez GC, Moser TL, Bast RC Jr, Pizzo SV, Stack MS. Coordinate expression of urinary-type plasminogen activator and its receptor accompanies malignant transformation of the ovarian surface epithelium. Am J Obstet Gynecol. 1994;170:1285–96.

96. Sier CF, Stephens R, Bizik J, Mariani A, Bassan M, Pedersen N, Frigerio L, Ferrari A, Danø K, Brünner N, Blasi F. The level of urokinase-type plasminogen activator receptor is increased in serum of ovarian cancer patients. Cancer Res. 1998;58:1843–9.

97. Sier CF, Nicoletti I, Santovito ML, Frandsen T, Aletti G, Ferrari A, Lissoni A, Giavazzi R, Blasi F, Sidenius N. Metabolism of tumour-derived urokinase receptor and receptor fragments in cancer patients and xenografted mice. Thromb Haemost. 2004;91:403–11.

98. Chambers SK, Gertz RE Jr, Ivins CM, Kacinski BM. The significance of urokinase- type plasminogen activator, its inhibitors, and its receptor in ascites of patients with epithelial ovarian cancer. Cancer. 1995;75:1627–33.

99. Price FV, Chambers SK, Chambers JT, Carcangiu ML, Schwartz PE, Kohorn EI, Stanley ER, Kacinski BM. Colony-stimulating factor-1 in primary ascites of ovarian cancer is a significant predictor of survival. Am J Obstet Gynecol. 1993;168:520–7.

100. Kobayashi H, Hirashima Y, Sun GW, Ohi H, Fujie M, Terao T. Identification and characterization of a Kunitz-type protease inhibitor in ascites fluid from patients with ovarian carcinoma. Int J Cancer. 2000;87:44–54.

101. Avgeris M, Scorilas A. Kallikrein-related peptidases (KLKs) as emerging therapeutic targets: focus on prostate cancer and skin pathologies. Expert Opin Ther Targets. 2016;20:801–18.

102. Shih IM, Salani R, Fiegl M, Wang TL, Soosaipillai A, Marth C, Müller-Holzner E, Gastl G, Zhang Z, Diamandis EP. Ovarian cancer specific kallikrein profile in effusions. Gynecol Oncol. 2007;105:501–7.

103. Davidson B, Xi Z, Klokk TI, Tropé CG, Dørum A, Scheistrøen M, Saatcioglu F. Kallikrein 4 expression is upregulated in ovarian carcinoma cells in effusions. Am J Clin Pathol. 2005;123:360–8.

104. Dong Y, Tan OL, Loessner D, Stephens C, Walpole C, Boyle GM, Parsons PG, Clements JA. Kallikrein-related peptidase 7 promotes multicellular aggregation via the alpha(5)beta(1) integrin pathway and paclitaxel chemoresistance in serous epithelial ovarian carcinoma. Cancer Res. 2010;70:2624–33.

105. Trackman PC. Lysyl oxidase isoforms and potential therapeutic opportunities for fibrosis and cancer. Expert Opin Ther Targets. 2016;20:935–45.
106. Sebban S, Davidson B, Reich R. Lysyl oxidase-like 4 is alternatively spliced in an anatomic site-specific manner in tumors involving the serosal cavities. Virchows Arch. 2009;454:71–9.
107. Sebban S, Golan-Gerstl R, Karni R, Vaksman O, Davidson B, Reich R. Alternatively spliced lysyl oxidase-like 4 isoforms have a pro-metastatic role in cancer. Clin Exp Metastasis. 2013;30:103–17.
108. Kassis J, Klominek J, Kohn EC. Tumor microenvironment: what can effusions teach us? Diagn Cytopathol. 2005;33:316–9.
109. Li H, Batth IS, Qu X, Xu L, Song N, Wang R, Liu Y. IGF-IR signaling in epithelial to mesenchymal transition and targeting IGF-IR therapy: overview and new insights. Mol Cancer. 2017;16:6.
110. Bach LA, Headey SJ, Norton RS. IGF-binding proteins—the pieces are falling into place. Trends Endocrinol Metab. 2005;16:228–34.
111. Firth SM, Baxter RC. Cellular actions of the insulin-like growth factor binding proteins. Endocr Rev. 2002;23:824–54.
112. Slipicevic A, Øy GF, Askildt IC, Holth A, Hellesylt E, Flørenes VA, Davidson B. The diagnostic and prognostic role of the insulin growth factor pathway members IGF-II and IGFBP3 in serous effusions. Hum Pathol. 2009;40:527–37.
113. Fidler IJ, Ellis LM. The implications of angiogenesis for the biology and therapy of cancer metastasis. Cell. 1994;79:185–8.
114. Folkman J, Klagsbrun M. Angiogenic factors. Science. 1987;235:442–7.
115. Roy H, Bhardwaj S, Yla-Herttuala S. Biology of vascular endothelial growth factors. FEBS Lett. 2006;580:2879–87.
116. Matulonis UA, Sood AK, Fallowfield L, Howitt BE, Sehouli J, Karlan BY. Ovarian cancer. Nat Rev Dis Primers. 2016;2:16061.
117. Presta M, Chiodelli P, Giacomini A, Rusnati M, Ronca R. Fibroblast growth factors (FGFs) in cancer: FGF traps as a new therapeutic approach. Pharmacol Ther. 2017;179:171–87.
118. Clayton NS, Wilson AS, Laurent EP, Grose RP, Carter EP. Fibroblast growth factor-mediated crosstalk in cancer etiology and treatment. Dev Dyn. 2017;246:493–501.
119. Alfaro C, Sanmamed MF, Rodríguez-Ruiz ME, Teijeira Á, Oñate C, González Á, Ponz M, Schalper KA, Pérez-Gracia JL, Melero I. Interleukin-8 in cancer pathogenesis, treatment and follow-up. Cancer Treat Rev. 2017;60:24–31.
120. Olson TA, Mohanraj D, Carson LF, Ramakrishnan S. Vascular permeability factor gene expression in normal and neoplastic human ovaries. Cancer Res. 1994;54:276–80.
121. Boocock CA, Charnock-Jones DS, Sharkey AM, McLaren J, Barker PJ, Wright KA, Twentyman PR, Smith SK. Expression of vascular endothelial growth factor and its receptors flt and KDR in ovarian carcinoma. J Natl Cancer Inst. 1995;87:506–16.
122. Barton DP, Cai A, Wendt K, Young M, Gamero A, De Cesare S. Angiogenic protein expression in advanced epithelial ovarian cancer. Clin Cancer Res. 1997;3:1579–86.
123. Santin AD, Hermonat PL, Ravaggi A, Cannon MJ, Pecorelli S, Parham GP. Secretion of vascular endothelial growth factor in ovarian cancer. Eur J Gynaecol Oncol. 1999;20:177–81.
124. Kraft A, Weindel K, Ochs A, Marth C, Zmija J, Schumacher P, Unger C, Marmé D, Gastl G. Vascular endothelial growth factor in the sera and effusions of patients with malignant and nonmalignant disease. Cancer. 1999;85:178–87.
125. Steele IA, Edmondson RJ, Bulmer JN, Bolger BS, Leung HY, Davies BR. Induction of FGF receptor 2-IIIb expression and response to its ligands in epithelial ovarian cancer. Oncogene. 2001;20:5878–87.
126. Davidson B, Reich R, Kopolovic J, Berner A, Nesland JM, Kristensen GB, Tropé CG, Bryne M, Risberg B, van de Putte G, Goldberg I. Interleukin-8 and vascular endothelial growth factor mRNA levels are down-regulated in ovarian carcinoma cells in serous effusions. Clin Exp Metastasis. 2002;19:135–44.
127. Parish CR, Freeman C, Hulett MD. Heparanase: a key enzyme involved in cell invasion. Biochim Biophys Acta. 2001;1471:M99–M108.
128. Sanderson RD, Elkin M, Rapraeger AC, Ilan N, Vlodavsky I. Heparanase regulation of cancer, autophagy and inflammation: new mechanisms and targets for therapy. FEBS J. 2017;284:42–55.
129. Davidson B, Shafat I, Ilan N, Tropé CG, Vlodavsky I, Reich R. Heparanase expression correlates with poor survival in metastatic ovarian carcinoma. Gynecol Oncol. 2007;104:311–9.
130. Ong CHP, Bateman A. Progranulin (Granulin-epithelin precursor, PC-cell derived growth factor, Acrogranin) in proliferation and tumorigenesis. Histol Histopathol. 2003;18:1275–88.
131. Kamrava M, Simpkins F, Alejandro E, Michener C, Meltzer E, Kohn EC. Lysophosphatidic acid and endothelin-induced proliferation of ovarian cancer cell lines is mitigated by neutralization of granulin-epithelin precursor (GEP), a prosurvival factor for ovarian cancer. Oncogene. 2005;24:7084–93.
132. Davidson B, Alejandro E, Flørenes VA, Goderstad JM, Risberg B, Kristensen GB, Tropé CG, Kohn EC. Granulin-epithelin precursor (GEP) is a novel prognostic marker in epithelial ovarian cancer. Cancer. 2004;100:2139–47.
133. Meulmeester E, Ten Dijke P. The dynamic roles of TGF-β in cancer. J Pathol. 2011;223:205–18.
134. Smith AL, Robin TP, Ford HL. Molecular pathways: targeting the TGF-β pathway for cancer therapy. Clin Cancer Res. 2012;18:4514–21.
135. Ikushima H, Miyazono K. TGFbeta signalling: a complex web in cancer progression. Nat Rev Cancer. 2010;10:415–24.
136. Derynck R, Zhang YE. Smad-dependent and Smad-independent pathways in TGF-beta family signalling. Nature. 2003;425:577–84.
137. Saltzman AK, Hartenbach EM, Carter JR, Contreras DN, Twiggs LB, Carson LF, Ramakrishnan S. Transforming growth factor-alpha levels in the serum and ascites of patients with advanced epithelial ovarian cancer. Gynecol Obstet Invest. 1999;47:200–4.
138. Gutgold N, Davidson B, Catane LJ, Holth A, Hellesylt E, Tropé CG, Dørum A, Reich R. TGFβ splicing and canonical pathway activation in high-grade serous carcinoma. Virchows Arch. 2017;470:665–78.
139. Bock AJ, Stavnes HT, Kempf T, Tropè CG, Berner A, Davidson B, Staff AC. Expression and clinical role of growth differentiation factor-15 in ovarian carcinoma effusions. Int J Gynecol Cancer. 2010;20:1448–55.
140. Dallas NA, Samuel S, Xia L, Fan F, Gray MJ, Lim SJ, Ellis LM. Endoglin (CD105): a marker of tumor vasculature and potential target for therapy. Clin Cancer Res. 2008;14:1931–7.
141. ten Dijke P, Goumans MJ, Pardali E. Endoglin in angiogenesis and vascular diseases. Angiogenesis. 2008;11:79–89.
142. Ollauri-Ibáñez C, López-Novoa JM, Pericacho M. Endoglin-based biological therapy in the treatment of angiogenesis-dependent pathologies. Expert Opin Biol Ther. 2017;17:1053–63.
143. Bock AJ, Tuft Stavnes H, Kærn J, Berner A, Staff AC, Davidson B. Endoglin (CD105) expression in ovarian serous carcinoma effusions is related to chemotherapy status. Tumour Biol. 2011;32:589–96.
144. Matei D, Emerson RE, Lai YC, Baldridge LA, Rao J, Yiannoutsos C, Donner DD. Autocrine activation of PDGFRalpha promotes the progression of ovarian cancer. Oncogene. 2006;25:2060–9.
145. Richardson M, Gunawan J, Hatton MW, Seidlitz E, Hirte HW, Singh G. Malignant ascites fluid (MAF), including ovarian-cancer-associated MAF, contains angiostatin and other factor(s) which inhibit angiogenesis. Gynecol Oncol. 2002;86:279–87.
146. Kleinberg L, Pradhan M, Tropé CG, Nesland JM, Davidson D, Risberg B. Ovarian carcinoma cells in effusions show increased

S-phase fraction compared to corresponding primary tumors. Diagn Cytopathol. 2008;36:637–44.

147. Deshpande A, Sicinski P, Hinds PW. Cyclins and cdks in development and cancer: a perspective. Oncogene. 2005;24:2909–15.

148. Cordon-Cardo C. Mutations of cell cycle regulators. Biological and clinical implications for human neoplasia. Am J Pathol. 1995;147:545–60.

149. Graña X, Reddy EP. Cell cycle control in mammalian cells: role of cyclins, cyclin dependent kinases (CDKs), growth suppressor genes and cyclin-dependent kinase inhibitors (CKIs). Oncogene. 1995;11:211–9.

150. Watson JE, Gabra H, Taylor KJ, Rabiasz GJ, Morrison H, Perry P, Smyth JF, Porteous DJ. Identification and characterization of a homozygous deletion found in ovarian ascites by representational difference analysis. Genome Res. 1999;9:226–33.

151. Goto T, Takano M, Hirata J, Kohno T, Ohtsuka S, Fujiwara K, Tsuda H. p16INK4a expression in cytology of ascites and response to chemotherapy in advanced ovarian cancer. Int J Cancer. 2009;125:339–44.

152. Davidson B, Risberg B, Berner A, Nesland JM, Tropé CG, Kristensen GB, Bryne M, van de Putte G, Flørenes VA. Expression of cell cycle proteins in ovarian carcinoma cells in serous effusions—biological and prognostic implications. Gynecol Oncol. 2001;83:249–56.

153. Davidson B, Skrede M, Silins I, Shih IM, Tropé CG, Flørenes VA. Low molecular weight cyclin E forms differentiate ovarian carcinoma from cells of mesothelial origin and are associated with poor survival in ovarian carcinoma. Cancer. 2007;110: 1264–71.

154. Salani R, Davidson B, Fiegl M, Marth C, Müller-Holzner E, Gastl G, Huang HY, Hsiao JC, Lin HS, Wang TL, Lin BL, Shih IM. Measurement of cyclin E genomic copy number and strand length in cell-free DNA distinguish malignant versus benign effusions. Clin Cancer Res. 2007;13:5805–9.

155. Provencher DM, Lounis H, Fink D, Drouin P, Mes-Masson AM. Discordance in p53 mutations when comparing ascites and solid tumors from patients with serous ovarian cancer. Tumour Biol. 1997;18:167–74.

156. Kappes S, Milde-Langosch K, Kressin P, Passlack B, Dockhorn-Dworniczak B, Röhlke P, Löning T. p53 mutations in ovarian tumors, detected by temperature-gradient gel electrophoresis, direct sequencing and immunohistochemistry. Int J Cancer. 1995;64:52–9.

157. Angelopoulou K, Diamandis EP. Detection of the TP53 tumour suppressor gene product and p53 auto-antibodies in the ascites of women with ovarian cancer. Eur J Cancer. 1997;33:115–21.

158. Abendstein B, Marth C, Müller-Holzner E, Widschwendter M, Daxenbichler G, Zeimet AG. Clinical significance of serum and ascitic p53 autoantibodies in epithelial ovarian carcinoma. Cancer. 2000;88:1432–7.

159. Montenarh M, Harlozińska A, Bar JK, Kartarius S, Günther J, Sedlaczek P. p53 autoantibodies in the sera, cyst and ascitic fluids of patients with ovarian cancer. Int J Oncol. 1998;13:605–10.

160. Ashkenazi A. Targeting death and decoy receptors of the tumor-necrosis factor superfamily. Nat Rev Cancer. 2002;2: 420–30.

161. Wajant H, Pfizenmaier K, Scheurich P. Tumor necrosis factor signaling. Cell Death Differ. 2003;10:45–65.

162. Twomey JD, Kim SR, Zhao L, Bozza WP, Zhang B. Spatial dynamics of TRAIL death receptors in cancer cells. Drug Resist Updat. 2015;19:13–21.

163. Reichmann E. The biological role of the Fas/FasL system during tumor formation and progression. Semin Cancer Biol. 2002;12:309–15.

164. Siegmund D, Lang I, Wajant H. Cell death-independent activities of the death receptors CD95, TRAILR1, and TRAILR2. FEBS J. 2017;284:1131–59.

165. Lane D, Goncharenko-Khaider N, Rancourt C, Piché A. Ovarian cancer ascites protects from TRAIL-induced cell death through alphavbeta5 integrin-mediated focal adhesion kinase and Akt activation. Oncogene. 2010;29:3519–31.

166. Lane D, Matte I, Rancourt C, Piché A. The prosurvival activity of ascites against TRAIL is associated with a shorter disease-free interval in patients with ovarian cancer. J Ovarian Res. 2010;3:1.

167. Connor JP, Felder M. Ascites from epithelial ovarian cancer contain high levels of functional decoy receptor 3 (DcR3) and is associated with platinum resistance. Gynecol Oncol. 2008;111: 330–5.

168. Abrahams VM, Straszewski SL, Kamsteeg M, Hanczaruk B, Schwartz PE, Rutherford TJ, Mor G. Epithelial ovarian cancer cells secrete functional Fas ligand. Cancer Res. 2003;63:5573–81.

169. Ciaravino G, Bhat M, Manbeian CA, Teng NN. Differential expression of CD40 and CD95 in ovarian carcinoma. Eur J Gynaecol Oncol. 2004;25:27–32.

170. Dong HP, Kleinberg L, Silins I, Flørenes VA, Tropé CG, Risberg B, Nesland JM, Davidson B. Death receptor expression is associated with poor response to chemotherapy and shorter survival in metastatic ovarian carcinoma. Cancer. 2008;112:84–93.

171. Igney FH, Krammer PH. Death and anti-death: tumour resistance to apoptosis. Nat Rev Cancer. 2002;2:277–88.

172. Taylor RC, Cullen SP, Martin SJ. Apoptosis: controlled demolition at the cellular level. Nat Rev Mol Cell Biol. 2008;9:231–41.

173. Dong HP, Kleinberg L, Davidson B, Risberg B. Methods for simultaneous measurement of apoptosis and cell surface phenotype of epithelial cells in effusions by flow cytometry. Nat Protoc. 2008;3:955–64.

174. Kleinberg L, Dong HP, Holth A, Risberg B, Tropé CG, Nesland JM, Flørenes VA, Davidson B. Cleaved caspases and NF-κB are prognostic factors in metastatic ovarian carcinoma. Hum Pathol. 2009;40:795–806.

175. Dong HP, Holth A, Kleinberg L, Ruud MG, Elstrand MB, Tropé CG, Davidson B, Risberg B. Evaluation of cell surface expression of phosphatidylserine in ovarian carcinoma effusions using the Annexin-V/7-AAD assay - Clinical relevance and comparison to other apoptosis parameters. Am J Clin Pathol. 2009;132: 756–62.

176. Dong HP, Ree Rosnes AK, Bock AJ, Holth A, Flørenes VA, Tropé CG, Risberg B, Davidson B. Flow cytometric measurement of cellular FLICE-inhibitory protein (c-FLIP) in ovarian carcinoma effusions. Cytopathology. 2011;22:373–82.

177. Fulda S. Molecular pathways: targeting inhibitor of apoptosis proteins in cancer—from molecular mechanism to therapeutic application. Clin Cancer Res. 2014;20:289–95.

178. Peery RC, Liu JY, Zhang JT. Targeting survivin for therapeutic discovery: past, present, and future promises. Drug Discov Today. 2017;22:1466–77.

179. Wu M, Yuan S, Szporn AH, Gan L, Shtilbans V, Burstein DE. Immunohistochemical detection of XIAP in body cavity effusions and washes. Mod Pathol. 2005;18:1618–22.

180. Kleinberg L, Flørenes VA, Silins I, Haug K, Tropé CG, Nesland JM, Davidson B. Nuclear expression of survivin is associated with improved survival in metastatic ovarian carcinoma. Cancer. 2007;109:228–38.

181. Danial NN. Bcl-2 family proteins: critical checkpoints of apoptotic cell death. Clin Cancer Res. 2007;13:7254–63.

182. Ashkenazi A, Fairbrother WJ, Leverson JD, Souers AJ. From basic apoptosis discoveries to advanced selective BCL-2 family inhibitors. Nat Rev Drug Discov. 2017;16:273–84.

183. Liu JR, Fletcher B, Page C, Hu C, Nunez G, Baker V. Bcl-xL is expressed in ovarian carcinoma and modulates chemotherapy-induced apoptosis. Gynecol Oncol. 1998;70:398–403.

184. Bunkholt Elstrand M, Kleinberg L, Kohn EC, Tropé CG, Davidson B. Expression and clinical role of anti-apoptotic proteins of the Bag, heat shock and Bcl-2 families in effusions, primary tumors

and solid metastases in ovarian carcinoma. Int J Gynecol Pathol. 2009;28:211–21.

185. Ciocca DR, Calderwood SK. Heat shock proteins in cancer: diagnostic, prognostic, predictive and treatment implications. Cell Stress Chaperones. 2005;10:86–103.

186. Garrido C, Brunet M, Didelot C, Zermati Y, Schmitt E, Kroemer G. Heat shock proteins 27 and 70: anti-apoptotic proteins with tumorigenic properties. Cell Cycle. 2006;5:2592–601.

187. Beere HM. "The stress of dying": the role of heat shock proteins in the regulation of apoptosis. J Cell Sci. 2004;117:2641–51.

188. Wu J, Liu T, Rios Z, Mei Q, Lin X, Cao S. Heat shock proteins and cancer. Trends Pharmacol Sci. 2017;38:226–56.

189. Schopf FH, Biebl MM, Buchner J. The HSP90 chaperone machinery. Nat Rev Mol Cell Biol. 2017;18:345–60.

190. Elstrand MB, Stavnes HT, Trope CG, Davidson B. Heat shock protein 90 is a putative therapeutic target in patients with recurrent advanced-stage ovarian carcinoma with serous effusions. Hum Pathol. 2012;43:529–35.

191. Behl C. Breaking BAG: the Co-Chaperone BAG3 in health and disease. Trends Pharmacol Sci. 2016;37:672–88.

192. Ma HT, Poon RY. How protein kinases co-ordinate mitosis in animal cells. Biochem J. 2011;435:17–31.

193. Damodaran AP, Vaufrey L, Gavard O, Prigent C. Aurora A Kinase is a priority pharmaceutical target for the treatment of cancers. Trends Pharmacol Sci. 2017;38:687–700.

194. Marumoto T, Zhang D, Saya H. Aurora-A—a guardian of poles. Nat Rev Cancer. 2005;5:42–50.

195. Vader G, Lens SM. The Aurora kinase family in cell division and cancer. Biochim Biophys Acta. 2008;1786:60–72.

196. Hetland TE, Nymoen DA, Holth A, Brusegard K, Florenes VA, Kærn J, Trope CG, Davidson B. Aurora B expression in metastatic effusions from advanced-stage ovarian serous carcinoma is predictive of intrinsic chemotherapy resistance. Hum Pathol. 2013;44:777–85.

197. Davidson B, Nymoen DA, Elgaaen BV, Staff AC, Trope CG, Kærn J, Reich R, Falkenthal TE. BUB1 mRNA is significantly co-expressed with AURKA and AURKB mRNA in advanced-stage ovarian serous carcinoma. Virchows Arch. 2014;464:701–7.

198. Matheson CJ, Backos DS, Reigan P. Targeting WEE1 Kinase in Cancer. Trends Pharmacol Sci. 2016;37:872–81.

199. Slipicevic A, Holth A, Hellesylt E, Trope CG, Davidson B, Florenes VA. Wee1 is a novel independent prognostic marker of poor survival in post-chemotherapy ovarian carcinoma effusions. Gynecol Oncol. 2014;135:118–24.

200. Pakish JB, Jazaeri AA. Immunotherapy in gynecologic cancers: are we there yet? Curr Treat Options Oncol. 2017;18:59.

201. Gaillard SL, Secord AA, Monk B. The role of immune checkpoint inhibition in the treatment of ovarian cancer. Gynecol Oncol Res Pract. 2016;24:3–11.

202. Ventriglia J, Paciolla I, Pisano C, Cecere SC, Di Napoli M, Tambaro R, Califano D, Losito S, Scognamiglio G, Setola SV, Arenare L, Pignata S, Della Pepa C. Immunotherapy in ovarian, endometrial and cervical cancer: state of the art and future perspectives. Cancer Treat Rev. 2017;59:109–16.

203. Fumita Y, Tanaka F, Saji F, Nakamuro K. Immunosuppressive factors in ascites fluids from ovarian cancer patients. Am J Reprod Immunol. 1984;6:175–8.

204. Akyol S, Gercel-Taylor C, Reynolds LC, Taylor DD. HSP-10 in ovarian cancer: expression and suppression of T-cell signaling. Gynecol Oncol. 2006;101:481–6.

205. Taylor DD, Gerçel-Taylor C. Tumour-derived exosomes and their role in cancer-associated T-cell signalling defects. Br J Cancer. 2005;92:305–11.

206. Gordon IO, Freedman RS. Defective antitumor function of monocyte-derived macrophages from epithelial ovarian cancer patients. Clin Cancer Res. 2006;12:1515–24.

207. Lai P, Rabinowich H, Crowley-Nowick PA, Bell MC, Mantovani G, Whiteside TL. Alterations in expression and function of signal-transducing proteins in tumor-associated T and natural killer cells in patients with ovarian carcinoma. Clin Cancer Res. 1996;2:161–73.

208. Loercher AE, Nash MA, Kavanagh JJ, Platsoucas CD, Freedman RS. Identification of an IL-10-producing HLA-DR-negative monocyte subset in the malignant ascites of patients with ovarian carcinoma that inhibits cytokine protein expression and proliferation of autologous T cells. J Immunol. 1999;163:6251–60.

209. Takaishi K, Komohara Y, Tashiro H, Ohtake H, Nakagawa T, Katabuchi H, Takeya M. Involvement of M2-polarized macrophages in the ascites from advanced epithelial ovarian carcinoma in tumor progression via Stat3 activation. Cancer Sci. 2010;101:2128–36.

210. Webb TJ, Giuntoli RL 2nd, Rogers O, Schneck J, Oelke M. Ascites specific inhibition of CD1d-mediated activation of natural killer T cells. Clin Cancer Res. 2008;14:7652–8.

211. Wischhusen J, Waschbisch A, Wiendl H. Immune-refractory cancers and their little helpers—an extended role for immunetolerogenic MHC molecules HLA-G and HLA-E. Semin Cancer Biol. 2007;17:459–68.

212. Morandi F, Rizzo R, Fainardi E, Rouas-Freiss N, Pistoia V. Recent advances in our understanding of HLA-G biology: lessons from a wide spectrum of human diseases. J Immunol Res. 2016;2016:4326495.

213. Singer G, Rebmann V, Chen YC, Liu HT, Ali SZ, Reinsberg J, McMaster MT, Pfeiffer K, Chan DW, Wardelmann E, Grosse-Wilde H, Cheng CC, Kurman RJ, Shih IM. HLA-G is a potential tumor marker in malignant ascites. Clin Cancer Res. 2003;9:4460–4.

214. Davidson B, Bukholt Elstrand M, McMaster MT, Berner A, Kurman RJ, Risberg B, Trope' CG, Shih IM. HLA-G expression in effusions is a possible marker of tumor susceptibility to chemotherapy in ovarian carcinoma. Gynecol Oncol. 2005;96:42–7.

215. Naylor MS, Stamp GW, Foulkes WD, Eccles D, Balkwill FR. Tumor necrosis factor and its receptors in human ovarian cancer. Potential role in disease progression. J Clin Invest. 1993;91:2194–206.

216. Stadlmann S, Amberger A, Pollheimer J, Gastl G, Offner FA, Margreiter R, Zeimet AG. Ovarian carcinoma cells and IL-1beta-activated human peritoneal mesothelial cells are possible sources of vascular endothelial growth factor in inflammatory and malignant peritoneal effusions. Gynecol Oncol. 2005;97:784–9.

217. Hurteau JA, Simon HU, Kurman C, Rubin L, Mills GB. Levels of soluble interleukin-2 receptor-alpha are elevated in serum and ascitic fluid from epithelial ovarian cancer patients. Am J Obstet Gynecol. 1994;170:918–28.

218. Barton DP, Blanchard DK, Michelini-Norris B, Nicosia SV, Cavanagh D, Djeu JY. High serum and ascitic soluble interleukin-2 receptor alpha levels in advanced epithelial ovarian cancer. Blood. 1993;81:424–9.

219. Garg R, Wollan M, Galic V, Garcia R, Goff BA, Gray HJ, Swisher E. Common polymorphism in interleukin 6 influences survival of women with ovarian and peritoneal carcinoma. Gynecol Oncol. 2006;103:793–6.

220. Schröder W, Ruppert C, Bender HG. Concomitant measurements of interleukin-6 (IL-6) in serum and peritoneal fluid of patients with benign and malignant ovarian tumors. Eur J Obstet Gynecol Reprod Biol. 1994;56:43–6.

221. Moradi MM, Carson LF, Weinberg B, Haney AF, Twiggs LB, Ramakrishnan S. Serum and ascitic fluid levels of interleukin-1, interleukin-6, and tumor necrosis factor-alpha in patients with ovarian epithelial cancer. Cancer. 1993;72:2433–40.

222. Plante M, Rubin SC, Wong GY, Federici MG, Finstad CL, Gastl GA. Interleukin-6 level in serum and ascites as a prognostic factor in patients with epithelial ovarian cancer. Cancer. 1994;73:1882–8.

223. Ripley D, Shoup B, Majewski A, Chegini N. Differential expression of interleukins IL-13 and IL-15 in normal ovarian tissue and ovarian carcinomas. Gynecol Oncol. 2004;92:761–8.

224. Zeimet AG, Widschwendter M, Knabbe C, Fuchs D, Herold M, Müller-Holzner E, Daxenbichler G, Offner FA, Dapunt O, Marth C. Ascitic interleukin-12 is an independent prognostic factor in ovarian cancer. J Clin Oncol. 1998;16:1861–8.

225. Mustea A, Pirvulescu C, Könsgen D, Braicu EI, Yuan S, Sun P, Lichtenegger W, Sehouli J. Decreased IL-1 RA concentration in ascites is associated with a significant improvement in overall survival in ovarian cancer. Cytokine. 2008;42:77–84.

226. Matte I, Lane D, Laplante C, Rancourt C, Piché A. Profiling of cytokines in human epithelial ovarian cancer ascites. Am J Cancer Res. 2012;2:566–80.

227. Kolomeyevskaya N, Eng KH, Khan AN, Grzankowski KS, Singel KL, Moysich K, Segal BH. Cytokine profiling of ascites at primary surgery identifies an interaction of tumor necrosis factor-α and interleukin-6 in predicting reduced progression-free survival in epithelial ovarian cancer. Gynecol Oncol. 2015;138:352–7.

228. Naldini A, Morena E, Belotti D, Carraro F, Allavena P, Giavazzi R. Identification of thrombin-like activity in ovarian cancer associated ascites and modulation of multiple cytokine networks. Thromb Haemost. 2011;106:705–11.

229. Lazennec G, Richmond A. Chemokines and chemokine receptors: new insights into cancer-related inflammation. Trends Mol Med. 2010;16:133–44.

230. Nagarsheth N, Wicha MS, Zou W. Chemokines in the cancer microenvironment and their relevance in cancer immunotherapy. Nat Rev Immunol. 2017;17:559–72.

231. Scotton CJ, Wilson JL, Milliken D, Stamp G, Balkwill FR. Epithelial cancer cell migration: a role for chemokine receptors? Cancer Res. 2001;61:4961–5.

232. Scotton CJ, Wilson JL, Scott K, Stamp G, Wilbanks GD, Fricker S, Bridger G, Balkwill FR. Multiple actions of the chemokine CXCL12 on epithelial tumor cells in human ovarian cancer. Cancer Res. 2002;62:5930–8.

233. Milliken D, Scotton C, Raju S, Balkwill F, Wilson J. Analysis of chemokines and chemokine receptor expression in ovarian cancer ascites. Clin Cancer Res. 2002;8:1108–14.

234. Dong HP, Bunkholt Elstrand M, Holth A, Silins I, Berner A, Tropé CG, Davidson B, Risberg B. NK and B cell infiltration correlates with worse outcome in metastatic ovarian carcinoma. Am J Clin Pathol. 2006;125:451–8.

235. Schutyser E, Struyf S, Proost P, Opdenakker G, Laureys G, Verhasselt B, Peperstraete L, Van de Putte I, Saccani A, Allavena P, Mantovani A, Van Damme J. Identification of biologically active chemokine isoforms from ascitic fluid and elevated levels of CCL18/pulmonary and activation-regulated chemokine in ovarian carcinoma. J Biol Chem. 2002;277:24584–93.

236. Bamias A, Tsiatas ML, Kafantari E, Liakou C, Rodolakis A, Voulgaris Z, Vlahos G, Papageorgiou T, Tsitsilonis O, Bamia C, Papatheodoridis G, Politi E, Archimandritis A, Antsaklis A, Dimopoulos MA. Significant differences of lymphocytes isolated from ascites of patients with ovarian cancer compared to blood and tumor lymphocytes. Association of CD3+CD56+ cells with platinum resistance. Gynecol Oncol. 2007;106:75–81.

237. Bamias A, Koutsoukou V, Terpos E, Tsiatas ML, Liakos C, Tsitsilonis O, Rodolakis A, Voulgaris Z, Vlahos G, Papageorgiou T, Papatheodoridis G, Archimandritis A, Antsaklis A, Dimopoulos MA. Correlation of NK T-like CD3+CD56+ cells and CD4+CD25+(hi) regulatory T cells with VEGF and TNFalpha in ascites from advanced ovarian cancer: Association with platinum resistance and prognosis in patients receiving first-line, platinum-based chemotherapy. Gynecol Oncol. 2008;108:421–7.

238. Melichar B, Nash MA, Lenzi R, Platsoucas CD, Freedman RS. Expression of costimulatory molecules CD80 and CD86

and their receptors CD28, CTLA-4 on malignant ascites CD3+ tumour-infiltrating lymphocytes (TIL) from patients with ovarian and other types of peritoneal carcinomatosis. Clin Exp Immunol. 2000;119:19–27.

239. Landskron J, Helland Ø, Torgersen KM, Aandahl EM, Gjertsen BT, Bjørge L, Taskén K. Activated regulatory and memory T-cells accumulate in malignant ascites from ovarian carcinoma patients. Cancer Immunol Immunother. 2015;64:337–47.

240. Reijnhart RM, Bieber MM, Teng NN. FACS analysis of peritoneal lymphocytes in ovarian cancer and control patients. Immunobiology. 1994;191:1–8.

241. Condeelis J, Pollard JW. Macrophages: obligate partners for tumor cell migration, invasion, and metastasis. Cell. 2006;124:263–6.

242. Lewis CE, Pollard JW. Distinct role of macrophages in different tumor microenvironments. Cancer Res. 2006;66:605–12.

243. Risberg B, Davidson B, Nielsen S, Dong HP, Christensen J, Johansen P, Asschenfeldt P, Berner A. Detection of monocyte/macrophage cell populations in effusions: a comparative study using flow cytometric immunophenotyping and immunocytochemistry. Diagn Cytopathol. 2001;25:214–9.

244. Wang R, Zhang T, Ma Z, Wang Y, Cheng Z, Xu H, Li W, Wang X. The interaction of coagulation factor XII and monocyte/macrophages mediating peritoneal metastasis of epithelial ovarian cancer. Gynecol Oncol. 2010;117:460–6.

245. Reinartz S, Schumann T, Finkernagel F, Wortmann A, Jansen JM, Meissner W, Krause M, Schwörer AM, Wagner U, Müller-Brüsselbach S, Müller R. Mixed-polarization phenotype of ascites-associated macrophages in human ovarian carcinoma: correlation of CD163 expression, cytokine levels and early relapse. Int J Cancer. 2014;134:32–42.

246. Adhikary T, Wortmann A, Finkernagel F, Lieber S, Nist A, Stiewe T, Wagner U, Müller-Brüsselbach S, Reinartz S, Müller R. Interferon signaling in ascites-associated macrophages is linked to a favorable clinical outcome in a subgroup of ovarian carcinoma patients. BMC Genomics. 2017;18:243.

247. Wagner EF, Nebreda AR. Signal integration by JNK and p38 MAPK pathways in cancer development. Nat Rev Cancer. 2009;9:537–49.

248. Kim EK, Choi EJ. Pathological roles of MAPK signaling pathways in human diseases. Biochim Biophys Acta. 2010;1802:396–405.

249. Rauch N, Rukhlenko OS, Kolch W, Kholodenko BN. MAPK kinase signalling dynamics regulate cell fate decisions and drug resistance. Curr Opin Struct Biol. 2016;41:151–8.

250. Givant-Horwitz V, Davidson B, Lazarovici P, Schaefer E, Nesland JM, Tropé CG, Reich R. Mitogen-activated protein kinases (MAPK) as predictors of clinical outcome in serous ovarian carcinoma in effusions. Gynecol Oncol. 2003;91:160–72.

251. Givant-Horwitz V, Davidson B, Goderstad JM, Nesland JM, Tropé CG, Reich R. The PAC-1 dual specificity phosphatase predicts poor outcome in serous ovarian carcinoma. Gynecol Oncol. 2004;93:517–23.

252. Davidson B, Espina V, Flørenes VA, Liotta LA, Kristensen GB, Trope' CG, Berner A, Kohn EC. Proteomic profiling of malignant ovarian cancer effusions: survival and injury pathways discriminate clinical outcome. Clin Cancer Res. 2006;12:791–9.

253. Dokianakis DN, Varras MN, Papaefthimiou M, Apostolopoulou J, Simiakaki H, Diakomanolis E, Spandidos DA. Ras gene activation in malignant cells of human ovarian carcinoma peritoneal fluids. Clin Exp Metastasis. 1999;17:293–7.

254. Fruman DA, Chiu H, Hopkins BD, Bagrodia S, Cantley LC, Abraham RT. The PI3K pathway in human disease. Cell. 2017;170:605–35.

255. Manning BD, Toker A. AKT/PKB signaling: navigating the network. Cell. 2017;169:381–405.

256. Davidson B, Hadar R, Schlossberg A, Sternlicht T, Slipicevic A, Skrede M, Risberg B, Flørenes VA, Kopolovic J, Reich

R. Expression and clinical role of DJ-1, a negative regulator of PTEN, in ovarian carcinoma. Hum Pathol. 2008;39:87–95.

257. Cao J, Lou S, Ying M, Yang B. DJ-1 as a human oncogene and potential therapeutic target. Biochem Pharmacol. 2015;93:241–50.

258. Bunkholt Elstrand M, Dong HP, Ødegaard E, Holth A, Elloul S, Reich R, Tropé CG, Davidson B. Mammalian target of rapamycin is a biomarker of poor survival in metastatic ovarian carcinoma. Hum Pathol. 2010;41:794–804.

259. Perkins ND, Gilmore TD. Good cop, bad cop: the different faces of NF-kappaB. Cell Death Differ. 2006;13:759–72.

260. Neumann M, Naumann M. Beyond IkappaBs: alternative regulation of NF-kappaB activity. FASEB J. 2007;21:2642–54.

261. Perkins ND. Integrating cell-signalling pathways with NF-kappaB and IKK function. Nat Rev Mol Cell Biol. 2007;8:49–62.

262. Seth A, Watson DK. Ets transcription factors and their emerging roles in human cancer. Eur J Cancer. 2005;41:2462–78.

263. Verger A, Duterque-Coquillaud M. When Ets transcription factors meet their partners. Bioessays. 2002;24:362–70.

264. Sharrocks AD. The ETS-domain transcription factor family. Nat Rev Mol Cell Biol. 2001;2:827–37.

265. Sizemore GM, Pitarresi JR, Balakrishnan S, Ostrowski MC. The ETS family of oncogenic transcription factors in solid tumours. Nat Rev Cancer. 2017;17:337–51.

266. Davidson B, Risberg B, Goldberg I, Nesland JM, Berner A, Tropé CG, Kristensen GB, Bryne M, Reich R. Ets-1 mRNA expression in effusions of serous ovarian carcinoma patients is a marker of poor outcome. Am J Surg Pathol. 2001;25:1493–500.

267. Davidson B, Goldberg I, Reich R, Tell L, Baekelandt M, Kristensen GB, Berner A, Kopolovic J. The clinical role of the PEA3 transcription factor in ovarian and breast carcinoma in effusions. Clin Exp Metastasis. 2004;21:191–9.

268. Brenne K, Nymoen DA, Hetland TE, Trope' CG, Davidson B. Expression of the Ets transcription factor EHF in serous ovarian carcinoma effusions is a marker of poor survival. Hum Pathol. 2012;43:496–505.

269. Sertznig P, Seifert M, Tilgen W, Reichrath J. Present concepts and future outlook: function of peroxisome proliferator-activated receptors (PPARs) for pathogenesis, progression, and therapy of cancer. J Cell Physiol. 2007;212:1–12.

270. Michalik L, Desvergne B, Wahli W. Peroxisome-proliferator-activated receptors and cancers: complex stories. Nat Rev Cancer. 2004;4:61–70.

271. Davidson B, Hadar R, Tuft Stavnes H, Trope' CG, Reich R. Expression of the peroxisome proliferator-activated receptors (PPAR)-α, -β and -γ in ovarian carcinoma effusions is associated with poor chemoresponse and shorter survival. Hum Pathol. 2009;40:705–13.

272. Gorovetz M, Baekelandt M, Berner A, Trope' CG, Davidson B, Reich R. The clinical role of phospholipase A$_2$ isoforms in advanced-stage ovarian carcinoma. Gynecol Oncol. 2006;103:831–40.

273. Denkert C, Köbel M, Pest S, Koch I, Berger S, Schwabe M, Siegert A, Reles A, Klosterhalfen B, Hauptmann S. Expression of cyclooxygenase 2 is an independent prognostic factor in human ovarian carcinoma. Am J Pathol. 2002;160:893–903.

274. Westermann AM, Havik E, Postma FR, Beijnen JH, Dalesio O, Moolenaar WH, Rodenhuis S. Malignant effusions contain lysophosphatidic acid (LPA)-like activity. Ann Oncol. 1998;9:437–42.

275. Xiao YJ, Schwartz B, Washington M, Kennedy A, Webster K, Belinson J, Xu Y. Electrospray ionization mass spectrometry analysis of lysophospholipids in human ascitic fluids: comparison of the lysophospholipid contents in malignant vs nonmalignant ascitic fluids. Anal Biochem. 2001;290:302–13.

276. Lee MJ, Jeon ES, Lee JS, Cho M, Suh DS, Chang CL, Kim JH. Lysophosphatidic acid in malignant ascites stimulates

277. Harel-Dassa K, Yedgar S, Tropé CG, Davidson B, Reich R. Phospholipase D messenger RNA expression and clinical role in high-grade serous carcinoma. Hum Pathol. 2017;62:115–21.

278. Melnikova VO, Bar-Eli M. Transcriptional control of the melanoma malignant phenotype. Cancer Biol Ther. 2008;7:997–1003.

279. Pellikainen JM, Kosma VM. Activator protein-2 in carcinogenesis with a special reference to breast cancer—a mini review. Int J Cancer. 2007;120:2061–7.

280. Ødegaard E, Staff AC, Kærn J, Flørenes VA, Kopolovic J, Tropé CG, Abeler VM, Reich R, Davidson B. AP-2γ is a marker of tumor progression in ovarian carcinoma. Gynecol Oncol. 2006;100:462–8.

281. St Pierre R, Kadoch C. Mammalian SWI/SNF complexes in cancer: emerging therapeutic opportunities. Curr Opin Genet Dev. 2017;42:56–67.

282. Shih IM, Sheu JJ, Santillan A, Nakayama K, Yen MJ, Bristow RE, Vang R, Parmigiani G, Kurman RJ, Trope CG, Davidson B, Wang TL. Amplification of a chromatin remodeling gene, Rsf-1/HBXAP, in ovarian carcinoma. Proc Natl Acad Sci U S A. 2005;102:14004–9.

283. Davidson B, Trope' CG, Wang TL, Shih IM. Expression of the chromatin remodeling factor Rsf-1 in effusions is a novel predictor of poor survival in ovarian carcinoma. Gynecol Oncol. 2006;103:814–9.

284. Collins T, Stone JR, Williams AJ. All in the family: the BTB/POZ, KRAB, and SCAN domains. Mol Cell Biol. 2001;21:3609–15.

285. Stogios PJ, Downs GS, Jauhal JJ, Nandra SK, Prive GG. Sequence and structural analysis of BTB domain proteins. Genome Biol. 2005;6:R82.

286. Cha XY, Pierce RC, Kalivas PW, Mackler SA. NAC-1, a rat brain mRNA, is increased in the nucleus accumbens three weeks after chronic cocaine self-administration. J Neurosci. 1997;17:6864–71.

287. Nakayma K, Nakayma N, Davidson B, Sheu J, Jinawath N, Santillan A, Salani R, Bristow RE, Morin PJ, Kurman RJ, Wang TL, Shih IM. A BTB/POZ protein, NAC-1, is related to tumor recurrence and is essential for tumor growth and survival. Proc Natl Acad Sci U S A. 2006;103:18739–44.

288. Davidson B, Berner A, Tropé CG, Wang TL, IeM S. Expression and clinical role of the BTB/POZ protein NAC-1 in ovarian carcinoma effusions. Hum Pathol. 2007;38:1030–6.

289. Ueda SM, Yap KL, Davidson B, Tian Y, Murthy V, Wang TL, Visvanathan K, Kuhajda FP, Bristow RE, Zhang H, Shih IM. Expression of fatty acid synthase depends on NAC1 and is associated with recurrent ovarian serous carcinomas. J Oncol. 2010;2010:285191.

290. D'Souza B, Meloty-Kapella L, Weinmaster G. Canonical and non-canonical Notch ligands. Curr Top Dev Biol. 2010;92:73–129.

291. Artavanis-Tsakonas S, Muskavitch MA. Notch: the past, the present, and the future. Curr Top Dev Biol. 2010;92:1–29.

292. Koch U, Radtke F. Notch signaling in solid tumors. Curr Top Dev Biol. 2010;92:411–55.

293. Takebe N, Harris PJ, Warren RQ, Ivy SP. Targeting cancer stem cells by inhibiting Wnt, Notch, and Hedgehog pathways. Nat Rev Clin Oncol. 2011;8:97–106.

294. Nowell CS, Radtke F. Notch as a tumour suppressor. Nat Rev Cancer. 2017;17:145–59.

295. Park JT, Li M, Nakayama K, Mao TL, Davidson B, Zhang Z, Kurman RJ, Eberhart CG, Shih IM, Wang TL. Notch3 gene amplification in ovarian cancer. Cancer Res. 2006;66:6312–8.

296. Choi JH, Park JT, Davidson B, Morin PJ, Shih IM, Wang TL. Jagged-1 and notch3 juxtacrine loop regulates ovarian tumor growth and adhesion. Cancer Res. 2008;68:5716–23.

297. Park J, Chen X, Tropé CG, Davidson B, Shih IM, Wang TL. Notch3 overexpression is related to the recurrence of ovarian cancer

and confers resistance to carboplatin. Am J Pathol. 2010;177: 1087–94.

298. Burleson KM, Casey RC, Skubitz KM, Pambuccian SE, Oegema TR Jr, Skubitz AP. Ovarian carcinoma ascites spheroids adhere to extracellular matrix components and mesothelial cell monolayers. Gynecol Oncol. 2004;93:170–81.

299. Burleson KM, Boente MP, Pambuccian SE, Skubitz AP. Disaggregation and invasion of ovarian carcinoma ascites spheroids. J Transl Med. 2006;4:6.

300. Alvero AB, Chen R, Fu HH, Montagna M, Schwartz PE, Rutherford T, Silasi DA, Steffensen KD, Waldstrom M, Visintin I, Mor G. Molecular phenotyping of human ovarian cancer stem cells unravels the mechanisms for repair and chemoresistance. Cell Cycle. 2009;8:158–66.

301. Runz S, Keller S, Rupp C, Stoeck A, Issa Y, Koensgen D, Mustea A, Sehouli J, Kristiansen G, Altevogt P. Malignant ascites-derived exosomes of ovarian carcinoma patients contain CD24 and EpCAM. Gynecol Oncol. 2007;107:563–71.

302. Davidson B. CD24 is highly useful in differentiating high-grade serous carcinoma from benign and malignant mesothelial cells. Hum Pathol. 2016;58:123–7.

303. Meng E, Long B, Sullivan P, McClellan S, Finan MA, Reed E, Shevde L, Rocconi RP. CD44+/CD24- ovarian cancer cells demonstrate cancer stem cell properties and correlate to survival. Clin Exp Metastasis. 2012;29:939–48.

304. Meng E, Mitra A, Tripathi K, Finan MA, Scalici J, McClellan S, Madeira da Silva L, Reed E, Shevde LA, Palle K, Rocconi RP. ALDH1A1 maintains ovarian cancer stem cell-like properties by altered regulation of cell cycle checkpoint and DNA repair network signaling. PLoS One. 2014;9:e107142.

305. Latifi A, Luwor RB, Bilandzic M, Nazaretian S, Stenvers K, Pyman J, Zhu H, Thompson EW, Quinn MA, Findlay JK, Ahmed N. Isolation and characterization of tumor cells from the ascites of ovarian cancer patients: molecular phenotype of chemoresistant ovarian tumors. PLoS One. 2012;7:e46858.

306. Abubaker K, Luwor RB, Zhu H, McNally O, Quinn MA, Burns CJ, Thompson EW, Findlay JK, Ahmed N. Inhibition of the JAK2/STAT3 pathway in ovarian cancer results in the loss of cancer stem cell-like characteristics and a reduced tumor burden. BMC Cancer. 2014;14:317.

307. Rizzo S, Hersey JM, Mellor P, Dai W, Santos-Silva A, Liber D, Luk L, Titley I, Carden CP, Box G, Hudson DL, Kaye SB, Brown R. Ovarian cancer stem cell-like side populations are enriched following chemotherapy and overexpress EZH2. Mol Cancer Ther. 2011;10:325–35.

308. Neradil J, Veselska R. Nestin as a marker of cancer stem cells. Cancer Sci. 2015;106:803–11.

309. Zhang S, Balch C, Chan MW, Lai HC, Matei D, Schilder JM, Yan PS, Huang TH, Nephew KP. Identification and characterization of ovarian cancer-initiating cells from primary human tumors. Cancer Res. 2008;68:4311–20.

310. Hetland TE, Hellesylt E, Flørenes VA, Tropé C, Davidson B, Kærn J. Class III β-tubulin expression in advanced-stage serous ovarian carcinoma effusions is associated with poor survival and primary chemoresistance. Hum Pathol. 2011;42:1019–26.

311. Salazar MD, Ratnam M. The folate receptor: what does it promise in tissue-targeted therapeutics? Cancer Metastasis Rev. 2007;26:141–52.

312. Kelemen LE. The role of folate receptor α in cancer development, progression and treatment: cause, consequence or innocent bystander? Int J Cancer. 2006;119:243–50.

313. Cheung A, Bax HJ, Josephs DH, Ilieva KM, Pellizzari G, Opzoomer J, Bloomfield J, Fittall M, Grigoriadis A, Figini M, Canevari S, Spicer JF, Tutt AN, Karagiannis SN. Targeting folate receptor alpha for cancer treatment. Oncotarget. 2016;7:52553–74.

314. Mantovani LT, Miotti S, Ménard S, Canevari S, Raspagliesi F, Bottini C, Bottero F, Colnaghi MI. Folate binding protein distribution in normal tissues and biological fluids from ovarian carcinoma patients as detected by the monoclonal antibodies MOv18 and MOv19. Eur J Cancer. 1994;30A: 363–9.

315. Corona G, Toffoli G, Fabris M, Viel A, Zarrelli A, Donada C, Boiocchi M. Homocysteine accumulation in human ovarian carcinoma ascitic/cystic fluids possibly caused by metabolic alteration of the methionine cycle in ovarian carcinoma cells. Eur J Cancer. 1997;33:1284–90.

316. Forster MD, Ormerod MG, Agarwal R, Kaye SB, Jackman AL. Flow cytometric method for determining folate receptor expression on ovarian carcinoma cells. Cytometry A. 2007;71:945–50.

317. Yuan Y, Nymoen DA, Dong HP, Bjørang O, Shih IM, Low PS, Trope' CG, Davidson B. Expression of the folate receptor genes FOLR1 and FOLR3 differentiates ovarian carcinoma from breast carcinoma and malignant mesothelioma in serous effusions. Hum Pathol. 2009;40:1453–60.

318. Orr GA, Verdier-Pinard P, McDaid H, Horwitz SB. Mechanisms of Taxol resistance related to microtubules. Oncogene. 2003;22:7280–95.

319. Parker AL, Teo WS, McCarroll JA, Kavallaris M. An emerging role for tubulin isotypes in modulating cancer biology and chemotherapy resistance. Int J Mol Sci. 2017;18. pii: E1434.

320. Kavallaris M, Kuo DY, Burkhart CA, Regl DL, Norris MD, Haber M, Band Horwitz S. Taxol-resistant epithelial ovarian tumors are associated with altered expression of specific beta-tubulin isotypes. J Clin Invest. 1997;100:1282–93.

321. Chu TM, Lin TH, Kawinski E. Detection of soluble P-glycoprotein in culture media and extracellular fluids. Biochem Biophys Res Commun. 1994;203:506–12.

322. Kerr EH, Frederick PJ, Egger ME, Stockard CR, Sellers J, DellaManna D, Oelschlager DK, Amm HM, Eltoum IE, Straughn JM, Buchsbaum DJ, Grizzle WE, McNally LR. Lung resistance-related protein (LRP) expression in malignant ascitic cells as a prognostic marker for advanced ovarian serous carcinoma. Ann Surg Oncol. 2013;20:3059–65.

323. Huang H, Li Y, Liu J, Zheng M, Feng Y, Hu K, Huang Y, Huang Q. Screening and identification of biomarkers in ascites related to intrinsic chemoresistance of serous epithelial ovarian cancers. PLoS One. 2012;7:e51256.

324. Kase H, Kodama S, Nagai E, Tanaka K. Glutathione S-transferase pi immunostaining of cisplatin-resistant ovarian cancer cells in ascites. Acta Cytol. 1998;42:1397–402.

325. Brown JS, O'Carrigan B, Jackson SP, Yap TA. Targeting DNA repair in cancer: beyond PARP inhibitors. Cancer Discov. 2017;7:20–37.

326. Ibanez de Caceres I, Battagli C, Esteller M, Herman JG, Dulaimi E, Edelson MI, Bergman C, Ehya H, Eisenberg BL, Cairns P. Tumor cell-specific BRCA1 and RASSF1A hypermethylation in serum, plasma, and peritoneal fluid from ovarian cancer patients. Cancer Res. 2004;64:6476–81.

327. Ercoli A, Ferrandina G, Raspaglio G, Marone M, Maggiano N, Del Mastro P, Benedetti Panici P, Mancuso S, Scambia G. hMSH2 and GTBP expression in advanced stage epithelial ovarian cancer. Br J Cancer. 1999;80:1665–71.

328. Stevens EV, Raffeld M, Espina V, Kristensen GB, Tropé CG, Kohn EC, Davidson B. Expression of Xeroderma Pigmentosum A protein predicts improved outcome in metastatic ovarian carcinoma. Cancer. 2005;103:2313–9.

329. Counter CM, Hirte HW, Bacchetti S, Harley CB. Telomerase activity in human ovarian carcinoma. Proc Natl Acad Sci U S A. 1994;91:2900–4.

330. Tseng CJ, Jain S, Hou HC, Liu W, Pao CC, Lin CT, Horng SG, Soong YK, Hsueh S. Applications of the telomerase assay in peritoneal washing fluids. Gynecol Oncol. 2001;81:420–3.

331. Murakami J, Nagai N, Ohama K. Telomerase activity in body cavity fluid and peritoneal washings in uterine and ovarian cancer. J Int Med Res. 1998;26:129–39.

332. Elg SA, Mayer AR, Carson LF, Twiggs LB, Hill RB, Ramakrishnan S. Alpha-1 acid glycoprotein is an immunosuppressive factor found in ascites from ovaria carcinoma. Cancer. 1997;80:1448–56.

333. Elg SA, Carson LF, Fowler JM, Twiggs LB, Moradi MM, Ramakrishnan S. Ascites levels of haptoglobin in patients with ovarian cancer. Cancer. 1993;71:3938–41.

334. Gericke B, Raila J, Sehouli J, Haebel S, Könsgen D, Mustea A, Schweigert FJ. Microheterogeneity of transthyretin in serum and ascitic fluid of ovarian cancer patients. BMC Cancer. 2005;5:133.

335. Schweigert FJ, Raila J, Sehouli J, Buscher U. Accumulation of selected carotenoids, alpha-tocopherol and retinol in human ovarian carcinoma ascitic fluid. Ann Nutr Metab. 2004;48:241–5.

336. Gillan L, Matei D, Fishman DA, Gerbin CS, Karlan BY, Chang DD. Periostin secreted by epithelial ovarian carcinoma is a ligand for alpha(V)beta(3) and alpha(V)beta(5) integrins and promotes cell motility. Cancer Res. 2002;62:5358–64.

337. Hofmann M, Ruschenburg I. mRNA detection of tumor-rejection genes BAGE, GAGE, and MAGE in peritoneal fluid from patients with ovarian carcinoma as a potential diagnostic tool. Cancer. 2002;96:187–93.

338. Jeschke U, Mylonas I, Kunert-Keil C, Stahn R, Scholz C, Janni W, Kuhn C, Schröder E, Mayr D, Friese K. Immunohistochemistry, glycosylation and immunosuppression of glycodelin in human ovarian cancer. Histochem Cell Biol. 2009;131:283–95.

339. Kajiyama H, Kikkawa F, Maeda O, Suzuki T, Ino K, Mizutani S. Increased expression of dipeptidyl peptidase IV in human mesothelial cells by malignant ascites from ovarian carcinoma patients. Oncology. 2002;63:158–65.

340. Masiakos PT, MacLaughlin DT, Maheswaran S, Teixeira J, Fuller AF Jr, Shah PC, Kehas DJ, Kenneally MK, Dombkowski DM, Ha TU, Preffer FI, Donahoe PK. Human ovarian cancer, cell lines, and primary ascites cells express the human Mullerian inhibiting substance (MIS) type II receptor, bind, and are responsive to MIS. Clin Cancer Res. 1999;5:3488–99.

341. Simon I, Zhuo S, Corral L, Diamandis EP, Sarno MJ, Wolfert RL, Kim NW. B7-h4 is a novel membrane-bound protein and a candidate serum and tissue biomarker for ovarian cancer. Cancer Res. 2006;66:1570–5.

342. Thomsen LL, Sargent JM, Williamson CJ, Elgie AW. Nitric oxide synthase activity in fresh cells from ovarian tumour tissue: relationship of enzyme activity with clinical parameters of patients with ovarian cancer. Biochem Pharmacol. 1998;56:1365–70.

343. Jandu N, Richardson M, Singh G, Hirte H, Hatton MW. Human ovarian cancer ascites fluid contains a mixture of incompletely degraded soluble products of fibrin that collectively possess an antiangiogenic property. Int J Gynecol Cancer. 2006;16:1536–44.

344. Wilhelm S, Schmitt M, Parkinson J, Kuhn W, Graeff H, Wilhelm OG. Thrombomodulin, a receptor for the serine protease thrombin, is decreased in primary tumors and metastases but increased in ascitic fluids of patients with advanced ovarian cancer FIGO IIIc. Int J Oncol. 1998;13:645–51.

345. Hough CD, Sherman-Baust CA, Pizer ES, Montz FJ, Im DD, Rosenshein NB, Cho KR, Riggins GJ, Morin PJ. Large-scale serial analysis of gene expression reveals genes differentially expressed in ovarian cancer. Cancer Res. 2000;60:6281–7.

346. Chen YC, Pohl G, Wang TL, Morin PJ, Risberg B, Kristensen GB, Yu A, Davidson B, Shih IM. Apolipoprotein E is required for cell proliferation and survival in ovarian cancer. Cancer Res. 2005;65:331–7.

347. Chen YC, Davidson B, Cheng CC, Maitra A, Giuntoli RL II, Hruban RH, Wang TL, Shih IM. Identification and characterization of membralin, a novel tumor-associated gene, in ovarian carcinoma. Biochim Biophys Acta. 2005;1730:96–102.

348. Nakayama K, Nakayama N, Davidson B, Katabuci H, Kurman RJ, Velculescu VE, Shih IM, Wang TL. Homozygous deletion of MKK4 in ovarian serous carcinomas. Cancer Biol Ther. 2006;5:630–4.

349. Rayhman O, Klipper E, Muller L, Davidson B, Reich R, Meidan R. Small interfering RNA molecules targeting endothelin-converting enzyme-1 inhibit endothelin-1 synthesis and the invasive phenotype of ovarian carcinoma cells. Cancer Res. 2008;68:9265–73.

350. Mælandsmo GM, Flørenes VA, Nguyen MTP, Flatmark K, Davidson B. Different expression and clinical role of S100A4 in ovarian carcinoma at different anatomic sites. Tumor Biol. 2009;30:15–25.

351. Davidson B, Holth A, Moripen L, Trope' CG, Shih IM. Osteopontin expression in ovarian carcinoma effusions is related to improved clinical outcome. Hum Pathol. 2011;42:991–7.

352. Reich R, Hadar S, Davidson B. Expression and clinical role of protein of regenerating liver (PRL) phosphatases in ovarian carcinoma. Int J Mol Sci. 2011;12:1133–45.

353. Becker MA, Haluska P Jr, Bale LK, Oxvig C, Conover CA. A novel neutralizing antibody targeting pregnancy-associated plasma protein-a inhibits ovarian cancer growth and ascites accumulation in patient mouse tumorgrafts. Mol Cancer Ther. 2015;14:973–81.

354. Bock AJ, Dong HP, Tropé CG, Staff AC, Risberg B, Davidson B. Nucleoside transporters are widely expressed in ovarian carcinoma effusions. Cancer Chemother Pharmacol. 2012;69:467–75.

355. Vaksman O, Davidson B, Tropé C, Reich R. Calreticulin expression is reduced in high-grade ovarian serous carcinoma effusions compared with primary tumors and solid metastases. Hum Pathol. 2013;44:2677–83.

356. Hetland TE, Nymoen DA, Emilsen E, Kærn J, Tropé CG, Flørenes VA, Davidson B. MGST1 expression in serous ovarian carcinoma differs at various anatomic sites, but is unrelated to chemoresistance or survival. Gynecol Oncol. 2012;126:460–5.

357. Hetland TE, Holth A, Kærn J, Flørenes VA, Tropé CG, Davidson B. HMGA2 protein expression in ovarian serous carcinoma effusions, primary tumors, and solid metastases. Virchows Arch. 2012;460:505–13.

358. Davidson B, Holth A, Hellesylt E, Hadar R, Katz B, Tropé CG, Reich R. HUR mRNA expression in ovarian high-grade serous carcinoma effusions is associated with poor survival. Hum Pathol. 2016;48:95–101.

359. Horwitz V, Davidson B, Stern D, Tropé CG, Tavor Re'em T, Reich R. Ezrin is associated with disease progression in ovarian carcinoma. PLoS One. 2016;11:e0162502.

360. Ioakim-Liossi A, Gagos S, Athanassiades P, Athanassiadou P, Gogas J, Davaris P, Markopoulos C. Changes of chromosomes 1, 3, 6, and 11 in metastatic effusions arising from breast and ovarian cancer. Cancer Genet Cytogenet. 1999;110:34–40.

361. Chang HW, Ali SZ, Cho SK, Kurman RJ, Shih IM. Detection of allelic imbalance in ascitic supernatant by digital single nucleotide polymorphism analysis. Clin Cancer Res. 2002;8:2580–5.

362. Lounis H, Mes-Masson AM, Dion F, Bradley WE, Seymour RJ, Provencher D, Tonin PN. Mapping of chromosome 3p deletions in human epithelial ovarian tumors. Oncogene. 1998;17:2359–65.

363. Nagel H, Schulten HJ, Gunawan B, Brinck U, Füzesi L. The potential value of comparative genomic hybridization analysis in effusion-and fine needle aspiration cytology. Mod Pathol. 2002;15:818–25.

364. Brenne K, Nymoen DA, Reich R, Davidson B. PRAME (preferentially expressed antigen of melanoma) is a novel marker for

differentiating serous carcinoma from malignant mesothelioma. Am J Clin Pathol. 2012;137:240–7.

365. Brusegard K, Stavnes HT, Nymoen DA, Flatmark K, Trope CG, Davidson B. Rab25 is overexpressed in Müllerian serous carcinoma compared to malignant mesothelioma. Virchows Arch. 2012;460:193–202.

366. Davidson B, Stavnes HT, Hellesylt E, Hager T, Zeppa P, Pinamonti M, Wohlschlaeger J. MMP-7 is a highly specific negative marker for benign and malignant mesothelial cells in serous effusions. Hum Pathol. 2016;47:104–8.

367. Yuan Y, Dong HP, Nymoen DA, Nesland JM, Wu C, Davidson B. PINCH-2 expression in cancers involving the serosal cavities using quantitative PCR. Cytopathology. 2011;22:22–9.

368. Yuan Y, Nymoen DA, Tuft Stavnes H, Rossnes AK, Bjørang O, Wu C, Nesland JM, Davidson B. Tenascin-X is a novel diagnostic marker of malignant mesothelioma. Am J Surg Pathol. 2009;33:1673–82.

369. Davidson B, Stavnes HT, Holth A, Chen X, Yang Y, Shih IM, Wang TL. Gene expression signatures differentiate ovarian/peritoneal serous carcinoma from breast carcinoma in effusions. J Cell Mol Med. 2011;15:535–44.

370. Bock AJ, Nymoen DA, Brenne K, Kærn J, Davidson B. SCARA3 mRNA is overexpressed in ovarian carcinoma compared with breast carcinoma effusions. Hum Pathol. 2012;43:669–74.

371. Tuft Stavnes H, Nymoen DA, Hetland Falkenthal TE, Kærn J, Tropé CG, Davidson B. APOA1 mRNA expression in ovarian serous carcinoma effusions is a marker of longer survival. Am J Clin Pathol. 2014;142:51–7.

372. Stavnes HT, Holth A, Don T, Kærn J, Vaksman O, Reich R, Trope' CG, Davidson B. HOXB8 expression in ovarian serous carcinoma effusions is associated with shorter survival. Gynecol Oncol. 2013;129:358–63.

373. Stavnes HT, Nymoen DA, Langerød A, Holth A, Børresen Dale AL, Davidson B. AZGP1 and SPDEF mRNA expression differentiates breast carcinoma from ovarian serous carcinoma. Virchows Arch. 2013;462:163–73.

374. Schaner ME, Davidson B, Skrede M, Reich R, Flørenes VA, Risberg B, Berner A, Goldberg I, Givant-Horwitz V, Tropé CG, Kristensen GB, Nesland JM, Børresen-Dale AL. Variation in gene expression patterns in effusions and primary tumors from serous ovarian cancer patients. Mol Cancer. 2005;4:26.

375. Vaksman O, Stavnes HT, Kærn J, Trope CG, Davidson B, Reich R. miRNA profiling along tumor progression in ovarian carcinoma. J Cell Mol Med. 2011;15:1593–602.

376. Vaksman O, Hetland TE, Tropé CG, Reich R, Davidson B. Argonaute, Dicer, and Drosha are up-regulated along tumor progression in serous ovarian carcinoma. Hum Pathol. 2012;43:2062–9.

377. Nymoen DA, Slipicevic A, Holth A, Emilsen E, Hetland Falkenthal TE, Tropé CG, Reich R, Flørenes VA, Davidson B. MiR-29a is a candidate biomarker of better survival in metastatic high-grade serous carcinoma. Hum Pathol. 2016;54:74–81.

378. Valadi H, Ekström K, Bossios A, Sjöstrand M, Lee JJ, Lötvall JO. Exosome-mediated transfer of mRNAs and microRNAs is a novel mechanism of genetic exchange between cells. Nat Cell Biol. 2007;9:654–9.

379. Siravegna G, Marsoni S, Siena S, Bardelli A. Integrating liquid biopsies into the management of cancer. Nat Rev Clin Oncol. 2017;14:531–48.

380. Moore C, Kosgodage U, Lange S, Inal JM. The emerging role of exosome and microvesicle- (EMV-) based cancer therapeutics and immunotherapy. Int J Cancer. 2017;141:428–36.

381. Vaksman O, Tropé C, Davidson B, Reich R. Exosome-derived miRNAs and ovarian carcinoma progression. Carcinogenesis. 2014;35:2113–20.

382. Cappellesso R, Tinazzi A, Giurici T, Simonato F, Guzzardo V, Ventura L, Crescenzi M, Chiarelli S, Fassina A. Programmed cell death 4 and microRNA 21 inverse expression is maintained in cells and exosomes from ovarian serous carcinoma effusions. Cancer Cytopathol. 2014;122:685–93.

383. Broner EC, Tropé CG, Reich R, Davidson B. TSAP6 is a novel candidate marker of poor survival in metastatic high-grade serous carcinoma. Hum Pathol. 2017;60:180–7.

384. Gillet JP, Wang J, Calcagno AM, Green LJ, Varma S, Bunkholt Elstrand M, Trope CG, Ambudkar SV, Davidson B, Gottesman MM. Clinical relevance of multidrug resistance gene expression in ovarian serous carcinoma effusions. Mol Pharm. 2011;8: 2080–8.

385. Nymoen DA, Holth A, Hetland Falkenthal TE, Tropé CG, Davidson B. CIAPIN1 and ABCA13 are markers of poor survival in metastatic ovarian serous carcinoma. Mol Cancer. 2015;14:44.

386. Gortzak-Uzan L, Ignatchenko A, Evangelou AI, Agochiya M, Brown KA, St Onge P, Kireeva I, Schmitt-Ulms G, Brown TJ, Murphy J, Rosen B, Shaw P, Jurisica I, Kislinger T. A proteome resource of ovarian cancer ascites: integrated proteomic and bioinformatic analyses to identify putative biomarkers. J Proteome Res. 2008;7:339–51.

387. Gunawardana CG, Memari N, Diamandis EP. Identifying novel autoantibody signatures in ovarian cancer using high-density protein microarrays. Clin Biochem. 2009;42:426–9.

388. Puiffe ML, Le Page C, Filali-Mouhim A, Zietarska M, Ouellet V, Tonin PN, Chevrette M, Provencher DM, Mes-Masson AM. Characterization of ovarian cancer ascites on cell invasion, proliferation, spheroid formation, and gene expression in an in vitro model of epithelial ovarian cancer. Neoplasia. 2007;9:820–9.

389. Jinawath N, Vasoontara C, Jinawath A, Fang X, Zhao K, Yap KL, Guo T, Lee CS, Wang W, Balgley BM, Davidson B, Wang TL, Shih IM. Oncoproteomic analysis reveals co-upregulation of RELA and STAT5 in carboplatin resistant ovarian carcinoma. PLoS One. 2010;5:e11198.

390. Saini U, Naidu S, Elnaggar AC, Bid HK, Wallbillich JJ, Bixel K, Bolyard C, Suarez AA, Kaur B, Kuppusamy P, Hays J, Goodfellow PJ, Cohn DE, Selvendiran K. Elevated STAT3 expression in ovarian cancer ascites promotes invasion and metastasis: a potential therapeutic target. Oncogene. 2017;36:168–81.

391. Vettukattil R, Hetland TE, Flørenes VA, Kærn J, Davidson B, Bathen TF. Proton magnetic resonance metabolomic characterization of ovarian serous carcinoma effusions: chemotherapy-related effects and comparison with malignant mesothelioma and breast carcinoma. Hum Pathol. 2013;44:1859–66.

392. Zennaro L, Vanzani P, Nicolè L, Cappellesso R, Fassina A. Metabonomics by proton nuclear magnetic resonance in human pleural effusions: a route to discriminate between benign and malignant pleural effusions and to target small molecules as potential cancer biomarkers. Cancer. 2017;125:341–8.

393. Liu JF, Palakurthi S, Zeng Q, Zhou S, Ivanova E, Huang W, Zervantonakis IK, Selfors LM, Shen Y, Pritchard CC, Zheng M, Adleff V, Papp E, Piao H, Novak M, Fotheringham S, Wulf GM, English J, Kirschmeier PT, Velculescu VE, Paweletz C, Mills GB, Livingston DM, Brugge JS, Matulonis UA, Drapkin R. Establishment of patient-derived tumor xenograft models of epithelial ovarian cancer for preclinical evaluation of novel therapeutics. Clin Cancer Res. 2017;23:1263–73.

394. Patch AM, Christie EL, Etemadmoghadam D, Garsed DW, George J, Fereday S, Nones K, Cowin P, Alsop K, Bailey PJ, Kassahn KS, Newell F, Quinn MC, Kazakoff S, Quek K, Wilhelm-Benartzi C, Curry E, Leong HS, Australian Ovarian Cancer Study Group, Hamilton A, Mileshkin L, Au-Yeung G, Kennedy C, Hung J, Chiew YE, Harnett P, Friedlander M, Quinn M, Pyman J, Cordner

S, O'Brien P, Leditschke J, Young G, Strachan K, Waring P, Azar W, Mitchell C, Traficante N, Hendley J, Thorne H, Shackleton M, Miller DK, Arnau GM, Tothill RW, Holloway TP, Semple T, Harliwong I, Nourse C, Nourbakhsh E, Manning S, Idrisoglu S, Bruxner TJ, Christ AN, Poudel B, Holmes O, Anderson M, Leonard C, Lonie A, Hall N, Wood S, Taylor DF, Xu Q, Fink JL, Waddell N, Drapkin R, Stronach E, Gabra H, Brown R, Jewell A, Nagaraj SH, Markham E, Wilson PJ, Ellul J, McNally O, Doyle MA, Vedururu R, Stewart C, Lengyel E, Pearson JV, Waddell N, deFazio A, Grimmond SM, Bowtell DD. Whole-genome characterization of chemoresistant ovarian cancer. Nature. 2015;521(7553):489–94.

395. Shah RH, Scott SN, Brannon AR, Levine DA, Lin O, Berger MF. Comprehensive mutation profiling by next-generation sequencing of effusion fluids from patients with high-grade serous ovarian carcinoma. Cancer Cytopathol. 2015;123:289–97.

396. Penner-Goeke S, Lichtensztejn Z, Neufeld M, Ali JL, Altman AD, Nachtigal MW, McManus KJ. The temporal dynamics of chromosome instability in ovarian cancer cell lines and primary patient samples. PLoS Genet. 2017;13:e1006707.

397. Lund RJ, Huhtinen K, Salmi J, Rantala J, Nguyen EV, Moulder R, Goodlett DR, Lahesmaa R, Carpén O. DNA methylation and transcriptome changes associated with Cisplatin resistance in ovarian cancer. Sci Rep. 2017;7:1469.

398. Castellarin M, Milne K, Zeng T, Tse K, Mayo M, Zhao Y, Webb JR, Watson PH, Nelson BH, Holt RA. Clonal evolution of high-grade serous ovarian carcinoma from primary to recurrent disease. J Pathol. 2013;229:515–24.

# Breast Cancer

## Ben Davidson and Fernando Schmitt

## Introduction

Breast cancer is the most commonly diagnosed malignancy in women in the majority of countries, with an estimated 1.7 million new cases and 521,900 deaths in 2012, with highest incidence in developed countries [1]. As discussed in Chap. 4, despite the relatively small percentage of patients diagnosed with distant metastasis, involvement of the serosal cavities, particularly the pleural space, is not a rare condition [2–9].

Malignant pleural effusion may occur at diagnosis, occasionally as the presenting sign of breast carcinoma, or at disease recurrence, alone or in the presence of metastasis to other organs [3, 4, 10, 11]. The time interval from diagnosis to the development of effusion for breast carcinoma patients is longer than in other malignancies affecting the serosal cavities, such as carcinoma of the lung and ovary [12].

The prognosis of breast cancer is relatively good, with 5-year relative survival at 90% for all stages in the United States [1]. However, the presence of pleural effusion is associated with poor prognosis, with median survival of 5–13 months reported in four series [3, 4, 13, 14]. A study of 233 patients with advanced recurrent breast cancer did not show association between the presence of malignant effusion and survival in this patient group, while liver metastasis was associated with shorter survival in univariate analysis [15]. The formation of spheroids by breast carcinoma cells in pleural effusions was reported to be associated with less atypia, lower mitotic activity, and longer survival compared to other morphological patterns [13].

In a more recent study of 49 patients, van Galen and co-workers found significant association between survival and HER2 status, presence of metastases at other sites, antihormonal therapy, and the interval from diagnosis to development of malignant effusion (cutoff at 5 years). Median and mean survival were 9.3 and 19 months, respectively [16].

Bielsa et al. measured the levels of the tumor markers carcinoembryonic antigen (CEA), CA 15–3, cytokeratin fragment 19 (CYFRA 21-1), and CA 125 by immunoassay in 224 malignant effusions, including 63 breast carcinoma metastases, and found that CA 125 and CYFRA 21-1 levels of $\geq 1000$ U/mL and $\geq 100$ ng/mL, respectively, were associated with significantly shorter patient survival [17]. Measurement of cancer antigens in supernatants and sediments of malignant ($n = 103$) and benign ($n = 32$) pleural effusions, the former including 37 breast carcinoma effusions, showed higher levels of CEA and CA 15–3 in breast carcinoma effusions compared to benign specimens [18].

In view of the dismal clinical outcome of breast carcinoma patients with effusions, there is an urgent need to study the molecular profile of tumor cells in the serosal cavities in order to design effective therapeutic approaches to extend survival and improve their life quality. To date, the extensive research effort focusing on primary breast carcinoma and metastases to solid organs, primarily to lymph nodes, has not been matched by similar efforts toward understanding the biology of breast carcinoma cells in effusions. Nevertheless, some data that have emerged in recent years expand our understanding of the molecular characteristics of breast carcinoma cells at this unique anatomic site. The following paragraphs detail these studies.

## Cytogenetics

Several studies have investigated genetic events in breast carcinoma effusions. Comparative analysis of three serial effusions from a single patient showed mutation of the *KRAS*

B. Davidson, M.D., Ph.D. (✉)
Department of Pathology, The Norwegian Radium Hospital, Oslo University Hospital, Oslo, Norway

Faculty of Medicine, Institute of Clinical Medicine, University of Oslo, Oslo, Norway
e-mail: bend@medisin.uio.no; bdd@ous-hf.no

F. Schmitt, M.D., Ph.D., F.I.A.C.
Molecular Pathology Unit, Department of Pathology and Oncology, Medical Faculty of Porto University, Institute of Pathology and Molecular Immunology of Porto University, IPATIMUP, Porto, Portugal
e-mail: fernando.schmitt@ipatimup.pt

© Springer International Publishing AG, part of Springer Nature 2018
B. Davidson et al. (eds.), *Serous Effusions*, https://doi.org/10.1007/978-3-319-76478-8_10

gene and a loss of heterozygosity at the *HRAS* locus only in the last specimen, providing molecular evidence of tumor progression in this case [19].

Driouch et al. analyzed 122 primary breast carcinomas and 62 distant metastases, the latter consisting of 44 pleural effusions and 18 solid metastases, for amplification of the *MYC*, *ERBB2*, *INT2/FGF3*, and *CCND1* genes using restriction fragment length polymorphism (RFLP) [20]. *MYC* and *ERBB2* gene amplification was less frequent in metastases compared to primary carcinomas, significantly so for the former gene, with no differences observed for *INT2/FGF3* and *CCND1*. However, amplification of all four genes was more frequently found in effusions compared to solid metastases, significantly so for *INT2/FGF3* and *CCND1* at the 11q13 chromosome band. The percentage of effusions with MYC, ERBB2 and INT2/FGF3-CCND1 gene amplifications was 9.1%, 11.8%, and 25%, respectively.

Roka and co-workers analyzed 86 specimens from breast carcinoma patients, including 30 primary carcinomas, 5 lymph node metastases, and 51 pleural ($n = 36$) and peritoneal ($n = 15$) effusions, of which 40 were malignant and 11 reactive, for chromosome 8 status using FISH [21]. Aneuploidy with gain of chromosome 8 was found in 30/40 (75%) malignant effusions. One specimen had chromosome 8 monosomy. Ten of 11 benign effusions did not show aneusomy, whereas 1 specimen had few positive cells and was suspected of being malignant. The authors suggested that this assay may be used as a diagnostic assay for the identification of small populations of malignant cells in effusions.

A subsequent study by the same group applied interphase cytogenetics using FISH with chromosome 11 and 17 probes to a series of 55 breast carcinoma and 39 non-small cell lung carcinoma effusions [22]. Aneuploidy for chromosome 11 and/or 17 was found in 47 breast carcinoma and 35 lung carcinoma effusions. The overall chromosome number did not predict survival in the two patient groups. However, absence of aneuploidy at chromosome 11 was associated with shorter overall survival for breast carcinoma patients.

An additional cytogenetic study of 15 pleural effusions from 11 breast carcinoma patients, as well as 27 peritoneal effusions from 16 ovarian carcinoma patients, showed frequent tumor aneuploidy. Near-triploid DNA content was found in breast carcinomas, with 52–72 chromosomes in the major clone. Ovarian and breast carcinoma cells had frequent alteration of chromosomes 1, 3, 6, 7, 8, 9, 11, 12, and 17 [23].

De Matos Granja studied 41 effusions from patients previously diagnosed with breast carcinoma for loss of heterozygosity (LOH) at 1p32, 7q31, and 17q21 [24]. Effusions consisted of 24 specimens diagnosed as malignant by morphology, 14 diagnosed as suspicious, and 3 that were morphologically benign. LOH at chromosomes 1, 7, and 17 was found in 22%, 27%, and 32% of informative cases, respectively. LOH was found in 38% and 36% of the morphologically malignant and suspicious specimens, respectively, and

was absent in the benign effusions, suggesting that this assay may be a useful adjunct to morphology in the diagnosis of breast carcinoma effusions.

## Cytokines, Growth Factors, and Growth Factor Receptors

The proliferative and survival-promoting capacity of cancer cells is dependent of their ability to activate and utilize multiple pathways mediating these actions. Studies of breast carcinoma effusions have consequently focused on this aspect of cell biology from the very beginning of molecular research in this area. As analysis of HER2 status is part of the routine diagnostic and clinical management of breast cancer, this issue is briefly discussed in Chap. 4.

## Transforming Growth Factors (TGFs)

TGFs consist of two proteins, TGF-$\alpha$ and TGF-$\beta$. TGF-$\alpha$, member of the epidermal growth factor (EGF) family, is synthesized as pro-TGF-$\alpha$ and is cleaved to its mature form by the protease TGF-$\alpha$-converting enzyme (TACE), forming a 5–20-kDa protein, variation being due to different glycosylation. It is produced by a variety of normal tissues, the majority of which are epithelia, and has a role in embryogenesis, wound healing, and bone reabsorption. TGF-$\alpha$ is additionally produced by different cancers, including breast carcinoma, and its binding to the EGF receptor (EGFR) mediates cell proliferation and survival [25].

Arteaga et al. measured the levels of TGF-$\alpha$ in 130 malignant effusions, including 34 breast carcinomas, using radioimmunoassay. TGF-$\alpha$ was detected in 38% of breast carcinoma effusions, as well as 50% and 42% of lung and ovarian carcinoma effusions, respectively. In breast carcinoma, it was more frequently found in hormone receptor-negative cases. The presence of TGF-$\alpha$ was associated with larger tumor burden, as evaluated by the number of metastatic sites, as well as with poor survival in univariate and multivariate analysis [26].

In another study, TGF-$\alpha$ levels were measured in 100 effusions, comprising 63 malignant and 37 benign specimens, including 13 breast carcinomas, applying the same method. Levels ranged from 0.2 to 26 ng/mL in both specimen types, but were significantly higher in malignant effusions, with particularly high levels in breast carcinoma effusions [27].

Endoglin (CD105) is a transmembrane glycoprotein composed of two 95-kDa subunits that form a homodimeric 180-kDa protein and is an auxiliary receptor for several TGF-$\beta$ family proteins. There are two splice isoforms of the protein, termed short (S)-endoglin and long (L)-endoglin based on differences in its cytoplasmic part. In addition, a soluble form of the protein (sEng) is probably formed by proteolytic shedding. Endoglin is primarily expressed on endothelial cells but has been detected in mesenchymal and hematopoietic cells, as well as in different cancers. TGF-β binding results in activin-like kinase (ALK) recruitment and signaling propagation to the nucleus via Smad proteins that act as transcription repressors or activators. Mutations in endoglin or ALK-1 are the molecular cause for hereditary hemorrhagic telangiectasia (Osler-Weber-Rendu disease), a condition that is characterized by vascular malformations and severe bleeding episodes [28, 29]. Its involvement in multiple pathologic conditions related to altered angiogenesis led to its identification as a potential therapeutic target of a range of diseases, including cancer [30].

Endoglin was detected in 36/36 breast carcinoma effusion supernatants by ELISA and was shown to be expressed by both carcinoma cells and reactive mesothelium using immunohistochemistry. Tumor cell expression was significantly higher in effusions compared to patient-matched primary carcinoma (Fig. 10.1), as well as in post-chemotherapy compared to pre-chemotherapy effusions. Higher tumor endoglin expression was associated with poor overall and disease-free survival in univariate and multivariate survival analysis, suggesting that endoglin may be an important therapeutic target in metastatic breast cancer [31].

## Vascular Endothelial Growth Factor (VEGF)

Malignant tumors are highly dependent on the formation of new vessels (angiogenesis), a process in which VEGF plays a central role. The VEGF family comprises seven secreted glycoproteins: VEGF-A, VEGF-B, VEGF-C, VEGF-D, and VEGF-E and placenta growth factors (PlGFs) PlGF-1 and PlGF-2. VEGF family members bind several receptors, including VEGFR-1 (fms-like tyrosine kinase-1, Flt-1), VEGFR-2 (kinase insert domain-containing receptor, KDR), and VEGFR-3, the latter expressed in endothelial cells of lymphatic vessels.

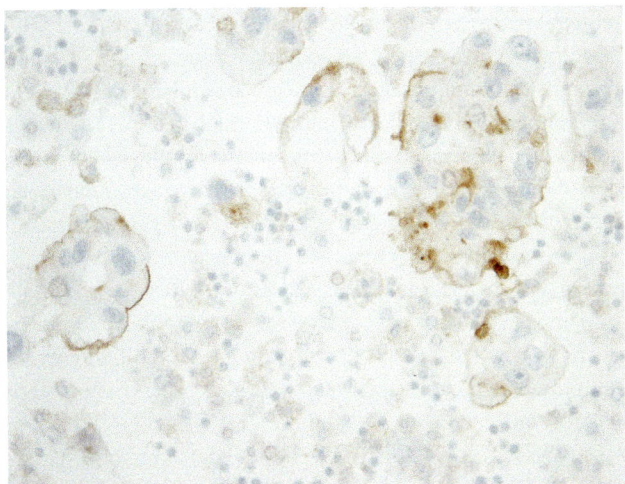

**Fig. 10.1** Endoglin (CD105) membrane expression in breast carcinoma cells in effusion

Two additional VEGF receptors, neuropilin 1 (NRP-1) and neuropilin 2 (NRP-2), are coreceptors of VEGFRs, increasing the binding of VEGF to its receptors [32]. In addition to its role in angiogenesis, VEGF has autocrine tumor effects on survival, migration, and invasion and mediates immunosuppression and homing of bone marrow progenitors to prepare an organ for subsequent metastasis. In the context of the serosal cavities, VEGF (previously also termed vascular permeability factor) increases vessel permeability, thereby contributing to the accumulation of effusions [33, 34]. The therapeutic role of bevacizumab (Avastin), a monoclonal antibody against VEGF, as well as other anti-angiogenic drugs, has been investigated in several clinical trials of patients with breast cancer, including those with metastatic disease, in recent years [35].

VEGF levels were previously measured in 445 serum samples and 56 effusions, the latter including 12 breast carcinomas, by sandwich enzyme-linked immunoadsorbent assay. Serum VEGF levels were not significantly higher in breast carcinoma patients compared to controls. However, serum levels were higher in patients with metastatic compared to localized disease. Effusion VEGF levels were higher in malignant compared to reactive effusions and were up to tenfold higher than in the malignant effusions compared to serum samples [36]. VEGF was similarly shown to be elevated in 39 malignant effusions, including 7 breast carcinomas, compared to controls consisting of 4 effusions from patients with cirrhosis and serum from healthy subjects, a difference that was significant also in analysis of breast carcinoma effusions alone vs. controls. Levels of two other angiogenic factors, interleukin-8 (IL-8) and angiogenin, did not differ between malignant effusions and controls [37].

Angiogenic molecule expression was studied in effusions (n = 49) and patient-matched solid primary and metastatic tumors (n = 68) [38]. mRNA in situ hybridization (ISH) showed the presence of *VEGF*, *IL-8*, and *FGF2* (encoding basic fibroblast growth factor, bFGF) mRNA in the majority of specimens, irrespective of anatomic site (Fig. 10.2a–c), and *KDR* mRNA was detected in 6/22 effusions using RT-PCR. However, whereas VEGF protein expression by immunohistochemistry was comparable at all anatomic sites, IL-8 and bFGF protein expression was significantly lower in effusions compared to primary tumors. The difference in bFGF expression was additionally seen in comparative analysis of effusions and lymph node metastases. *IL-8* and *VEGF* mRNA in tumor cells in effusions was co-expressed with mRNA of the ETS family transcription factors ETS1 and PEA3, which regulate angiogenesis (see below). bFGF protein expression in effusions predicted shorter disease-free survival in univariate survival analysis.

## Nerve Growth Factor (NGF) and Its Receptors

Nerve growth factor (NGF) is the prototype molecule of the neurotrophin family, which in addition comprises brain-derived

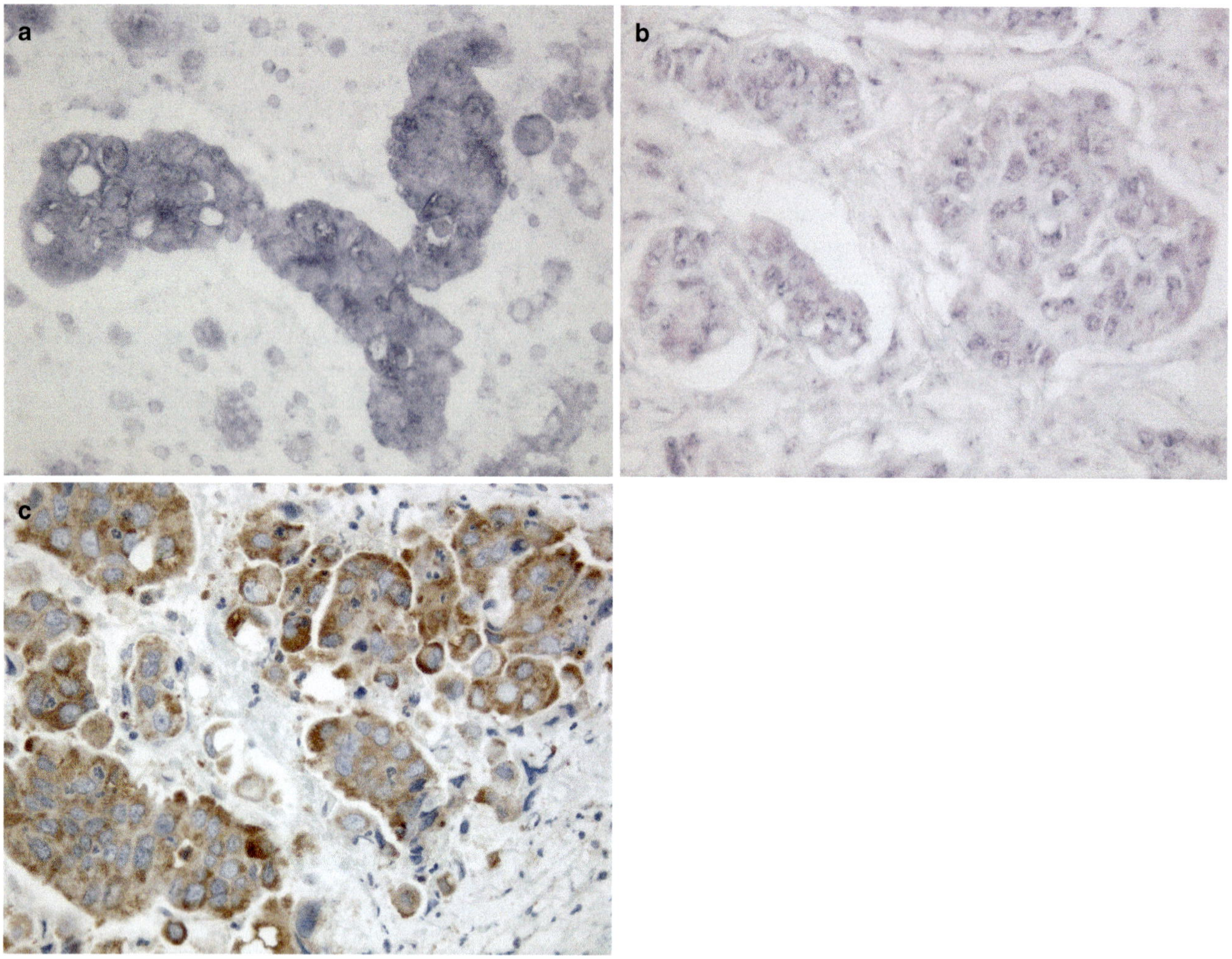

**Fig. 10.2** (**a–c**) Angiogenic molecules; (**a**) in situ hybridization for *FGF2* mRNA in effusion; (**b**) in situ hybridization for *IL-8* mRNA in a local recurrence; (**c**) VEGF protein in a primary carcinoma; (**a**, **b**) NBT-BCIP as chromogen, nuclear fast red as counterstain

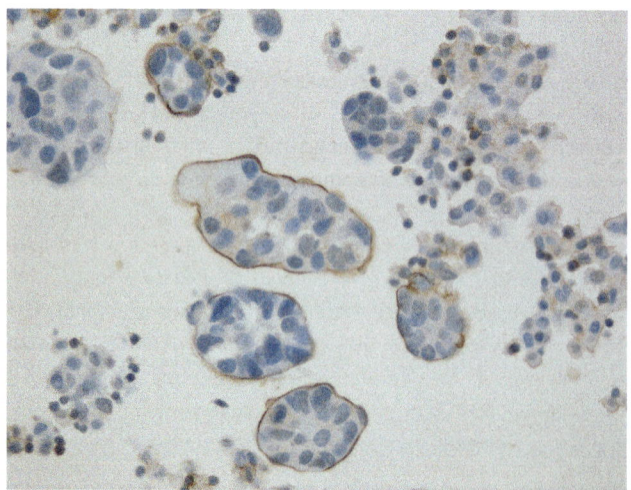

**Fig. 10.3** Expression of the activated nerve growth factor receptor p-TrkA at the membrane in breast carcinoma cells in effusion

neurotrophic factor (BDNF) and neurotrophin-3 (NT-3) and NT-4/NT-5. NGF binds to the tyrosine kinase high-affinity receptor TrkA, resulting in activation of the mitogen-activated protein kinase (MAPK) and phosphoinositide 3-kinase (PI3K) signaling pathways. p75, an additional neurotrophin receptor, belongs to the tumor necrosis receptor family, has a different structure from TrkA, lacks intrinsic catalytic activity, and is able to bind all neurotrophins [39, 40]. Rearrangement or mutation of the TrkA gene, resulting in constitutive activation of the receptor, has been reported in papillary thyroid carcinomas and in acute myeloid leukemia, and the receptor is expressed in various neural and nonneural cancers [41, 42].

The expression of activated TrkA (phospho-TrkA, p-TrkA) was studied in 42 breast carcinoma effusions and 65 patient-matched solid tumors [43]. The majority of lesions were additionally studied for NGF and p75 expression. p-TrkA was found in 93% and 92% of effusions (Fig. 10.3) and locoregional recurrences, respectively, val-

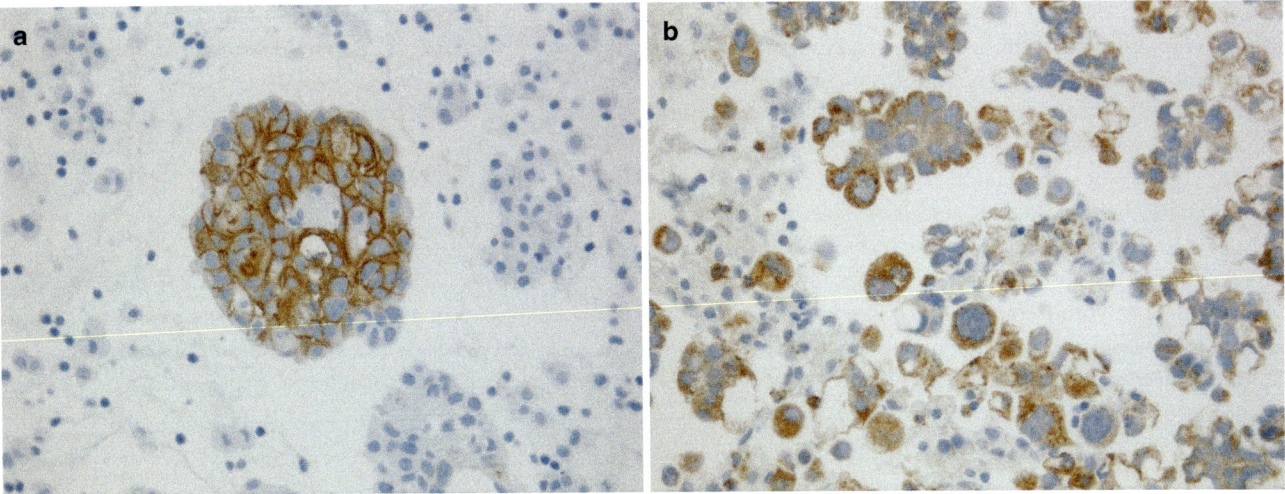

**Fig. 10.4** IGF system. Breast carcinoma cells in effusion express IGFBP3 (**a**) and IGF-II (**b**)

ues that were significantly higher than in primary carcinomas (41%) and lymph node metastases (44%). In contrast, p75 expression was less frequent in effusions compared to both primary tumors and lymph node metastases. NGF was expressed at all anatomic sites, but its presence in tumor cells in effusions was observed exclusively in specimens from patients who developed effusions within 5 years from primary operation. These data document upregulation of p-TrkA during the progression from primary tumor and lymph node metastasis to effusion in breast carcinoma. The co-expression of TrkA and NGF suggests the presence of an autocrine NGF-TrkA signaling pathway in this cancer.

## The Insulin-Like Growth Factor (IGF) System

The IGF system consists of the peptide hormones insulin, IGF-I and IGF-II; the cell surface insulin receptor (IR), IGF-1R, IGF-2R, and hybrid IGF-1R/IR receptors; and a family of circulating high-affinity IGF-binding proteins (IGFBP). IGF-I and IGF-II are 7.6-kDa and 7.5-kDa peptides that share about 50% homology with proinsulin and 62% among themselves. These three ligands bind with different affinity to IGF system receptors, of which all except IGF-2R possess tyrosine kinase activity. Activation of IGF receptors leads to phosphorylation of adaptor proteins of the IRS family or SHC, with subsequent activation of several signaling pathways regulating cell proliferation and survival, differentiation, metabolism, adhesion, migration, and metastasis, as well as epithelial-to-mesenchymal transition (EMT) [44–47]. Inhibitors of the IGF system are under investigation for their potential as targeted therapy in different cancer types, including breast cancer, though results have to date been disappointing [47].

A previous study of IGF-1R protein expression in 90 breast carcinoma effusions and 36 benign effusions using immunohistochemistry showed that expression of this receptor is limited to carcinoma cells, with a sensitivity of 91.1% [48]. In an additional study, the diagnostic and clinical role of IGF-II and IGFBP3 was immunohistochemically analyzed in 327 effusions, including 48 breast carcinomas. IGFBP3 and IGF-II expression was significantly higher in carcinomas, including those of breast origin (Fig. 10.4a, b), compared to malignant mesothelioma. However, breast carcinomas expressed these two proteins less frequently than tumors of the lower genital tract (ovary, endometrium, and cervix), with predominantly focal expression of IGFBP3 [49].

## Adhesion and Other Cell Membrane Molecules

One of the biological properties enabling cancer cells to invade and metastasize is the ability to undergo dynamic changes in their adhesive phenotype. Several important families, including cadherins, integrins, and claudins, and the immunoglobulin superfamily, among others, are involved in these processes.

## Integrins

Integrins are a family of heterodimeric glycoproteins composed of α and β subunits. Eighteen α and 8 β subunits are known to date, forming at least 24 different receptors. Intracellular signaling through integrins affects proliferation, apoptosis, and synthesis of cancer-associated molecules in response to cues originating from other cells (e.g., stromal myofibroblasts) or from ECM proteins, including laminin, fibronectin, collagen, vitronectin, entactin, tenascin, and fibrinogen [50]. Other binding partners of integrins include matrix metalloproteinases (MMPs) and their inhibitor TIMP2, urokinase-type plasminogen activator (uPA), osteopontin, IRS1, thrombospondin-1, integrin-linked kinase (ILK), von Willebrand factor, and the cytoskeletal proteins talin, actinin, and tensin [51]. Integrins have been shown to regulate multiple critical cellular processes involved in cancer, including cell proliferation, survival, migration, invasion and metastasis, stemness, and drug resistance [52].

Expression of the $\alpha$V integrin subunit was previously studied as part of the above-discussed analysis of angiogenic molecule expression, in view of the role of this integrin subunit in cell migration, invasion, and angiogenesis. Breast carcinoma cells in effusions had significantly higher expression of $\alpha$V integrin compared to both primary tumors and lymph node metastases, suggesting that this molecule is involved in metastasis and disease progression in breast carcinoma (Fig. 10.5a) [38]. A subsequent study of 55 malignant and 12 reactive effusions, including 7 breast carcinomas, using flow cytometry demonstrated frequent expression of the $\alpha$V, $\alpha$6, and $\beta$1 subunits, with no expression of the $\beta$3 integrin subunit. The proteoglycan syndecan-1 (CD138) was additionally detected (Fig. 10.5b–d) [53].

These three subunits form the $\alpha v \beta 1$ fibronectin receptor and the $\alpha 6 \beta 1$ laminin receptor. Fibronectin was shown to be an important migratory protein for tumor cells in effusions in analysis of cancer cells of various origins, including breast carcinoma [54].

The interaction with laminin, the major component of all basement membranes, was further analyzed in another study, in which expression of the non-integrin 67-kDa laminin receptor (67-kDa LR) was studied. This protein has a highly conserved mRNA sequence with a predicted product size of 37 kDa, and its expression has been shown to be upregulated by cytokines, inflammatory agents, and ECM proteins such as laminin and fibronectin. The receptor has been postulated to be co-regulated and co-expressed with the $\alpha 6 \beta 4$ integrin, another laminin receptor, in vitro. It is expressed in a wide range of malignancies, including in breast carcinoma, in many of which its presence has been shown to correlate with poor differentiation, disease progression, and poor survival [55, 56].

The expression of the 67-kDa LR was immunohistochemically studied in 86 effusions, consisting of 24 ovarian and 38 breast carcinomas, as well as 24 malignant mesotheliomas [57]. The 67-kDa LR was detected in 15/38 (39%) breast carcinomas, compared to 79% and 8% of ovarian carcinomas and malignant mesotheliomas, respectively. Nine benign effusions that were additionally studied were uniformly negative, as were all reactive mesothelial cells in malignant effusions. This suggested a biological difference in the expression

of laminin receptors between cells of epithelial and mesothelial origin, which may additionally have a potential diagnostic role in their differential diagnosis.

## E-Cadherin and Its Regulators

The biological role of cadherins is discussed in detail in Chap. 9. These membrane glycoproteins mediate homophilic cell-cell adhesion and are involved in differentiation during embryogenesis and in maintaining tissue structure in the mature organism. E-cadherin, expressed in epithelia, is an invasion inhibitor and tumor suppressor that is inactivated or downregulated through genetic (mutations) and epigenetic (CpG promoter hypermethylation, transcriptional regulation, and posttranslational modification) mechanisms, resulting in tumor progression in several cancers. Its loss may occur concomitantly to the upregulation of proinvasive mesenchymal markers, including N-cadherin, vimentin, and collagens, resulting in EMT. During EMT, E-cadherin is epigenetically silenced by its negative transcriptional regulators Snail and Slug, members of the Snail superfamily, as well as Twist, Zeb, and Smad interacting protein 1 (Sip1), member of the crystallin enhancer binding factor 1 family. Several of the mechanisms that negatively regulate E-cadherin expression have been shown to operate in breast carcinoma [58–60].

mRNA expression of Snail, Slug, SIP1, and E-cadherin was studied in 78 ovarian and 23 breast carcinoma effusions using RT-PCR. Lower E-cadherin mRNA expression was found in breast carcinomas compared to ovarian carcinomas, while Snail expression was higher, as were the Snail/E-cadherin and Sip1/E-cadherin ratios. High Snail mRNA expression in breast carcinoma effusions was associated with shorter effusion-free, disease-free, and overall survival, suggesting that further analysis of EMT mediators in this tumor may be of clinical and therapeutic value [61].

## Claudins

Claudins are a family of 24 transmembrane tight junction proteins. Tight junctions are located in the apical aspect of epithelial or endothelial cells, where they maintain cell polarity and regulate the paracellular transport of solutes and the diffusion of proteins and lipids. Claudins contain intracellular amino and carboxyl termini, four transmembrane domains, and two extracellular loops mediating intercellular interactions between claudins. The second extracellular loop serves as a binding site for *Clostridium perfringens* enterotoxin in claudin-3 and claudin-4. Claudins have been associated with metastasis, disease progression, and poor survival in a range of cancers [62].

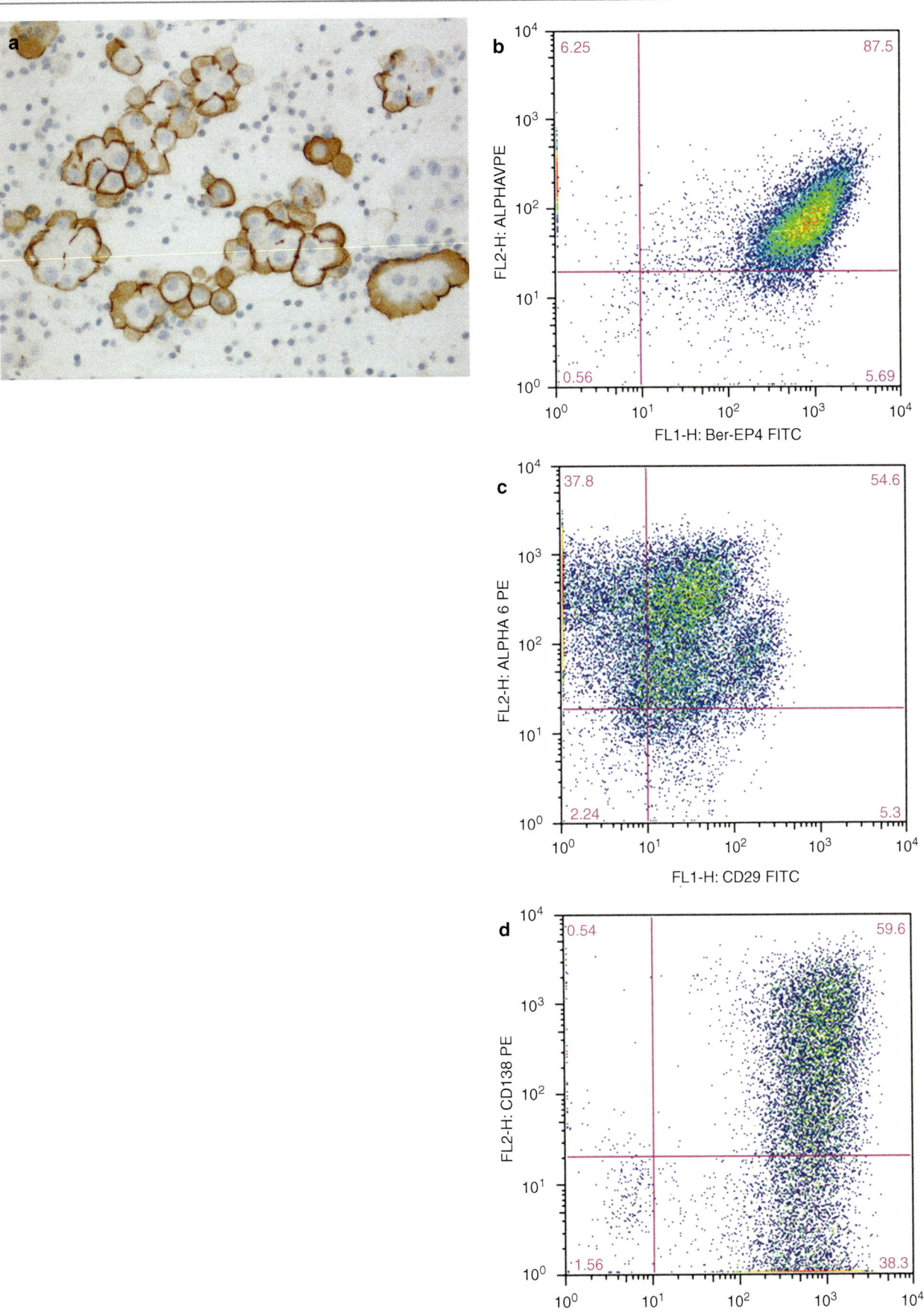

**Fig. 10.5** Membrane receptors. Breast carcinoma cells express the αV integrin chain by immunohistochemistry (**a**); co-expression of Ber-EP4 and αV integrin (**b**), α6 and β1 integrin (**c**), and Ber-EP4 and CD138 (syndecan-1, **d**) by flow cytometry is shown

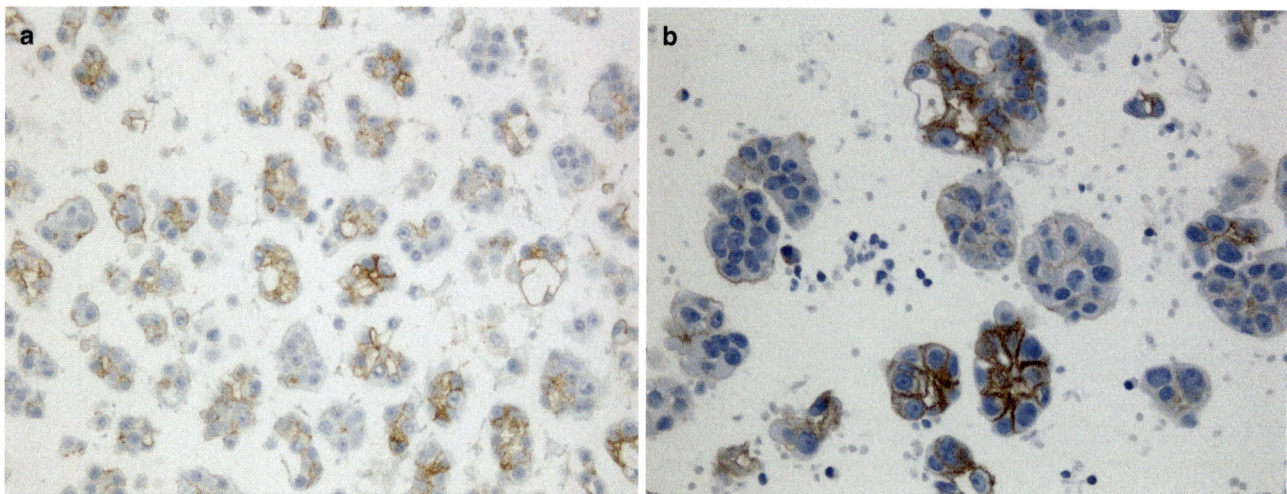

**Fig. 10.6** Claudins in breast carcinoma effusions. (**a**) claudin-3, (**b**) claudin-4

Analysis of breast carcinoma effusions showed expression of claudins 1, 3 and 7 in 51%, 82% and 69% of cases (Fig. 10.6a), with significantly lower expression of claudin-1 and claudin-7 compared to ovarian carcinomas. Claudin-3 and claudin-7 were rarely expressed on cells of mesothelial origin, suggesting a diagnostic role for these proteins in effusions [63]. In an additional study, claudin-4 expression was shown to be upregulated in breast carcinoma effusions compared to non-matched primary carcinomas by gene expression array analysis, and this finding was validated in immunohistochemistry analysis of patient-matched primary carcinomas and effusions (Fig. 10.6b, see below) [64].

## Others

Chondroitin sulfate proteoglycan-4 (CSPG4), a cell surface proteoglycan overexpressed in tumor cells in different cancers, has been implicated in tumor progression and metastasis and is consequently under consideration as therapeutic target [65]. Its expression has been documented in both primary breast carcinoma and malignant effusions in this disease [66].

## Proteases

Invasion and metastasis are critical events during tumor progression. They occur as a multistep process requiring degradation of the subepithelial and subendothelial basement membranes, ECM modification, the ability to enter and exit the circulation, and establishment of metastases in distant organs. Several protease families mediate these events, the

most important of which are the MMPs, zinc- and calcium-dependent enzymes that degrade a large variety of basement membrane and ECM components. Twenty-three MMPs have been identified in humans, with no functional redundancy among them. MMPs have been shown to have an important role in normal tissue homeostasis, as well as in a range of pathological conditions, including cancer. Their role in invasion, metastasis, and angiogenesis is now supplemented by data documenting their participation in other processes, such as regulation of cytokines and chemokines, intracellular signaling, and transcriptional regulation. Although attempts to target MMPs therapeutically have been disappointing to date, efforts in this direction are still being made [67, 68].

MMP-2 (gelatinase A, 72 kD type IV collagenase) and MMP-9 (gelatinase B, 92 kD type IV collagenase), the only enzymes with a gelatin-binding domain, are crucial for tumor metastasis due to their ability to degrade collagen type IV, a component of all basement membranes. MMP-2 and MMP-9 gelatinolytic activity was studied in 32 malignant and 10 benign effusions (5 from patients with pleurisy, 5 cirrhosis cases), the former including 20 breast carcinomas, using zymography. MMP-2 activity was more pronounced compared to MMP-9 and was higher in benign compared to malignant effusions. MMP-9 similarly showed higher activity in five pleurisy specimens compared to malignant specimens [69]. TIMP2 was reported to be expressed in 23/30 malignant effusions, including 1/3 breast carcinomas [70].

Analysis of MMP expression in 49 effusions and 68 patient-matched solid primary and metastatic lesions showed MMP-2 protein expression in 48/49 effusions by immunohistochemistry, with significantly higher expression at this anatomic site compared to both primary carcinomas and

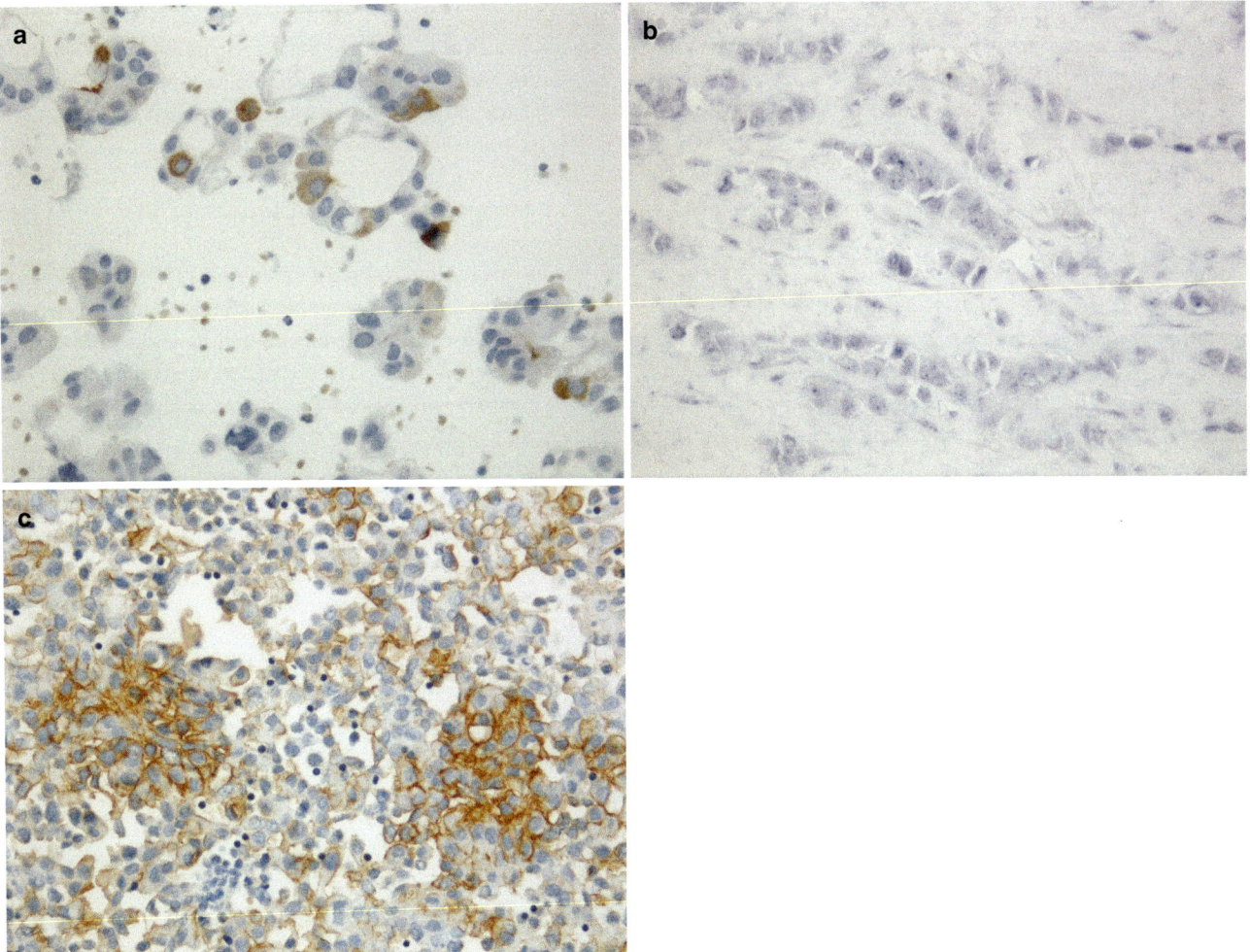

**Fig. 10.7** Proteases and related molecules. (**a**) MMP-2 protein expression in breast carcinoma cells in effusion; (**b**) In situ hybridization for *MMP2* mRNA in a primary carcinoma; (**c**) EMMPRIN protein in a primary carcinoma. (**b**) NBT-BCIP as chromogen, nuclear fast red as counterstain

lymph node metastases (Fig. 10.7a). MMP-1 and MMP-9 were less frequently expressed. *MMP2* mRNA was localized to carcinoma cells using in situ hybridization in both effusions (*n* = 33) and patient-matched primary carcinomas (*n* = 20; Fig. 10.7b), but as for MMP-2 protein, expression was significantly higher in effusions compared to primary carcinomas. This assay also detected *TIMP2* mRNA in 27/33 effusions. Zymography documented gelatinolytic activity of MMP-2 and MMP-9 in the majority of effusions, with significant correlation between MMP-2 protein expression and activity. MMP-1 expression in effusions was associated with shorter time to progression [71].

MMP-7 was recently reported to be selectively expressed in adenocarcinoma cells in effusion while absent in benign and malignant mesothelial cells. However, expression was more frequent in ovarian carcinoma, with only 9/55 breast carcinoma effusions staining for this marker [72].

EMMPRIN (extracellular matrix metalloproteinase inducer; CD147), a glycoprotein adhesion molecule belonging to the immunoglobulin superfamily, positively regulates the expression and secretion of several MMP members, including MMP-1, MMP-2, MMP-3, and MMP-9. It additionally interacts with other surface molecules, including integrins and monocarboxylate transporters, and is implicated in chemoresistance. EMMPRIN has been associated with aggressive clinical course in several cancers [73].

As MMP-2, EMMPRIN protein is upregulated in breast carcinoma effusions compared to primary carcinomas (Fig. 10.7c) and is co-expressed with MMP-9, and *EMMPRIN* mRNA is co-expressed with both *MMP2* and *MMP9* mRNA [72].

Few additional studies have focused on proteases and their activation pathways in breast carcinoma effusions. Gieseler et al. studied 136 effusions, of which 21.3% were breast carcinomas, for expression of proteins that form part of the tissue factor-induced thrombin activation pathway. Activity of factors II, V, VII, and X, as well as tissue factor and antithrombin, was found, though with lower levels than in normal plasma [74].

Human tissue kallikreins are a family of serine proteases, currently consisting of 15 different members, all encoded by a single gene cluster located at chromosome region 19q13.4. Their biological roles include regulation of blood pressure, seminal fluid liquefaction, skin desquamation, and synaptic neuronal plasticity. Kallikreins have been shown to be deregulated in several cancers [75]. Analysis of kallikrein-4 expression in 21 effusions and 44 solid primary and metastatic lesions detected this protease in 91% of solid lesions compared to 71% of effusions, a difference that was statistically significant. Comparative analysis of different tumor affecting the serosal cavities demonstrated higher kallikrein-4 expression in ovarian and breast adenocarcinoma compared to malignant mesothelioma [76].

The lysyl oxidase (LOX) family consists of 5 copper-binding secreted enzymes, LOX and LOX-like (LOXL)1-4. LOX is required the synthesis of elastin and collagen. Expression of LOX family members has been reported in multiple cancers [77]. The author's group studied the expression of LOXL2, LOXL3 and LOXL4 in breast carcinoma, ovarian carcinoma and malignant mesothelioma using RT-PCR. Two new alternative splice variants of LOXL4 were found, of which one was expressed only in effusions and absent from solid lesions. In breast carcinoma, LOXL4 was expressed only in effusions and these specimens additionally had significantly higher LOXL2 and lower LOXL3 expression compared to primary carcinomas, suggesting changes in the LOX profile of effusions compared to solid tumors [78].

## The Immune System

The immune system and its modulation in cancer have been assuming an increasing role in management of this disease in recent years. Data regarding the role of this system in the context of breast cancer effusions is nevertheless limited to date.

Kan et al. reported a retrospective series of 67 breast cancer patients with cytologically confirmed malignant pleural effusion who received intrapleural therapy. Twenty-nine patients underwent intrapleural administration of the streptococcal preparation OK-432, followed by transfer of autologous pleural effusion lymphocytes cultured with IL-2. The remaining patients, with the exception of one, were treated by OK-432 alone, chemotherapy alone, or a combination of OK-432 and chemotherapy. Patients treated with OK-432 plus cultured effusion lymphocytes had significantly higher

response rate compared to those who received other treatments (26/29 vs. 15/38) and had median survival of 12 months and 5-year survival at 36%, compared to 3 months and 0% in the other group. In multivariate analysis, treatment (adoptive immunotherapy) was the most significant prognostic factor for survival [79].

The therapeutic benefit and toxicity of IL-2 were analyzed in an additional series of 100 patients with malignant effusions, including 26 breast carcinomas [80]. Complete or partial response of 1–11 months (median = 5) was observed in 27 and 45 cases, respectively, with little toxicity. Response rate was particularly high in breast carcinoma and mesothelioma. Patients with peritoneal disease responded less than those with pleural or pericardial disease.

Spyridonidis et al. studied the potential role of ex vivo expansion of CD34(+) blood progenitor cells in eliminating tumor cells from autografts [81]. Breast carcinoma cells were identified in 6/11 pleural and peritoneal effusions and cultured in the presence of stem cell factor (SCF), interleukin-1β (IL-1β), IL-3, IL-6, and erythropoietin (EPO), cytokines that facilitate ex vivo expansion of CD34(+) blood progenitor cells. Hematopoietic growth factors had no effect on breast carcinoma cells in the presence of serum, although addition of TGF-β1 resulted in reduced tumor cell proliferation and suppressed clonogenic tumor growth. In contrast, culture under serum-free conditions resulted in death of the majority of tumor cells even in the presence of hematopoietic growth factors. The authors therefore recommended ex vivo expansion of CD34+ blood progenitor cells in serum-free medium, which may favor the elimination of carcinoma cells, when autologous progenitor cell transplantation is a therapeutic option.

Large numbers of lymphocytes and other leukocyte classes are frequently observed in breast carcinoma effusions, but their presence does not translate to longer survival, implying ineffective immune response in this disease. One of the cellular mechanisms that may be responsible for this failure is tumor cell evasion of the immune response by downregulation of classic HLA antigens, normally found on all cells, or by expression of non-classic antigens such as HLA-G and HLA-E. Natural killer (NK)- and T-cell-mediated lysis of target cells is inhibited by HLA-G through interaction with the inhibitory receptors immunoglobulin-like transcript (ILT)2 and ILT4, and the differential expression of inhibitory and activating NK receptors, such as NKG2 family members, may decide the effectiveness of the immune response in certain conditions. Two other receptors HLA-G interacts with are KIR2DL4 on NK cells and CD160 on T lymphocytes, NK cells, and endothelial cells. HLA-G is present as a membrane-bound or a soluble form, and its expression in normal tissues is limited to trophoblastic cells, where it is postulated to mediate immune tolerance during pregnancy. However,

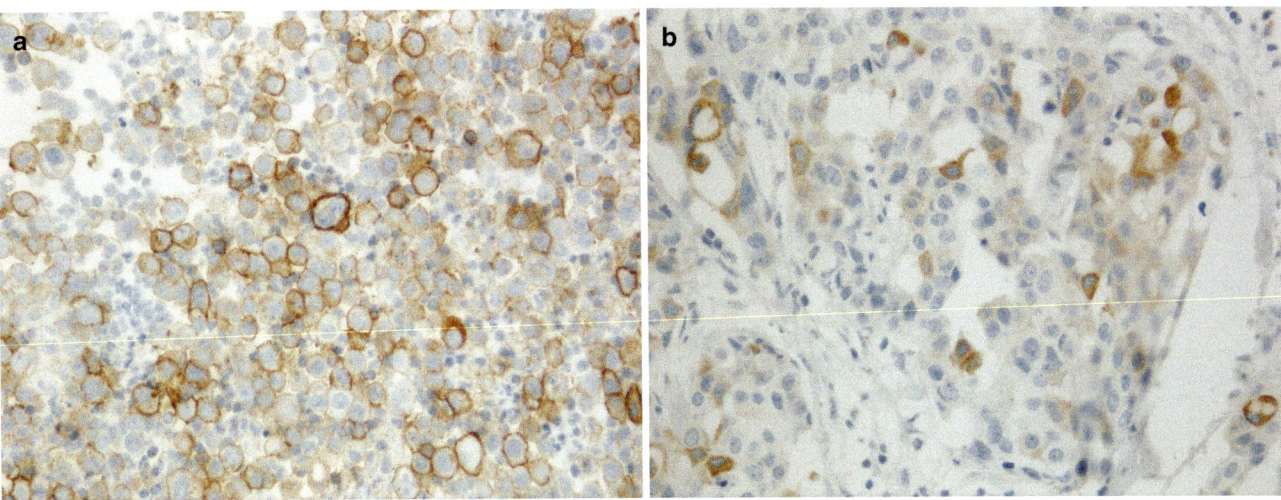

**Fig. 10.8** HLA-G. Combined membrane and cytoplasmic expression in effusion (**a**) and lymph node metastasis (**b**)

HLA-G is expressed in multiple tumor types, comprising carcinomas of different origin, including breast carcinoma, as well as lymphoma and melanoma [82, 83].

Analysis of 46 breast carcinoma effusions and 39 corresponding solid tumors using immunohistochemistry showed predominantly focal HLA-G expression in 12/46 (26%) breast carcinoma effusions and 16/39 (41%) solid lesions (Fig. 10.8a, b) [84]. Immunoblotting analysis showed some HLA-G expression in breast carcinoma effusions, and RT-PCR demonstrated the presence of HLA-G mRNA in tumor cells. Patients with HLA-G-positive tumor cells had shorter disease-free survival, though not significantly. These data suggest that minor populations of breast carcinoma cells express HLA-G and may use it as a means to escape the immune system. However, this does not appear to be a central biological mechanism in this disease.

Chemokines are a family of small secreted proteins that regulate the immune response and are produced by multiple cell classes in the tumor microenvironment, including cancer and stromal cells, endothelial cells, macrophages, and neutrophils. They are divided into four classes, C-C, C-X-C, C, and C-$X_3$-C, depending on the location of the first two cysteines in their sequence. Chemokines exert their biologic role through 18 G protein-coupled chemokine receptors expressed on tumor cells, creating an autocrine loop that mediates proliferation, regulates angiogenesis and cancer stemlike cell properties, and promotes invasion and metastasis [85, 86].

Thomachot et al. studied dendritic cell characteristics in breast carcinoma [87]. CCL20/MIP3α, a chemokine that attracts immature dendritic cells, was detected in breast carcinoma effusions using ELISA, and its levels were higher than those in other malignant or reactive effusions. Effusion fluid containing CCL20/MIP3α attracted immature dendritic cells, but not mature ones in vitro. Irradiated breast carcinoma cell lines and their conditioned media promoted CD34+ cell differentiation into CD1a+ Langerhans cells and immature dendritic cells that failed to mature in response to sCD40L or lipopolysaccharide (LPS) and had a reduced T-cell stimulatory capacity. The absolute number of CD4+ or CD8+ cells was also reduced, and T cells had lower CD25 and produced less IFNγ. These results show that breast carcinoma cells produce soluble factors, which may attract DC and their precursors in vivo, and promote the differentiation of the latter into LC and immature DC with altered functional capacities. The infiltration of breast cancer by these altered DC may contribute to the impaired immune response against the tumor.

Further insight regarding the role of chemokines in breast carcinoma is gained by the study of Soria et al., in which expression of the chemokines RANTES (CCL5) and MCP-1 (CCL2) was analyzed in tumor specimens, including eight pleural effusions [88]. RANTES and MCP-1 were minimally expressed in normal duct epithelium, but were frequently detected in DCIS and invasive ductal carcinoma, as well as in solid metastases and effusions, and their presence was associated with advanced stage. MCP-1 promoted the release of RANTES from endogenous premade vesicles, in breast carcinoma cell lines in vitro. These data show that breast carcinoma cells produce chemokines and suggest their role in tumor progression.

In an additional study, the presence of chemokine receptors in tumor cells and leukocytes in 21 breast carcinoma effusions was investigated using flow cytometry [89]. Breast carcinoma cells expressed CXCR4 in 7/21 effusions, with less frequent or absent expression of other receptors (CXCR1, CCR5, CCR7, CXCR2, and CCR2) (Fig. 10.9a, b). Lymphocytes frequently expressed CXCR4, CCR5, and CCR7; macrophages expressed all six receptors. Higher numbers of CD8-positive lymphocytes and higher CCR7

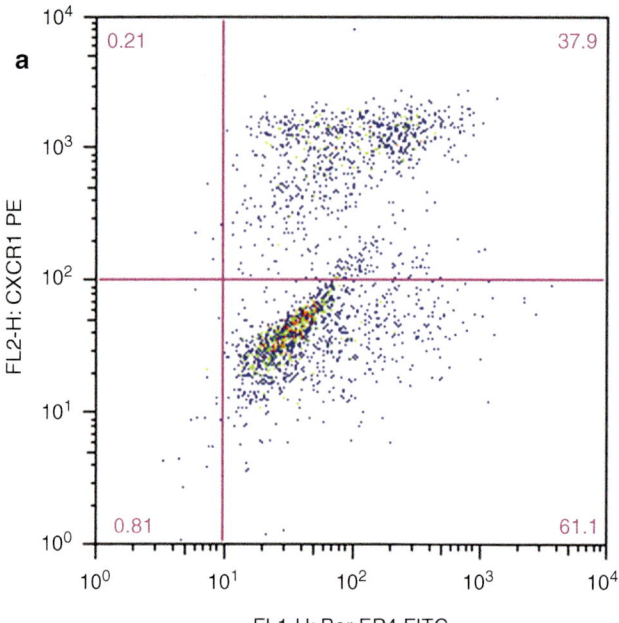

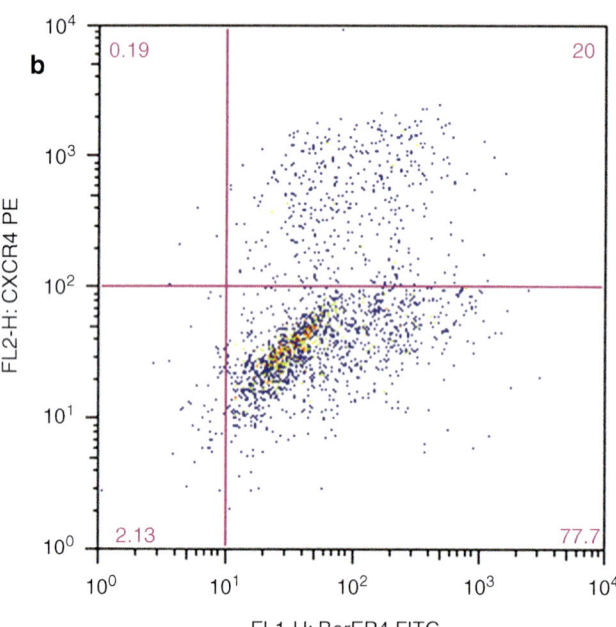

**Fig. 10.9** Chemokine receptors. Co-expression of Ber-EP4 and the chemokine receptors CXCR1 (**a**) and CXCR4 (**b**) in carcinoma cells. The former receptor was rarely expressed by tumor cells

The prognostic role of CCR7 expression in monocytes and CD8 counts in breast carcinoma effusions remains to be explored in a larger cohort.

Two additional studies focused on the leukocyte cell populations and cytokine content in breast carcinoma effusions. DeLong et al. analyzed 44 effusions, including 26 breast carcinoma specimens, and found high numbers of functionally suppressive CD4+/CD25+ T cells in breast carcinoma effusions. The effusions additionally contained the immunosuppressive cytokine TGF-β, though at lower concentrations than those found in mesothelioma effusions [90]. Desfrançois and co-workers found higher levels of double-positive CD4+/CD8+ lymphocytes in breast carcinoma pleural effusions (*n* = 16) compared to tumor specimens from other anatomic sites, and these cells produced higher levels of IL-5 and IL-13 compared to CD4(+) or CD8(+) cells. The significance of this observation is uncertain at present [91].

## Intracellular Signaling and Transcriptional Regulation

The signaling pathways activated in breast carcinoma cells in effusions and their clinical relevance are largely unknown. Among the two major intracellular signaling pathways, the MAPK and PI3K pathways, only the former was studied to date [92].

The MAPK pathway is a four-level cascade, in which each kinase activates the following kinase substrate through a complex network, enabling the cell to maintain diversity and specificity while responding to various extracellular cues. MAPK double phosphorylation at tyrosine and threonine residues at the final level of the cascade occurs in an enzyme-specific manner by the MEK family of MAPK kinases. Two MAPK family members, c-Jun amino-terminal kinase (JNK) and the high osmolarity glycerol response kinase (p38), are activated by stress-related stimuli, whereas the extracellular-regulated kinase (ERK) is largely activated by growth factor signals. MAPK activation leads to phosphorylation of a variety of cytosolic substrates, and to their own translocation to the nucleus, where they activate a large number of transcription factors, including AP-1 and ETS1. p38 and JNK activation may result in apoptosis or cell survival, depending on the nature of the signal, as well as in proliferation, differentiation, and inflammation, while ERK promotes differentiation, proliferation, and migration. MAPK activity is negatively regulated by dual specificity phosphatases (DUSP) that deactivate the enzymes [93, 94]. Activation of the RAS/RAF/MEK/ERK cascade is involved in chemoresistance [95].

monocyte expression were associated with a trend for shorter disease-free survival. The presence of CXCR4 in breast carcinoma cells in effusions is in agreement with previous observations in solid lesions and in vitro data, in which this receptor and its ligand CXCL12 were co-expressed, documenting the presence of an autocrine tumor-promoting loop.

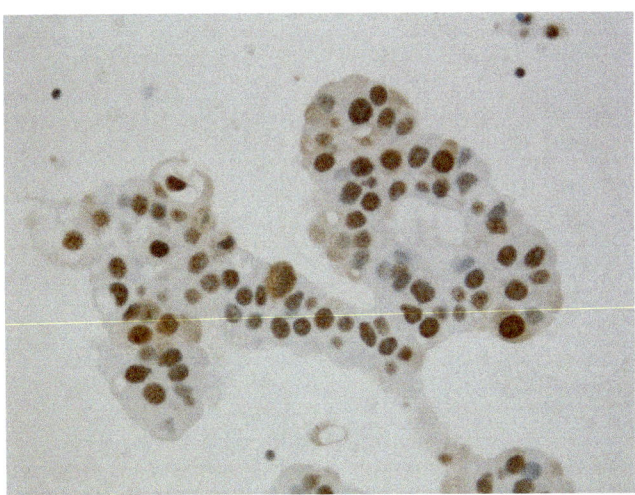

**Fig. 10.10** Signaling molecules. Expression of p-ERK in the nuclei of breast carcinoma cells in effusion

Expression of the activated phosphorylated MAPK members p-ERK, p-JNK, and p-p38 was studied in 42 breast carcinoma effusions and 51 patient-matched solid tumors (23 primary carcinomas, 28 metastases) using immunohistochemistry [92]. Quantitative analysis of MAPK levels using immunoblotting was performed in 19 effusions. Nuclear expression of p-p38 and p-JNK was found in 32 and 40 effusions, respectively, and was significantly higher than in primary carcinomas and lymph node metastases. p-ERK expression, found in 41 effusions (Fig. 10.10), was similar at all anatomic sites. Immunoblotting similarly showed MAPK expression and activation in the majority of effusions. Apoptosis, as measured using a p85-PARP fragment antibody, was minimal, whereas proliferation (by Ki-67 score) was high, exceeding 25% of cells in 14 effusions. MAPK expression by immunohistochemistry did not correlate with survival. However, higher p38 activation ratio (p-p38/total p38) correlated with shorter overall survival. The p38 and JNK upregulation in breast carcinoma effusions suggests a biological role in promoting tumor cell survival at this anatomic site.

The ETS family of transcriptional factors consists of 28 members in humans and is highly conserved across different species. All family members contain an 85 amino acid DNA-binding domain (the ETS domain) that confers the ability to bind to DNA sequences having the core motif GGAA/T (ETS-binding site, EBS). Another conserved area that is present in 11 members is the pointed (PNT) domain, which mediates protein-protein interactions and oligomerization. ETS factors have 200 known target genes, including proteases (MMP-1, MMP-3, and MMP-9, cathepsin) and their inhibitors (TIMP1), cell cycle mole-

cules (cyclin D1, p21), apoptosis promoters and inhibitors (Fas, PARP, Bcl-2, Bcl-xL), adhesion molecules (E-cadherin, integrins), immune response mediators (interleukins, immunoglobulins), and angiogenesis mediators (the VEGF receptors Flt-1 and flk-1, Tie-1 and Tie-2). In these multiple target genes, ETS factors can mediate transcriptional activation or repression according to the binding factor and the DNA sequence involved [96–98]. ETS members are aberrantly expressed in a range of solid tumors, including breast cancer, through gene amplification, overexpression of gene products, or creation of fusion genes with multiple partners [99].

Breast carcinoma cells in effusions frequently express *ETS1* and *PEA3* mRNA using *in situ* hybridization (22/33 and 24/33 specimens, respectively) (Fig. 10.11a, b), and *PEA3* is significantly upregulated compared to patient-matched primary carcinomas. They additionally express mRNA for AP-2, another transcription factor known to regulate MMP synthesis, by RT-PCR [71]. The coordinated upregulation of MMP-2, EMMPRIN and PEA3 in breast carcinoma effusions compared to primary carcinomas suggests that Ets transcription factors may regulate MMP expression at this site.

Genetic material in human cells is stored in the form of chromatin, which consists of nucleoprotein complexes containing DNA and protein. DNA is wrapped around an octamer core of histones whose position and density are regulated through chromatin remodeling complexes, consisting in eukaryotes of the SWI/SNF2, ISWI, CHD, and INO80 families. Among these families, mSWI/SNF2, consisting of BAF (BRG1 or BRM-associated factors) and PBAF (Polybromo-associated BAF), is the most commonly associated with disease, and 20% of cancers harbor mutations in genes belonging to this family [100].

RSF is a chromatin-remodeling complex that is composed of two subunits, hSNF2H and p325 (Rsf-1), and is involved in the formation of RNA polymerase II complexes. A truncated form of RSF-p325 codes for the hepatitis B virus transcription repressor HBXAP. Rsf-1 is amplified in ovarian carcinoma, and its protein expression in ovarian carcinoma effusions is associated with poor survival [101, 102].

Rsf-1 protein expression was found in tumor cells in 34/47 breast carcinoma effusions, significantly less than in patient-matched primary carcinomas and metastases (24/30 and 24/26 positive specimens, respectively). Rsf-1 immunoreactivity in effusions showed no association with HER2 or hormone receptor status or with patient survival. The observation that Rsf-1 expression is downregulated in breast carcinoma cells in effusions and has no prognostic role at this anatomic site suggests it has no major biological role in this context [103].

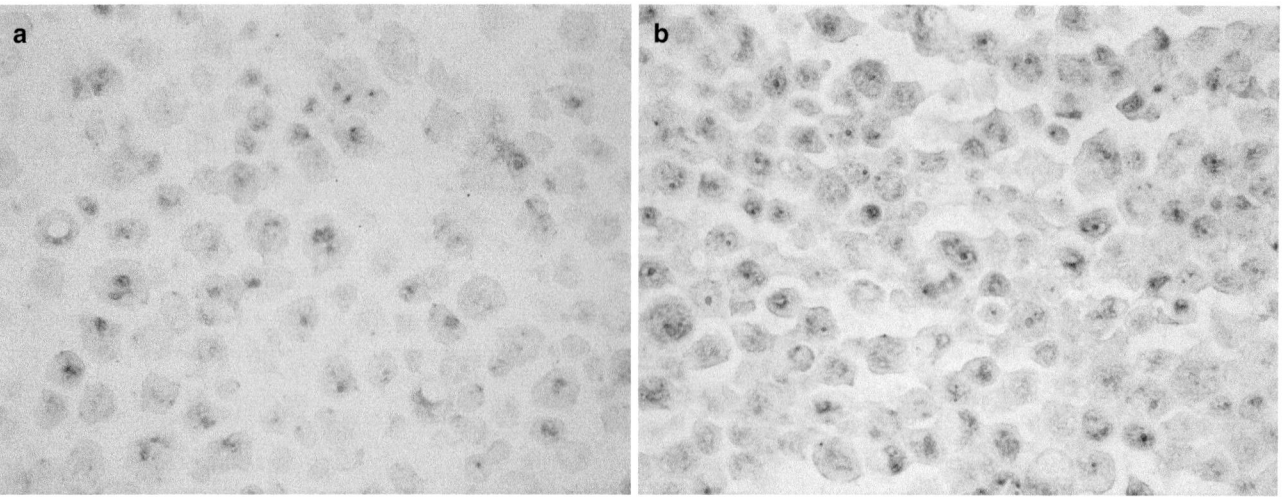

**Fig. 10.11** ETS transcription factors. In situ hybridization for *ETS1* (**a**) and *PEA3* (**b**) mRNA in a breast carcinoma effusion, showing co-expression of these two mRNAs. NBT-BCIP as chromogen, nuclear fast red as counterstain

## High-Throughput Analyses

Only a few studies analyzing the genomic profile of breast carcinoma cells have been published to date.

Dupont et al. analyzed the gene expression signature of 19 effusions and compared them to 4 primary carcinomas, eight cell lines, and four specimens consisting of benign breast tissue. Cells in effusions were purified using EpCAM-coated beads. Based on the array analysis, effusions could be differentiated into two categories, one resembling cell lines and expressing CD24, CD44, and cytokeratins 8, 18, and 19 and the other expressing metastasis-associated genes, such as S100A4, uPA receptor, vimentin, and CXCR4 [104].

The role of cancer stem cell markers in this context was assessed in two other studies. Grimshaw et al. studied the presence of breast cancer stem cells in pleural effusions based on their expression of CD24 and CD44. The majority (20/27) of effusions tested contained cells capable of forming mammospheres that could be passaged, and differentiated upon plating, as determined by the increased expression of cytokeratins and MUC1. Surface expression of CD24 and CD44 was found in some, but not all, uncultured effusions and did not correlate with the ability to form mammospheres or with their size. In contrast, the ability to form tumors in severe combined immunodeficiency disease (SCID) mice correlated with the ability to produce the larger mammospheres, but not with CD24 and CD44 expression [105].

Deng et al. recently investigated the role of the tamoxifen analog N,N-diethyl-2-[4-(phenylmethyl)phenoxy]ethanamine (DPPE, tesmilifene) in targeting breast tumor-initiating cells (TICs) [106]. Analysis of TICs from ten pleural effusions, identified as having a CD44+/CD24−/low phenotype by flow cytometry and the ability to form nonadherent

spheres in culture, showed that treatment with DPPE reduced spheroid formation and the viability of CD44+/CD24−/low breast cancer cells. In combination with doxorubicin, DPPE aided in completely eradicating tumorigenic cells, suggesting that combination of these drugs may be beneficial for targeting metastatic breast carcinoma.

The gene array signatures of breast carcinoma cells in primary carcinomas and effusions were compared in an additional study [64]. Array analysis identified 255 significantly downregulated and 96 upregulated genes in the effusions compared to primary carcinomas, the majority of which consisted of genes that are part of pathways involved in focal adhesion, extracellular matrix-cell interaction, and the regulation of actin cytoskeleton. Genes that were upregulated in effusions included *KRT8*, *BCAR1*, *CLDN4*, and *VIL2*, while *DCN*, *CLDN19*, *ITGA7*, and *ITGA5* were downregulated at this anatomic site. PCR, Western blotting, and immunohistochemistry confirmed the array findings for *BCAR1*, *CLDN4*, *VIL2*, and *DCN* (Figs. 10.6b and 10.12a, b). The differential expression of the *NTN4* gene product Netrin-4 at these two anatomic sites was confirmed in a separate study (Fig. 10.12c) [107].

The role of gene expression arrays in differentiating carcinomas affecting the serosal cavities was investigated in a comparative analysis of ovarian/primary peritoneal serous carcinoma ($n = 10$) and breast infiltrating duct carcinoma ($n = 8$) [108]. Unsupervised hierarchical clustering separated ovarian from breast carcinomas. A total of 288 unique probes were significantly differentially expressed in the 2 cancers, of which 81 and 207 were overexpressed in breast and ovarian/peritoneal carcinoma, respectively. Genes overexpressed in breast carcinoma included *TFF1*, *TFF3*, *FOXA1*, *CA12*, *GATA3*, *SDC1*, *PITX1*, *TH*, *EHFD1*, *EFEMP1*, *TOB1*, and

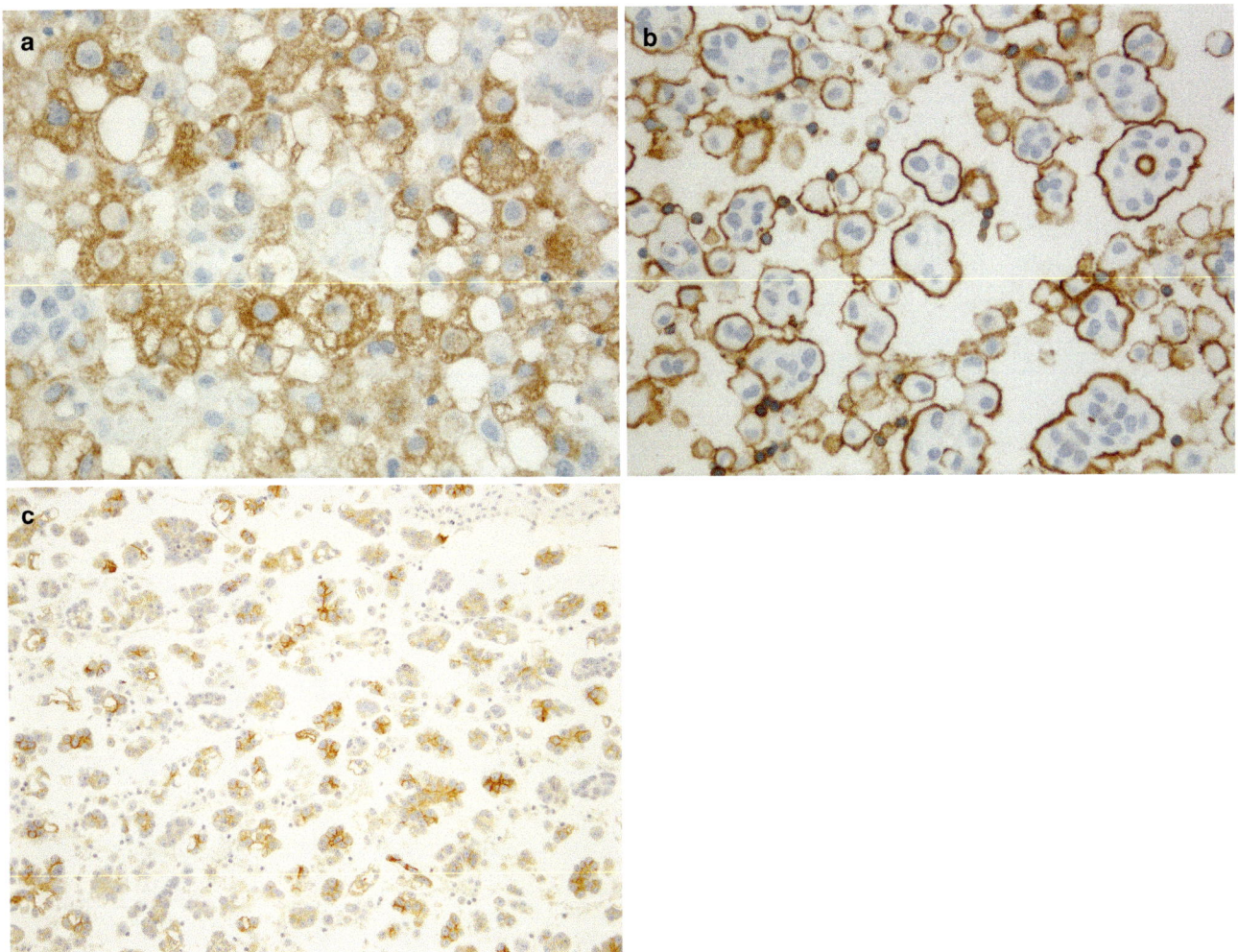

**Fig. 10.12** Validation of gene expression array analysis comparing primary breast carcinoma and effusions from this cancer. Tumor cells in effusion express p130Cas (**a**), p-ezrin (**b**), and Netrin-4 (**c**)

*KLF2.* Genes overexpressed in ovarian/peritoneal carcinoma included *SPON1, RBP1, MFGE8, TM4SF12, MMP7, KLK5/6/7, FOLR1/3, PAX8, APOL2,* and *NRCAM.* Results for 14 genes and 5 proteins were validated by quantitative real-time PCR and immunohistochemistry, respectively (Fig. 10.13a–d).

Three of the genes that were overexpressed in breast carcinoma effusions, consisting of *ANPEP, AZGP1,* and *SPDEF,* were studied in a follow-up study [109], in which 83 breast carcinomas (57 primary carcinomas and 26 effusions) and 40 ovarian carcinomas (20 primary carcinomas and 20 effusions) were analyzed using qPCR. ANPEP protein expression was additionally studied using immunohistochemistry. *AZGP1* and *SPDEF* mRNA was overexpressed in breast compared to ovarian carcinoma, whereas ANPEP protein was overexpressed in breast carcinoma effusions compared to primary tumors and lymph node metastases (Fig. 10.14). None of these molecules were informative of disease outcome based on expression in effusions. In another

follow-up study based on the same gene expression array analysis, scavenger receptor class A member 3 (SCARA3) was confirmed to be overexpressed in ovarian compared to breast carcinoma effusions [110].

The same array platform used for comparing breast and ovarian/peritoneal serous carcinoma was applied to comparative analysis of breast and lung carcinoma effusions [111]. A total of 289 unique probes were significantly differentially expressed in the 2 cancers, of which 65 and 224 were overexpressed in breast and lung adenocarcinoma, respectively. Genes overexpressed in breast adenocarcinoma included *TFF1, TFF3, FOXA1, CA12, PITX1, RARRES1, CITED4, MYC, TFAP2A, EFHD1, TOB1, SPDEF, FASN,* and *TH.* Genes overexpressed in lung adenocarcinoma included *TITF1, SFTPG, MMP7, EVA1, GPR116, HOP, SCGB3A2,* and *MET.* Results for 15 genes and 8 gene products were validated by quantitative real-time PCR and immunohistochemistry, respectively, with good agreement.

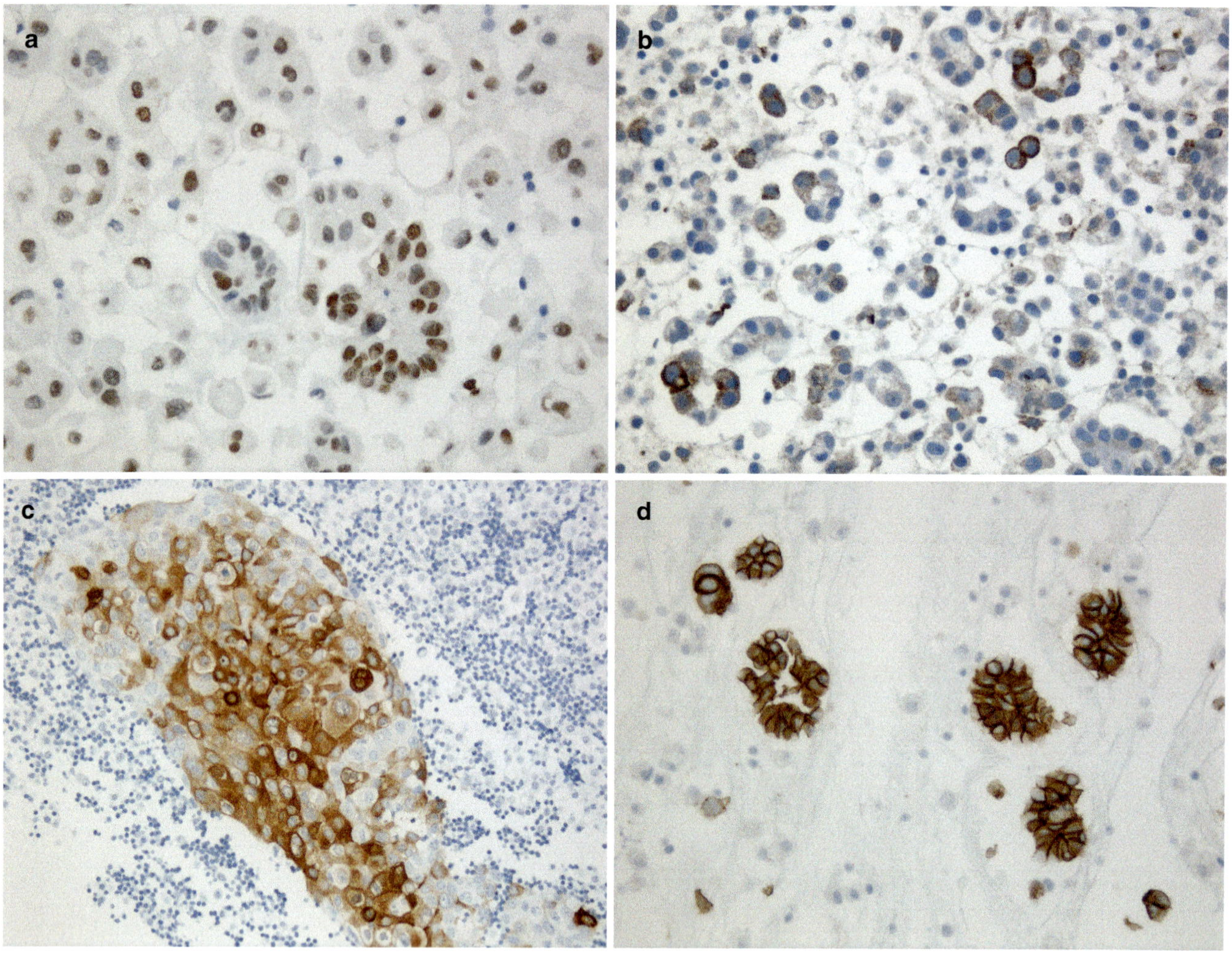

**Fig. 10.13** Validation of gene expression array analysis comparing ovarian/peritoneal serous carcinoma and infiltrating duct carcinoma of the breast in effusions. Breast carcinoma cells in effusion express FOXA1 (**a**), TFF1 (**b**), TFF3 (**c**), and CA12 (**d**)

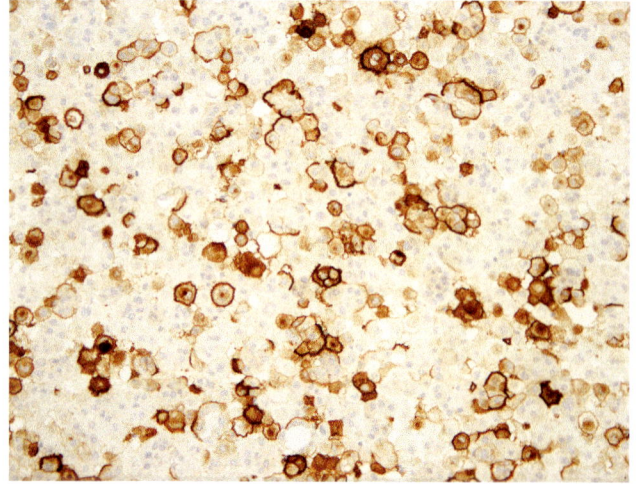

**Fig. 10.14** ANPEP protein expression in a breast carcinoma effusion

## Future Directions

Breast carcinoma is one of few cancer types in which targeted therapy has an undisputed therapeutic role, as evidenced by the use of hormone receptor and HER2 inhibitors. Nevertheless, breast carcinoma metastasis to the serosal cavities constitutes a significant medical problem to which no effective cure exists to date. As with many cancers, resistance to apoptosis is a major impediment to successful therapy. One of the molecular mechanisms behind this resistance may be the high expression of members of the inhibitors of apoptosis (IAP) family members XIAP and survivin [112], but there is little doubt that multiple molecules are involved in breast carcinoma chemoresistance in effusions.

New therapeutic approaches to this clinical condition should focus on targeting proteins that are essential for the survival of breast carcinoma cells. Two previous studies focused on the use of antibodies MT110 and catumaxomab against the cell surface protein EpCAM ex vivo [113] and in a phase 1–2 trial [114]. In the latter study, clinical response was observed in 5/7 patients, but serious side effects in two patients caused the investigators to question whether this treatment is indicated for patients with malignant effusions [114]. Molecular research and assessment of experimental therapy focused on breast carcinoma effusions have nevertheless been sparse in recent years, with ovarian and lung cancer, as well as mesothelioma, receiving considerably more attention (see relevant chapters). Designing ways to optimize the diagnosis of breast carcinoma in effusions, understanding the biological pathways that mediate the aggressive behavior of tumor cells at this anatomic site, and segregating patients into prognostic groups based on molecular markers are important tasks that are critically needed in order to attempt improving the outcome of patients suffering from this grievous condition.

# References

1. DeSantis CE, Bray F, Ferlay J, Lortet-Tieulent J, Anderson BO, Jemal A. International variation in female breast cancer incidence and mortality rates. Cancer Epidemiol Biomarkers Prev. 2015;24:1495–506.
2. Siegel RL, Miller KD, Jemal A. Cancer statistics, 2017. CA Cancer J Clin. 2017;67:7–30.
3. Fentiman IS, Millis R, Sexton S, Hayward JL. Pleural effusion in breast cancer: a review of 105 cases. Cancer. 1981;47:2087–92.
4. Raju RN, Kardinal CG. Pleural effusion in breast carcinoma: analysis of 122 cases. Cancer. 1981;48:2524–7.
5. Wilkes JD, Fidias P, Vaickus L, Perez RP. Malignancy-related pericardial effusion. 127 cases from the Roswell Park Center Institute. Cancer. 1995;76:1377–87.
6. Buck M, Ingle JN, Giuliani ER, Gordon JR, Therneau TM. Pericardial effusion in women with breast cancer. Cancer. 1987;60:263–9.
7. DiBonito L, Falconieri G, Colautti I, Bonifacio D, Dudine S. The positive peritoneal effusion. A retrospective study of cytopathologic diagnoses with autopsy confirmation. Acta Cytol. 1993;37:483–8.
8. Johnston WW. The malignant pleural effusion. A review of cytopathologic diagnoses of 584 specimens from 472 consecutive patients. Cancer. 1985;56:905–9.
9. Pokieser W, Cassik P, Fischer G, Vesely M, Ulrich W, Peters-Engl C. Malignant pleural and pericardial effusion in invasive breast cancer: impact of the site of the primary tumor. Breast Cancer Res Treat. 2004;83:139–42.
10. Kamby C, Vejborg I, Kristensen B, Olsen LO, Mouridsen HT. Metastatic pattern in recurrent breast cancer. Special reference to intrathoracic recurrences. Cancer. 1988;62:2226–33.
11. DeCamp MM Jr, Mentzer SJ, Swanson SJ, Sugarbaker DJ. Malignant effusive disease of the pleura and pericardium. Chest. 1997;112(4 Suppl):291S–5S.
12. van de Molengraft FJ, Vooijs GP. The interval between the diagnosis of malignancy and the development of effusions, with reference to the role of cytologic diagnosis. Acta Cytol. 1988;32:183–7.
13. Dieterich M, Goodman SN, Rojas-Corona RR, Emralino AB, Jimenez-Joseph D, Sherman ME. Multivariate analysis of prognostic features in malignant pleural effusions from breast cancer patients. Acta Cytol. 1994;38:945–52.
14. Sanchez-Armengol A, Rodriguez-Panadero F. Survival and talc pleurodesis in metastatic pleural carcinoma, revisited. Report of 125 cases. Chest. 1993;104:1482–5.
15. Inoue K, Ogawa M, Horikoshi N, Aiba K, Mukaiyama T, Mizunuma N, Itami S, Hirano A, Matsuoka A, Matsumura T. Evaluation of prognostic factors for 233 patients with recurrent advanced breast cancer. Jpn J Clin Oncol. 1991;21:334–9.
16. van Galen KP, Visser HP, van der Ploeg T, Smorenburg CH. Prognostic factors in patients with breast cancer and malignant pleural effusion. Breast J. 2010;16:675–7.
17. Bielsa S, Esquerda A, Salud A, Montes A, Arellano E, Rodríguez-Panadero F, Porcel JM. High levels of tumor markers in pleural fluid correlate with poor survival in patients with adenocarcinomatous or squamous malignant effusions. Eur J Intern Med. 2009;20:383–6.
18. Terracciano D, Mazzarella C, Cicalese M, Galzerano S, Apostolico G, DI Carlo A, Mariano A, Cecere C, Macchia V. Diagnostic value of carbohydrate antigens in supernatants and sediments of pleural effusions. Oncol Lett. 2010;1:465–71.
19. Liu E, Dollbaum C, Scott G, Rochlitz C, Benz C, Smith HS. Molecular lesions involved in the progression of a human breast cancer. Oncogene. 1988;3:323–7.
20. Driouch K, Champème MH, Beuzelin M, Bièche I, Lidereau R. Classical gene amplifications in human breast cancer are not associated with distant solid metastases. Br J Cancer. 1997;76:784–7.
21. Roka S, Fiegl M, Zojer N, Filipits M, Schuster R, Steiner B, Jakesz R, Huber H, Drach J. Aneuploidy of chromosome 8 as detected by interphase fluorescence in situ hybridization is a recurrent finding in primary and metastatic breast cancer. Breast Cancer Res Treat. 1998;48:125–33.
22. Massoner A, Augustin F, Duba HC, Zojer N, Fiegl MFISH. cytogenetics and prognosis in breast and non-small cell lung cancers. Cytometry B Clin Cytom. 2004;62:52–6.
23. Ioakim-Liossi A, Gagos S, Athanassiades P, Athanassiadou P, Gogas J, Davaris P, Markopoulos C. Changes of chromosomes 1, 3, 6, and 11 in metastatic effusions arising from breast and ovarian cancer. Cancer Genet Cytogenet. 1999;110:34–40.
24. de Matos Granja N, Soares R, Rocha S, Paredes J, Longatto Filho A, Alves VA, Wiley E, Schmitt FC, Bedrossian C. Evaluation of breast cancer metastases in pleural effusions by molecular biology techniques. Diagn Cytopathol. 2002;27:210–3.
25. Booth BW, Smith GH. Roles of transforming growth factor-alpha in mammary development and disease. Growth Factors. 2007;25:227–35.
26. Arteaga CL, Hanauske AR, Clark GM, Osborne CK, Hazarika P, Pardue RL, Tio F, Von Hoff DD. Immunoreactive alpha transforming growth factor activity in effusions from cancer patients as a marker of tumor burden and patient prognosis. Cancer Res. 1988;48:5023–8.
27. Ciardiello F, Kim N, Liscia DS, Bianco C, Lidereau R, Merlo G, Callahan R, Greiner J, Szpak C, Kidwell W, Schlom J, Salomon DS. mRNA expression of transforming growth factor alpha in human breast carcinomas and its activity in effusions of breast cancer patients. J Natl Cancer Inst. 1989;81:1165–71.
28. Dallas NA, Samuel S, Xia L, Fan F, Gray MJ, Lim SJ, Ellis LM. Endoglin (CD105): a marker of tumor vasculature and potential target for therapy. Clin Cancer Res. 2008;14:1931–7.
29. ten Dijke P, Goumans MJ, Pardali E. Endoglin in angiogenesis and vascular diseases. Angiogenesis. 2008;11:79–89.

30. Ollauri-Ibáñez C, López-Novoa JM, Pericacho M. Endoglin-based biological therapy in the treatment of angiogenesis-dependent pathologies. Expert Opin Biol Ther. 2017;17:1053–63.

31. Davidson B, Tuft Stavnes H, Førsund M, Berner A, Stafe AC. CD105 (Endoglin) expression in breast carcinoma effusions is a marker of poor survival. Breast. 2010;19:493–8.

32. Ellis LM, Hicklin DJ. VEGF-targeted therapy: mechanisms of anti-tumour activity. Nat Rev Cancer. 2008;8:579–91.

33. Dvorak HF, Brown LF, Detmar M, Dvorak AM. Vascular permeability factor/vascular endothelial growth factor, microvascular hyperpermeability, and angiogenesis. Am J Pathol. 1995;146:1029–39.

34. Nagy JA, Masse EM, Herzberg KT, Meyers MS, Yeo KT, Yeo TK, Sioussat TM, Dvorak HF. Pathogenesis of ascites tumor growth: vascular permeability factor, vascular hyperpermeability, and ascites tumor accumulation. Cancer Res. 1995;55:360–8.

35. Aalders KC, Tryfonidis K, Senkus E, Cardoso F. Anti-angiogenic treatment in breast cancer: facts, successes, failures and future perspectives. Cancer Treat Rev. 2017;53:98–110.

36. Kraft A, Weindel K, Ochs A, Marth C, Zmija J, Schumacher P, Unger C, Marmé D, Gastl G. Vascular endothelial growth factor in the sera and effusions of patients with malignant and nonmalignant disease. Cancer. 1999;85:178–87.

37. Zebrowski BK, Yano S, Liu W, Shaheen RM, Hicklin DJ, Putnam JBJ, Ellis LM. Vascular endothelial growth factor levels and induction of permeability in malignant pleural effusions. Clin Cancer Res. 1999;5:3364–8.

38. Konstantinovsky S, Nielsen S, Vyberg M, Kvalheim G, Nesland JM, Reich R, Davidson B. Angiogenic molecule expression is downregulated in effusions from breast cancer patients. Breast Cancer Res Treat. 2005;94:71–80.

39. Kaplan DR, Miller FD. Signal transduction by the neurotrophin receptors. Curr Opin Cell Biol. 1997;9:213–21.

40. Teng KK, Hempstead BL. Neurotrophins and their receptors: signaling trios in complex biological systems. Cell Mol Life Sci. 2004;61:35–48.

41. Nakagawara A. Trk receptor tyrosine kinases: a bridge between cancer and neural development. Cancer Lett. 2001;169:107–14.

42. Demir IE, Tieftrunk E, Schorn S, Friess H, Ceyhan GO. Nerve growth factor & TrkA as novel therapeutic targets in cancer. Biochim Biophys Acta. 2016;1866:37–50.

43. Davidson B, Reich R, Lazarovici P, Flørenes VA, Nielsen S, Nesland JM. Altered expression and activation of the nerve growth factor receptors TrkA and p75 provides the first evidence of tumor progression to effusion in breast carcinoma. Breast Cancer Res Treat. 2004;83:119–28.

44. Sachdev D, Yee D. Disrupting insulin-like growth factor signaling as a potential cancer therapy. Mol Cancer Ther. 2007;6:1–12.

45. Guvakova MA. Insulin-like growth factors control cell migration in health and disease. Int J Biochem Cell Biol. 2007;39:890–909.

46. Denley A, Cosgrove LJ, Booker GW, Wallace JC, Forbes BE. Molecular interactions of the IGF system. Cytokine Growth Factor Rev. 2005;16:421–39.

47. Li H, Batth IS, Qu X, Xu L, Song N, Wang R, Liu Y. IGF-IR signaling in epithelial to mesenchymal transition and targeting IGF-IR therapy: overview and new insights. Mol Cancer. 2017;16:6.

48. Athanassiadou P, Athanassiades P, Petrakakou E, Mavrikakis M, Konstantopoulos K, Kyrkou K. Expression of insulin-like growth factor-I receptor and transferrin receptor by breast cancer cells in pleural effusion smears. Cytopathology. 1996;7:400–5.

49. Slipicevic A, Øy GF, Askildt IC, Holth A, Hellesylt E, Flørenes VA, Davidson B. The diagnostic and prognostic role of the insulin growth factor pathway members IGF-II and IGFBP3 in serous effusions. Hum Pathol. 2009;40:527–37.

50. Hood JD, Cheresh DA. Role of integrins in cell invasion and migration. Nat Rev Cancer. 2002;2:91–100.

51. Rathinam R, Alahari SK. Important role of integrins in the cancer biology. Cancer Metastasis Rev. 2010;29:223–37.

52. Seguin L, Desgrosellier JS, Weis SM, Cheresh DA. Integrins and cancer: regulators of cancer stemness, metastasis, and drug resistance. Trends Cell Biol. 2015;25:234–40.

53. Sigstad E, Dong HP, Nielsen S, Berner A, Davidson B, Risberg B. Quantitative analysis of integrin expression in effusions using flow cytometric immunophenotyping. Diagn Cytopathol. 2005;33:321–31.

54. Kohn EC, Travers LA, Kassis J, Broome U, Klominek J. Malignant effusions are sources of fibronectin and other promigratory and proinvasive components. Diagn Cytopathol. 2005;33:300–8.

55. Menard S, Castronovo V, Tagliabue E, Sobel ME. New insights into the metastasis-associated 67 kD laminin receptor. J Cell Biochem. 1997;67:155–65.

56. Menard S, Tagliabue E, Colnaghi MI. The 67 kDa laminin receptor as a prognostic factor in human cancer. Breast Cancer Res Treat. 1998;52:137–45.

57. Reich R, Vintman L, Nielsen S, Kærn J, Bedrossian C, Berner A, Davidson B. Differential expression of the 67 kilodalton laminin receptor in malignant mesothelioma and carcinomas that spread to serosal cavities. Diagn Cytopathol. 2005;33:332–7.

58. Bruner HC, Derksen PWB. Loss of E-cadherin-dependent cell-cell adhesion and the development and progression of cancer. Cold Spring Harb Perspect Biol. 2017. pii: a029330. https://doi.org/10.1101/cshperspect.a029330. [Epub ahead of print].

59. Thiery JP, Acloque H, Huang RY, Nieto MA. Epithelial-mesenchymal transitions in development and disease. Cell. 2009;139:871–90.

60. Kalluri R, Weinberg RA. The basics of epithelial-mesenchymal transition. J Clin Invest. 2009;119:1420–8.

61. Elloul S, Bukholt Elstrand M, Nesland JM, Trope CG, Kvalheim G, Goldberg I, Reich R, Davidson B. Snail, Slug, and Smad-interacting protein 1 as novel parameters of disease aggressiveness in metastatic ovarian and breast carcinoma. Cancer. 2005;103:1631–43.

62. Tabariès S, Siegel PM. The role of claudins in cancer metastasis. Oncogene. 2017;36:1176–90.

63. Kleinberg L, Holth A, Fridman E, Schwartz I, Shih IM, Davidson B. The diagnostic role of claudins in serous effusions. Am J Clin Pathol. 2007;127:928–37.

64. Konstantinovsky S, Smith Y, Zilber S, Tuft Stavnes H, Becker AM, Nesland JM, Reich R, Davidson B. Breast carcinoma cells in primary tumors and effusions have different gene array profiles. J Oncol. 2010;2010:969084.

65. Rolih V, Barutello G, Iussich S, De Maria R, Quaglino E, Buracco P, Cavallo F, Riccardo F. CSPG4: a prototype oncoantigen for translational immunotherapy studies. J Transl Med. 2017;15:151.

66. Wang X, Osada T, Wang Y, Yu L, Sakakura K, Katayama A, McCarthy JB, Brufsky A, Chivukula M, Khoury T, Hsu DS, Barry WT, Lyerly HK, Clay TM, Ferrone S. CSPG4 protein as a new target for the antibody-based immunotherapy of triple-negative breast cancer. J Natl Cancer Inst. 2010;102:1496–512.

67. Levin M, Udi Y, Solomonov I, Sagi I. Next generation matrix metalloproteinase inhibitors - Novel strategies bring new prospects. Biochim Biophys Acta. 1864;2017:1927–39.

68. Jobin PG, Butler GS, Overall CM. New intracellular activities of matrix metalloproteinases shine in the moonlight. Biochim Biophys Acta. 1864;2017:2043–55.

69. Di Carlo A, Mariano A, Terracciano D, Mazzarella C, Galzerano S, Cicalese M, Cecere C, Macchia V. Gelatinolytic activities (matrix metalloproteinase-2 and -9) and soluble extracellular domain of Her-2/neu in pleural effusions. Oncol Rep. 2007;18:425–31.

70. Giarnieri E, Alderisio M, Mancini R, Falasca C, Ricci A, Mariotta S, Giovagnoli MR. Tissue inhibitor of metalloproteinase 2 (TIMP-2) expression in adenocarcinoma pleural effusions. Oncol Rep. 2008;19:483–7.

71. Davidson B, Konstantinovsky S, Nielsen S, Dong HP, Berner A, Vyberg M, Reich R. Altered expression of metastasis-associated and regulatory molecules in effusions from breast cancer patients- a novel model for tumor progression. Clin Cancer Res. 2004;10:7335–46.

72. Davidson B, Stavnes HT, Hellesylt E, Hager T, Zeppa P, Pinamonti M, Wohlschlaeger J. MMP-7 is a highly specific negative marker for benign and malignant mesothelial cells in serous effusions. Hum Pathol. 2016;47:104–8.

73. Xin X, Zeng X, Gu H, Li M, Tan H, Jin Z, Hua T, Shi R, Wang H. CD147/EMMPRIN overexpression and prognosis in cancer: A systematic review and meta-analysis. Sci Rep. 2016;6:32804.

74. Gieseler F, Lühr I, Kunze T, Mundhenke C, Maass N, Erhart T, Denker M, Beckmann D, Tiemann M, Schulte C, Dohrmann P, Cavaillé F, Godeau F, Gespach C. Activated coagulation factors in human malignant effusions and their contribution to cancer cell metastasis and therapy. Thromb Haemost. 2007;97:1023–30.

75. Avgeris M, Scorilas A. Kallikrein-related peptidases (KLKs) as emerging therapeutic targets: focus on prostate cancer and skin pathologies. Expert Opin Ther Targets. 2016;20:801–18.

76. Davidson B, Xi Z, Saatcioglu F. Kallikrein 4 is expressed in malignant mesothelioma—further evidence for the histogenetic link between mesothelial and epithelial cells. Diagn Cytopathol. 2007;35:80–4.

77. Trackman PC. Lysyl oxidase isoforms and potential therapeutic opportunities for fibrosis and cancer. Expert Opin Ther Targets. 2016;20:935–45.

78. Sebban S, Davidson B, Reich R. Lysyl oxidase-like 4 is alternatively spliced in an anatomic site-specific manner in tumors involving the serosal cavities. Virchows Arch. 2009;454:71–9.

79. Kan N, Kodama H, Hori T, Takenaka A, Yasumura T, Kato H, Ogawa H, Mukaihara S, Kudo T, Ohsumi K, Mise K. Intrapleural adaptive immunotherapy for breast cancer patients with cytologically-confirmed malignant pleural effusions: an analysis of 67 patients in Kyoto and Shiga Prefecture, Japan. Breast Cancer Res Treat. 1993;27:203–10.

80. Lissoni P, Mandalà M, Curigliano G, Ferretti G, Moro C, Ardizzoia A, Malugani F, Tancini G, Tisi E, Arrigoni C, Barni S. Progress report on the palliative therapy of 100 patients with neoplastic effusions by intracavitary low-dose interleukin-2. Oncology. 2001;60:308–12.

81. Spyridonidis A, Bernhardt W, Behringer D, Köhler G, Azemar M, Pflug A, Henschler R. Proliferation and survival of mammary carcinoma cells are influenced by culture conditions used for ex vivo expansion of CD34(+) blood progenitor cells. Blood. 1999;93:746–55.

82. Wischhusen J, Waschbisch A, Wiendl H. Immune-refractory cancers and their little helpers—an extended role for immunetolerogenic MHC molecules HLA-G and HLA-E. Semin Cancer Biol. 2007;17:459–68.

83. Morandi F, Rizzo R, Fainardi E, Rouas-Freiss N, Pistoia V. Recent advances in our understanding of HLA-G biology: lessons from a wide spectrum of human diseases. J Immunol Res. 2016;2016:4326495.

84. Kleinberg L, Flørenes VA, Skrede M, Dong HP, Nielsen S, McMaster MT, Nesland JM, Shih IM, Davidson B. Expression of HLA-G in malignant mesothelioma and clinically aggressive breast carcinoma. Virchows Arch. 2006;449:31–9.

85. Lazennec G, Richmond A. Chemokines and chemokine receptors: new insights into cancer-related inflammation. Trends Mol Med. 2010;16:133–44.

86. Nagarsheth N, Wicha MS, Zou W. Chemokines in the cancer microenvironment and their relevance in cancer immunotherapy. Nat Rev Immunol. 2017;17:559–72.

87. Thomachot MC, Bendriss-Vermare N, Massacrier C, Biota C, Treilleux I, Goddard S, Caux C, Bachelot T, Blay JY, Menetrier-Caux C. Breast carcinoma cells promote the differentiation of CD34+ progenitors towards 2 different subpopulations of dendritic cells with CD1a(high)CD86(−)Langerin- and CD1a(+)CD86(+)Langerin+ phenotypes. Int J Cancer. 2004;110:710–20.

88. Soria G, Yaal-Hahoshen N, Azenshtein E, Shina S, Leider-Trejo L, Ryvo L, Cohen-Hillel E, Shtabsky A, Ehrlich M, Meshel T, Keydar I, Ben-Baruch A. Concomitant expression of the chemokines RANTES and MCP-1 in human breast cancer: a basis for tumor-promoting interactions. Cytokine. 2008;44:191–200.

89. Davidson B, Dong HP, Holth A, Berner A, Risberg B. The chemokine receptor CXCR4 is more frequently expressed in breast compared to other metastatic adenocarcinomas in effusions. Breast J. 2008;14:476–82.

90. DeLong P, Carroll RG, Henry AC, Tanaka T, Ahmad S, Leibowitz MS, Sterman DH, June CH, Albelda SM, Vonderheide RH. Regulatory T cells and cytokines in malignant pleural effusions secondary to mesothelioma and carcinoma. Cancer Biol Ther. 2005;4:342–6.

91. Desfrançois J, Derré L, Corvaisier M, Le Mével B, Catros V, Jotereau F, Gervois N. Increased frequency of nonconventional double positive CD4CD8 alphabeta T cells in human breast pleural effusions. Int J Cancer. 2009;125:374–80.

92. Davidson B, Konstantinovsky S, Kleinberg L, Nguyen MTP, Bassarova A, Kvalheim G, Nesland JM, Reich R. The mitogen-activated protein kinases (MAPK) p38 and JNK are markers of tumor progression in breast carcinoma. Gynecol Oncol. 2006;102:453–61.

93. Wagner EF, Nebreda AR. Signal integration by JNK and p38 MAPK pathways in cancer development. Nat Rev Cancer. 2009;9:537–49.

94. Kim EK, Choi EJ. Pathological roles of MAPK signaling pathways in human diseases. Biochim Biophys Acta. 2010;1802:396–405.

95. Rauch N, Rukhlenko OS, Kolch W, Kholodenko BN. MAPK kinase signalling dynamics regulate cell fate decisions and drug resistance. Curr Opin Struct Biol. 2016;41:151–8.

96. Seth A, Watson DK. Ets transcription factors and their emerging roles in human cancer. Eur J Cancer. 2005;41:2462–78.

97. Verger A, Duterque-Coquillaud M. When Ets transcription factors meet their partners. Bioessays. 2002;24:362–70.

98. Sharrocks AD. The ETS-domain transcription factor family. Nat Rev Mol Cell Biol. 2001;2:827–37.

99. Sizemore GM, Pitarresi JR, Balakrishnan S, Ostrowski MC. The ETS family of oncogenic transcription factors in solid tumours. Nat Rev Cancer. 2017;17:337–51.

100. St Pierre R, Kadoch C. Mammalian SWI/SNF complexes in cancer: emerging therapeutic opportunities. Curr Opin Genet Dev. 2017;42:56–67.

101. Shih IM, Davidson B. Pathogenesis of ovarian cancer: clues from selected overexpressed genes. Future Oncol. 2009;5:1641–57.

102. Davidson B, Trope' CG, Wang TL, Shih IM. Expression of the chromatin remodeling factor Rsf-1 in effusions is a novel predictor of poor survival in ovarian carcinoma. Gynecol Oncol. 2006;103:814–9.

103. Davidson B, Wang TL, Shih IM, Berner A. Expression of the chromatin remodeling factor Rsf-1 in down-regulated in breast carcinoma effusions. Hum Pathol. 2008;39:616–22.

104. Dupont VN, Gentien D, Oberkampf M, De Rycke Y, Blin N. A gene expression signature associated with metastatic cells in effusions of breast carcinoma patients. Int J Cancer. 2007;121:1036–46.

105. Grimshaw MJ, Cooper L, Papazisis K, Coleman JA, Bohnenkamp HR, Chiapero-Stanke L, Taylor-Papadimitriou J, Burchell JM. Mammosphere culture of metastatic breast cancer cells enriches for tumorigenic breast cancer cells. Breast Cancer Res. 2008;10:R52.

106. Deng T, Liu JC, Pritchard KI, Eisen A, Zacksenhaus E. Preferential killing of breast tumor initiating cells by N,N-diethyl-2-[4-(phenylmethyl)phenoxy]ethanamine/tesmilifene. Clin Cancer Res. 2009;15:119–30.

107. Yuan Y, Leszczynska M, Konstantinovsky S, Tropé CG, Reich R, Davidson B. Netrin 4 is upregulated in breast carcinoma effusions compared to corresponding solid tumors. Diagn Cytopathol. 2011;39:562–6.
108. Davidson B, Tuft Stavnes H, Holth A, Chen X, Yang Y, Shih IM, Wang TL. Gene expression signatures differentiate ovarian/peritoneal serous carcinoma from breast carcinoma in effusions. J Cell Mol Med. 2011;15:535–44.
109. Stavnes HT, Nymoen DA, Langerød A, Holth A, Børresen Dale AL, Davidson B. AZGP1 and SPDEF mRNA expression differentiates breast carcinoma from ovarian serous carcinoma. Virchows Arch. 2013;462:163–73.
110. Bock AJ, Nymoen DA, Brenne K, Kærn J, Davidson B. SCARA3 mRNA is overexpressed in ovarian carcinoma compared with breast carcinoma effusions. Hum Pathol. 2012;43:669–74.
111. Davidson B, Stavnes HT, Nesland JM, Wohlschlaeger J, Yang Y, Shih IM, Wang TL. Gene expression signatures differentiate adenocarcinoma of lung and breast origin in effusions. Hum Pathol. 2012;43:684–94.
112. Kleinberg L, Flørenes VA, Nesland JM, Davidson B. Survivin, a member of the inhibitors of apoptosis (IAP) family, is downregulated in breast carcinoma effusions. Am J Clin Pathol. 2007;128:389–97.
113. Witthauer J, Schlereth B, Brischwein K, Winter H, Funke I, Jauch KW, Baeuerle P, Mayer B. Lysis of cancer cells by autologous T cells in breast cancer pleural effusates treated with anti-EpCAM BiTE antibody MT110. Breast Cancer Res Treat. 2009;117:471–81.
114. Sebastian M, Kiewe P, Schuette W, Brust D, Peschel C, Schneller F, Rühle KH, Nilius G, Ewert R, Lodziewski S, Passlick B, Sienel W, Wiewrodt R, Jäger M, Lindhofer H, Friccius-Quecke H, Schmittel A. Treatment of malignant pleural effusion with the trifunctional antibody catumaxomab (Removab) (anti-EpCAM x Anti-CD3): results of a phase 1/2 study. J Immunother. 2009;32:195–202.

# Malignant Mesothelioma

## Katalin Dobra and Anders Hjerpe

## Introduction

Malignant mesothelioma (MM) is the primary tumor of the serous cavities caused by exposure to fibrous minerals such as asbestos and erionite [1, 2]. The most frequent location for MM is the pleura, followed by the peritoneum, pericardium, and *tunica vaginalis testis*. Environmental factors, genetic predisposition, and various cofactors alone or together contribute the development of MM [3].

The development of MM occurs after a long latency period, typically 20–40 years from the time of initial asbestos exposure to diagnosis, suggesting that multiple genetic events are required for tumorigenic conversion of mesothelial cells. Malignant mesotheliomas are characteristically highly heterogeneous in terms of differentiation, which is also mirrored in variable biological behavior and prognosis. Median survival ranges from 4 to 12 months, but there is a changing trend as current studies report better survival than historical controls, particularly in the peritoneal subtype [4]. Survival time also depends on the tumor stage at diagnosis and on the histological subtype [3, 5]. The typical clinical manifestations of MM are dyspnea, chest pain, and a pleural effusion, which often is the first material available for diagnosis.

## Histogenesis

MM arises from the mesothelial cells lining the serosal cavities. The mesothelium is of mesodermal origin and consists of a single layer of flat mesothelial cells resting on a basement membrane and a sub-mesothelial layer of connective tissue of variable thickness. Mesothelial cells play a dynamic role in the homeostasis and immunoregulation of the serosal membranes. They synthesize hyaluronan, various growth factors, matrix proteins, proteoglycans, and cytokines that are essential to restore the integrity and the normal function of the serosal membrane after injury [6–10]. The renewal of surface mesothelium following injury is intriguing and comprises at least two different mechanisms, depending on whether the basement membrane is injured or not. Electron microscopic studies of the healing of the mesothelium showed that the mesothelial cells can be replaced by the sub-serosal mesenchymal cells [11] but also through reattachment of desquamated mesothelial cells to the denuded surfaces [12–14]. Mesothelial cells possess unique characteristics and may be regarded as pluripotential cells. Mesothelial progenitor cells are able to switch between different cell phenotypes depending on the local environment and may achieve endothelial-, myocyte-, osteoblast-, and adipocyte-like cell characteristics [15–18]. This plasticity of mesothelial cells has opened new perspectives in tissue engineering and regenerative medicine [15, 17] and may at least partly explain the characteristic heterogeneity of MM.

Poorly differentiated tumor components gradually lose their epithelial characteristics in a process termed epithelial-mesenchymal transition (EMT). Loss of specific differentiation markers, adoption of a spindle-like morphology, invasive growth, and progressive replacement of the cytokeratin network by vimentin intermediate filaments characterize this transition. This switch from epithelial markers (E-cadherin, β-catenin, and cytokeratins 5/6) to mesenchymal markers (N-cadherin, vimentin, α-smooth muscle actin, Snail, Slug, Twist, ZEB1, ZEB2, S100A4, MMP2, and MMP9) between epithelioid, biphasic, and sarcomatoid histotypes was demonstrated in 109 mesothelioma specimens [19].

Mesothelioma cells show a remarkable capacity to transdifferentiate in both directions along the mesenchymal-epithelial axis also in vitro. This can be seen in mesothelioma cells obtained from a pleural effusion, which show diverging differentiation potential and inducible growth pattern. Similar to the in vivo situation, they possess a characteristic biphasic growth potential and can be induced by serum growth factors to differentiate into stable epithelioid or fibro-

K. Dobra, M.D., Ph.D. (✉) · A. Hjerpe, M.D., Ph.D.
Division of Pathology, Department of Laboratory Medicine,
Karolinska Institute, Stockholm, Sweden
e-mail: katalin.dobra@ki.se

© Springer International Publishing AG, part of Springer Nature 2018
B. Davidson et al. (eds.), *Serous Effusions*, https://doi.org/10.1007/978-3-319-76478-8_11

blast-like phenotypes [20]. Similarly, epithelioid cells of mesothelial origin undergo a reversible morphological transition after exposure to several growth factors. This EMT involves transient cytoskeleton remodeling, and it is accompanied by changes in the adhesive status of these cells. In this way, the unique properties of mesothelioma cells provide an excellent model for identifying the critical changes in the regulation of cell differentiation and tumor cell progression, and they may also serve as valuable instruments for drug sensitivity testing.

## Etiology and Pathogenesis

### Asbestos Exposure

Epidemiological studies have established exposure to asbestos or asbestos-like mineral fibers as a main primary cause of MM [1, 21]. Malignant mesothelioma is frequently associated with occupational exposure, but there are also nonoccupational, domestic cases and geographic areas with environmental exposure [22–28]. Despite a ban on asbestos use in Western countries, MM is still of great international concern due to the long latency period between asbestos exposure and diagnosis. Moreover, asbestos is still used in developing countries, and therefore the incidence of mesothelioma is expected to further increase during the next decades [29, 30]. Experimental studies suggest that the carcinogenicity of asbestos fibers is related to its fibrous structure rather than to chemical characteristics. Furthermore, differences in the structure of various types of asbestos fibers may explain the variability in their carcinogenicity. The curly white asbestos is therefore considered less oncogenic than other types of fibers, and fibers less than 0.25 μm in diameter and more than 8 μm in length are more potent than shorter, thicker ones.

Erionite, a naturally occurring volcanic mineral, is causing extremely high incidence of mesothelioma in Cappadocia region in Turkey, and it is more potent than asbestos in causing mesothelioma [2, 23].

### Asbestos-Induced Molecular Alterations

Two different oncogenic mechanisms have been proposed. Firstly, asbestos fibers deform the cytoskeleton in mesothelial cells more efficiently than in airway epithelial cells [31]. In tissue culture, asbestos physically interacts with the mitotic spindle apparatus [32] and can interfere with normal chromosome segregation, leading to aneuploidy [33]. Secondly, asbestos fibers have been shown to induce chronic inflammation and the enzymatic activity of the mammalian DNA repair enzyme, apurinic/apyrimidinic (AP)-

endonuclease, suggesting that the release of reactive oxygen species (ROS) generated by asbestos can damage DNA double strands [34, 35]. AKT, ERK, AP-1, and NF-κB are frequently activated by the oxidative stress elicited by asbestos fibers in mesothelial cells [35, 36]. In addition, the hypoxic microenvironment of mesotheliomas [37] may alter the DNA damage repair pathways [38] and reprogram the metabolism by switching from oxidative phosphorylation to anaerobic glycolysis [39].

## Chromosomal Damage Induced by Asbestos

A hallmark of mesotheliomas is the large number of nonrandom cytogenic alterations [22, 27–33]. These include monosomy or frequent deletions at specific sites within chromosomes 1p, 3p, 4q, 6q, 9p, 10p, 13q, 14q, 15q, 18q, 19, and 22q, trisomy, polysomy, or gains of specific regions on chromosomes 1q, 5p, 7p, 8q, 11, 12, 20p, and 22. Chromosome losses are more common, and the most frequent recurrent changes involve chromosomes 3, 9, and 22. This array of nonrandom chromosome deletions in human mesotheliomas contributes to alterations in several tumor suppressor genes (TSGs) and oncogenes including *P16/CDKN2A, BAP1, NF2, P15 (INK4b), p14ARF, TP53, WT1* [40], *RASSF1, CTNNB1,* and *MAP3K3,* respectively [41, 42].

Karyotypic studies show multiple clonal chromosomal abnormalities in most human MM specimens [43–48]. Deletions of specific chromosomal sites in the short (p) arms of chromosomes 1, 3, and 9 and long (q) arm of chromosome 6 occur frequently, and loss of a copy of chromosome 22 was the single most consistent numerical cytogenetic change [48]. It is noteworthy that most of the changes described above occur in combination in a given MM. Comparative genomic hybridization (CGH) and array CGH also reveals multiple genomic imbalances [41]. In accord with previous karyotypic data, chromosomal losses were more frequent than gains with this approach.

## Inactivation of Tumor Suppressor Genes (TSGs)

The major feature of malignant mesothelioma is the loss of tumor suppressor genes. They are inactivated due to chromosomal deletions and mutations or epigenetic changes such as CpG methylation that result in loss of function. The accumulated loss and/or inactivation of multiple TSGs at chromosomes 1p, 3p, 6q, 9p, and 22q appear to play a critical role in the pathogenesis of MM. TSGs within these regions, i.e., $p16^{INK4A}$-$p14^{ARF}$ at 9p21, *NF2* at 22q12, *CTNNB1* at 3p22.1, *RASSF1A* at 3p21.3, and *BAP1* at 3p21.31-p21.2, are frequently altered in MM.

## P16 (INK4a)

The gene coding for p16 (INK4a) was identified as the 9p21 putative TSG [49–51]. It is particularly interesting because of its location in the region that is often deleted in MM. The protein encoded by p16 (INK4a) binds to the cyclin-dependent kinase CDK4 and thereby inhibits the catalytic activity of the CDK4/cyclin D enzymes. Abnormal p16 protein levels were observed in most, if not all, MM and MM-derived cell lines [52]. The product of the p16 (INK4a) gene induces a G1 cell cycle arrest by inhibiting the phosphorylation of the retinoblastoma protein, pRb. Thus, homozygous loss of *p16 (INK4a)* and *p14*ARF would together affect both Rb- and p53-dependent growth regulatory pathways. Homozygous deletion of *p16/CDKN2A* is found in a majority of mesotheliomas (>80%), and it is one of the most common genetic alterations in MM [41]. Loss of *p16/CDKN2A* is associated with more aggressive clinical behavior and non-epithelioid differentiation [53], and it may also serve as an independent adverse prognostic factor [54–57].

## BAP1

*BAP1* (BRCA1-associated protein 1) is located at chromosome 3p21.1, and it acts as a tumor suppressor gene that encodes for a nuclear deubiquitinase involved in regulation of gene transcription, control of G1/S phase transition of the cell cycle, cellular differentiation, and DNA damage response and repair [58]. *BAP1* is frequently lost by chromosomal deletion in several tumors and predisposes to development of malignant mesothelioma and uveal melanoma [59–61], often being part of a cancer syndrome. In addition to deletions, the spectrum of alterations in *BAP1* gene comprises inactivating mutations, including insertions, deletions, frameshift, and nonsense and missense mutations [62]. The tumor suppressor effect of *BAP1* requires both its deubiquitinating activity and its nuclear translocation, functions that can be lost by missense and truncated mutations [62], leading to cytoplasmic sequestration and inactivation.

Familial occurrence of mesothelioma has been described in the literature since long [63, 64]. Clustering of MM in families suggested that genetic susceptibility could be a contributory factor [65], and there was also an inherited component described in the development of mesothelioma in erionite-exposed Turkish patients in the Cappadocia region [66]. *BAP1* has early been associated in this context with tumor predisposition syndrome and malignant mesothelioma; for review, see [67].

Various studies describe different frequencies for *BAP1* mutations, germline mutations being rather infrequent, ranging between 1 and 2%, leading to familial accumulation of mesothelioma and being associated with certain geographic areas [66]. The germline mutation of *BAP1* is inherited in an autosomal dominant way and renders affected individuals an earlier onset of mesothelioma, also when exposed to lower level of asbestos fibers [59]. Somatic mutations and losses of *BAP1* are more frequent; deletions, somatic mutations, or other alterations have been reported in up to 60% of sporadic mesothelioma cases [68, 69]. *BAP1* mutations are associated with female gender, earlier onset, epithelioid differentiation, and a less aggressive disease with longer survival [70, 71]. Germline mutation carriers have slightly more frequently peritoneal localization of mesothelioma [72], a localization which per se has a particular biology and in general better survival. A recent report underscores the importance of matching germline and tumor DNA for correct assessment and interpretation of somatic versus germline mutations and highlights the risk of overreporting somatic mutations and underestimating the frequency of germline mutations if only tumors are tested [73]. Genetic testing for *BAP1* of high-risk individuals with family history of malignant mesothelioma might be beneficial for prevention, early detection, and treatment purposes.

In addition to *BAP1* mutations, asbestos-exposed individuals harboring germline mutations in DNA repair genes are highly predisposed to malignant mesothelioma as shown in a next-generation sequencing-based study on a cohort of 93 mesothelioma patients [74]. Among 94 germline pathogenic truncating variants tested, ten genes, predominantly involved in homologous recombination DNA repair (i.e., *PALB2, BRCA1, FANC1, ATM, SLX4, BRCA2; FANCC, FANCF, PMS1,* and *XPC*), were associated with asbestos exposure.

## NF2

The neurofibromatosis type 2 (*NF2*), autosomal dominant tumor suppressor gene, resides on chromosome 22q12 and is frequently altered in malignant mesothelioma. Approximately 30–50% of mesothelioma patients show mutation and/or allelic loss of *NF2*, suggesting that inactivation of this gene occurs via a two-hit mechanism [75]. Loss of chromosome 22q is more frequently associated with epithelioid differentiation [53] than to other histological subtypes.

*NF2* codes for a protein called merlin, which plays a role in cell surface dynamics and structure by linking the cytoskeleton to the plasma membrane [76] and interacts with many downstream proteins and signaling pathways. Merlin exerts its tumor suppressor and negative growth regulatory functions through a plethora of signaling pathways comprising phosphatidylinositol 3-kinase (PI3K)-AKT, RAS-ERK, and mTOR. The Hippo pathway is also a downstream target of merlin, and several elements of this pathway have been shown to be altered or lost in MM, including the serine/threonine kinase large tumor suppressor homolog 2 (*LATS2*) [77] and (*LATS1*) genes [78], the latter being fused to presenilin-1 (*PSEN1*) forming a fusion transcript (*LATS1-PSEN1*) leading to lost tumor suppressor function and lack of kinase activity. The loss of tumor suppression function liberates downstream growth-promoting factors or putative oncogenes such as the Yes-associated protein (YAP) [79] that translocates to the nucleus and co-activates various transcription factors. Merlin negatively regulates YAP by initiating its phosphorylation and thereby hampering its nuclear translocation and activity.

## Activation of Proto-Oncogenes

The nonrandom rearrangements and polysomy of chromosomes 1, 7, and 22 may generate growth-promoting oncogenes. Oncogenes often cause inappropriate expression of growth factors (GFs), growth factor receptors, and other compounds involved in the signaling mechanisms. In consequence, normal growth control mechanisms are abrogated. It has also been suggested that autocrine production of the platelet-derived growth factor-B (PDGF-B) chain may stimulate autoreplication of tumor cells, also when there are no or low levels of $\beta$ receptors [80–82].

Asbestos can also induce the proto-oncogenes *c-fos* and *c-jun*, which encode transcription factors that activate various genes critical in the initiation of DNA synthesis [83]. The induction of these transcription activators may enhance cellular proliferation and could render cells more susceptible to subsequent mutations. Several investigators found JUN located at chromosome 1p32 to be amplified [41, 42, 84]. JUN is a transcription factor that has role in cell division. Such activation of proto-oncogenes, together with inactivation of tumor suppressor genes, may cooperate in a multistep series of critical events in the development of MM.

Taken together, MM results from the accumulation of numerous acquired genetic events, mainly chromosome deletions, indicating a multistep cascade involving the inactivation of multiple TSGs. Future targeted therapeutic approaches have to take this into account and target downstream molecules or concomitantly several different signaling pathways.

## The Molecular Signature of MM by Next-Generation Sequencing

New techniques, such as next-generation DNA sequencing, have enabled more precise definition of the cancer genome and identified tumor-specific rearrangements and mutations related to asbestos exposure. Exome sequencing revealed novel asbestos-related mutations in *BAP1* and a frameshift mutation in *NF2*, along with *MRPL1* (a gene encoding for mitochondrial ribosome), *SDK1* (an adhesion molecule

activated by reactive oxygen species), and *COPG1* (a subunit of a protein complex involved in vesicular protein transport) [85]. This method also identified novel rearrangements; point mutations; large-scale, inter- and intra-chromosomal deletions; inversions; and translocations, disrupting gene-encoding regions, including kinases, transcription factors, and growth factors [86].

Extensive efforts of massively parallel sequencing and genome-wide screening comprising whole genome, exome [85, 87, 88], and transcriptome sequencing [89, 90] verified the earlier identified genetic alterations [87, 91] but also added novel mutations to the spectrum of mesothelioma-associated molecular signature such as cullin 1 (*CUL1*), an essential component of the ubiquitin ligase complex. Recurrent mutations have been seen at lower frequency in *SF3B1* and *TRAF7* in approximately 2% of the studied 216 MPMs along with recurrent fusions and splice alterations in *NF2*, *BAP1*, *PTEN*, and 8 other genes. Although MM tumors showed a low protein-altering mutation rate compared to other cancer types, integrated bioinformatic approach identified several signaling pathway alterations including the Hippo pathway, mTOR, histone methylation, RNA helicase, and p53 [91].

The involvement of the Hippo pathway, *TP53*/DNA, and cell cycle regulators such as CDKN2A was repeatedly described. New elements of the MAPK pathway, including *KIT* and kinase insert domain receptor gene (*KDR*); several members of the PI3K-AKT pathway comprising *PIK3CA/B*, *AKT*, and *mTOR*; microRNA 31 (*MIR31*); semaphorin 5B gene (*SEMA5*); and serine/threonine kinase 11 gene (*STK11*) were all affected. For a comprehensive review, see [92].

Genetic variations of advanced-stage MM revealed two major pathways involving the p53/DNA repair and the PI3K-AKT pathways. Several elements of these pathways offer diagnostic, therapeutic, and prognostic information [93].

Genomic profiling of peritoneal mesotheliomas revealed recurrent alterations in *BAP1*, *SETD2*, and *DDX3X* [94]. The mutational spectrum of peritoneal mesothelioma is very similar to the pleural one, but it occurs at different frequencies and is associated with prognosis [94, 95]. For instance, *BAP1* alterations are present in 85% of peritoneal and 20–30% of pleural tumors [94], whereas alterations in *CDKN2A* and *NF2* are less frequent [96]. Homozygous deletion of *CDKN2A* and heterozygous loss of *NF2* correlated with shorter progression-free and overall survival, and alterations in both had a cumulative effect [97]. In multicystic mesothelioma, two fusion genes were identified by RNA sequencing corresponding to translocation t(7;17)(p12;q23) *TNS3-MAP 3K3* and t(8;11)(q23;p13) *ZFPM2-ELF5*, respectively [98].

Many of the molecular alterations detected in MM can also be found in other cancers, but their clustering and arrangement in distinct pathways with several perturbations in the same or parallel pathway delineate a complex pattern of alterations that could at least partly explain why MM is such a therapy-refractory malignancy.

As the genomic landscape of MM is emerging, simultaneous occurrence of loss of several tumor suppressor genes and other genetic aberrations is obvious. Kato et al. found 116 different aberrations in 42 mesothelioma patients of which in median 3 (range 1–5) potentially actionable alterations were identified in each patient [99]. Moreover, the authors postulate that 96.6% of the studied individuals harbored at least one potentially targetable molecular alteration where an FDA-approved drug or therapies included in clinical trials were available. In mesothelioma no single driver mutation has been found, and many alterations cluster together; the variations are almost infinite, so each individual has a unique setting of alterations, motivating an individualized choice of treatment matched to the unique setup of genetic alterations for each patient.

Understanding of the molecular landscape of mesothelioma and recognition of co-activation of several receptor tyrosine kinases such as epidermal growth factor (*EGFR*) and *MET* in a subgroup of mesothelioma patients [100] imply simultaneous targeting of several pathways that might render more effective treatments in the future. This also underscores the need for diagnostic molecular testing and biomarker-guided clinical studies and personalized treatment strategies.

## Gene Expression Profiling

A significant number of studies have used gene microarrays to examine the gene expression profile of MM, comprising both mesothelioma-derived cell lines and patient samples, in the purpose of finding molecular fingerprints connected to differentiation, diagnosis, prediction of treatment response, or prognostication. Major pathways and molecular signatures were identified in this way, involving DNA damage, cell cycle regulation, cytoskeletal organization, extracellular matrix components, the ubiquitin-proteasome system [101, 102], redox regulation [103, 104], and regulation of apoptosis [105, 106].

Data from several experimental setups are converging and highlight the involvement of RARRES1, thioredoxin, and several members of the insulin growth factor (IGF) family in the development and differentiation of MM [101, 104, 107]. Retinoic acid receptor responder 1 (RARRES1) is a retinoid-regulated gene, frequently downregulated through DNA hypermethylation in several types of malignant tissues. Several reports have implicated RARRES1 as a putative tumor suppressor gene. Studies involving the re-expression of RARRES1 have also pointed to its tumor suppressive function, as it decreased the growth and greatly reduced the in vitro invasiveness of cancer cells [108].

Various elements of the redox system are differentially deregulated in MM, comprising the thioredoxin system and superoxide dismutase. Thioredoxin (trx) is a small ubiqui-

tous redox-active protein [109] originally discovered as a hydrogen donor to ribonucleotide reductase, an enzyme essential for DNA synthesis. This protein, present in human plasma, is secreted by normal and neoplastic cells via a leaderless secretory pathway [110]. It operates with the FAD-selenoenzyme thioredoxin reductase (TR) and NADPH (the Trx-system) as an efficient general protein disulfide reductase system [109]. Mammalian TR is a homodimeric flavoenzyme with a selenocysteine, a FAD, and a functional dithiol/disulfide in each subunit [111, 112]. Trx binds to a variety of proteins and selectively activates the DNA binding of certain transcription factors, such as NF-κB and AP-1 [113]. Trx stimulates cell growth and is an inhibitor of apoptosis. An increase in thioredoxin levels seen in many human primary cancers, unlike in normal tissues, appears to contribute to an increase in cancer cell growth and resistance to chemotherapy.

Distinct expression pattern signatures characterize the epithelioid and sarcomatoid tumor subtypes [101]. Sarcomatoid tumors contain elevated levels of growth factor receptors and associated binding proteins such as PDGF receptor β (PDGFRβ), fibroblast growth factor receptor 1 (FGFR1), and transforming growth factor β1 (TGFβ1), whereas epithelioid mesothelioma cells overexpress tumor-promoting factors involved in differentiation, metabolism, and proteasome activation. Overall, the expression profile of the epithelioid cell line reflects a more differentiated tumor. The fibroblast-like cell line had a profile more commonly associated with growth factors and genes that may contribute to the particularly unfavorable prognosis of sarcomatoid tumors. These factors are present at significant levels also in patient samples and pleural effusions [114, 115].

## Epigenetic Alterations

Gene silencing by DNA methylation at CpG dinucleotides in promoter regions is a well-recognized mechanism of gene inactivation. Epidermal growth factor receptor (EGFR) and c-Met are often epigenetically modulated in mesothelioma [116, 117]. A characteristic epigenetic profile characterizes MM, corresponding to 387 (6.3%) hypermethylated genes. An integrated evaluation of epigenetic and genetic alterations revealed that 11% of heterozygously deleted genes were affected by DNA methylation in MM [118]. Others argue for a strong association between global genetic and global epigenetic deregulation in mesothelioma, rather than local correlation of gene inactivation [119].

## Classification and Morphology

MM may be restricted to a small area as a localized tumor, or it may involve the serosal membrane multifocally or grow in a diffuse manner. Four main morphological differentiation patterns are recognized: epithelial (tubulopapillary and nonglandular or epithelioid), sarcomatous (including desmoplastic), biphasic (mixed), and poorly differentiated (or undifferentiated). It has been stated that 50% of pleural and 75% of peritoneal diffuse malignant mesotheliomas are of epithelial type [120]; 25% and 15%, respectively, are of biphasic or sarcomatous type; and the remaining cases are poorly differentiated or unclassifiable. Sufficient sampling, however, often shows both epithelial and fibroblastic components. Consequently, the proportion of mixed type increases with the amount of tissue available for diagnosis [121].

The clinical outcome of patients depends largely on the phenotype of the tumor. In pleural effusions, which are often the first diagnostic material, sarcomatoid tumor components are not recognized, and it has been debated if a correct diagnosis can be based on cytology alone. Modern diagnostic approaches, however, will make the accurate diagnosis possible in the majority of epithelioid and mixed-type MMs, involving a spectrum of adjuvant methods. The positive predictive value of such a cytological diagnosis is as high as of one obtained by histology [122] and therefore provides a sufficient basis for initiation of treatment. As described in published international guidelines [123, 124], the diagnosis cannot be based on routine morphology only and necessitates the use of ancillary techniques.

## Adjuvant Diagnostic Methods

The major diagnostic challenges for cytopathologists are the distinction between reactive mesothelium—so-called mesotheliosis—and malignancy on one hand and between pleural epithelioid mesothelioma and metastatic adenocarcinoma involving the pleura on the other hand. The diagnostic accuracy can be improved by the use of a number of ancillary methods, including optimized immunocytochemical panels [125–128], electron microscopy (EM) [129, 130], molecular biology [48, 50, 83], and chemical analyses of soluble biomarkers such as hyaluronan (HA) [131] and mesothelin [132].

## Immunocytochemistry

Immunocytochemistry (ICC) is the most established adjuvant technique used to expand the diagnostic value of effusion cytology. The vast number of different epitopes claimed to be more or less specific merely reflects the need for supporting diagnostic adjuvant methods. Although ICC has been in use for more than two decades, new antibodies still add to the available reagent arsenal. Although different in different centers, the use of ICC in effusion cytology is well established. Different antibodies/epitopes useful for these

diagnostic situations have been thoroughly reviewed [126] and will be described elsewhere in this book.

Since most of the antibodies recommended for the distinction of MM from an adenocarcinoma are not completely specific for or against any of the diagnostic alternatives, the risk of an aberrant outcome of a single reaction necessitates further diagnostic support and the use of additional reactions, which has developed into the use of variously sized immunocytochemical batteries. However, the risk for at least one reaction to be aberrant, and therefore confusing, increases with the number of reactions performed. This problem can be resolved on two principally different ways: when the case is analyzed with a larger number of ICC reactions; the diagnosis can be based on a dominating reaction pattern. A more precise way is to use optimized batteries, where a limited number of defined antibodies have been evaluated and an interpretation algorithm defined. The statistical power during such optimization of batteries is, however, limited by the size of the material. Thus, a histological material containing 119 mesotheliomas and 57 adenocarcinomas allowed the calculation of a battery of 8 parameters [127]. A similar study based on effusions, including 36 mesotheliomas and 53 adenocarcinomas, allowed a similar battery of 3 antibodies to be calculated [133]. The sensitivity of these batteries is limited; the latter based on ICC of effusions identifies around 50% of the mesotheliomas only. Combination of ICC with independent parameters, such as the concentration of soluble biomarkers, can be more successful. Thus, the addition of hyaluronan analysis to effusion ICC increased the sensitivity for MM to almost 80% [134]. This sensitivity is, however, not validated externally, and the true sensitivity when routinely used is probably somewhat lower.

ICC is a useful adjunct to the diagnosis of a MM, and a multitude of diagnostic markers may be helpful [135, 136]. There are, however, no sufficiently specific individual antibodies that always will distinguish malignant from benign mesothelial cells. A common event when the mesothelial cell turns malignant is that it loses its expression of desmin, and loss of reactivity to this epitope is a sensitive marker for MM [137, 138]. Desmin is, however, since long known to be sensitive to formalin fixation [139], and the use of this marker necessitates titrated antibody concentration and positive controls. More recently, BAP1 immunocytochemistry combined with homozygous deletion of p16 by FISH analysis has been recommended as an alternative, yielding high specificity but low sensitivity [140–144].

Expression of EMA with membrane accentuation is useful to differentiate MM from reactive mesothelium [137, 138, 145, 146]. Such expressions can, however, occasionally be seen in scattered reactive mesothelial cells. Other markers described to distinguish malignant from reactive mesothelium are IMP3, CD146, and Glut1 [147]. In case

ICC will remain inconclusive as to the problem of malignancy, this can often be solved by ploidy analysis using FISH ([56, 148] see below).

## Electron Microscopy

The ultrastructural examination of cells recovered from effusions adds diagnostic information to the distinction of MM. It is indeed a most reliable diagnostic tool and is sometimes considered the gold standard for this diagnosis [90]. The criteria for malignancy and mesothelial origin of cells are well-defined for epithelioid mesothelioma cells [81, 91]. Purely sarcomatoid and fibroblast-like tumor cells cannot be recognized in the effusion, either due to lack of their exfoliation or because they lose their characteristic morphology and take a rounded epithelioid shape when in suspension. EM is erroneously considered to be a too expensive diagnostic tool. In fact, the cost is in the same order as a moderately sized set of immunocytochemical reactions. The preparation of the material, however, is time-consuming, and the examination often takes 2–3 weeks with standard preparation procedures.

To make this analysis a useful diagnostic tool, it is necessary to have the cells adequately fixed. Therefore, to have the possibility to use electron microscopy on demand, material should be taken care of already when the fresh effusion is centrifuged to prepare routine smears. One aliquot of the cell pellet is then directly transferred to a glutaraldehyde-based EM fixative and kept at 4°C until further processing. Because of the time needed, the ultrastructural examination is best performed as an adjuvant analysis, when routine morphology and immunocytochemistry raise the suspicion of mesothelioma without allowing a definite diagnosis.

## Criteria Indicating Malignancy

It is important first to establish that there is a malignant condition, i.e., that the examined cells are neoplastic and not reactive. Ultrastructural criteria for malignancy include those in effusion cytology (as seen in light microscopy of the semithin sections), together with some entirely ultrastructural ones. Thus, ultrathin sections of MM often show cells with nuclei that are highly irregular and carry large nucleoli (Figs. 11.1 and 11.2), changes that sometimes can be seen already in the glutaraldehyde-fixed and plastic-embedded semithin sections stained with toluidine blue. These nuclear irregularities are more pronounced than can be seen in routine Giemsa- or Papanicolaou-stained smears, and they are even more apparent in the ultrathin sections, with deep indentions of the nuclear envelope.

The ultrastructural criteria for malignancy, analyzing an effusion cell pellet from a mesothelioma, are mainly based on the presence of cell groups. One of the major criteria for

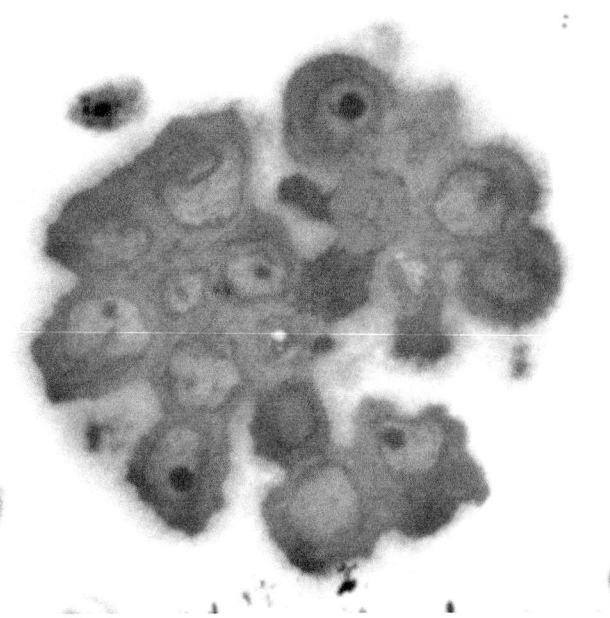

**Fig. 11.1** Light microscopy of a plastic embedded papillary mesothelioma fragment from an effusion. The irregular cell nuclei contain macronucleoli. Note also the villi surrounding the cells, here merely seen as a haze

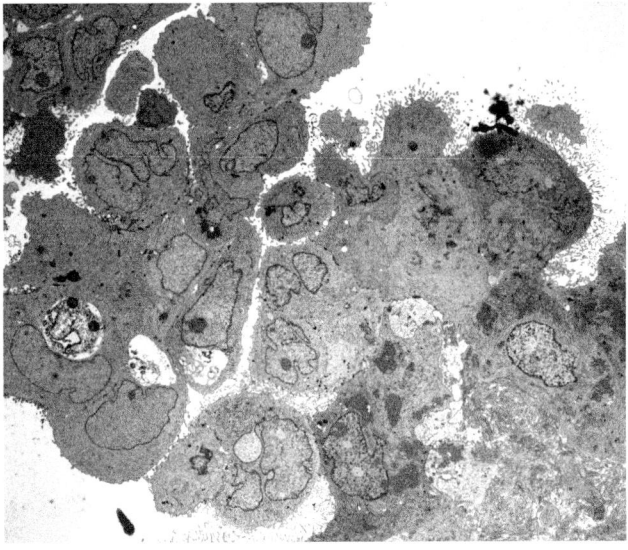

**Fig. 11.2** Groups of malignant mesothelioma cells, showing highly irregular nuclei, some of which contain large nucleoli

malignancy is the finding of neolumina (Fig. 11.3). A neolumen is a vesicular structure formed by an apical cell membrane (best characterized by presence of microvilli). These can be found in basolateral location, limited by two adjacent cells, or as an intracellular vesicle. In both cases, it represents a disordered organization of the cytoplasmic membrane, and this is considered a specific sign of malignancy, as long as oblique sectioning of tumor tissue surface can be excluded. The irregular occurrence of basement membrane-

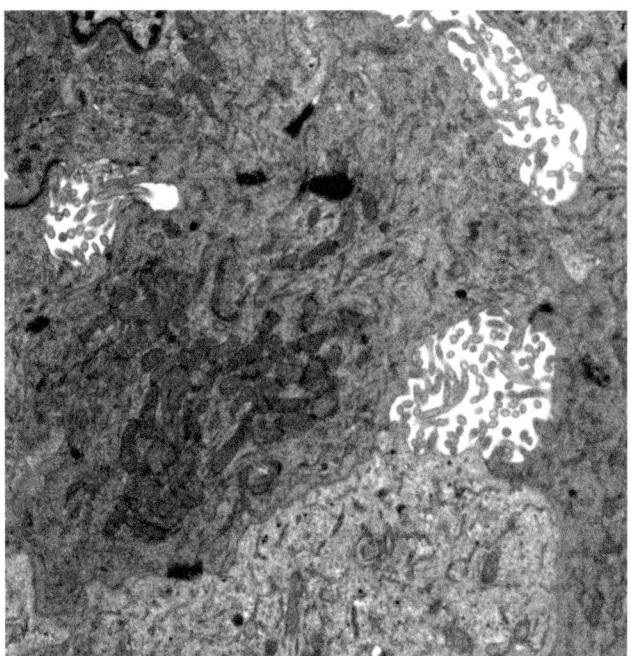

**Fig. 11.3** Neolumina containing slender microvilli in a papillary mesothelioma fragment

like material within the group is a similar indication of disturbed organization in a malignant tumor.

The ultrastructural examination sometimes also reveals the presence of specific markers for epithelial tumors, such as secretory granules in adenocarcinoma cells. Such findings definitely indicate malignancy, and at the same time, they exclude that this is a malignant mesothelioma.

An ultrastructural diagnosis of malignancy can be difficult when the tumor cells are dissociated without presence of cell groups. The diagnosis must then be obtained in other ways, ploidy analysis by FISH (see below) often being an accurate way to solve this diagnostic dilemma.

### Criteria Indicating Mesothelial Origin of Tumor Cells

The ultrastructure of the MM cell has been known for decades [129, 149]. One problem, however, is that an activated benign mesothelial cell may develop similar characteristics, although most often not to the same extent. In the individual case, this may cause considerable interpretation problems, and it is therefore important that the malignant nature of examined cells is beyond any doubt.

Already in semithin sections, light microscopy of these well-fixed tumor cells can show a broad zone of microvilli at the cell membrane (Figs. 11.1 and 11.4), indicating their mesothelial origin. Furthermore, common cytological criteria such as raspberry-like and poorly coherent tumor cell groups indicate that the tumor is a mesothelioma.

The groups of epithelioid mesothelioma cells show desmosomes between adjacent cells, excluding artificial cell cohesion (Fig. 11.5). The tumor cell cytoplasm often contains glycogen deposits (Fig. 11.6), and microtubule typically surrounds the nucleus like a scarf (Fig. 11.7). The most important diagnostic findings are associated with the cell membrane. The typical microvilli of a mesothelioma cell are numerous and slender (Fig. 11.4). They lack core rootlets and have an appearance of long jelly snakes rather than stiff rods, the latter being more typical of an adenocarcinoma. Particularly, when these slender villi are packed between two adjacent cells (Fig. 11.3), this indicates a neolumen diagnostic of MM.

It is important also to look for the presence of the glycocalyx at the cell membrane. Presence of this is diagnostic for an adenocarcinoma (Fig. 11.8), whereas a malignant mesothelioma cell should have a smooth "denuded" surface.

When using electron microscopy as an adjuvant to inconclusive effusion cytology, we could correctly suggest a malignant diagnosis in 77 (53%) out of 146 malignant cases with no false positives (Table 11.1), while the remaining 47% remained inconclusive, mainly because of the lack of preserved diagnostic cells. A correct distinction between mesothelioma and adenocarcinoma could be possible in all cases with diagnostic material.

For further reading, see [150, 151].

## Molecular Biology

One way to establish a malignant condition in an effusion cell pellet is the determination of ploidy by fluorescence in situ hybridization (FISH). A commercially available kit, Urovysion® (Abbott), contains three centromeric probes specific for chromosomes number 3, 7, and 17 and one probe labelling the 9p21 band, containing the locus for p16. The kit vas originally presented as a tool to diagnose urothelial cancers. When applied to effusion cytology [148] and with the interpretation algorithm presented by the manufacturer (at least four cells with gains of at least two chromosomes or homozygous deletion of the 9p21 in at least 12 cells), this could correctly identify 49 out of 50 cancers as aneuploid with no false-positive reaction (Fig. 11.9).

Two interpretation problems can appear when using this test in clinical routine. The first is when the signals from one probe appear as a group of dots. This is most likely a "signal split" from a single target sequence due to degeneration and should not be taken as an indication of chromosomal gain. A second problem relates to tri- and tetraploidization during the S and G2 phases of the cell cycle. Reactive mesothelium is characterized by an

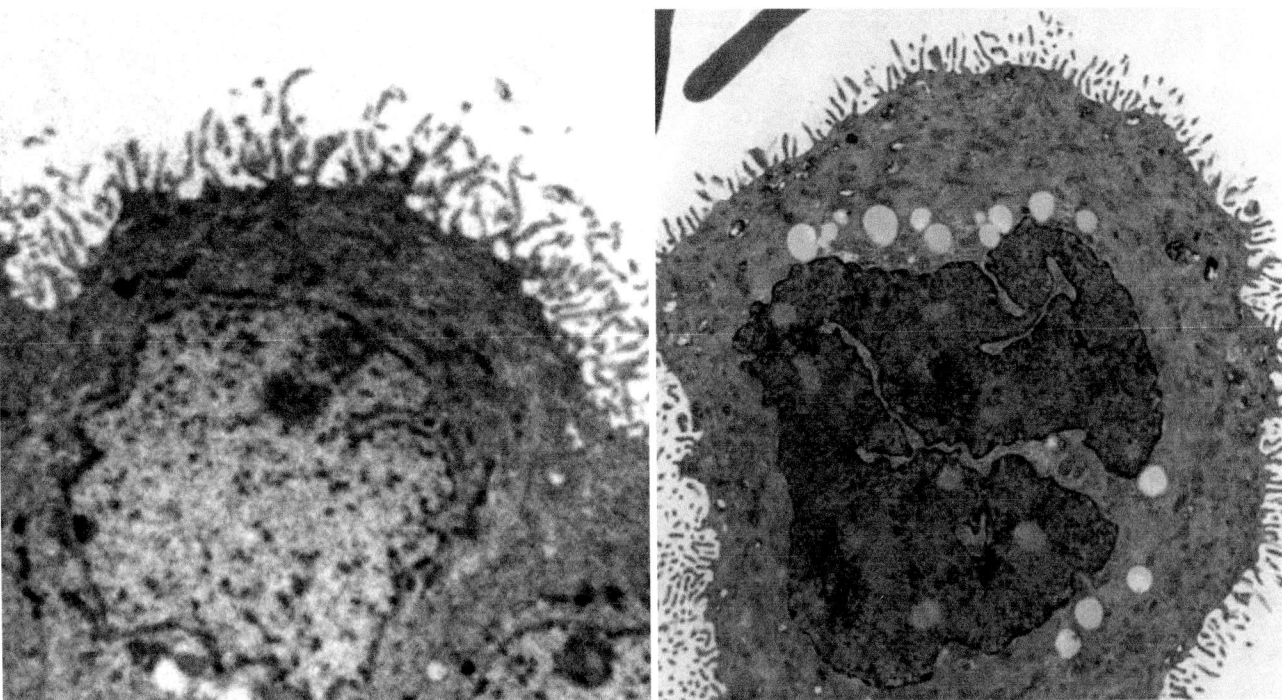

**Fig. 11.4** Mesothelioma cells (left) have long slender microvilli, while those in adenocarcinoma (right) are fewer and more rigidly straight

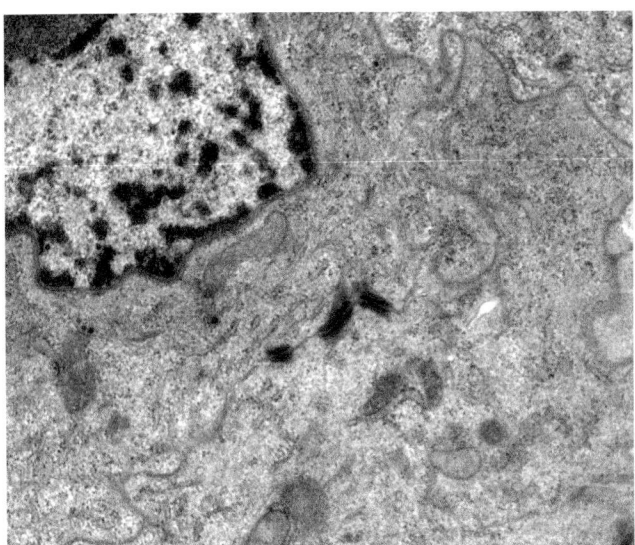

**Fig. 11.5** One typical finding in mesothelioma fragments recovered from an effusion is the presence of desmosomes, joining the tumor cells

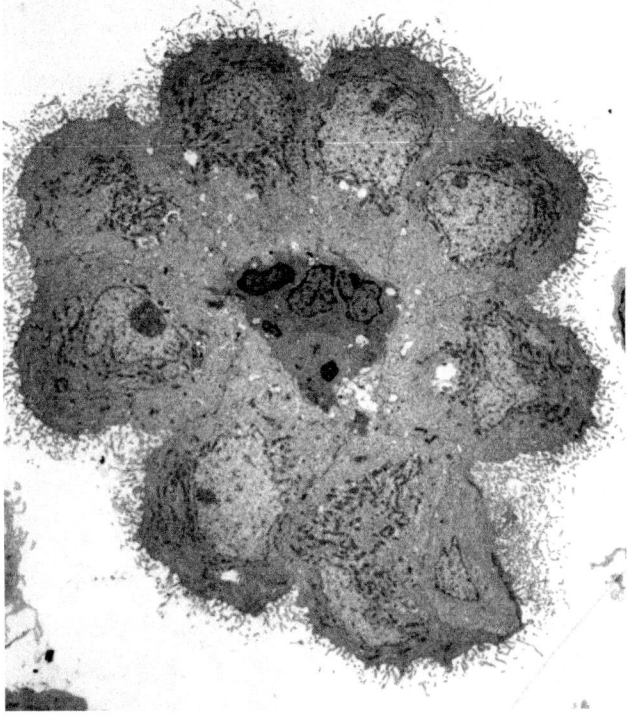

**Fig. 11.6** Raspberry-like papillary group of mesothelioma cells rich in electron-dense glycogen deposits

increased number of proliferating cells, i.e., cells duplicating their chromosomes. These cells are hyperchromatic with the DAPI stain and are often selected for counting of signals. A general finding of 3–4 signals from all three centromeric probes and from the 9p21 probe most likely represents a reactive condition. Cautious interpretation, with the possibility of reactive tetraploidization in mind, will, however, solve many of these cases.

The second criterion for malignancy, homozygous deletion of the 9p21 band, is easier to define when present. Of interest in this context is that 12 out of 21 MM presented

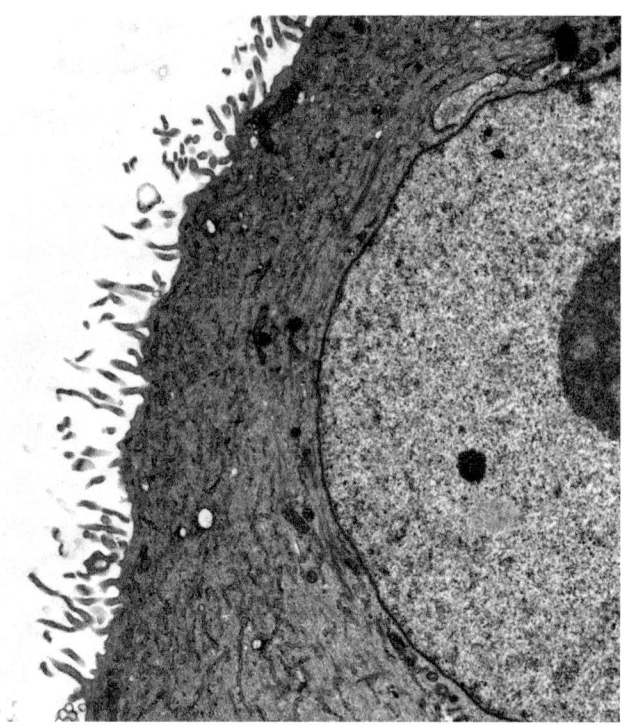

**Fig. 11.7** The perinuclear area of mesothelioma cells contains microfilaments, oriented parallel to the nuclear envelope

with homozygous deletions of 9p21, while this only was seen in 2 out of 29 cancers of other origin (Fig. 11.10). This is in line with previous studies by Knuutila S and coworkers [41]. In fact, their results indicate that deletions in this region are even more common in mesothelioma. The minimal size of the deletions may, however, be much less than the 200 kB covered by the commercial probe.

## Soluble Biomarkers for Mesothelioma

MM represents a group of tumors that is unique in many aspects. The biology of the mesothelium, with its intermediate differentiation pattern in between epithelial and mesenchymal phenotypes, is also reflected immunocytochemically and biochemically (see the above paragraph on immunocytochemistry).

Several attempts have been made to use possible chemical fingerprints of these tumors to establish the diagnosis, predict prognosis and sensitivity to drugs, and follow effects of a given treatment. In clinical practice, only a few such biochemical markers have been established for diagnostic use, while attempts to predict drug sensitivity are still under development. The diagnostic biomarker analyses have been performed either on sera/plasma or on effusions, as an adjuvant to cytology.

The most natural way for biomarkers to enter the effusion is by secretion directly from the tumor cell, by disintegration of tumor cells, or indirectly as a result of paracrine stimulation of

the tumor stroma. Biomarkers may be secreted directly to the bloodstream, and those present in the effusion will also reach the blood via the pleural stomata, which drain the effusion fluid to the lymphatic system. The concentration of biomarkers in the two kinds of fluids depends on both the rate of synthesis and the rate of elimination. Generally, the concentration of such a biomarker is 10–100 times higher in the effusion than in serum, indicating that the transport via pleural stomata is more important than direct secretion into tumor blood vessels.

Case studies and genome-wide screenings have identified several biomarkers associated with MPM. Some of the more scrutinized to date are hyaluronan (HA), mesothelin, and osteopontin (OPN). The first diagnostic marker shown to have importance for the diagnosis of MM was HA (previously named "hyaluronic acid"). Several authors have described high HA concentrations in effusions associated with MM [152, 153]. HA is a linear glycosaminoglycan composed of repeated N-acetyl glucosamine-glucuronic acid disaccharides, and it interacts with various extracellular and intracellular components. The chain is synthesized in the cell membrane by any of three HA synthases. The released macromolecule is water soluble, which makes it difficult to demonstrate by immunocytochemistry.

It has been discussed whether the elevated levels seen in mesothelioma effusions relate to synthesis by the tumor cells themselves or if there is paracrine stimulation by PDGF, increasing HA synthesis by tumor stromal fibroblasts. Staining with alcian blue before and after treatment with *Streptomyces* hyaluronidase definitely indicates synthesis by the tumor cells, but both alternatives are possible and may work side by side [154, 155].

In effusions, HA is best demonstrated by biochemical means. The analysis became available for routine analysis with the use of a simple ion suppression HPLC separation following enzymatic digestion of precipitated glycosaminoglycans [131, 156]. The sensitivity of this analysis allows accurate determinations based on HA in effusions, while the concentration of this compound in serum often is too low. Later techniques, employing HA-binding proteins [157], have improved the sensitivity to enable also analysis of blood samples. These reagents are now commercially available. A limitation of using this latter method for the analysis of effusions is, however, that the reagents in few cases may cross-react with some bacterial sugars, particularly in connection to bacterial pleuritis, causing false-positive results. When the analysis is combined with simultaneous measurement of mesothelin, acting as a marker of malignancy, the combination of these two biomarkers yields high specificity [158].

Since completely dry HA standards are difficult to prepare, the concentration is sometimes expressed as HA-derived uronic acid per volume. Such value in an effusion exceeding 75 μg/mL, corresponding to 150 μg/mL of "dry" HA (without crystal water), is a strong argument in favor of a MM [131]. The standards provided in the commercial kits are

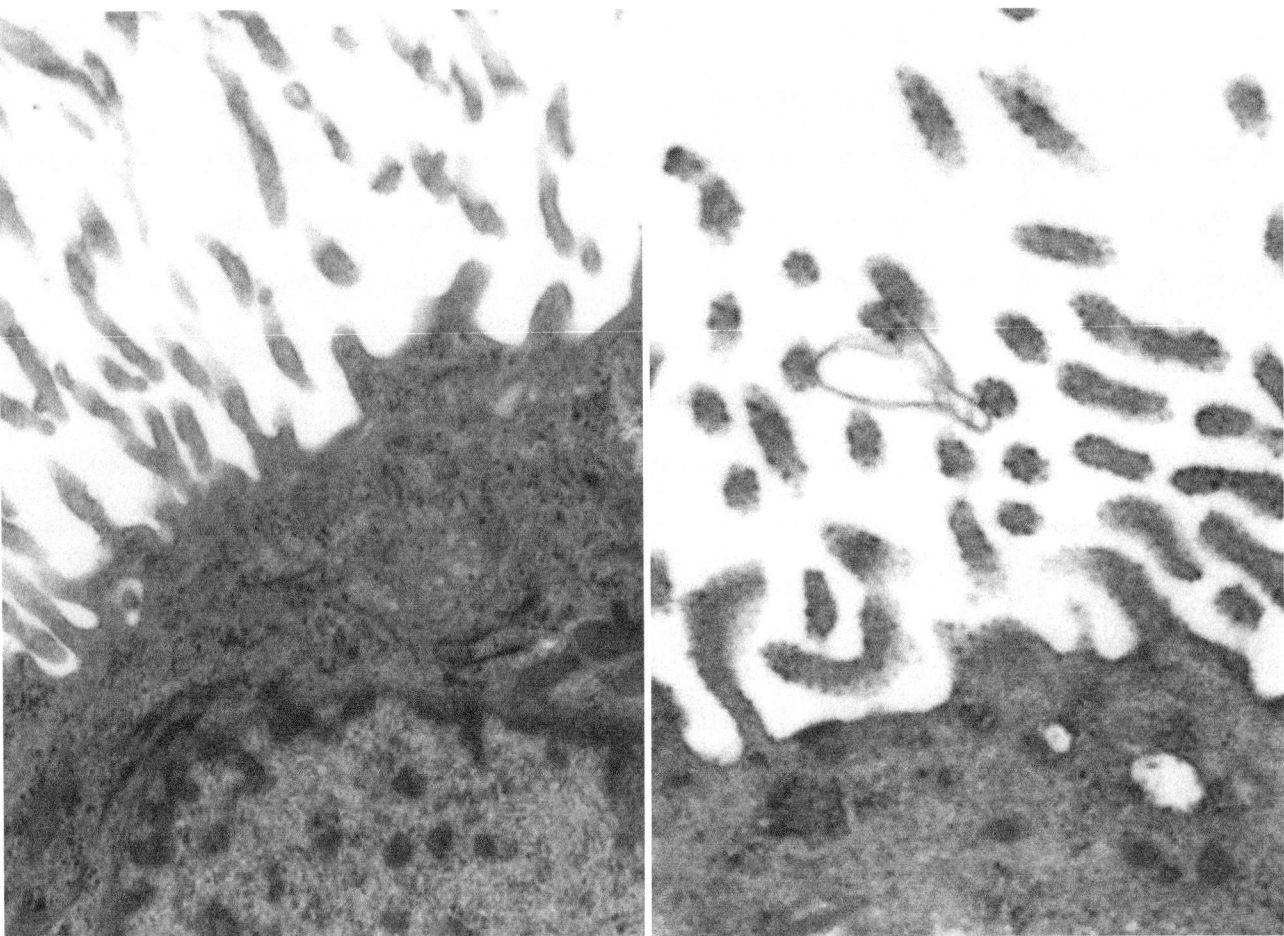

**Fig. 11.8** The cell membrane on adenocarcinoma cells (right) is often covered with glycocalyx, while that of mesothelioma cells (left) is smooth, devoid of such precipitates

**Table 11.1** Outcome of electron microscopy (EM) diagnosis on effusion cell pellets in 295 cases with inconclusive routine *cytology*

| | | EM diagnosis | | | |
| --- | --- | --- | --- | --- | --- |
| | | Benign or inconclusive | MM | ADCA | Total |
| Final diagnosis | Benign | 149 | 0 | 0 | 149 |
| | MM | 31 | 38 | 0 | 69 |
| | ADCA | 38 | 0 | 39 | 77 |
| | Total | 218 | 38 | 39 | 295 |

given as concentration of "wet" HA, corresponding to a cut-off around 230 μg/mL. Such diagnostic values are seen in 50–60% of MM. In case the thoracocentesis is repeated, HA concentrations tend to be lower in the second sample when this is obtained within a few weeks. It seems as if the fluid and HA enter the pleural cavity at different rates.

Attempts have also been made to trace HA in serum. The diagnostic utility, however, seems to be less. This can be related to two circumstances. First, HA can enter the bloodstream in other conditions, such as inflammation [159] or liver cirrhosis [160]. Secondly, the turnover of HA in the serum is fast, half of the amount being eliminated within a few minutes [161]. Despite this, results have indicated that the serum concentration reflects the tumor burden, when fol-lowed over time, and it has been suggested that serum HA content can be used to follow the effects of treatment given [162].

*Mesothelin/ERC* is a membrane-bound precursor protein that more recently has been presented as a possible marker for MM [132]. The newly synthesized mesothelin/ERC is transported to the cell membrane, where it sheds a 31 kD fragment (N-ERC, also called megakaryocyte potentiating factor, MPF), the remaining 40 kD C-ERC fragment persisting in the cell membrane, where it normally is involved in cell signaling and cell adhesion and responsible for binding to the cancer antigen CA 125 [163]. In addition, mesothelin also presents as various splice variants, including soluble mesothelin-related protein (SMRP).

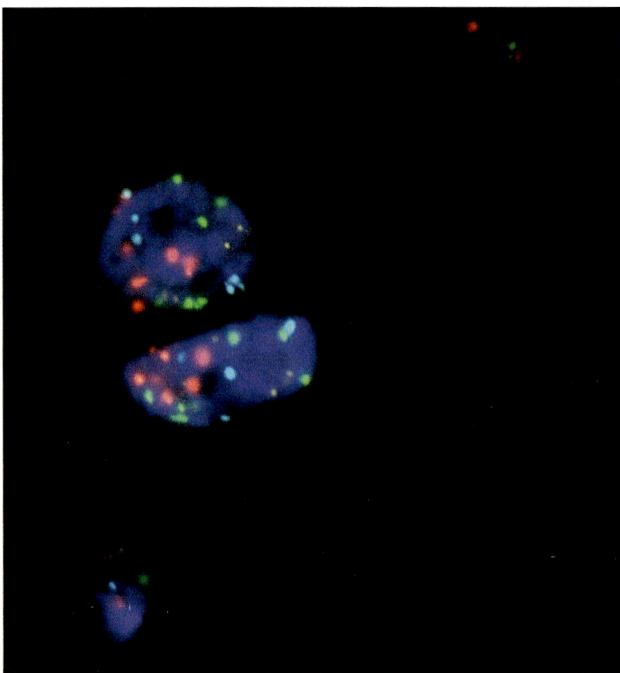

**Fig. 11.9** Highly aneuploid cells in effusion shown by the Urovysion® FISH test (Red = chromosome 3 centromere, green = chromosome 7 centromere, blue = chromosome 17 centromere, yellow = 9p21 band)

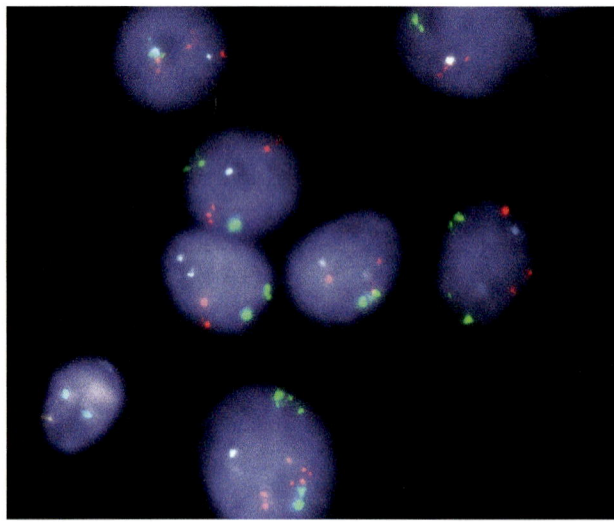

**Fig. 11.10** Mesothelioma cells lacking both yellow signals, indicating homozygous deletion of the 9p21 band (Urovysion® FISH test)

Both ERC fragments have been proposed as biomarkers, although their occurrence in the effusion may be of different diagnostic value, and they are both commercially available as ELISA tests. While HA seems to be specific for MM, some other cancers, such as ovarian and pancreatic carcinomas, also produce mesothelin. The first available set of reagents "Mesomark" will label the C-ERC fragment and perhaps also SMRP. Other necessary concerns when using ERC as biomarker is the risk for elevated values in patients

with renal failure [164]. Thorough studies showed that levels exceeding those in benign effusions are found in 84% of patients with mesothelioma [132]. The positive predictive value is high, but ERC is expressed also in some other cancers, and the same study reports high values in 2% of patients with other malignancies. When the test was performed on blood samples preceding the mesothelioma diagnosis, the average level was somewhat elevated, although only 15% of the samples showed diagnostically high values [165].

ELISA reagents demonstrating the shed N-ERC peptide are now also commercially available. As a diagnostic biomarker for mesothelioma, the N-ERC fragment performs similar to C-ERC [166], both when analyzing effusions and serum. As can be anticipated, these two reactions correlate closely when analyzing effusions (Fig. 11.11), with a marginally better performance of the N-ERC peptide [158]. There is, however, a principal difference in the mechanism for how the two ERC fragments reach the effusion, and their respective diagnostic importance may differ when analyzing effusions and sera. Analysis of the mesothelin peptides have also been recommended as a way of following changes in the tumor burden, i.e., as a tool to monitor the effects of given therapy.

*Osteopontin* (OPN) is a phosphoglycoprotein that is normally expressed by different cell types. It facilitates cell-matrix interactions by binding the HA receptor CD44 and various integrins. As a biomarker, OPN has not only been associated with MM, as well as carcinomas in the breast, lung, colon and prostate, but has also been shown to be upregulated in other diseases, such as psoriasis. OPN has been recommended as a biomarker to diagnose mesothelioma. The sensitivity for detecting mesothelioma or monitoring tumor burden over time varies in different reports [167, 168].

*Other suggested biomarkers* for the diagnosis of mesothelioma include calretinin [169], WT1 [170], trx1, syndecan-1 [170–172] and syndecan-2 [173], intelectin-1 [174], and high mobility group box protein-1 (HMGB-1) [175]. The *TXN* gene, which codes for the 12 kDa redox-enzyme Trx1, is upregulated in mesothelioma cell lines, and the protein is readily stained in sections from this tumor [176]. The Syndecans constitute a four-member family of transmembrane proteoglycan co-receptors, associated with a multitude of functions such as differentiation, adhesion, migration, and proliferation. Syndecan-1 (CD138) is more abundant in different cancers, especially in epithelial tumors, while syndecan-2 seems to dominate in mesotheliomas. The concentration of these proteoglycans also depends on the rate of secretion, which is the result of enzymatic shedding of the extracellular domain. The shed syndecan-1 ectodomain differentiates malignant conditions in effusion fluid from reactive hyperplasia and inflammation, and it carries also prognostic information [177].

At present, there are a few established biomarkers for MM. Particularly, HA and mesothelin seem to be diagnos-

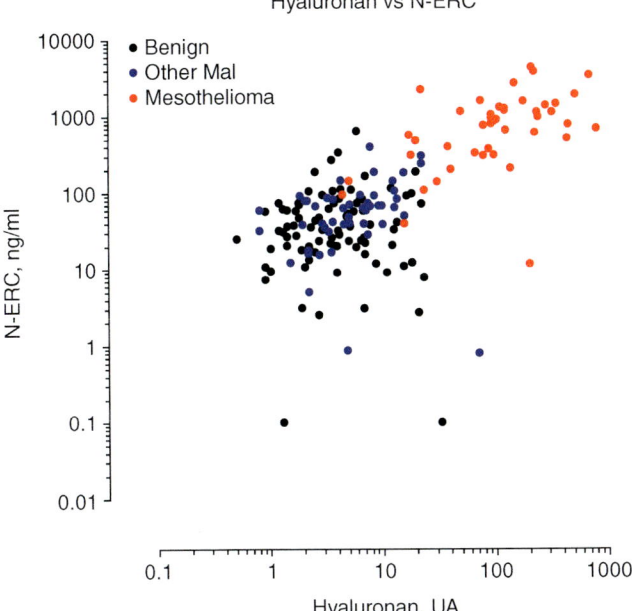

**Fig. 11.11** Hyaluronan and N-ERC concentrations in effusions correlate, i.e., to a large extent, they detect the same mesothelioma cases. Their combination in a battery will improve the test to a limited extent

tically most useful. To incorporate the information from multiple markers is a strategy to improve diagnostic sensitivity. The levels of these two markers however seem to correlate, and their combination will only give a minor improvement in sensitivity compared to the respective single analyses. The specificity will, however, be improved, more or less eliminating the problems with cross-reactivity that is sometimes seen in bacterial pleuritis [158].

The development of additional biomarkers could be one way toward obtaining the mesothelioma diagnosis at a stage early enough to change its poor prognosis. Broad screening strategies, studying gene expression and proteomics patterns, can be one way to find new possible markers. Based on proteomic screening galectin 1, aldo-keto reductase 1B10, and apolipoprotein C-I were identified as potential prognostic biomarkers for MM [178]. Another promising example is Tenascin-X, which is overexpressed in mesotheliomas [179]. The diagnostic value of such compounds awaits biochemical validation in effusions or serum.

When these analyses are used to screen effusions, it will, together with routine cytology and other ancillary analyses, quite often allow an accurate mesothelioma diagnosis already with the first effusion. Still the number of cases representing early disease remains highly limited, indicating that an effusion, in fact, is a sign of a more advanced disease. The detection of a mesothelioma early enough to improve the chance for curative treatment would need the screening of blood samples, employing new biomarkers, yet to be defined.

## How to Combine These Adjuncts in Diagnostic Cytopathology

This paragraph describes one way to handle the material to optimize the possibilities for reaching a conclusive mesothelioma diagnosis.

If possible, the effusions should be sent without fixatives to the laboratory. In most cases, viable cells can be grown out in cell cultures and are suitable for drug sensitivity testing. Thus, handling of effusion without fixatives can be recommended when transport to the laboratory takes less than 48 h. It is then important that the fluid is particularly labeled when the patient has infectious disease such as hepatitis or HIV.

In the laboratory, the material should be taken care of without delay. In cases with the abovementioned biohazards, formalin fixation for 24 h at 4°C will inactivate possible viral contents. Such fixation will, however, interfere with some ancillary analyses. In case the sample is bloody, one aliquot is hemolyzed, preparing both this and non-hemolyzed cell pellets for subsequent morphology. Routine preparations can then be made by any of the commercial liquid-based techniques or just as a conventional smear of a cell pellet. In all cases an aliquot of the fresh cell pellet is directly transferred to a glutaraldehyde fixative to allow electron microscopy if needed. When there is a clinical suspicion of mesothelioma, it can be wise to analyze the effusion supernatant for biomarkers. In case the material has been fixed in formalin, its HA content can still be analyzed, providing the ethanol precipitate is carefully washed to remove free aldehydes.

When cell morphology indicates a malignancy that could be a mesothelioma, a limited ICC battery (calretinin, Ber-Ep4 or MOC31, EMA, desmin or BAP1, and monoclonal CEA or WT1) will distinguish most mesotheliomas from secondary cancers. When four of the five ICC reactions and the biomarker analysis are in favor of a mesothelioma, then a mesothelioma is the most probable diagnosis. Including epitopes such as TTF-1 and PAX8 can, of course, expand the limited ICC battery mentioned here. In case the ICC is inconclusive, the analysis of soluble biomarkers such as HA and mesothelin [158] can be helpful.

In malignant cases where the tumor type still is equivocal, the true diagnosis can in many cases be reached by electron microscopy of the cell pellet. When the routine cytology is inconclusive regarding malignancy, then a FISH analysis will in most cases be helpful. The above battery of ancillary techniques can then be used to specify tumor type.

This diagnostic approach will allow the diagnosis of a mesothelioma in most cases, based on effusion material. The sensitivity is in these cases mainly limited by the cytopathologist's awareness for the possibility of a mesothelioma. Therefore, sensitivity will be further improved if the analysis of HA concentrations is performed on all effusions. In those few cases where the diagnosis is still inconclusive after immunocytochemistry, FISH, and biomarker analyses, the material taken for electron microscopy may provide the necessary basis for diagnosis.

These ancillary analyses will not allow a specific diagnosis in every case, and biopsies for histopathology will then be needed. The techniques can, however, enable a correct diagnosis of a MM in a majority of cases, and this is possible already with the first effusion drawn from the patient [180].

## Further Developments of Ancillary Analyses

### Predictive Biomarkers

A predictive biomarker will give information if a defined prerequisite for a therapy is at hand. Among predictive biomarkers, supporting choice of therapy, positive immunohistochemical reaction for the death receptor pathway (PD-1/PDL1) is associated with a greater likelihood of response to immune checkpoint inhibitors in various cancer types. PD-L1 is present in up to 63% of both pleural and peritoneal MM (range 5–80%) [181, 182], and it associates to higher extent to non-epithelial phenotype and poor prognosis [181, 183]. Moreover, the lymphocytes present in MM effusions induce the PD-L1 expression of tumor cells and render them sensitive to anti-PD-L1 antibody treatment [182].

Several clinical trials are ongoing [184, 185], and in a recent nonrandomized study (KEYNOTE-028) using Pembrolizumab, a PD1 inhibitor, the overall radiological response rate was 20% in MM according to the modified RECIST criteria which together with 52% stable disease resulted in 72% disease control [186]. An optimized combined integrative strategy of different treatment modalities might be even more effective as sensitization of MM by radiation therapy and/or chemotherapy [187, 188] may give complementary immunological benefits that enhance the antitumor response. Radiation therapy may itself be immunomodulatory and maximize tumor immunity, as it upregulates the tumor-infiltrating lymphocytes (TILs) and low-dose irradiation can program macrophage differentiation and potentiate T-cell-mediated immunotherapy [189]. Apart from effusions, in a recent study, material from fine needle aspiration was also successfully used for flow cytometry to provide a diagnostic tool for immunophenotyping MMs with regard to the presence and activation of T-cell lineage and biomarker assessment for immunotherapy [190].

Predictive markers involved in the uptake or effect of various drugs may offer help to further individualize therapy. Thus, thymidylate synthase (TS) [191], glycinamide ribonucleotide formyltransferase (GARFT), and dihydrofolatereductase (DHFR) have been suggested as predictors of response to pemetrexed [192], although results are divergent in this respect. Similarly, excision repair cross complementation group 1 (ERCC1) and copper transporter 2 (CTR2) are supposed to predict sensitivity to platinum drugs, but these are not yet routinely used [193]. Our recent PD-L1 testing reveals similar frequency of PD-L1 positivity in pleural effusions as previously reported for histological sections [194].

### In Vitro Analysis of Drug Sensitivity

An alternate way of individualizing therapy is to isolate cells from the individual tumor and test their reaction to different drugs in primary cultures. This is possible in most cases when the effusion is obtained unfixed. Such in vitro testing of drug sensitivity of mesothelioma cell cultures has indicated considerable variability from one patient to another [195]. The development of high-throughput systems for such testing is also a prerequisite for simultaneously testing a sufficient number of drugs to provide meaningful guidance for designing therapy [196–198]. One problem with such analyses is the varying admixture of different benign cells in the effusion, cells that also react to the drug exposure. Tumor cell-specific determination of drug sensitivity is possible by FACS analysis or magnetic separation of these cells. Although very promising, such techniques need further optimization before they can be applied to clinical samples.

### Genome-Wide Screening Combined with Biological Chemotherapy Response Profiles

Chemosensitivity testing combined with genome-wide analysis of cells derived from pleural effusions has the potential to improve the basis for rational selection of personalized treatment options. A high-throughput drug screen using a panel of targeted therapeutic agents was combined with extensive whole exome sequencing and transcriptome profiling of pleural MM cell lines and primary early passage lines. A subgroup of mesotheliomas demonstrated high sensitivity to FGFR inhibition. Loss of *BAP1* could be associated with this sensitivity, being a potential biomarker for FGFR inhibitor efficacy [199].

In a recent study, a novel resistance signature to pemetrexed/carboplatin treatment was established by microarray analysis [200]. In another study, the microarray data revealed that the mitotic spindle assembly checkpoint pathway was most significantly altered. This analysis was followed by cell viability assays to assess sensitivity to specific small molecule inhibitors targeting microtubules and a nontaxane small molecule inhibitor, epothilone B. Targeting the microtubules was identified as a potential therapeutic approach [201].

The increasing number of actionable mutations and expanding number of experimental drugs warrant further improvement of response prediction. As a consequence, multiple biological pathways have to be integrated with drug sensitivity prediction algorithms [202, 203]. To convert these in vitro data to clinically reliable drug predictions requires accurate validation, in a prospective and randomized setting. A major challenge is to find optimal drug sensitivity algorithms and to match therapeutic interventions to the individual genomic context of each patient.

## Treatment Options

Traditional strategies for the treatment of MM include surgery, radiotherapy, and chemotherapy. Single modality therapy using traditional approaches alone has failed to improve patient survival compared to supportive care. Multimodality approaches, in particular, cytoreductive surgery (pleuropneumonectomy), followed by sequential chemotherapy and radiotherapy, are more promising [204], especially for patients with epithelioid histology, negative resection margins, and no metastases to extrapleural lymph nodes.

During the past two decades, much effort has been invested in using gene therapy in preclinical and clinical settings. These trials have been safe but had only intermittent effect. Gene transfer was achievable, but with the currently available vectors, only a small proportion of tumor cells could be affected [205–207].

Many cases of MM are diagnosed late during the disease, and radical surgery is only possible in about 10% of cases. Chemotherapy is in these cases the main therapeutic option. However, the advanced tumor stage makes these tumors generally highly resistant to chemotherapeutic agents [208]. This may be related to overexpression of detoxification proteins associated with drug resistance [209, 210], yet the mechanisms by which resistance occurs are still poorly understood. Defects in apoptotic signaling also account for much of the therapy resistance of mesothelioma, comprising various members of the antiapoptotic Bcl-2 family [211] and inhibitors of apoptosis IAP family such as XIAP, IAP1, Survivin, and Livin [212–215].

About 40% of the patients can be expected to respond to the combination of pemetrexed and cisplatinum [216], and similar results can be obtained by combining liposomized doxorubicin, carboplatin, and gemcitabine [217]. Use of predictive markers and in vitro testing of chemosensitivity in primary mesothelioma cell cultures could provide opportunities for a more individualized choice of drugs, but this has not yet been established in clinical routines.

## Targeted Therapy and Clinical Trials

The key regulators involved in the biology of mesothelioma all contribute to a better understanding of molecular mechanisms, which may be used to tailor personalized targeted therapies. During the past decade, several high-throughput analytical methods for gene expression profiling have been applied in the field of mesothelioma

research to select groups of genes able to predict the prognosis of the patients and their response to chemotherapy. Together with the analysis of specific predictive markers and in vitro testing of resistance patterns, these technologies provide an opportunity to refine the antineoplastic treatment.

A multitude of novel treatment strategies are currently in clinical trials for mesothelioma [218, 219], comprising immunotherapy, vaccines, and targeted therapy [184, 185, 220, 221]. Among others, several angiogenesis inhibitors are tested as first-line or second-line treatment [222]. Targeted treatment options require accurate selection of patients, and they will be successful only for a subset of patients [223]. These clinical trials demonstrate the need for more effective treatment for mesothelioma patients and that apart from the standard treatment option there might be other more effective combinations for the individual patient. Recent studies also indicate that treatment outcome might be predicted by biomarkers [224, 225].

Future treatment options are preferably based on rational drug combinations that target various pathways. Molecular fingerprints of MM provide a rationale for targeted interventions, some of which are already under evaluation as new potential therapeutic options for mesothelioma patients. Approaches based on inhibitors of the ubiquitin-proteasome pathway and of histone deacetylases share the ability to modulate a wide variety of pathways and are currently investigated for management of MM. These targeted therapy approaches had so far failed or had only modest effect on patient outcome, the most likely cause of treatment failure being unselected patients and high toxicity.

Growth factor receptors, ligands, and intracellular effectors, in particular vascular endothelial growth factor (VEGF) signaling, are also intensively studied, due to the involvement of this pathway both in tumor angiogenesis and autocrine stimulation of mesothelioma cell growth [226]. A recent randomized phase 3 clinical trial showed prolonged survival in patients treated with bevacizumab in addition to standard chemotherapy [227].

## Prognosis

The prognosis of MM varies greatly because of differences in growth potential and difficulties in obtaining an early diagnosis. High degree of chronic stromal inflammation correlates with improved prognosis and prolonged survival to 19 months versus 14 months [228]. Independent indicators of poor prognosis include male gender, disease stage, non-epithelial cell type, poor performance status, anemia, leukocytosis [229], and increased angiogenesis, assessed by microvessel density [230].

Differentiation into epithelioid and sarcomatoid phenotypes seen in routinely stained histological sections remains one of the best predictors of survival time. Markers of mesothelial phenotype such as WT1 [231]; high calretinin and podoplanin (D2-40) expression [232]; elevated HA content in pleural effusion [233, 234]; epithelial markers comprising E-cadherin [19] and syndecan-1 [171]; the presence of cell membrane molecules such as EGFR [235], c-MET [236], tetraspanin (CD9) [237], CD26 [238], and CD74 [239]; high cytoplasmic expression of ILK and PTEN; as well as high nuclear expression of p21 and p27 [236, 240] are all associated with good prognosis. In contrast, mesothelin [168, 241, 242], osteopontin [168, 243, 244], fibulin-3 [245], and caveolin-1 [246] indicate poor prognosis. Elevated levels of cytokines and growth factors are generally associated with poor prognosis, comprising CD34 [247], FGF-2 [114], serum VEGF [248], and serum Ang-1 [249], as well as DNA repair and chemotherapy response-related proteins such as excision repair cross-complementing group 1 (ERCCC) [225], thymidylate synthase (TS) [250–252], and class III β- tubulin [224]. For a comprehensive review of prognostic factors in MPM, see [253].

Apart from histological subtypes, stage, and clinicopathologic characteristics, loss of tumor suppressor genes and the molecular signature of MM are also important and shows a gender-related profile. Thus, *CDKN2A* is more often represented in non-epithelioid MMs, particularly in men, and it correlates with shorter overall survival [53], whereas *TP53* is more often mutated in women. A subgroup of patients that has a strikingly long survival is most often of female gender and has a peritoneal localization of their tumor.

Regardless of the type of therapy used, MM is almost invariably a fatal disease, the 5-year survival rate being estimated at less than 5% [254]. However, some patients survive several years without treatment [255]. The average survival of patients with MM is, however, only modestly improved by today's chemotherapy regimens, and patients responding to treatment have the longest survival time [256].

Interestingly, our ongoing evaluation of the mean survival following treatment of patients with cytologically diagnosed MM is longer than those with epithelioid and mixed-type MM diagnosed by histology [257]. The improvement is independent of other clinical parameters or asbestos exposure, and it seems that cases detected by cytology include less aggressive tumors.

Survival after multimodality treatment, involving radical surgery, intensive postoperative radiotherapy, and chemotherapy, is reported to be considerably longer. This is, however, only possible in less advanced cancers, and an improved survival is not definitely proven. Future possibilities for targeted and individualized therapies may fundamentally improve the possibility to treat mesothelioma patients, but the complex molecular feature and rarity of MM require multicenter studies, biomarker-based well-defined selection criteria, and joint efforts to gain sufficient insight and statistical power for a more successful therapy.

# References

1. Wagner JC, Sleggs CA, Marchand P. Diffuse pleural mesothelioma and asbestos exposure in the North Western Cape Province. Br J Ind Med. 1960;17:260–71.
2. Wagner JC, Skidmore JW, Hill RJ, Griffiths DM. Erionite exposure and mesotheliomas in rats. Br J Cancer. 1985;51(5):727–30.
3. Carbone M, Ly BH, Dodson RF, Pagano I, Morris PT, Dogan UA, Gazdar AF, Pass HI, Yang H. Malignant mesothelioma: facts, myths, and hypotheses. J Cell Physiol. 2012;227(1):44–58.
4. Faig J, Howard S, Levine EA, Casselman G, Hesdorffer M, Ohar JA. Changing pattern in malignant mesothelioma survival. Transl Oncol. 2015;8(1):35–9.
5. Ai J, Stevenson JP. Current issues in malignant pleural mesothelioma evaluation and management. Oncologist. 2014;19(9):975–84.
6. Mutsaers SE. Mesothelial cells: their structure, function and role in serosal repair. Respirology. 2002;7(3):171–91.
7. Mutsaers SE. The mesothelial cell. Int J Biochem Cell Biol. 2004;36(1):9–16.
8. Mutsaers SE, Kalomenidis I, Wilson NA, Lee YC. Growth factors in pleural fibrosis. Curr Opin Pulm Med. 2006;12(4):251–8.
9. Mutsaers SE, Di Paolo N. Future directions in mesothelial transplantation research. Int J Artif Organs. 2007;30(6):557–61.
10. Dobra K, Andang M, Syrokou A, Karamanos NK, Hjerpe A. Differentiation of mesothelioma cells is influenced by the expression of proteoglycans. Exp Cell Res. 2000;258(1):12–22.
11. Bolen JW, Hammar SP, McNutt MA. Reactive and neoplastic serosal tissue. A light-microscopic, ultrastructural, and immunocytochemical study. Am J Surg Pathol. 1986;10(1):34–47.
12. Whitaker D, Papadimitriou J. Mesothelial healing: morphological and kinetic investigations. J Pathol. 1985;145(2):159–75.
13. Foley-Comer AJ, Herrick SE, Al-Mishlab T, Prele CM, Laurent GJ, Mutsaers SE. Evidence for incorporation of free-floating mesothelial cells as a mechanism of serosal healing. J Cell Sci. 2002;115(Pt 7):1383–9.
14. Warn R, Harvey P, Warn A, Foley-Comer A, Heldin P, Versnel M, Arakaki N, Daikuhara Y, Laurent GJ, Herrick SE, et al. HGF/SF induces mesothelial cell migration and proliferation by autocrine and paracrine pathways. Exp Cell Res. 2001;267(2):258–66.
15. Herrick SE, Mutsaers SE. Mesothelial progenitor cells and their potential in tissue engineering. Int J Biochem Cell Biol. 2004;36(4):621–42.
16. Chua F, Dunsmore SE, Clingen PH, Mutsaers SE, Shapiro SD, Segal AW, Roes J, Laurent GJ. Mice lacking neutrophil elastase are resistant to bleomycin-induced pulmonary fibrosis. Am J Pathol. 2007;170(1):65–74.
17. Herrick SE, Mutsaers SE. The potential of mesothelial cells in tissue engineering and regenerative medicine applications. Int J Artif Organs. 2007;30(6):527–40.
18. Lansley SM, Searles RG, Hoi A, Thomas C, Moneta H, Herrick SE, Thompson PJ, Newman M, Sterrett GF, Prele CM, et al. Mesothelial cell differentiation into osteoblast- and adipocyte-like cells. J Cell Mol Med. 2011;15(10):2095–105.
19. Fassina A, Cappellesso R, Guzzardo V, Dalla Via L, Piccolo S, Ventura L, Fassan M. Epithelial-mesenchymal transition in malignant mesothelioma. Mod Pathol. 2012;25(1):86–99.
20. Klominek J, Robert KH, Hjerpe A, Wickstrom B, Gahrton G. Serum-dependent growth patterns of two, newly established human mesothelioma cell lines. Cancer Res. 1989;49(21):6118–22.
21. Craighead JE, Mossman BT. The pathogenesis of asbestos-associated diseases. N Engl J Med. 1982;306(24):1446–55.
22. Sebastien P, Gaudichet A, Bignon J, Baris YI. Zeolite bodies in human lungs from Turkey. Lab Invest. 1981;44(5):420–5.

23. Carbone M, Emri S, Dogan AU, Steele I, Tuncer M, Pass HI, Baris YI. A mesothelioma epidemic in Cappadocia: scientific developments and unexpected social outcomes. Nat Rev Cancer. 2007;7(2):147–54.

24. Baumann F, Rougier Y, Ambrosi JP, Robineau BP. Pleural mesothelioma in New Caledonia: an acute environmental concern. Cancer Detect Prev. 2007;31(1):70–6.

25. Metintas M, Ozdemir N, Hillerdal G, Ucgun I, Metintas S, Baykul C, Elbek O, Mutlu S, Kolsuz M. Environmental asbestos exposure and malignant pleural mesothelioma. Respir Med. 1999;93(5):349–55.

26. Hillerdal G. Mesothelioma: cases associated with non-occupational and low dose exposures. Occup Environ Med. 1999;56(8):505–13.

27. Maher B. Epidemiology: fear in the dust. Nature. 2010;468(7326):884–5.

28. Baris YI, Grandjean P. Prospective study of mesothelioma mortality in Turkish villages with exposure to fibrous zeolite. J Natl Cancer Inst. 2006;98(6):414–7.

29. McDonald JC. Epidemiology of malignant mesothelioma—an outline. Ann Occup Hyg. 2010;54(8):851–7.

30. Lotti M, Bergamo L, Murer B. Occupational toxicology of asbestos-related malignancies. Clin Toxicol (Phila). 2010;48(6):485–96.

31. Lechner JF, Tokiwa T, LaVeck M, Benedict WF, Banks-Schlegel S, Yeager H Jr, Banerjee A, Harris CC. Asbestos-associated chromosomal changes in human mesothelial cells. Proc Natl Acad Sci U S A. 1985;82(11):3884–8.

32. Ault JG, Cole RW, Jensen CG, Jensen LC, Bachert LA, Rieder CL. Behavior of crocidolite asbestos during mitosis in living vertebrate lung epithelial cells. Cancer Res. 1995;55(4):792–8.

33. Hesterberg TW, Barrett JC. Induction by asbestos fibers of anaphase abnormalities: mechanism for aneuploidy induction and possibly carcinogenesis. Carcinogenesis. 1985;6(3):473–5.

34. Fung H, Kow YW, Van Houten B, Taatjes DJ, Hatahet Z, Janssen YM, Vacek P, Faux SP, Mossman BT. Asbestos increases mammalian AP-endonuclease gene expression, protein levels, and enzyme activity in mesothelial cells. Cancer Res. 1998;58(2):189–94.

35. Sekido Y. Molecular pathogenesis of malignant mesothelioma. Carcinogenesis. 2013;34(7):1413–9.

36. Chew SH, Toyokuni S. Malignant mesothelioma as an oxidative stress-induced cancer: an update. Free Radic Biol Med. 2015;86:166–78.

37. Francis RJ, Segard T, Morandeau L, Lee YC, Millward MJ, Segal A, Nowak AK. Characterization of hypoxia in malignant pleural mesothelioma with FMISO PET-CT. Lung Cancer. 2015;90(1):55–60.

38. Bristow RG, Hill RP. Hypoxia and metabolism. Hypoxia, DNA repair and genetic instability. Nat Rev Cancer. 2008;8(3):180–92.

39. Nabavi N, Bennewith KL, Churg A, Wang Y, Collins CC, Mutti L. Switching off malignant mesothelioma: exploiting the hypoxic microenvironment. Genes Cancer. 2016;7(11-12):340–54.

40. Lechner JF, Tesfaigzi J, Gerwin BI. Oncogenes and tumor-suppressor genes in mesothelioma—a synopsis. Environ Health Perspect. 1997;105(Suppl 5):1061–7.

41. Lindholm PM, Salmenkivi K, Vauhkonen H, Nicholson AG, Anttila S, Kinnula VL, Knuutila S. Gene copy number analysis in malignant pleural mesothelioma using oligonucleotide array CGH. Cytogenet Genome Res. 2007;119(1-2):46–52.

42. Musti M, Kettunen E, Dragonieri S, Lindholm P, Cavone D, Serio G, Knuutila S. Cytogenetic and molecular genetic changes in malignant mesothelioma. Cancer Genet Cytogenet. 2006;170(1):9–15.

43. Gibas Z, Li FP, Antman KH, Bernal S, Stahel R, Sandberg AA. Chromosome changes in malignant mesothelioma. Cancer Genet Cytogenet. 1986;20(3-4):191–201.

44. Popescu NC, Chahinian AP, DiPaolo JA. Nonrandom chromosome alterations in human malignant mesothelioma. Cancer Res. 1988;48(1):142–7.

45. Tiainen M, Tammilehto L, Mattson K, Knuutila S. Nonrandom chromosomal abnormalities in malignant pleural mesothelioma. Cancer Genet Cytogenet. 1988;33(2):251–74.

46. Flejter WL, Li FP, Antman KH, Testa JR. Recurring loss involving chromosomes 1, 3, and 22 in malignant mesothelioma: possible sites of tumor suppressor genes. Genes Chromosomes Cancer. 1989;1(2):148–54.

47. Hagemeijer A, Versnel MA, Van Drunen E, Moret M, Bouts MJ, van der Kwast TH, Hoogsteden HC. Cytogenetic analysis of malignant mesothelioma. Cancer Genet Cytogenet. 1990;47(1):1–28.

48. Taguchi T, Jhanwar SC, Siegfried JM, Keller SM, Testa JR. Recurrent deletions of specific chromosomal sites in 1p, 3p, 6q, and 9p in human malignant mesothelioma. Cancer Res. 1993;53(18):4349–55.

49. Kamb A, Shattuck-Eidens D, Eeles R, Liu Q, Gruis NA, Ding W, Hussey C, Tran T, Miki Y, Weaver-Feldhaus J, et al. Analysis of the p16 gene (CDKN2) as a candidate for the chromosome 9p melanoma susceptibility locus. Nat Genet. 1994;8(1):23–6.

50. Cheng JQ, Jhanwar SC, Klein WM, Bell DW, Lee WC, Altomare DA, Nobori T, Olopade OI, Buckler AJ, Testa JR. p16 alterations and deletion mapping of 9p21-p22 in malignant mesothelioma. Cancer Res. 1994;54(21):5547–51.

51. Nobori T, Miura K, Wu DJ, Lois A, Takabayashi K, Carson DA. Deletions of the cyclin-dependent kinase-4 inhibitor gene in multiple human cancers. Nature. 1994;368(6473):753–6.

52. Kratzke RA, Otterson GA, Lincoln CE, Ewing S, Oie H, Geradts J, Kaye FJ. Immunohistochemical analysis of the p16INK4 cyclin-dependent kinase inhibitor in malignant mesothelioma. J Natl Cancer Inst. 1995;87(24):1870–5.

53. De Rienzo A, Archer MA, Yeap BY, Dao N, Sciaranghella D, Sideris AC, Zheng Y, Holman AG, Wang YE, Dal Cin PS, et al. Gender-specific molecular and clinical features underlie malignant pleural mesothelioma. Cancer Res. 2016;76(2):319–28.

54. Illei PB, Ladanyi M, Rusch VW, Zakowski MF. The use of CDKN2A deletion as a diagnostic marker for malignant mesothelioma in body cavity effusions. Cancer. 2003;99(1):51–6.

55. Ladanyi M. Implications of P16/CDKN2A deletion in pleural mesotheliomas. Lung Cancer. 2005;49(Suppl 1):S95–8.

56. Savic S, Franco N, Grilli B, Barascud Ade V, Herzog M, Bode B, Loosli H, Spieler P, Schonegg R, Zlobec I, et al. Fluorescence in situ hybridization in the definitive diagnosis of malignant mesothelioma in effusion cytology. Chest. 2010;138(1):137–44.

57. Lopez-Rios F, Chuai S, Flores R, Shimizu S, Ohno T, Wakahara K, Illei PB, Hussain S, Krug L, Zakowski MF, et al. Global gene expression profiling of pleural mesotheliomas: overexpression of aurora kinases and P16/CDKN2A deletion as prognostic factors and critical evaluation of microarray-based prognostic prediction. Cancer Res. 2006;66(6):2970–9.

58. Testa JR, Cheung M, Pei J, Below JE, Tan Y, Sementino E, Cox NJ, Dogan AU, Pass HI, Trusa S, et al. Germline BAP1 mutations predispose to malignant mesothelioma. Nat Genet. 2011;43(10):1022–5.

59. Carbone M, Yang H, Pass HI, Krausz T, Testa JR, Gaudino G. BAP1 and cancer. Nat Rev Cancer. 2013;13(3):153–9.

60. Cheung M, Talarchek J, Schindeler K, Saraiva E, Penney LS, Ludman M, Testa JR. Further evidence for germline BAP1 mutations predisposing to melanoma and malignant mesothelioma. Cancer Genet. 2013;206(5):206–10.

61. Wang A, Papneja A, Hyrcza M, Al-Habeeb A, Ghazarian D. Gene of the month: BAP1. J Clin Pathol. 2016;69(9):750–3.

62. Bhattacharya S, Hanpude P, Maiti TK. Cancer associated missense mutations in BAP1 catalytic domain induce amyloidogenic aggregation: a new insight in enzymatic inactivation. Sci Rep. 2015;5:18462.

63. Dawson A, Gibbs A, Browne K, Pooley F, Griffiths M. Familial mesothelioma. Details of 17 cases with histopathologic findings and mineral analysis. Cancer. 1992;70(5):1183–7.

64. Attanoos RL, Gibbs AR. Pathology of malignant mesothelioma. Histopathology. 1997;30(5):403–18.

65. Ascoli V, Aalto Y, Carnovale-Scalzo C, Nardi F, Falzetti D, Mecucci C, Knuutila S. DNA copy number changes in familial malignant mesothelioma. Cancer Genet Cytogenet. 2001;127(1):80–2.

66. Roushdy-Hammady I, Siegel J, Emri S, Testa JR, Carbone M. Genetic-susceptibility factor and malignant mesothelioma in the Cappadocian region of Turkey. Lancet. 2001;357(9254): 444–5.

67. Pilarski R, Rai K, Cebulla C, Abdel-Rahman M. BAP1 tumor predisposition syndrome. In: Pagon RA, Adam MP, Ardinger HH, Wallace SE, Amemiya A, Bean LJH, Bird TD, Ledbetter N, Mefford HC, Smith RJH, et al., editors. GeneReviews(R). Seattle, WA; 1993.

68. Cheung M, Testa JR. BAP1, a tumor suppressor gene driving malignant mesothelioma. Transl Lung Cancer Res. 2017;6(3):270–8.

69. Nasu M, Emi M, Pastorino S, Tanji M, Powers A, Luk H, Baumann F, Zhang YA, Gazdar A, Kanodia S, et al. High incidence of somatic BAP1 alterations in sporadic malignant mesothelioma. J Thorac Oncol. 2015;10(4):565–76.

70. Farzin M, Toon CW, Clarkson A, Sioson L, Watson N, Andrici J, Gill AJ. Loss of expression of BAP1 predicts longer survival in mesothelioma. Pathology. 2015;47(4):302–7.

71. Rai K, Pilarski R, Cebulla CM, Abdel-Rahman MH. Comprehensive review of BAP1 tumor predisposition syndrome with report of two new cases. Clin Genet. 2016;89(3):285–94.

72. Ohar JA, Cheung M, Talarchek J, Howard SE, Howard TD, Hesdorffer M, Peng H, Rauscher FJ, Testa JR. Germline BAP1 mutational landscape of asbestos-exposed malignant mesothelioma patients with family history of cancer. Cancer Res. 2016;76(2):206–15.

73. Abdel-Rahman MH, Rai K, Pilarski R, Davidorf FH, Cebulla CM. Germline BAP1 mutations misreported as somatic based on tumor-only testing. Fam Cancer. 2016;15(2):327–30.

74. Betti M, Casalone E, Ferrante D, Aspesi A, Morleo G, Biasi A, Sculco M, Mancuso G, Guarrera S, Righi L et al. Germline mutations in DNA repair genes predispose asbestos-exposed patients to malignant pleural mesothelioma. Cancer Lett. 2017.

75. Cheng JQ, Lee WC, Klein MA, Cheng GZ, Jhanwar SC, Testa JR. Frequent mutations of NF2 and allelic loss from chromosome band 22q12 in malignant mesothelioma: evidence for a two-hit mechanism of NF2 inactivation. Genes Chromosomes Cancer. 1999;24(3):238–42.

76. Bianchi AB, Mitsunaga SI, Cheng JQ, Klein WM, Jhanwar SC, Seizinger B, Kley N, Klein-Szanto AJ, Testa JR. High frequency of inactivating mutations in the neurofibromatosis type 2 gene (NF2) in primary malignant mesotheliomas. Proc Natl Acad Sci U S A. 1995;92(24):10854–8.

77. Murakami H, Mizuno T, Taniguchi T, Fujii M, Ishiguro F, Fukui T, Akatsuka S, Horio Y, Hida T, Kondo Y, et al. LATS2 is a tumor suppressor gene of malignant mesothelioma. Cancer Res. 2011;71(3):873–83.

78. Miyanaga A, Masuda M, Tsuta K, Kawasaki K, Nakamura Y, Sakuma T, Asamura H, Gemma A, Yamada T. Hippo pathway gene mutations in malignant mesothelioma: revealed by RNA and targeted exon sequencing. J Thorac Oncol. 2015;10(5):844–51.

79. Yokoyama T, Osada H, Murakami H, Tatematsu Y, Taniguchi T, Kondo Y, Yatabe Y, Hasegawa Y, Shimokata K, Horio Y, et al. YAP1 is involved in mesothelioma development and negatively regulated by Merlin through phosphorylation. Carcinogenesis. 2008;29(11):2139–46.

80. Langerak AW, De Laat PA, Van Der Linden-Van Beurden CA, Delahaye M, Van Der Kwast TH, Hoogsteden HC, Benner R,
Versnel MA. Expression of platelet-derived growth factor (PDGF) and PDGF receptors in human malignant mesothelioma in vitro and in vivo. J Pathol. 1996;178(2):151–60.

81. Langerak AW, van der Linden-van Beurden CA, Versnel MA. Regulation of differential expression of platelet-derived growth factor alpha- and beta-receptor mRNA in normal and malignant human mesothelial cell lines. Biochim Biophys Acta. 1996;1305(1-2):63–70.

82. Gerwin BI. Cytokine signaling in mesothelial cells: receptor expression closes the autocrine loop. Am J Respir Cell Mol Biol. 1996;14(6):505–7.

83. Heintz NH, Janssen YM, Mossman BT. Persistent induction of c-fos and c-jun expression by asbestos. Proc Natl Acad Sci U S A. 1993;90(8):3299–303.

84. Sekido Y. Molecular biology of malignant mesothelioma. Environ Health Prev Med. 2008;13(2):65–70.

85. Maki-Nevala S, Sarhadi VK, Knuuttila A, Scheinin I, Ellonen P, Lagstrom S, Ronty M, Kettunen E, Husgafvel-Pursiainen K, Wolff H, et al. Driver gene and novel mutations in asbestos-exposed lung adenocarcinoma and malignant mesothelioma detected by exome sequencing. Lung. 2016;194(1):125–35.

86. Bueno R, De Rienzo A, Dong L, Gordon GJ, Hercus CF, Richards WG, Jensen RV, Anwar A, Maulik G, Chirieac LR, et al. Second generation sequencing of the mesothelioma tumor genome. PLoS One. 2010;5(5):e10612.

87. Guo G, Chmielecki J, Goparaju C, Heguy A, Dolgalev I, Carbone M, Seepo S, Meyerson M, Pass HI. Whole-exome sequencing reveals frequent genetic alterations in BAP1, NF2, CDKN2A, and CUL1 in malignant pleural mesothelioma. Cancer Res. 2015;75(2):264–9.

88. Kang HC, Kim HK, Lee S, Mendez P, Kim JW, Woodard G, Yoon JH, Jen KY, Fang LT, Jones K, et al. Whole exome and targeted deep sequencing identify genome-wide allelic loss and frequent SETDB1 mutations in malignant pleural mesotheliomas. Oncotarget. 2016;7(7):8321–31.

89. Sugarbaker DJ, Richards WG, Gordon GJ, Dong L, De Rienzo A, Maulik G, Glickman JN, Chirieac LR, Hartman ML, Taillon BE, et al. Transcriptome sequencing of malignant pleural mesothelioma tumors. Proc Natl Acad Sci U S A. 2008;105(9):3521–6.

90. Dong L, Jensen RV, De Rienzo A, Gordon GJ, Xu Y, Sugarbaker DJ, Bueno R. Differentially expressed alternatively spliced genes in malignant pleural mesothelioma identified using massively parallel transcriptome sequencing. BMC Med Genet. 2009;10:149.

91. Bueno R, Stawiski EW, Goldstein LD, Durinck S, De Rienzo A, Modrusan Z, Gnad F, Nguyen TT, Jaiswal BS, Chirieac LR, et al. Comprehensive genomic analysis of malignant pleural mesothelioma identifies recurrent mutations, gene fusions and splicing alterations. Nat Genet. 2016;48(4):407–16.

92. Hylebos M, Van Camp G, van Meerbeeck JP, Op de Beeck K. The genetic landscape of malignant pleural mesothelioma: results from massively parallel sequencing. J Thorac Oncol. 2016;11(10):1615–26.

93. Lo Iacono M, Monica V, Righi L, Grosso F, Libener R, Vatrano S, Bironzo P, Novello S, Musmeci L, Volante M, et al. Targeted next-generation sequencing of cancer genes in advanced stage malignant pleural mesothelioma: a retrospective study. J Thorac Oncol. 2015;10(3):492–9.

94. Joseph NM, Chen YY, Nasr A, Yeh I, Talevich E, Onodera C, Bastian BC, Rabban JT, Garg K, Zaloudek C, et al. Genomic profiling of malignant peritoneal mesothelioma reveals recurrent alterations in epigenetic regulatory genes BAP1, SETD2, and DDX3X. Mod Pathol. 2017;30(2):246–54.

95. Chirac P, Maillet D, Lepretre F, Isaac S, Glehen O, Figeac M, Villeneuve L, Peron J, Gibson F, Galateau-Salle F, et al. Genomic copy number alterations in 33 malignant peritoneal mesothelioma analyzed by comparative genomic hybridization array. Hum Pathol. 2016;55:72–82.

96. Alakus H, Yost SE, Woo B, French R, Lin GY, Jepsen K, Frazer KA, Lowy AM, Harismendy O. BAP1 mutation is a frequent somatic event in peritoneal malignant mesothelioma. J Transl Med. 2015;13:122.

97. Singhi AD, Krasinskas AM, Choudry HA, Bartlett DL, Pingpank JF, Zeh HJ, Luvison A, Fuhrer K, Bahary N, Seethala RR, et al. The prognostic significance of BAP1, NF2, and CDKN2A in malignant peritoneal mesothelioma. Mod Pathol. 2016;29(1):14–24.

98. Panagopoulos I, Gorunova L, Davidson B, Heim S. Novel TNS3-MAP 3K3 and ZFPM2-ELF5 fusion genes identified by RNA sequencing in multicystic mesothelioma with t(7,17)(p12;q23) and t(8,11)(q23;p13). Cancer Lett. 2015;357(2):502–9.

99. Kato S, Tomson BN, Buys TP, Elkin SK, Carter JL, Kurzrock R. Genomic landscape of malignant mesotheliomas. Mol Cancer Ther. 2016;15(10):2498–507.

100. Brevet M, Shimizu S, Bott MJ, Shukla N, Zhou Q, Olshen AB, Rusch V, Ladanyi M. Coactivation of receptor tyrosine kinases in malignant mesothelioma as a rationale for combination targeted therapy. J Thorac Oncol. 2011;6(5):864–74.

101. Sun X, Wei L, Liden J, Hui G, Dahlman-Wright K, Hjerpe A, Dobra K. Molecular characterization of tumour heterogeneity and malignant mesothelioma cell differentiation by gene profiling. J Pathol. 2005;207(1):91–101.

102. Gordon GJ, Rockwell GN, Jensen RV, Rheinwald JG, Glickman JN, Aronson JP, Pottorf BJ, Nitz MD, Richards WG, Sugarbaker DJ, et al. Identification of novel candidate oncogenes and tumor suppressors in malignant pleural mesothelioma using large-scale transcriptional profiling. Am J Pathol. 2005;166(6):1827–40.

103. Rihn BH, Mohr S, McDowell SA, Binet S, Loubinoux J, Galateau F, Keith G, Leikauf GD. Differential gene expression in mesothelioma. FEBS Lett. 2000;480(2-3):95–100.

104. Sun X, Dobra K, Bjornstedt M, Hjerpe A. Upregulation of 9 genes, including that for thioredoxin, during epithelial differentiation of mesothelioma cells. Differentiation. 2000;66(4-5):181–8.

105. Singhal S, Wiewrodt R, Malden LD, Amin KM, Matzie K, Friedberg J, Kucharczuk JC, Litzky LA, Johnson SW, Kaiser LR, et al. Gene expression profiling of malignant mesothelioma. Clin Cancer Res. 2003;9(8):3080–97.

106. Roe OD, Anderssen E, Helge E, Pettersen CH, Olsen KS, Sandeck H, Haaverstad R, Lundgren S, Larsson E. Genome-wide profile of pleural mesothelioma versus parietal and visceral pleura: the emerging gene portrait of the mesothelioma phenotype. PLoS One. 2009;4(8):e6554.

107. Gray SG, Fennell DA, Mutti L, O'Byrne KJ. In arrayed ranks: array technology in the study of mesothelioma. J Thorac Oncol. 2009;4(3):411–25.

108. Sahab ZJ, Hall MD, Zhang L, Cheema AK, Byers SW. Tumor suppressor RARRES1 regulates DLG2, PP2A, VCP, EB1, and Ankrd26. J Cancer. 2010;1:14–22.

109. Holmgren A, Bjornstedt M. Thioredoxin and thioredoxin reductase. Methods Enzymol. 1995;252:199–208.

110. Rubartelli A, Bajetto A, Allavena G, Wollman E, Sitia R. Secretion of thioredoxin by normal and neoplastic cells through a leaderless secretory pathway. J Biol Chem. 1992;267(34):24161–4.

111. Williams CH Jr. Thioredoxin-thioredoxin reductase—a system that has come of age. Eur J Biochem. 2000;267(20):6101.

112. Williams CH, Arscott LD, Muller S, Lennon BW, Ludwig ML, Wang PF, Veine DM, Becker K, Schirmer RH. Thioredoxin reductase two modes of catalysis have evolved. Eur J Biochem. 2000;267(20):6110–7.

113. Hayashi T, Ueno Y, Okamoto T. Oxidoreductive regulation of nuclear factor kappa B. Involvement of a cellular reducing catalyst thioredoxin. J Biol Chem. 1993;268(15):11380–8.

114. Kumar-Singh S, Weyler J, Martin MJ, Vermeulen PB, Van Marck E. Angiogenic cytokines in mesothelioma: a study of VEGF, FGF-1 and -2, and TGF beta expression. J Pathol. 1999;189(1):72–8.

115. DeLong P, Carroll RG, Henry AC, Tanaka T, Ahmad S, Leibowitz MS, Sterman DH, June CH, Albelda SM, Vonderheide RH. Regulatory T cells and cytokines in malignant pleural effusions secondary to mesothelioma and carcinoma. Cancer Biol Ther. 2005;4(3):342–6.

116. Jagadeeswaran R, Ma PC, Seiwert TY, Jagadeeswaran S, Zumba O, Nallasura V, Ahmed S, Filiberti R, Paganuzzi M, Puntoni R, et al. Functional analysis of c-Met/hepatocyte growth factor pathway in malignant pleural mesothelioma. Cancer Res. 2006;66(1):352–61.

117. Destro A, Ceresoli GL, Falleni M, Zucali PA, Morenghi E, Bianchi P, Pellegrini C, Cordani N, Vaira V, Alloisio M, et al. EGFR overexpression in malignant pleural mesothelioma. An immunohistochemical and molecular study with clinico-pathological correlations. Lung Cancer. 2006;51(2):207–15.

118. Goto Y, Shinjo K, Kondo Y, Shen L, Toyota M, Suzuki H, Gao W, An B, Fujii M, Murakami H, et al. Epigenetic profiles distinguish malignant pleural mesothelioma from lung adenocarcinoma. Cancer Res. 2009;69(23):9073–82.

119. Christensen BC, Houseman EA, Poage GM, Godleski JJ, Bueno R, Sugarbaker DJ, Wiencke JK, Nelson HH, Marsit CJ, Kelsey KT. Integrated profiling reveals a global correlation between epigenetic and genetic alterations in mesothelioma. Cancer Res. 2010;70(14):5686–94.

120. Kannerstein M, Churg J. Mesothelioma in man and experimental animals. Environ Health Perspect. 1980;34:31–6.

121. Johansson L, Linden CJ. Aspects of histopathologic subtype as a prognostic factor in 85 pleural mesotheliomas. Chest. 1996;109(1):109–14.

122. Segal A, Sterrett GF, Frost FA, Shilkin KB, Olsen NJ, Musk AW, Nowak AK, Robinson BW, Creaney J. A diagnosis of malignant pleural mesothelioma can be made by effusion cytology: results of a 20 year audit. Pathology. 2013;45(1):44–8.

123. Hjerpe A, Ascoli V, Bedrossian CW, Boon ME, Creaney J, Davidson B, Dejmek A, Dobra K, Fassina A, Field A, et al. Guidelines for the cytopathologic diagnosis of epithelioid and mixed-type malignant mesothelioma. Complementary statement from the International Mesothelioma Interest Group, also endorsed by the International Academy of Cytology and the Papanicolaou Society of Cytopathology. Acta Cytol. 2015;59(1):2–16.

124. Husain AN, Colby TV, Ordonez NG, Allen TC, Attanoos RL, Beasley MB, Butnor KJ, Chirieac LR, Churg AM, Dacic S et al. Guidelines for pathologic diagnosis of malignant mesothelioma: 2017 update of the Consensus Statement from the International Mesothelioma Interest Group. Arch Pathol Lab Med. 2017.

125. Dejmek A, Hjerpe A. Immunohistochemical reactivity in mesothelioma and adenocarcinoma: a stepwise logistic regression analysis. Apmis. 1994;102(4):255–64.

126. Ordonez NG. Role of immunohistochemistry in differentiating epithelial mesothelioma from adenocarcinoma. Review and update. Am J Clin Pathol. 1999;112(1):75–89.

127. Brockstedt U, Gulyas M, Dobra K, Dejmek A, Hjerpe A. An optimized battery of eight antibodies that can distinguish most cases of epithelial mesothelioma from adenocarcinoma. Am J Clin Pathol. 2000;114(2):203–9.

128. Carella R, Deleonardi G, D'Errico A, Salerno A, Egarter-Vigl E, Seebacher C, Donazzan G, Grigioni WF. Immunohistochemical panels for differentiating epithelial malignant mesothelioma from lung adenocarcinoma: a study with logistic regression analysis. Am J Surg Pathol. 2001;25(1):43–50.

129. Warhol MJ, Hickey WF, Corson JM. Malignant mesothelioma: ultrastructural distinction from adenocarcinoma. Am J Surg Pathol. 1982;6(4):307–14.

130. Stoebner P, Brambilla E. Ultrastructural diagnosis of pleural tumors. Pathol Res Pract. 1982;173(4):402–16.

131. Nurminen M, Dejmek A, Martensson G, Thylen A, Hjerpe A. Clinical utility of liquid-chromatographic analysis of effusions for hyaluronate content. Clin Chem. 1994;40(5):777–80.

132. Robinson BW, Creaney J, Lake R, Nowak A, Musk AW, de Klerk N, Winzell P, Hellstrom KE, Hellstrom I. Mesothelin-family proteins and diagnosis of mesothelioma. Lancet. 2003;362(9396):1612–6.

133. Dejmek A, Brockstedt U, Hjerpe A. Optimization of a battery using nine immunocytochemical variables for distinguishing between epithelial mesothelioma and adenocarcinoma. Apmis. 1997;105(11):889–94.

134. Dejmek A, Hjerpe A. The combination of CEA, EMA, and BerEp4 and hyaluronan analysis specifically identifies 79% of all histologically verified mesotheliomas causing an effusion. Diagn Cytopathol. 2005;32(3):160–6.

135. Davidson B. The diagnostic and molecular characteristics of malignant mesothelioma and ovarian/peritoneal serous carcinoma. Cytopathology. 2011;22(1):5–21.

136. Davidson B. New diagnostic and molecular characteristics of malignant mesothelioma. Ultrastruct Pathol. 2008;32(6):227–40.

137. Davidson B, Nielsen S, Christensen J, Asschenfeldt P, Berner A, Risberg B, Johansen P. The role of desmin and N-cadherin in effusion cytology: a comparative study using established markers of mesothelial and epithelial cells. Am J Surg Pathol. 2001;25(11):1405–12.

138. Attanoos RL, Griffin A, Gibbs AR. The use of immunohistochemistry in distinguishing reactive from neoplastic mesothelium. A novel use for desmin and comparative evaluation with epithelial membrane antigen, p53, platelet-derived growth factor-receptor, P-glycoprotein and Bcl-2. Histopathology. 2003;43(3):231–8.

139. Parham DM, Webber B, Holt H, Williams WK, Maurer H. Immunohistochemical study of childhood rhabdomyosarcomas and related neoplasms. Results of an Intergroup Rhabdomyosarcoma study project. Cancer. 1991;67(12):3072–80.

140. Sheffield BS, Hwang HC, Lee AF, Thompson K, Rodriguez S, Tse CH, Gown AM, Churg A. BAP1 immunohistochemistry and p16 FISH to separate benign from malignant mesothelial proliferations. Am J Surg Pathol. 2015;39(7):977–82.

141. McGregor SM, Dunning R, Hyjek E, Vigneswaran W, Husain AN, Krausz T. BAP1 facilitates diagnostic objectivity, classification, and prognostication in malignant pleural mesothelioma. Hum Pathol. 2015;46(11):1670–8.

142. Cigognetti M, Lonardi S, Fisogni S, Balzarini P, Pellegrini V, Tironi A, Bercich L, Bugatti M, Rossi G, Murer B, et al. BAP1 (BRCA1-associated protein 1) is a highly specific marker for differentiating mesothelioma from reactive mesothelial proliferations. Mod Pathol. 2015;28(8):1043–57.

143. Andrici J, Sheen A, Sioson L, Wardell K, Clarkson A, Watson N, Ahadi MS, Farzin M, Toon CW, Gill AJ. Loss of expression of BAP1 is a useful adjunct, which strongly supports the diagnosis of mesothelioma in effusion cytology. Mod Pathol. 2015;28(10):1360–8.

144. Hwang HC, Sheffield BS, Rodriguez S, Thompson K, Tse CH, Gown AM, Churg A. Utility of BAP1 immunohistochemistry and p16 (CDKN2A) FISH in the diagnosis of malignant mesothelioma in effusion cytology specimens. Am J Surg Pathol. 2016;40(1):120–6.

145. Shen J, Pinkus GS, Deshpande V, Cibas ES. Usefulness of EMA, GLUT-1, and XIAP for the cytologic diagnosis of malignant mesothelioma in body cavity fluids. Am J Clin Pathol. 2009;131(4):516–23.

146. Hasteh F, Lin GY, Weidner N, Michael CW. The use of immunohistochemistry to distinguish reactive mesothelial cells from malignant mesothelioma in cytologic effusions. Cancer Cytopathol. 2010;118(2):90–6.

147. Minato H, Kurose N, Fukushima M, Nojima T, Usuda K, Sagawa M, Sakuma T, Ooi A, Matsumoto I, Oda M, et al. Comparative immunohistochemical analysis of IMP3, GLUT1, EMA, CD146, and desmin for distinguishing malignant mesothelioma from reactive mesothelial cells. Am J Clin Pathol. 2014;141(1):85–93.

148. Flores-Staino C, Darai-Ramqvist E, Dobra K, Hjerpe A, et al. Lung cancer. 2010;68(1):39–43.

149. Legrand M, Pariente R. Ultrastructural study of pleural fluid in mesothelioma. Thorax. 1974;29(2):164–71.

150. Henderson DW, Papadimitriou JM, Coleman M. Ultrastructural appearances of tumours. Edinburgh: Churchill Livingstone; 1986.

151. Ghadially F. Diagnostic electron microscopy of tumours. London: Butterworth; 1985. p. 96–105.

152. Blix G. Hyaluronic acid in the pleural and peritoneal fluids from a case of mesothelioma. Acta Soc Med Ups. 1951;56(1-2):47–50.

153. Harington JS, Wagner JC, Smith M. The detection of hyaluronic acid in pleural fluids of cases with diffuse pleural mesotheliomas. Br J Exp Pathol. 1963;44:81–3.

154. Asplund T, Versnel MA, Laurent TC, Heldin P. Human mesothelioma cells produce factors that stimulate the production of hyaluronan by mesothelial cells and fibroblasts. Cancer Res. 1993;53(2):388–92.

155. Liu Z, Dobra K, Hauzenberger D, Klominek J. Expression of hyaluronan synthases and hyaluronan in malignant mesothelioma cells. Anticancer Res. 2004;24(2B):599–603.

156. Hjerpe A. Liquid-chromatographic determination of hyaluronic acid in pleural and ascitic fluids. Clin Chem. 1986;32(6):952–6.

157. Chichibu K, Matsuura T, Shichijo S, Yokoyama MM. Assay of serum hyaluronic acid in clinical application. Clin Chim Acta. 1989;181(3):317–23.

158. Mundt F, Nilsonne G, Arslan S, Csuros K, Hillerdal G, Yildirim H, Metintas M, Dobra K, Hjerpe A. Hyaluronan and N-ERC/mesothelin as key biomarkers in a specific two-step model to predict pleural malignant mesothelioma. PLoS One. 2013;8(8):e72030.

159. Engstrom-Laurent A, Hallgren R. Circulating hyaluronate in rheumatoid arthritis: relationship to inflammatory activity and the effect of corticosteroid therapy. Ann Rheum Dis. 1985;44(2):83–8.

160. Engstrom-Laurent A, Loof L, Nyberg A, Schroder T. Increased serum levels of hyaluronate in liver disease. Hepatology. 1985;5(4):638–42.

161. Fraser JR, Laurent TC, Engstrom-Laurent A, Laurent UG. Elimination of hyaluronic acid from the blood stream in the human. Clin Exp Pharmacol Physiol. 1984;11(1):17–25.

162. Thylen A, Wallin J, Martensson G. Hyaluronan in serum as an indicator of progressive disease in hyaluronan-producing malignant mesothelioma. Cancer. 1999;86(10):2000–5.

163. Rump A, Morikawa Y, Tanaka M, Minami S, Umesaki N, Takeuchi M, Miyajima A. Binding of ovarian cancer antigen CA125/MUC16 to mesothelin mediates cell adhesion. J Biol Chem. 2004;279(10):9190–8.

164. Hollevoet K, Bernard D, De Geeter F, Walgraeve N, Van den Eeckhaut A, Vanholder R, Van de Wiele C, Stove V, van Meerbeeck JP, Delanghe JR. Glomerular filtration rate is a confounder for the measurement of soluble mesothelin in serum. Clin Chem. 2009;55(7):1431–3.

165. Creaney J, Olsen NJ, Brims F, Dick IM, Musk AW, de Klerk NH, Skates SJ, Robinson BW. Serum mesothelin for early detection of asbestos-induced cancer malignant mesothelioma. Cancer Epidemiol Biomarkers Prev. 2010;19(9):2238–46.

166. Shiomi K, Miyamoto H, Segawa T, Hagiwara Y, Ota A, Maeda M, Takahashi K, Masuda K, Sakao Y, Hino O. Novel ELISA system for detection of N-ERC/mesothelin in the sera of mesothelioma patients. Cancer Sci. 2006;97(9):928–32.

167. Pass HI, Lott D, Lonardo F, Harbut M, Liu Z, Tang N, Carbone M, Webb C, Wali A. Asbestos exposure, pleural mesothelioma, and serum osteopontin levels. N Engl J Med. 2005;353(15):1564–73.

168. Grigoriu BD, Scherpereel A, Devos P, Chahine B, Letourneux M, Lebailly P, Gregoire M, Porte H, Copin MC, Lassalle P. Utility

of osteopontin and serum mesothelin in malignant pleural mesothelioma diagnosis and prognosis assessment. Clin Cancer Res. 2007;13(10):2928–35.

169. Raiko I, Sander I, Weber DG, Raulf-Heimsoth M, Gillissen A, Kollmeier J, Scherpereel A, Bruning T, Johnen G. Development of an enzyme-linked immunosorbent assay for the detection of human calretinin in plasma and serum of mesothelioma patients. BMC Cancer. 2010;10:242.

170. Gulyas M, Hjerpe A. Proteoglycans and WT1 as markers for distinguishing adenocarcinoma, epithelioid mesothelioma, and benign mesothelium. J Pathol. 2003;199(4):479–87.

171. Kumar-Singh S, Jacobs W, Dhaene K, Weyn B, Bogers J, Weyler J, Van Marck E. Syndecan-1 expression in malignant mesothelioma: correlation with cell differentiation, WT1 expression, and clinical outcome. J Pathol. 1998;186(3):300–5.

172. Saqi A, Yun SS, Yu GH, Alexis D, Taub RN, Powell CA, Borczuk AC. Utility of CD138 (syndecan-1) in distinguishing carcinomas from mesotheliomas. Diagn Cytopathol. 2005;33(2):65–70.

173. Seidel C, Gulyas M, David G, Dobra K, Theocharis AD, Hjerpe A. A sandwich ELISA for the estimation of human syndecan-2 and syndecan-4 in biological samples. J Pharm Biomed Anal. 2004;34(4):797–801.

174. Tsuji S, Tsuura Y, Morohoshi T, Shinohara T, Oshita F, Yamada K, Kameda Y, Ohtsu T, Nakamura Y, Miyagi Y. Secretion of intelectin-1 from malignant pleural mesothelioma into pleural effusion. Br J Cancer. 2010;103(4):517–23.

175. Chen Z, Gaudino G, Pass HI, Carbone M, Yang H. Diagnostic and prognostic biomarkers for malignant mesothelioma: an update. Transl Lung Cancer Res. 2017;6(3):259–69.

176. Rundlof AK, Fernandes AP, Selenius M, Babic M, Shariatgorji M, Nilsonne G, Ilag LL, Dobra K, Bjornstedt M. Quantification of alternative mRNA species and identification of thioredoxin reductase 1 isoforms in human tumor cells. Differentiation. 2007;75(2):123–32.

177. Mundt F, Heidari-Hamedani G, Nilsonne G, Metintas M, Hjerpe A, Dobra K. Diagnostic and prognostic value of soluble syndecan-1 in pleural malignancies. Biomed Res Int. 2014;2014:419853.

178. Mundt F, Johansson HJ, Forshed J, Arslan S, Metintas M, Dobra K, Lehtio J, Hjerpe A. Proteome screening of pleural effusions identifies galectin 1 as a diagnostic biomarker and highlights several prognostic biomarkers for malignant mesothelioma. Mol Cell Proteomics. 2014;13(3):701–15.

179. Yuan Y, Nymoen DA, Stavnes HT, Rosnes AK, Bjorang O, Wu C, Nesland JM, Davidson B. Tenascin-X is a novel diagnostic marker of malignant mesothelioma. Am J Surg Pathol. 2009;33(11):1673–82.

180. Aerts JG, Delahaye M, van der Kwast TH, Davidson B, Hoogsteden HC, van Meerbeeck JP. The high post-test probability of a cytological examination renders further investigations to establish a diagnosis of epithelial malignant pleural mesothelioma redundant. Diagn Cytopathol. 2006;34(8):523–7.

181. Cedres S, Ponce-Aix S, Zugazagoitia J, Sansano I, Enguita A, Navarro-Mendivil A, Martinez-Marti A, Martinez P, Felip E. Analysis of expression of programmed cell death 1 ligand 1 (PD-L1) in malignant pleural mesothelioma (MPM). PLoS One. 2015;10(3):e0121071.

182. Khanna S, Thomas A, Abate-Daga D, Zhang J, Morrow B, Steinberg SM, Orlandi A, Ferroni P, Schlom J, Guadagni F, et al. Malignant mesothelioma effusions are infiltrated by CD3+ T cells highly expressing PD-L1 and the PD-L1+ tumor cells within these effusions are susceptible to ADCC by the anti-PD-L1 antibody Avelumab. J Thorac Oncol. 2016;11(11):1993–2005.

183. Mansfield AS, Roden AC, Peikert T, Sheinin YM, Harrington SM, Krco CJ, Dong H, Kwon ED. B7-H1 expression in malignant pleural mesothelioma is associated with sarcomatoid histology and poor prognosis. J Thorac Oncol. 2014;9(7):1036–40.

184. Dozier J, Zheng H, Adusumilli PS. Immunotherapy for malignant pleural mesothelioma: current status and future directions. Transl Lung Cancer Res. 2017;6(3):315–24.

185. Bakker E, Guazzelli A, Ashtiani F, Demonacos C, Krstic-Demonacos M, Mutti L. Immunotherapy advances for mesothelioma treatment. Expert Rev Anticancer Ther. 2017;17:799–814.

186. Alley EW, Lopez J, Santoro A, Morosky A, Saraf S, Piperdi B, van Brummelen E. Clinical safety and activity of pembrolizumab in patients with malignant pleural mesothelioma (KEYNOTE-028): preliminary results from a non-randomised, open-label, phase 1b trial. Lancet Oncol. 2017;18(5):623–30.

187. Wu L, de Perrot M. Radio-immunotherapy and chemo-immunotherapy as a novel treatment paradigm in malignant pleural mesothelioma. Transl Lung Cancer Res. 2017;6(3):325–34.

188. Alley EW, Katz SI, Cengel KA, Simone CB II. Immunotherapy and radiation therapy for malignant pleural mesothelioma. Transl Lung Cancer Res. 2017;6(2):212–9.

189. Klug F, Prakash H, Huber PE, Seibel T, Bender N, Halama N, Pfirschke C, Voss RH, Timke C, Umansky L, et al. Low-dose irradiation programs macrophage differentiation to an iNOS(+)/M1 phenotype that orchestrates effective T cell immunotherapy. Cancer Cell. 2013;24(5):589–602.

190. Lizotte PH, Jones RE, Keogh L, Ivanova E, Liu H, Awad MM, Hammerman PS, Gill RR, Richards WG, Barbie DA, et al. Fine needle aspirate flow cytometric phenotyping characterizes immunosuppressive nature of the mesothelioma microenvironment. Sci Rep. 2016;6:31745.

191. Zucali PA, Giovannetti E, Assaraf YG, Ceresoli GL, Peters GJ, Santoro A. New tricks for old biomarkers: thymidylate synthase expression as a predictor of pemetrexed activity in malignant mesothelioma. Ann Oncol. 2010;21(7):1560–1.

192. Uramoto H, Onitsuka T, Shimokawa H, Hanagiri T. TS, DHFR and GARFT expression in non-squamous cell carcinoma of NSCLC and malignant pleural mesothelioma patients treated with pemetrexed. Anticancer Res. 2010;30(10):4309–15.

193. Vilmar A, Sorensen JB. Excision repair cross-complementation group 1 (ERCC1) in platinum-based treatment of non-small cell lung cancer with special emphasis on carboplatin: a review of current literature. Lung Cancer. 2009;64(2):131–9.

194. Mansour MSI, Seidal T, Mager U, Baigi A, Dobra K, Dejmek A. Determination of PD-L1 expression in effusions from mesothelioma by immuno-cytochemical staining. Cancer Cytopathol. 2017;125(12):908–17. https://doi.org/10.1002/cncy.21917.

195. Szulkin A, Nilsonne G, Mundt F, Wasik AM, Souri P, Hjerpe A, Dobra K. Variation in drug sensitivity of malignant mesothelioma cell lines with substantial effects of selenite and bortezomib, highlights need for individualized therapy. PLoS One. 2013;8(6):e65903.

196. Markasz L, Kis LL, Stuber G, Flaberg E, Otvos R, Eksborg S, Skribek H, Olah E, Szekely L. Hodgkin-lymphoma-derived cells show high sensitivity to dactinomycin and paclitaxel. Leuk Lymphoma. 2007;48(9):1835–45.

197. Flaberg E, Markasz L, Petranyi G, Stuber G, Dicso F, Alchihabi N, Olah E, Csizy I, Jozsa T, Andren O, et al. High throughput live cell imaging reveals differential inhibition of tumor cell proliferation by human fibroblasts. Int J Cancer. 2011;128(12):2793–802.

198. Szulkin A, Otvos R, Hillerdal CO, Celep A, Yousef-Fadhel E, Skribek H, Hjerpe A, Szekely L, Dobra K. Characterization and drug sensitivity profiling of primary malignant mesothelioma cells from pleural effusions. BMC Cancer. 2014;14:709.

199. Alifrangis C, Janssen JQ, Badhai J, Iorio F, Schunselaar L, Kolluri K, Baas P, Garnett M, McDermott U. High throughput therapeutic screening of malignant pleural mesothelioma (MPM) to identify correlation of sensitivity to FGFR inhibitors with BAP1 inactivation. J Clin Oncol. 2015;33(15).

200. Roe OD, Szulkin A, Anderssen E, Flatberg A, Sandeck H, Amundsen T, Erlandsen SE, Dobra K, Sundstrom SH. Molecular resistance fingerprint of pemetrexed and platinum in a long-term survivor of mesothelioma. PLoS One. 2012;7(8):e40521.

201. Takeuchi S, Seike M, Noro R, Soeno C, Sugano T, Zou F, Uesaka H, Nishijima N, Matsumoto M, Minegishi Y, et al. Significance of osteopontin in the sensitivity of malignant pleural mesothelioma to pemetrexed. Int J Oncol. 2014;44(6):1886–94.

202. Costello JC, Heiser LM, Georgii E, Gonen M, Menden MP, Wang NJ, Bansal M, Ammad-ud-din M, Hintsanen P, Khan SA, et al. A community effort to assess and improve drug sensitivity prediction algorithms. Nat Biotechnol. 2014;32(12):1202–12.

203. Khan SA, Faisal A, Mpindi JP, Parkkinen JA, Kalliokoski T, Poso A, Kallioniemi OP, Wennerberg K, Kaski S. Comprehensive data-driven analysis of the impact of chemoinformatic structure on the genome-wide biological response profiles of cancer cells to 1159 drugs. BMC Bioinform. 2012;13:112.

204. Jaklitsch MT, Grondin SC, Sugarbaker DJ. Treatment of malignant mesothelioma. World J Surg. 2001;25(2):210–7.

205. Molnar-Kimber KL, Sterman DH, Chang M, Kang EH, ElBash M, Lanuti M, Elshami A, Gelfand K, Wilson JM, Kaiser LR, et al. Impact of preexisting and induced humoral and cellular immune responses in an adenovirus-based gene therapy phase I clinical trial for localized mesothelioma. Hum Gene Ther. 1998;9(14):2121–33.

206. Sterman DH, Treat J, Litzky LA, Amin KM, Coonrod L, Molnar-Kimber K, Recio A, Knox L, Wilson JM, Albelda SM, et al. Adenovirus-mediated herpes simplex virus thymidine kinase/ganciclovir gene therapy in patients with localized malignancy: results of a phase I clinical trial in malignant mesothelioma. Hum Gene Ther. 1998;9(7):1083–92.

207. Caminschi I, Venetsanakos E, Leong CC, Garlepp MJ, Robinson BW, Scott B. Cytokine gene therapy of mesothelioma. Immune and antitumor effects of transfected interleukin-12. Am J Respir Cell Mol Biol. 1999;21(3):347–56.

208. McLaren BR, Whitaker D, Robinson BW, Lake RA. Expression and integrity of DNA topoisomerase II isoforms does not explain generic drug resistance in malignant mesothelioma. Cancer Chemother Pharmacol. 2001;48(1):1–8.

209. Segers K, Kumar-Singh S, Weyler J, Bogers J, Ramael M, Van Meerbeeck J, Van Marck E. Glutathione S-transferase expression in malignant mesothelioma and non-neoplastic mesothelium: an immunohistochemical study. J Cancer Res Clin Oncol. 1996;122(10):619–24.

210. Dejmek A, Brockstedt U, Hjerpe A. Immunoreactivity of pleural malignant mesotheliomas to glutathione S-transferases. Apmis. 1998;106(4):489–94.

211. Soini Y, Kinnula V, Kaarteenaho-Wiik R, Kurttila E, Linnainmaa K, Paakko P. Apoptosis and expression of apoptosis regulating proteins bcl-2, mcl-1, bcl-X, and bax in malignant mesothelioma. Clin Cancer Res. 1999;5(11):3508–15.

212. Gordon GJ, Appasani K, Parcells JP, Mukhopadhyay NK, Jaklitsch MT, Richards WG, Sugarbaker DJ, Bueno R. Inhibitor of apoptosis protein-1 promotes tumor cell survival in mesothelioma. Carcinogenesis. 2002;23(6):1017–24.

213. Xia C, Xu Z, Yuan X, Uematsu K, You L, Li K, Li L, McCormick F, Jablons DM. Induction of apoptosis in mesothelioma cells by anti-survivin oligonucleotides. Mol Cancer Ther. 2002;1(9):687–94.

214. Kleinberg L, Lie AK, Florenes VA, Nesland JM, Davidson B. Expression of inhibitor-of-apoptosis protein family members in malignant mesothelioma. Hum Pathol. 2007;38(7):986–94.

215. Zaffaroni N, Costa A, Pennati M, De Marco C, Affini E, Madeo M, Erdas R, Cabras A, Kusamura S, Baratti D, et al. Survivin is highly expressed and promotes cell survival in malignant perito-neal mesothelioma. Cell Oncol. 2007;29(6):453–66.

216. Vogelzang NJ, Rusthoven JJ, Symanowski J, Denham C, Kaukel E, Ruffie P, Gatzemeier U, Boyer M, Emri S, Manegold C, et al. Phase III study of pemetrexed in combination with cisplatin versus cisplatin alone in patients with malignant pleural mesothelioma. J Clin Oncol. 2003;21(14):2636–44.

217. Hillerdal G, Sorensen JB, Sundstrom S, Vikstrom A, Hjerpe A. Treatment of malignant pleural mesothelioma with lipo-somized doxorubicine: prolonged time to progression and good survival. A Nordic study. Clin Respir J. 2008;2(2):80–5.

218. Schunselaar LM, Quispel-Janssen JM, Neefjes JJ, Baas P. A catalogue of treatment and technologies for malignant pleural meso-thelioma. Expert Rev Anticancer Ther. 2016;16(4):455–63.

219. Remon J, Reguart N, Corral J, Lianes P. Malignant pleural meso-thelioma: new hope in the horizon with novel therapeutic strate-gies. Cancer Treat Rev. 2015;41(1):27–34.

220. Signorelli D, Macerelli M, Proto C, Vitali M, Cona MS, Agustoni F, Zilembo N, Platania M, Trama A, Gallucci R, et al. Systemic approach to malignant pleural mesothelioma: what news of chemotherapy, targeted agents and immunotherapy? Tumori. 2016;102(1):18–30.

221. Guazzelli A, Bakker E, Tian K, Demonacos C, Krstic-Demonacos M, Mutti L. Promising investigational drug candidates in phase I and phase II clinical trials for mesothelioma. Expert Opin Investig Drugs. 2017;26(8):933–44.

222. Christoph DC, Eberhardt WE. Systemic treatment of malignant pleural mesothelioma: new agents in clinical trials raise hope of relevant improvements. Curr Opin Oncol. 2014;26(2):171–81.

223. Papa S, Popat S, Shah R, Prevost AT, Lal R, McLennan B, Cane P, Lang-Lazdunski L, Viney Z, Dunn JT, et al. Phase 2 study of sorafenib in malignant mesothelioma previously treated with platinum-containing chemotherapy. J Thorac Oncol. 2013;8(6):783–7.

224. Zimling ZG, Sorensen JB, Gerds TA, Bech C, Andersen CB, Santoni-Rugiu E. A biomarker profile for predicting efficacy of cisplatin-vinorelbine therapy in malignant pleural mesothelioma. Cancer Chemother Pharmacol. 2012;70(5):743–54.

225. Ting S, Mairinger FD, Hager T, Welter S, Eberhardt WE, Wohlschlaeger J, Schmid KW, Christoph DC. ERCC1, MLH1, MSH2, MSH6, and betaIII-tubulin: resistance proteins asso-ciated with response and outcome to platinum-based chemo-therapy in malignant pleural mesothelioma. Clin Lung Cancer. 2013;14(5):558–67. e553

226. Palumbo C, Bei R, Procopio A, Modesti A. Molecular targets and targeted therapies for malignant mesothelioma. Curr Med Chem. 2008;15(9):855–67.

227. Zalcman G, Mazieres J, Margery J, Greillier L, Audigier-Valette C, Moro-Sibilot D, Molinier O, Corre R, Monnet I, Gounant V, et al. Bevacizumab for newly diagnosed pleural mesothelioma in the Mesothelioma Avastin Cisplatin Pemetrexed Study (MAPS): a randomised, controlled, open-label, phase 3 trial. Lancet. 2016;387(10026):1405–14.

228. Suzuki K, Kadota K, Sima CS, Sadelain M, Rusch VW, Travis WD, Adusumilli PS. Chronic inflammation in tumor stroma is an independent predictor of prolonged survival in epithelioid malig-nant pleural mesothelioma patients. Cancer Immunol Immunother. 2011;60(12):1721–8.

229. Campbell NP, Kindler HL. Update on malignant pleural mesothe-lioma. Semin Respir Crit Care Med. 2011;32(1):102–10.

230. Bongiovanni M, Cassoni P, De Giuli P, Viberti L, Cappia S, Ivaldi C, Chiusa L, Bussolati G. p27(kip1) immunoreactivity corre-lates with long-term survival in pleural malignant mesothelioma. Cancer. 2001;92(5):1245–50.

231. Cedres S, Montero MA, Zamora E, Martinez A, Martinez P, Farinas L, Navarro A, Torrejon D, Gabaldon A, Ramon YCS, et al. Expression of Wilms' tumor gene (WT1) is associated with survival in malignant pleural mesothelioma. Clin Transl Oncol. 2014;16(9):776–82.

232. Kao SC, Klebe S, Henderson DW, Reid G, Chatfield M, Armstrong NJ, Yan TD, Vardy J, Clarke S, van Zandwijk N, et al. Low cal-

retinin expression and high neutrophil-to-lymphocyte ratio are poor prognostic factors in patients with malignant mesothelioma undergoing extrapleural pneumonectomy. J Thorac Oncol. 2011;6(11):1923–9.

233. Thylen A, Hjerpe A, Martensson G. Hyaluronan content in pleural fluid as a prognostic factor in patients with malignant pleural mesothelioma. Cancer. 2001;92(5):1224–30.

234. Creaney J, Dick IM, Segal A, Musk AW, Robinson BW. Pleural effusion hyaluronic acid as a prognostic marker in pleural malignant mesothelioma. Lung Cancer. 2013;82(3):491–8.

235. Edwards JG, Swinson DE, Jones JL, Waller DA, O'Byrne KJ. EGFR expression: associations with outcome and clinicopathological variables in malignant pleural mesothelioma. Lung Cancer. 2006;54(3):399–407.

236. Levallet G, Vaisse-Lesteven M, Le Stang N, Ilg AG, Brochard P, Astoul P, Pairon JC, Bergot E, Zalcman G, Galateau-Salle F. Plasma cell membrane localization of c-MET predicts longer survival in patients with malignant mesothelioma: a series of 157 cases from the MESOPATH Group. J Thorac Oncol. 2012;7(3):599–606.

237. Amatya VJ, Takeshima Y, Aoe K, Fujimoto N, Okamoto T, Yamada T, Kishimoto T, Morimoto C, Inai K. CD9 expression as a favorable prognostic marker for patients with malignant mesothelioma. Oncol Rep. 2013;29(1):21–8.

238. Aoe K, Amatya VJ, Fujimoto N, Ohnuma K, Hosono O, Hiraki A, Fujii M, Yamada T, Dang NH, Takeshima Y, et al. CD26 overexpression is associated with prolonged survival and enhanced chemosensitivity in malignant pleural mesothelioma. Clin Cancer Res. 2012;18(5):1447–56.

239. Otterstrom C, Soltermann A, Opitz I, Felley-Bosco E, Weder W, Stahel RA, Triponez F, Robert JH, Serre-Beinier V. CD74: a new prognostic factor for patients with malignant pleural mesothelioma. Br J Cancer. 2014;110(8):2040–6.

240. Schramm A, Opitz I, Thies S, Seifert B, Moch H, Weder W, Soltermann A. Prognostic significance of epithelial-mesenchymal transition in malignant pleural mesothelioma. Eur J Cardiothorac Surg. 2010;37(3):566–72.

241. Cristaudo A, Foddis R, Vivaldi A, Guglielmi G, Dipalma N, Filiberti R, Neri M, Ceppi M, Paganuzzi M, Ivaldi GP, et al. Clinical significance of serum mesothelin in patients with mesothelioma and lung cancer. Clin Cancer Res. 2007;13(17):5076–81.

242. Schneider J, Hoffmann H, Dienemann H, Herth FJ, Meister M, Muley T. Diagnostic and prognostic value of soluble mesothelin-related proteins in patients with malignant pleural mesothelioma in comparison with benign asbestosis and lung cancer. J Thorac Oncol. 2008;3(11):1317–24.

243. Cappia S, Righi L, Mirabelli D, Ceppi P, Bacillo E, Ardissone F, Molinaro L, Scagliotti GV, Papotti M. Prognostic role of osteopontin expression in malignant pleural mesothelioma. Am J Clin Pathol. 2008;130(1):58–64.

244. Hollevoet K, Nackaerts K, Gosselin R, De Wever W, Bosquee L, De Vuyst P, Germonpre P, Kellen E, Legrand C, Kishi Y, et al. Soluble mesothelin, megakaryocyte potentiating factor, and osteopontin as markers of patient response and outcome in mesothelioma. J Thorac Oncol. 2011;6(11):1930–7.

245. Creaney J, Dick IM, Meniawy TM, Leong SL, Leon JS, Demelker Y, Segal A, Musk AW, Lee YC, Skates SJ, et al. Comparison of fibulin-3 and mesothelin as markers in malignant mesothelioma. Thorax. 2014;69(10):895–902.

246. Righi L, Cavallo MC, Gatti G, Monica V, Rapa I, Busso S, Albera C, Volante M, Scagliotti GV, Papotti M. Tumor/stromal caveolin-1 expression patterns in pleural mesothelioma define a subgroup of the epithelial histotype with poorer prognosis. Am J Clin Pathol. 2014;141(6):816–27.

247. Edwards JG, Cox G, Andi A, Jones JL, Walker RA, Waller DA, O'Byrne KJ. Angiogenesis is an independent prognostic factor in malignant mesothelioma. Br J Cancer. 2001;85(6):863–8.

248. Kao SC, Harvie R, Paturi F, Taylor R, Davey R, Abraham R, Clarke S, Marx G, Cullen M, Kerestes Z, et al. The predictive role of serum VEGF in an advanced malignant mesothelioma patient cohort treated with thalidomide alone or combined with cisplatin/gemcitabine. Lung Cancer. 2012;75(2):248–54.

249. Tabata C, Hirayama N, Tabata R, Yasumitsu A, Yamada S, Murakami A, Iida S, Tamura K, Fukuoka K, Kuribayashi K, et al. A novel clinical role for angiopoietin-1 in malignant pleural mesothelioma. Eur Respir J. 2010;36(5):1099–105.

250. Righi L, Papotti MG, Ceppi P, Bille A, Bacillo E, Molinaro L, Ruffini E, Scagliotti GV, Selvaggi G. Thymidylate synthase but not excision repair cross-complementation group 1 tumor expression predicts outcome in patients with malignant pleural mesothelioma treated with pemetrexed-based chemotherapy. J Clin Oncol. 2010;28(9):1534–9.

251. Zucali PA, Giovannetti E, Destro A, Mencoboni M, Ceresoli GL, Gianoncelli L, Lorenzi E, De Vincenzo F, Simonelli M, Perrino M, et al. Thymidylate synthase and excision repair cross-complementing group-1 as predictors of responsiveness in mesothelioma patients treated with pemetrexed/carboplatin. Clin Cancer Res. 2011;17(8):2581–90.

252. Christoph DC, Asuncion BR, Mascaux C, Tran C, Lu X, Wynes MW, Gauler TC, Wohlschlaeger J, Theegarten D, Neumann V, et al. Folylpoly-glutamate synthetase expression is associated with tumor response and outcome from pemetrexed-based chemotherapy in malignant pleural mesothelioma. J Thorac Oncol. 2012;7(9):1440–8.

253. Davidson B. Prognostic factors in malignant pleural mesothelioma. Hum Pathol. 2015;46(6):789–804.

254. Achatzy R, Beba W, Ritschler R, Worn H, Wahlers B, Macha HN, Morgan JA. The diagnosis, therapy and prognosis of diffuse malignant mesothelioma. Eur J Cardiothorac Surg. 1989;3(5):445–447; discussion 448.

255. Law MR, Gregor A, Hodson ME, Bloom HJ, Turner-Warwick M. Malignant mesothelioma of the pleura: a study of 52 treated and 64 untreated patients. Thorax. 1984;39(4):255–9.

256. Blayney JK, Ceresoli GL, Castagneto B, O'Brien ME, Hasan B, Sylvester R, Rudd R, Steele J, Busacca S, Porta C, et al. Response to chemotherapy is predictive in relation to longer overall survival in an individual patient combined-analysis with pleural mesothelioma. Eur J Cancer. 2012;48(16):2983–92.

257. Own SA, Hillerdal G, Dobra K, Hjerpe A. PP01.05: Early diagnosis by cytology improves survival. In: 13th International Conference of the International Mesothelioma Group, 2016, Birmingham.

# Cancer of Other Origin

# 12

## Ben Davidson

B. Davidson, M.D., Ph.D.
Department of Pathology, The Norwegian Radium Hospital, Oslo University Hospital, Oslo, Norway

Faculty of Medicine, Institute of Clinical Medicine, University of Oslo, Oslo, Norway
e-mail: bend@medisin.uio.no; bdd@ous-hf.no

## Introduction

The previous chapters in this section discussed our current knowledge of the biology and clinical relevance of lung, ovarian, and breast carcinoma metastasis in serous effusions, with similar analysis of the native cancer of the serosal cavities, malignant mesothelioma. As discussed in Chap. 7, a vast array of malignant tumors may additionally be diagnosed in serous effusions. The majority of these cancers are highly aggressive, and their detection in effusion specimens precludes any curative approach, underscoring the need to better characterize them with respect to the presence of potential molecular targets. However, the rarity of the majority of these entities has undoubtedly contributed to the scarceness of research aimed at better understanding their biology and improving therapy. The only obvious exception is cancer originating in the gastrointestinal (GI) tract, which has been the subject of a relatively large number of publications. This chapter will consequently focus on these tumors, followed by a brief discussion of the few published investigations of malignant melanoma and sarcomas in effusions. New diagnostic markers that are useful in the diagnosis of these cancers by immunohistochemistry are discussed in Chap. 7.

## GI Cancers

The sites of origin for gastrointestinal cancers disseminating to effusions are the stomach, pancreas, liver, biliary tract, colorectum, and esophagus. With the exception of colorectal carcinoma, all these organs give rise to highly aggressive tumors, which are associated with very poor 5-year survival, often in the range of 5–10% [1–9]. Not unexpectedly, the detection of carcinoma cells from these organs in effusions marks a subset of patients with a still worse outcome within this patient group [10–22]. The epidemiology of these malignancies and their clinical features are briefly discussed in Chap. 7.

While cancers originating from the GI tract are biologically different, two or more types have been analyzed together in several studies, making it logical to discuss these tumors as one group, focusing on a single site of origin where relevant. Generally, studies of GI tract cancers have focused on three issues:

1. Improving the diagnosis, especially in the differential diagnosis from benign effusions in conditions mimicking cancer (e.g., cirrhosis).
2. Understanding aspects of tumor biology.
3. Assessment of new therapeutic modalities.

## Diagnostic Approaches

Despite the central role of immunohistochemistry in effusion cytology, several other approaches have been evaluated in this context as an adjunct to morphology.

Cascinu et al. analyzed the levels of soluble carcinoembryonic antigen (CEA), CA 19.9, CA 15.3, CA 125, mucin-like carcinoma-associated antigen (MCA), α-fetoprotein (AFP), and prostate-specific antigen (PSA) in 89 effusion supernatants, including 30 gastric, 11 colorectal, and 6 liver carcinomas, as well as 5 prostate carcinomas, using an immunoradiometric assay. CEA, CA 19.9, and CA 125 levels were above cutoff levels in all colorectal and in the majority of gastric carcinomas. AFP and PSA identified all liver and prostate carcinomas, respectively, with high degree of specificity [23].

Yu and co-workers analyzed 112 effusions, consisting of malignant effusions, the majority of which were lung carcinomas, benign exudates, and cytology-negative effusions from cancer patients for mRNA levels of *MUC1*, *MUC2*, and *MUC5AC*. The malignant effusion group included four gas-

© Springer International Publishing AG, part of Springer Nature 2018
B. Davidson et al. (eds.), *Serous Effusions*, https://doi.org/10.1007/978-3-319-76478-8_12

tric carcinomas, whereas the cytology-negative group included five specimens from patients with liver carcinoma and one from pancreatic carcinoma. *MUC1* and *MUC5AC* levels were significantly higher in malignant compared to benign specimens. They were additionally higher in the cytology-negative group compared to benign effusions, and in the former group, 11/23 specimens were subsequently found to contain tumor cells which were not detected in the initial morphological examination [24].

An additional study investigated the presence of *KRAS* mutations in 34 malignant and 15 benign cytological specimens, including 41 effusion supernatants, using single-strand conformation polymorphism (SSCP) analysis. The majority of malignant specimens were from patients with GI cancers. *KRAS* mutations were found in 8/9 pancreatic carcinomas, as well as in 2 colorectal and 1 gastric carcinoma, and findings were similar in analysis of effusion cell pellets and solid lesions. The assay identified three false-negative specimens, including two pancreatic and one colorectal carcinomas [25].

Telomerase, the enzyme that synthesizes telomeric DNA and contributes to the ability of cancer cells to avoid aging and replicate endlessly, has been the subject of a large number of diagnostic studies, including two which focused on GI cancer effusions.

Analysis of telomerase expression using the telomeric repeat amplification protocol (TRAP) assay was performed on 95 ascites specimens, including 40 HCC, 31 non-HCC GI carcinomas (10 gastric, 10 pancreatic, 8 colon, 3 cholangiocarcinomas), and 24 cirrhosis samples. The assay was positive in 16/31 (52%) and 10/40 (25%) of non-HCC GI carcinomas and HCC, compared to 1/24 (4%) of cirrhosis specimens, performing better than morphology in both malignant entities [26].

In an additional study, 25 malignant, including 14 GI carcinomas (9 HCC, 2 colon, 2 gastric, and 1 pancreatic carcinoma), and 47 benign specimens, the majority from patients with cirrhosis, were analyzed using the same assay. The TRAP assay was positive in 6/9 HCC and 4/5 of the non-HCC tumors, compared to 2/47 benign specimens, performing better than cytology also in this series [27].

The diagnostic role of Newcastle disease virus expressing the enhanced green fluorescent protein (NDV-GFP) was studied in gastric carcinoma washings. GFP-positive cells were found in 6/6 cases in which laparoscopy showed the presence of metastatic disease, compared to 3/6 specimens diagnosed by cytology [28].

The diagnostic value of flow cytometry (FCM) in the diagnosis of serous effusions based on the presence of specific leukocyte populations was assessed in several studies. Cornfield and Gheith compared the natural killer (NK) and T-cell populations in 30 benign and 30 malignant effusions, the latter including 5 GI carcinomas [29]. CD16+/ CD56+ NK cell counts were significantly higher in malignant effusions, though only modestly ($p = 0.04$). Wang et al. found significantly higher numbers of CD14+/CD163+ tumor-infiltrating macrophages, considered tumor-promoting, in malignant compared to benign effusions [30]. Effector memory CD8+ T-cell levels were significantly higher in blood and pleural fluid from healthy controls compared to patients with malignant pleural effusion, pleural metastases, or benign asbestos-related lesions [31].

HCC deserves separate discussion in this context, as it expresses tumor markers shared by few other cancers, such as AFP, glypican-3, Hep-Par1, and arginase-1 [32]. In the last two decades, several diagnostic approaches were studied with the aim of differentiating HCC (or cancer in general) from cirrhosis.

The levels of α1-antitrypsin were reported to be higher in malignant ascites, including eight HCC specimens, compared to ascites from patients with cirrhosis, and this assay performed better than measurement of total protein ascitic concentration or the serum-ascites albumin gradient [33].

In an additional study of 149 ascites specimens, including 46 HCC, the concentrations of fibronectin, albumin, total protein, lactate dehydrogenase, and CEA were shown to be significantly higher in malignant non-HCC compared to benign specimens, whereas the opposite was true for the serum-ascites albumin gradient. However, none of these parameters differentiated chronic liver disease from HCC [34]. In contrast, fibronectin concentration was significantly higher in HCC ($n = 33$) compared to cirrhosis specimens ($n = 89$) in the series of Colli et al. [35].

Analysis of free fatty acid levels in 14 malignant (predominantly GI cancers, including HCC) and 19 cirrhotic ascites showed significantly higher levels in the former group. Free fatty acid and albumin levels were strongly interrelated [36]. Parenthetically, in situ hybridization for albumin mRNA using a digoxigenin-labeled oligonucleotide probe as complement to AFP immunohistochemistry was reported to be useful in HCC effusion cytology [37].

Miédougé and co-workers measured serum and ascites AFP in specimens from 125 patients, consisting of 31 HCC, 14 non-HCC cancers, and 80 benign cases. AFP serum levels were higher than ascites levels, but in both specimen types AFP, levels were significantly higher in HCC compared to the two other diagnostic categories. A diagnostic specificity of 95% was associated with a sensitivity of 67.7%, which was not improved by calculating the ratio between AFP and albumin or total protein [38].

Another marker suggested as useful in differentiating between HCC and cirrhosis is the nucleoside pseudouridine, product of RNA catabolism. In analysis of 54 cirrhosis and 17 HCC ascites specimens, this marker had a sensitivity of 88.2% and a specificity of 90.8% in diagnosing HCC [39].

The levels of vascular endothelial growth factor (VEGF) and the v6 isoform of the adhesion molecule CD44 (CD44v6) were significantly higher in malignant ascites (=23), including 14 GI carcinomas (6 gastric, 5 colonic, 2 HCC, 1 pancreatic) compared to cirrhotic ($n = 26$) or tuberculous ($n = 8$) ascites. There markers were consequently suggested as adjunct in this differential diagnosis [40]. Similar findings with respect to VEGF were reported in another study, in which 25 malignant ascites specimens, including 7 colon and 6 gastric carcinomas, were compared to 4 effusions from patients with cirrhosis [41].

Kraft and co-workers measured VEGF levels in 445 sera samples, including 212 samples from patients with cancer, among which 48 were of GI origin [42]. VEGF levels in sera from patients with GI or ovarian carcinomas were significantly higher compared to normal subjects. Analysis of 56 effusion specimens, including 9 from GI cancer patients, showed considerably higher VEGF levels in this material compared to matched serum samples.

## Tumor Biology

The majority of studies in which biological and clinical aspects of GI cancers have been studied focused on gastric carcinoma. Many of the molecules discussed in this section have already been introduced in previous chapters, where their biological role is discussed.

## Surface Molecules

Several studies analyzed the expression of cell surface molecules in gastric carcinoma. Tamai et al. analyzed 51 gastric carcinoma specimens for CEA expression by FCM. Tumor cell expression was unrelated to serum CEA levels or to patient survival, the latter available for 39 patients, although higher CEA expression was associated with shorter survival in the group of 8 patients with signet ring cell carcinoma [43]. In another study, serum and ascites CEA levels were measured in 119 patients with peritoneal carcinomatosis. Ascites CEA levels were higher than the corresponding serum levels, and higher levels in ascites were associated with shorter survival in univariate and multivariate analysis. In contrast, neither serum CEA nor the findings in cytological examination, in which 54.6% of specimens contained tumor cells, correlated with survival. Ascites CEA levels additionally correlated with treatment response in patients with serial measurements [44].

Analysis of the expression of the cell-cell adhesion molecule E-cadherin in 21 primary gastric carcinomas showed reduced or absent protein expression in poorly differentiated tumors with single-infiltrating cells compared

to better differentiated ones. Tumor cells from 11 malignant effusions, including 7 gastric, 2 pancreatic, and 2 pulmonary carcinomas, were E-cadherin-negative in all but one specimen by immunofluorescence [45].

Gastric carcinoma cells in ascites specimens ($n = 20$) were shown to frequently express epidermal growth factor receptor (EGFR) and the CD44v9 isoform, with little expression of the v6 isoform, using FCM. The latter finding differed from both normal gastric mucosa and primary gastric carcinomas, suggesting altered expression of this adhesion molecule along tumor progression in this malignancy [46].

Kitayama and co-workers analyzed 506 ascites and peritoneal washing specimens from 333 patients, of whom 300 had gastric cancer and 33 had liver cirrhosis, for CD45 and CD326 (EpCAM) expression by FCM. High tumor-to-leukocyte ratio using these markers was significantly associated with poor survival [47].

## Proteases

The expression and activity of proteases were analyzed in several studies, with focus on the matrix metalloproteinases (MMP) family (see Chap. 9). MMP-2 and MMP-9 expression was analyzed in the abovementioned material studied for VEGF expression [40] using zymography. Both enzymes were absent from cirrhotic or tuberculous specimens, whereas 20 and 18 of 23 malignant specimens were positive for MMP-2 and MMP-9, respectively [48]. Koyama reported on increased expression of MMP-2, MMP-7, MMP-9, membrane-type-1 MMP (MT1-MMP; MMP-14), and the MMP inhibitors TIMP-2 and TIMP-4 in both tumor cells and tumor-infiltrating lymphocytes from gastric carcinoma effusions ($n = 20$) compared to benign gastric mucosa (=20) and primary carcinomas (=15) using FCM [49]. A subsequent study by this author applying the same method documented the presence of these enzymes on α-smooth muscle actin-positive myofibroblasts from 20 gastric carcinoma effusions [50].

## The Immune Response

As in other cancers, the interaction between the host immune response and tumor cells has been the subject of a relatively large number of studies of GI cancers, with focus on gastric cancer. As in other tumor systems, many of these studies provide evidence for altered or deficient immune response in this setting.

Expression of Fas ligand (FasL) by FCM was found in benign gastric mucosa and in gastric carcinoma cells, with highest levels in effusions, whereas tumor cells had little Fas receptor (FasR) expression and little apoptosis. Tumor-infiltrating lymphocytes expressed both FasL and FasR and underwent apoptosis, suggesting that they may be attacked by carcinoma cells in the tumor environment [51]. Another study by the same group showed high expression of TRAIL and its receptors DR4, DR5, and DcR2 (see Chap. 9) on gastric carcinoma cells in primary carcinomas and effusions, with little apoptosis. Tumor-infiltrating CD3-positive T lymphocytes in effusions similarly expressed these molecules but underwent a greater degree of apoptosis [52]. The authors concluded that gastric carcinoma cells were resistant to Trail-mediated apoptosis, whereas lymphocytes were susceptible, probably through tumor-mediated attack on the immune system [52]. In a third paper by this author, expression of the apoptotic proteins caspase-3, caspase-8, and caspase-10, the anti-apoptotic proteins cFLIP and survivin, and the transcription factor NF-κB in tumor-infiltrating lymphocytes increased from benign mucosa through primary gastric carcinoma to malignant effusions. Tumor cells in primary and metastatic carcinomas had increased levels of cFLIP, survivin, and NF-κB, with highest level in carcinoma cells in effusions, suggesting their involvement in the inhibition of apoptosis in this cancer [53].

Analysis of 23 ascites specimens showed association between transforming growth factor-β1 (TGF-β1) mRNA expression in tumor cells and reduced activity of NK cells [54]. Of note, TGF-β1 serum levels were elevated in sera from patients with HCC, as well as in those with cirrhosis, compared to normal subjects, with similar findings for the TGF-β family member activin and its inhibitor follistatin. The levels of these molecules in 16 ascites specimens showed no relationship with those in matched sera [55].

Sasada et al. analyzed the presence of CD4 + CD25+ regulatory T cells, which have an immunosuppressive effect, in sera from 149 patients with GI malignancies. The proportion of this cell population was higher in samples from cancer patients compared to controls and was associated with shorter survival. CD4 + CD25+ regulatory T cells were additionally found in 7 ascites specimens that consisted of 6 gastric and 1 pancreatic carcinoma, with their percentage ranging from 30.3% to 75.9% of CD4+ T cells [56]. In agreement with these data, the percentage of CD4 + CD25 + CD127$^{low/-}$ regulatory T cells was higher in the blood of 57 gastric carcinoma patients compared with controls, and these cells were found in primary carcinomas, lymph nodes, and ascites from the studied patients [57].

Ormandy et al. found higher percentage of CD4 + CD25+ regulatory T cells in the blood of HCC patients compared with specimens from patients with cirrhosis, infection by the hepatitis viruses HBV and HCV, and healthy controls. Three analyzed ascites specimens had comparable presence of CD4 + CD25+ regulatory T cells. CD4 + CD25+ regulatory T cells were anergic toward T-cell stimulation and suppressed

proliferation and cytokine production in co-cultured CD4 + CD25- T cells in vitro [58].

In two studies, modification of the immune response against GI cancer was used as potential therapeutic approach. Kono et al. isolated tumor-associated lymphocytes from the effusion specimens of 11 gastric and 3 colon stage IV carcinoma patients. Cells were co-stimulated in the presence of autologous tumor with IL-2 and returned to the patients' effusions. Upregulation of T-cell receptor CD3-associated signal transducing ζ (zeta) molecules, which are often lost along tumor progression, was seen in 2 of 14 patients, but was unrelated to the minor clinical response observed in 3 patients [59].

In another study, immunotherapy for malignant ascites in gastric carcinoma with the streptococcal preparation OK-432 resulted in eight positive and four negative responses. TNF-α production in vitro by cells isolated from ascites was significantly higher in responders compared to nonresponders, and this was associated with mRNA expression of the Toll-like receptor *TLR4* and the presence of a CD11c + TLR-4+ cell population [60].

Chemokines, a family of cytokines that are mainly produced by and affect the function of leukocytes, promote tumor cell survival and tumor progression in non-hematological cancer (see Chap. 9). The chemokine CXCL12 and its receptor CXCR4, which have been shown to form an autocrine pathway in other carcinomas (e.g., breast carcinoma), were studied for their biological role in gastric carcinoma. In vitro and in vivo experiments showed a role for CXCL12 and CXCR4 in migration, tumor growth, and ascites formation, with activation of ERK and AKT signaling. CXCL12 mRNA and protein were detected in mesothelial cells from human tissues, and high levels of CXCL12 were measured in 19 ascites specimens from patients with gastric carcinoma. Comparison of CXCR4 expression in primary carcinomas from stage IV patients who had peritoneal carcinomatosis with tumors that metastasized to other organs showed significantly higher CXCR4 expression in the former group, supporting the role of this pathway in peritoneal metastasis in gastric cancer [61].

## Molecular/High-Throughput Analyses

Two early studies applying traditional cytogenetics have documented multiple chromosomal aberrations in gastric carcinoma effusions. Misawa et al. analyzed 6 peritoneal and 1 pleural effusions and observed changes in chromosome number and structure in 6 of 7 specimens, most frequently involving chromosomes 3, 5, 7, 13, and 17 [62]. Trigo studied 5 pleural effusions from gastric carcinoma patients and found frequent trisomy of chromosomes 1, 3, 16, and 19 and monosomy of chromosomes 5 and 21. Structural changes were most frequently found in chromosomes 1, 4, 5, 9, and 17 [63].

Zojer and co-workers studied the cytogenetic profile of 12 primary pancreatic carcinomas and 25 effusions (22 peritoneal, 3 pleural) from patients with metastatic pancreatic carcinoma using interphase fluorescence in situ hybridization (FISH). Cytological examination identified carcinoma cells in 12/25 effusions. Six of the primary carcinomas were hyperdiploid with no chromosomal imbalances, whereas imbalances, affecting mainly chromosome 8, were found in all effusions. Two of ten analyzed malignant effusions were found to have *MYC* mutations. FISH analysis identified aneuploid tumor cells in cytology-negative specimens [64].

Gene expression analysis was applied to compare the molecular profile of a gastric carcinoma cell line isolated from a primary carcinoma to that of five cell lines isolated from effusions. Upregulated genes in effusions included, among others, those encoding for proteins mediating the epithelial phenotype and adhesion (keratins 7, 8, and 14, CD44, integrin α3, occludin, desmoplakin), drug metabolism (aldehyde dehydrogenase, aldo-keto reductase family I), apoptosis (TGFβ-induced anti-apoptotic factor), and signaling (caveolin 3). Downregulated genes included those encoding death-associated protein (apoptosis), integrin β4 (adhesion), insulin growth factor binding protein-2 (IGFBP2, growth and metabolism), and p27$^{kip}$ and histone deacetylase 3 (signaling). The expression of three genes (*KRT7*, *ALDH*, and *IP3R*) was observed in clinical malignant effusions from gastric carcinoma patients and was absent in washings from patients with benign diseases [65].

Proteomics analysis of 3 ascites specimens from patients with pancreatic ductal adenocarcinoma identified 816 proteins, of which 493 were found in all 3 specimens. Little overlap with ovarian carcinoma ascites was seen. Twenty proteins were chosen as potential tumor biomarkers, including known cancer-associated proteins such as MMP-2, stathmin, osteopontin, and neural cell adhesion molecule-1 (NCAM1) [66].

Exosomes are 30–100 nm vesicles which contain cell-specific cargo, including various lipids, proteins, functional mRNA, microRNA (miRNA), and long noncoding RNA (see Chap. 9). Tokuhisa et al. analyzed the exosomal miRNA profiles of gastric cancer in 6 malignant ascites specimens, 24 peritoneal lavage samples, and culture supernatants of 2 gastric carcinoma cell lines, in the aim of identifying microRNAs related to peritoneal dissemination.

miR-1225-5p, miR-320c, miR-1202, miR-1207-5p, and miR-4270 were overexpressed in malignant ascites, lavage specimens from patients with serosa-invasive tumors, and the highly metastatic cell line OCUM-2MD3. PCR validation of the observed differences for miR-21, miR-320c, and miR-1225-5p confirmed the findings for miR-21 and miR-1225-5p [67].

The potential of next-generation sequencing (NGS) in defining the molecular profile of GI cancers in effusion specimens is beginning to gain research focus. Lim and co-workers compared normal gastric mucosa, the primary tumor (six diffuse-type and two intestinal-type adenocarcinomas), and malignant ascites from eight patients using whole-exome sequencing.

Analysis of base substitutions showed a mutational signature dominated by C-to-A substitutions in malignant ascites, whereas tumors from patients who received adjuvant chemotherapy had a high rate of C-to-T substitutions and hypermutation in malignant ascites. Recurrent mutations linked to carcinogenesis were observed in *COL4A6*, *INTS2*, and *PTPN13*. Mutations in druggable genes included those in *TEP1*, *PRKCD*, *BRAF*, *ERBB4*, *PIK3CA*, *HDAC9*, *FYN*, *FASN*, *BIRC2*, *FLT3*, *ROCK1*, *CD22*, and *PIK3C2B*, whereas mutations in metastasis-associated genes were observed in *TNFSF12*, *L1CAM*, *DIAPH3*, *ROCK1*, *TGFBR1*, *MYO9B*, *NR4A1*, and *RHOA*. Pathway analysis showed enrichment of mutations in the Rho-ROCK signaling pathway in malignant ascites [68].

## Other Cancers

Little data is available regarding the biology of non-GI cancers in effusions, with the majority of studies focusing on malignant melanoma.

Savoia and co-workers studied the diagnostic role of an RT-PCR assay for tyrosinase mRNA in detecting melanoma in biological fluids. Analysis of 17 specimens, including 8 effusions, identified tyrosinase mRNA in 12 cases, whereas cytology and immunocytochemistry detected tumor cells in 7 specimens. The five patients with positive tyrosinase assay and negative cytology and immunocytochemistry had radiological evidence of tumor and died within 4 months. The assay was additionally more sensitive than measurement of tyrosinase in peripheral blood [69].

Pirker studied the cytogenetic profile of melanoma cells in 48 samples from 46 patients, including 5 effusion specimens, using comparative genomic hybridization [70]. The most common alterations observed were gains within chromosomes 20q, 7q, 7p, 20p, 6p, and 17q and losses in 9p, 10q, 6q, 10p, 4q, and 11q. Amplification of the telomerase reverse transcriptase gene (*hTERT*) on 5p15.33 and the telomerase RNA component gene (*hTERC*) on 3q26 were found in 22% and 12%, respectively, and the former was common in effusion specimens. Chromosomes or chromosomal regions containing telomerase-suppressing activities at 3p, 4p, 6p, and 10p were frequently underrepresented in melanomas.

Andre analyzed 11 malignant effusions, including 2 melanomas, for the presence of exosomes. Melanoma exosomes contained the tetraspanin family member CD81 and HLA class I and II molecules, as well as the melanoma antigen

Mart1. The possibility of immunizing patients against tumor antigens in exosomes was investigated [71].

Mutation of the *b2m* gene, encoding for a component of the HLA class I machinery, was identified in two cell lines from one melanoma patient, isolated from a lymph node metastasis and pleural effusion, resulting in loss of HLA class I antigen presentation and postulated by the authors to be a mechanism mediating resistance to immunotherapy [72].

Research focusing on metastases from sarcomas or small round blue cell tumors in effusions is to date limited to a few case reports documenting the establishment of cell lines from these tumors [73–77]. However, these reports provide an example of how such cell lines may be useful for studying chromosomal aberrations and other biological characteristics of these tumors, thereby providing a possibility to test potential therapy.

## Targeted Therapy and Concluding Remarks

Patients diagnosed with malignant effusions have grim outlook, and prognosis is particularly poor for those who are diagnosed with one of the cancers discussed in this chapter, even when conventional therapy such as chemotherapy and radiotherapy is applied. Consequently, prolonging survival is critically dependent on the ability to offer more novel therapeutics.

Initial efforts in this direction in the context of malignant effusions included the use of catumaxomab, a trifunctional antibody that binds to EpCAM and CD3, in treating gastric cancer patients [78]. In an additional study, effusion specimens from patients with GI cancers were shown to be informative in identifying genes related to the metabolism of chemotherapy agents [79].

The feasibility of analyzing the expression of molecules relevant for targeted therapy in effusion specimens has been documented for HER2 [80, 81]. Recently, the ability to culture tumor cells from effusion specimens in the aim of testing novel therapeutics has been shown in several studies. Yoo et al. studied bile duct cancer specimens from 40 patients, of whom 20 had stage I–III and 20 had stage IV disease at diagnosis, using a NGS targeted sequencing kit including 381 genes. Ascites or pleural effusion was available in 24 cases. Fifteen mutations were found in primary tumor specimens, affecting *TP53*, *NRAS*, *KRAS*, *ERBB2*, and *PIK3CA*. Patient-derived cultures were successfully established from effusions in 22/24 cases [82].

Supporting the latter report, Golan et al. succeeded in establishing primary cultures from 93/101 ascites specimens obtained from 32 pancreatic carcinoma patients. Cultures were successfully assessed for invasion and migration and epithelial-mesenchymal transition (EMT) charac-

teristics, as well as for *KRAS* status and chemotherapy sensitivity [83].

Similarly, Lee and co-workers successfully established tumor cell cultures from 130/176 cancerous effusions, predominantly ascites specimens, the majority from patients with GI-cancers. Genomic profiling was successful in 116 cases, yielding detection of 181 mutations in 50 genes using the Ion AmpliSeq Cancer Panel v2 platform [84].

Although reports focusing on targeted therapy are currently limited to case studies, there is growing awareness that this approach is the way forward in treating these cancers. The benefit of targeting VEGF or of dual targeting of HER2 and MET was recently documented in metastatic gastric carcinoma [85, 86]. *CDK4* amplification was identified in refractory rhabdomyosarcoma diagnosed in a 27-year-old man, in whom metastatic tumor analyzed included ascites and pleural effusion specimens, suggesting this molecule may be a target for patient-tailored therapy [87]. A *BRAF* V600 K mutation was detected in a pleural effusion from a 74-year-old male with primary melanoma of the scalp in a recent report [88]. These reports suggest that malignant effusions may gain more relevance in the management of patients with metastatic cancer already in the near future.

## References

1. Torre LA, Bray F, Siegel RL, Ferlay J, Lortet-Tieulent J, Jemal A. Global cancer statistics, 2012. CA Cancer J Clin. 2015;65:87–108.
2. Ajani JA, Lee J, Sano T, Janjigian YY, Fan D, Song S. Gastric adenocarcinoma. Nat Rev Dis Primers. 2017;3:17036.
3. Chiaravalli M, Reni M, O'Reilly EM. Pancreatic ductal adenocarcinoma: state-of-the-art 2017 and new therapeutic strategies. Cancer Treat Rev. 2017;60:32–43.
4. Conroy T, Bachet JB, Ayav A, Huguet F, Lambert A, Caramella C, Maréchal R, Van Laethem JL, Ducreux M. Current standards and new innovative approaches for treatment of pancreatic cancer. Eur J Cancer. 2016;57:10–22.
5. Das KK, Early D. Pancreatic cancer screening. Curr Treat Options Gastroenterol. 2017;15(4):562–75. https://doi.org/10.1007/s11938-017-0149-8.
6. Kamisawa T, Wood LD, Itoi T, Takaori K. Pancreatic cancer. Lancet. 2016;388:73–85.
7. Dienstmann R, Vermeulen L, Guinney J, Kopetz S, Tejpar S, Tabernero J. Consensus molecular subtypes and the evolution of precision medicine in colorectal cancer. Nat Rev Cancer. 2017;17:79–92.
8. Forner A, Llovet JM, Bruix J. Hepatocellular carcinoma. Lancet. 2012;379:1245–55.
9. Lagergren J, Smyth E, Cunningham D, Lagergren P. Oesophageal cancer. Lancet. 2017;390(10110):2383–96.
10. Lee J, Lim T, Uhm JE, Park KW, Park SH, Lee SC, Park JO, Park YS, Lim HY, Sohn TS, Noh JH, Heo JS, Park CK, Kim S, Kang WK. Prognostic model to predict survival following first-line chemotherapy in patients with metastatic gastric adenocarcinoma. Ann Oncol. 2007;18:886–91.

11. Lello E, Furnes B, Edna TH. Short and long-term survival from gastric cancer. A population-based study from a county hospital during 25 years. Acta Oncol. 2007;46:308–15.

12. Ikeda M, Okusaka T, Ueno H, Morizane C, Kojima Y, Iwasa S, Hagihara A. Predictive factors of outcome and tumor response to systemic chemotherapy in patients with metastatic hepatocellular carcinoma. Jpn J Clin Oncol. 2008;38:675–82.

13. Carr BI, Pancoska P, Branch RA. Tumor and liver determinants of prognosis in unresectable hepatocellular carcinoma: a large case cohort study. Hepatol Int. 2009;4:396–405.

14. Ozyurtkan MO, Balci AE, Cakmak M. Predictors of mortality within three months in the patients with malignant pleural effusion. Eur J Intern Med. 2010;21:30–4.

15. Maeda H, Kobayashi M, Sakamoto J. Evaluation and treatment of malignant ascites secondary to gastric cancer. World J Gastroenterol. 2015;21:10936–47.

16. DeWitt J, Yu M, Al-Haddad MA, Sherman S, McHenry L, Leblanc JK. Survival in patients with pancreatic cancer after the diagnosis of malignant ascites or liver metastases by EUS-FNA. Gastrointest Endosc. 2010;71:260–5.

17. Zervos EE, Osborne D, Boe BA, Luzardo G, Goldin SB, Rosemurgy AS. Prognostic significance of new onset ascites in patients with pancreatic cancer. World J Surg Oncol. 2006;4:16.

18. Nakata B, Nishino H, Ogawa Y, Yokomatsu H, Kawasaki F, Kosaka K, Wada T, Suto R, Montani A, Hirakawa K. Prognostic predictive value of endoscopic ultrasound findings for invasive ductal carcinomas of pancreatic head. Pancreas. 2005;30:200–5.

19. Hicks AM, Chou J, Capanu M, Lowery MA, Yu KH, O'Reilly EM. Pancreas adenocarcinoma: ascites, clinical manifestations, and management implications. Clin Colorectal Cancer. 2016;15(4):360–8.

20. Shukuya T, Yasui H, Boku N, Onozawa Y, Fukutomi A, Yamazaki K, Taku K, Kojima T, Machida N. Weekly paclitaxel after failure of gemcitabine in pancreatic cancer patients with malignant ascites: a retrospective study. Jpn J Clin Oncol. 2010;40:1135–8.

21. Yonemori K, Okusaka T, Ueno H, Morizane C, Takesako Y, Ikeda M. FP therapy for controlling malignant ascites in advanced pancreatic cancer patients. Hepato-Gastroenterology. 2007;54:2383–6.

22. Warshaw AL. Implications of peritoneal cytology for staging of early pancreatic cancer. Am J Surg. 1991;161:26–9; Discussion 29–30.

23. Cascinu S, Del Ferro E, Barbanti I, Ligi M, Fedeli A, Catalano G. Tumor markers in the diagnosis of malignant serous effusions. Am J Clin Oncol. 1997;20:247–50.

24. Yu CJ, Shew JY, Liaw YS, Kuo SH, Luh KT, Yang PC. Application of mucin quantitative competitive reverse transcription polymerase chain reaction in assisting the diagnosis of malignant pleural effusion. Am J Respir Crit Care Med. 2001;164:1312–8.

25. Yamashita K, Kuba T, Shinoda H, Takahashi E, Okayasu I. Detection of K-ras point mutations in the supernatants of peritoneal and pleural effusions for diagnosis complementary to cytologic examination. Am J Clin Pathol. 1998;109:704–11.

26. Li CP, Huang TS, Chao Y, Chang FY, Whang-Peng J, Lee SD. Advantages of assaying telomerase activity in ascites for diagnosis of digestive tract malignancies. World J Gastroenterol. 2004;10:2468–71.

27. Tangkijvanich P, Tresukosol D, Sampatanukul P, Sakdikul S, Voravud N, Mahachai V, Mutirangura A. Telomerase assay for differentiating between malignancy-related and nonmalignant ascites. Clin Cancer Res. 1999;5:2470–5.

28. Wong J, Schulman A, Kelly K, Zamarin D, Palese P, Fong Y. Detection of free peritoneal cancer cells in gastric cancer using cancer-specific Newcastle disease virus. J Gastrointest Surg. 2010;14:7–14.

29. Cornfield DB, Gheith SM. Flow cytometric quantitation of natural killer cells and T lymphocytes expressing T-cell receptors alpha/ beta and gamma/delta is not helpful in distinguishing benign from malignant body cavity effusions. Cytometry B Clin Cytom. 2009;76:213–7.

30. Wang F, Yang L, Gao Q, Huang L, Wang L, Wang J, Wang S, Zhang B, Zhang Y. CD163+CD14+ macrophages, a potential immune biomarker for malignant pleural effusion. Cancer Immunol Immunother. 2015;64:965–76.

31. Scherpereel A, Grigoriu BD, Noppen M, Gey T, Chahine B, Baldacci S, Trauet J, Copin MC, Dessaint JP, Porte H, Labalette M. Defect in recruiting effector memory CD8+ T-cells in malignant pleural effusions compared to normal pleural fluid. BMC Cancer. 2013;13:324.

32. Yan BC, Gong C, Song J, Krausz T, Tretiakova M, Hyjek E, Al-Ahmadie H, Alves V, Xiao SY, Anders RA, Hart JA. Arginase-1: a new immunohistochemical marker of hepatocytes and hepatocellular neoplasms. Am J Surg Pathol. 2010;34:1147–54.

33. Villamil FG, Sorroche PB, Aziz HF, Lopez PM, Oyhamburu JM. Ascitic fluid alpha 1-antitrypsin. Dig Dis Sci. 1990;35:1105–9.

34. Lee CM, Changchien CS, Shyu WC, Liaw YF. Serum-ascites albumin concentration gradient and ascites fibronectin in the diagnosis of malignant ascites. Cancer. 1992;70:2057–60.

35. Colli A, Cocciolo M, Riva C, Marcassoli L, Pirola M, Di Gregorio P, Buccino G. Ascitic fluid analysis in hepatocellular carcinoma. Cancer. 1993;72:677–82.

36. Greco AV, Mingrone G, Gasbarrini G. Free fatty acid analysis in ascitic fluid improves diagnosis in malignant abdominal tumors. Clin Chim Acta. 1995;239:13–22.

37. Stephen MR, Oien K, Ferrier RK, Burnett RA. Effusion cytology of hepatocellular carcinoma with in situ hybridisation for human albumin. J Clin Pathol. 1997;50:442–4.

38. Miédougé M, Salama G, Barange K, Vincent C, Vinel JP, Serre G. Evaluation of alpha-fetoprotein assay in ascitic fluid for the diagnosis of hepatocellular carcinoma. Clin Chim Acta. 1999;280:161–71.

39. Castaldo G, Intrieri M, Calcagno G, Cimino L, Budillon G, Sacchetti L, Salvatore F. Ascitic pseudouridine discriminates between hepatocarcinoma-derived ascites and cirrhotic ascites. Clin Chem. 1996;42:1843–6.

40. Dong WG, Sun XM, Yu BP, Luo HS, Yu JP. Role of VEGF and CD44v6 in differentiating benign from malignant ascites. World J Gastroenterol. 2003;9:2596–600.

41. Zebrowski BK, Liu W, Ramirez K, Akagi Y, Mills GB, Ellis LM. Markedly elevated levels of vascular endothelial growth factor in malignant ascites. Ann Surg Oncol. 1999;6:373–8.

42. Kraft A, Weindel K, Ochs A, Marth C, Zmija J, Schumacher P, Unger C, Marmé D, Gastl G. Vascular endothelial growth factor in the sera and effusions of patients with malignant and nonmalignant disease. Cancer. 1999;85:178–87.

43. Tamai M, Tanimura H, Yamaue H, Iwahashi M, Tsunoda T, Tani M, Noguchi K, Mizobata S, Hotta T, Arii K, Terasawa H. Clinical significance of quantitative analysis of carcinoembryonic antigen assessed by flow cytometry in fresh human gastric cancer cells. Cancer Lett. 1995;90:111–7.

44. Jung M, Jeung HC, Lee SS, Park JY, Hong S, Lee SH, Noh SH, Chung HC, Rha SY. The clinical significance of ascitic fluid CEA in advanced gastric cancer with ascites. J Cancer Res Clin Oncol. 2010;136:517–26.

45. Matsuura K, Kawanishi J, Fujii S, Imamura M, Hirano S, Takeichi M, Niitsu Y. Altered expression of E-cadherin in gastric cancer tissues and carcinomatous fluid. Br J Cancer. 1992;66:1122–30.

46. Koyama S, Maruyama T, Adachi S. Expression of epidermal growth factor receptor and CD44 splicing variants sharing exons 6 and 9 on gastric and esophageal carcinomas: a two-color flow-cytometric analysis. J Cancer Res Clin Oncol. 1999;125:47–54.

47. Kitayama J, Emoto S, Yamaguchi H, et al. Flow cytometric quantification of Intraperitoneal free tumor cells is a useful

biomarker in gastric cancer patients with peritoneal metastasis. Ann Surg Oncol. 2015;22:2336–42.

48. Sun XM, Dong WG, Yu BP, Luo HS, Yu JP. Detection of type IV collagenase activity in malignant ascites. World J Gastroenterol. 2003;9:2592–5.

49. Koyama S. Enhanced cell surface expression of matrix metalloproteinases and their inhibitors, and tumor-induced host response in progression of human gastric carcinoma. Dig Dis Sci. 2004;49:1621–30.

50. Koyama S. Coordinate cell-surface expression of matrix metalloproteinases and their inhibitors on cancer-associated myofibroblasts from malignant ascites in patients with gastric carcinoma. J Cancer Res Clin Oncol. 2005;131:809–14.

51. Koyama S, Koike N, Adachi S. Fas receptor counterattack against tumor-infiltrating lymphocytes in vivo as a mechanism of immune escape in gastric carcinoma. J Cancer Res Clin Oncol. 2001;127:20–6.

52. Koyama S, Koike N, Adachi S. Expression of TNF-related apoptosis-inducing ligand (TRAIL) and its receptors in gastric carcinoma and tumor-infiltrating lymphocytes: a possible mechanism of immune evasion of the tumor. J Cancer Res Clin Oncol. 2002;128:73–9.

53. Koyama S. Differential expression of intracellular apoptotic signaling molecules in tumor and tumor-infiltrating lymphocytes during development of invasion and/or metastasis of gastric carcinoma. Dig Dis Sci. 2003;48:2290–300.

54. Yoon SJ, Heo DS, Kang SH, Lee KH, Kim WS, Kim GP, Lee JA, Lee KS, Bang YJ, Kim NK. Natural killer cell activity depression in peripheral blood and ascites from gastric cancer patients with high TGF-beta 1 expression. Anticancer Res. 1998;18:1591–6.

55. Yuen MF, Norris S, Evans LW, Langley PG, Hughes RD. Transforming growth factor-beta 1, activin and follistatin in patients with hepatocellular carcinoma and patients with alcoholic cirrhosis. Scand J Gastroenterol. 2002;37:233–8.

56. Sasada T, Kimura M, Yoshida Y, Kanai M, Takabayashi A. CD4+CD25+ regulatory T cells in patients with gastrointestinal malignancies: possible involvement of regulatory T cells in disease progression. Cancer. 2003;98:1089–99.

57. Shen LS, Wang J, Shen DF, Yuan XL, Dong P, Li MX, Xue J, Zhang FM, Ge HL, Xu D. CD4(+)CD25(+)CD127(low/-) regulatory T cells express Foxp3 and suppress effector T cell proliferation and contribute to gastric cancers progression. Clin Immunol. 2009;131:109–18.

58. Ormandy LA, Hillemann T, Wedemeyer H, Manns MP, Greten TF, Korangy F. Increased populations of regulatory T cells in peripheral blood of patients with hepatocellular carcinoma. Cancer Res. 2005;65:2457–64.

59. Kono K, Ichihara F, Iizuka H, Sekikawa T, Matsumoto Y. Expression of signal transducing T-cell receptor zeta molecules after adoptive immunotherapy in patients with gastric and colon cancer. Int J Cancer. 1998;78:301–5.

60. Hironaka K, Yamaguchi Y, Okita R, Okawaki M, Nagamine I. Essential requirement of toll-like receptor 4 expression on CD11c+ cells for locoregional immunotherapy of malignant ascites using a streptococcal preparation OK-432. Anticancer Res. 2006;26:3701–7.

61. Yasumoto K, Koizumi K, Kawashima A, Saitoh Y, Arita Y, Shinohara K, Minami T, Nakayama T, Sakurai H, Takahashi Y, Yoshie O, Saiki I. Role of the CXCL12/CXCR4 axis in peritoneal carcinomatosis of gastric cancer. Cancer Res. 2006;66:2181–7.

62. Misawa S, Horiike S, Taniwaki M, Tsuda S, Okuda T, Kashima K, Abe T, Sugihara H, Noriki S, Fukuda M. Chromosome abnormalities of gastric cancer detected in cancerous effusions. Jpn J Cancer Res. 1990;81:148–52.

63. Trigo MI, San Martín MV, Novales MA, Maraví J. Cytogenetic studies of five gastric carcinomas metastatic to the pleura. Cancer Genet Cytogenet. 1994;75:145–6.

64. Zojer N, Fiegl M, Müllauer L, Chott A, Roka S, Ackermann J, Raderer M, Kaufmann H, Reiner A, Huber H, Drach J. Chromosomal imbalances in primary and metastatic pancreatic carcinoma as detected by interphase cytogenetics: basic findings and clinical aspects. Br J Cancer. 1998;77:1337–42.

65. Sakakura C, Hagiwara A, Nakanishi M, Shimomura K, Takagi T, Yasuoka R, Fujita Y, Abe T, Ichikawa Y, Takahashi S, Ishikawa T, Nishizuka I, Morita T, Shimada H, Okazaki Y, Hayashizaki Y, Yamagishi H. Differential gene expression profiles of gastric cancer cells established from primary tumour and malignant ascites. Br J Cancer. 2002;87:1153–61.

66. Kosanam H, Makawita S, Judd B, Newman A, Diamandis EP. Mining the malignant ascites proteome for pancreatic cancer biomarkers. Proteomics. 2011;11:4551–8.

67. Tokuhisa M, Ichikawa Y, Kosaka N, Ochiya T, Yashiro M, Hirakawa K, Kosaka T, Makino H, Akiyama H, Kunisaki C, Endo I. Exosomal miRNAs from peritoneum lavage fluid as potential prognostic biomarkers of peritoneal metastasis in gastric cancer. PLoS One. 2015;10:e0130472.

68. Lim B, Kim C, Kim JH, Kwon WS, Lee WS, Kim JM, Park JY, Kim HS, Park KH, Kim TS, Park JL, Chung HC, Rha SY, Kim SY. Genetic alterations and their clinical implications in gastric cancer peritoneal carcinomatosis revealed by whole-exome sequencing of malignant ascites. Oncotarget. 2016;7:8055–66.

69. Savoia P, Quaglino P, Osella-Abate S, Comessatti A, Nardò T, Bernengo MG. Tyrosinase mRNA RT-PCR analysis as an additional diagnostic tool for the identification of melanoma cells in biological fluid samples other than blood: a preliminary report. Int J Biol Markers. 2005;20:11–7.

70. Pirker C, Holzmann K, Spiegl-Kreinecker S, Elbling L, Thallinger C, Pehamberger H, Micksche M, Berger W. Chromosomal imbalances in primary and metastatic melanomas: over-representation of essential telomerase genes. Melanoma Res. 2003;13:483–92.

71. Andre F, Schartz NE, Movassagh M, Flament C, Pautier P, Morice P, Pomel C, Lhomme C, Escudier B, Le Chevalier T, Tursz T, Amigorena S, Raposo G, Angevin E, Zitvogel L. Malignant effusions and immunogenic tumour-derived exosomes. Lancet. 2002;360:295–305.

72. Paschen A, Méndez RM, Jimenez P, Sucker A, Ruiz-Cabello F, Song M, Garrido F, Schadendorf D. Complete loss of HLA class I antigen expression on melanoma cells: a result of successive mutational events. Int J Cancer. 2003;103:759–67.

73. Schiavo R, Tullio C, La Grotteria M, Andreotti IC, Scarpati B, Romiti L, Bozzi F, Pedrazzoli P, Siena S. Establishment and characterization of a new Ewing's sarcoma cell line from a malignant pleural effusion. Anticancer Res. 2007;27:3273–8.

74. Nishio J, Iwasaki H, Ishiguro M, Ohjimi Y, Fujita C, Yanai F, Nibu K, Mitsudome A, Kaneko Y, Kikuchi M. Establishment and characterization of a novel human desmoplastic small round cell tumor cell line, JN-DSRCT-1. Lab Investig. 2002;82:1175–82.

75. Kudo N, Ogose A, Hotta T, Kawashima H, Gu W, Umezu H, Toyama T, Endo N. Establishment of novel human dedifferentiated chondrosarcoma cell line with osteoblastic differentiation. Virchows Arch. 2007;451:691–9.

76. Ikemoto S, Sugimura K, Yoshida N, Nakatani T. Chondrosarcoma of the urinary bladder and establishment of a human chondrosarcoma cell line (OCUU-6). Hum Cell. 2004;17:93–6.

77. Sonobe H, Manabe Y, Furihata M, Iwata J, Oka T, Ohtsuki Y, Mizobuchi H, Yamamoto H, Kumano O, Abe S. Establishment and characterization of a new human synovial sarcoma cell line, HS-SY-II. Lab Investig. 1992;67:498–505.

78. Heiss MM, Murawa P, Koralewski P, Kutarska E, Kolesnik OO, Ivanchenko VV, Dudnichenko AS, Aleknaviciene B, Razbadauskas A, Gore M, Ganea-Motan E, Ciuleanu T, Wimberger P, Schmittel A, Schmalfeldt B, Burges A, Bokemeyer C, Lindhofer H, Lahr A, Parsons SL. The trifunctional antibody

catumaxomab for the treatment of malignant ascites due to epithelial cancer: results of a prospective randomized phase II/III trial. Int J Cancer. 2010;127:2209–21.

79. Wang T, Wang L, Qian X, Yu L, Ding Y, Liu B. Relationship between gene expression of 5-fluorouracil metabolic enzymes and 5-fluorouracil sensitivity in primary cancer cells isolated from malignant ascites. Cancer Investig. 2011;29:130–6.

80. Bozzetti C, Negri FV, Lagrasta CA, Crafa P, Bassano C, Tamagnini I, Gardini G, Nizzoli R, Leonardi F, Gasparro D, Camisa R, Cavalli S, Silini EM, Ardizzoni A. Comparison of HER2 status in primary and paired metastatic sites of gastric carcinoma. Br J Cancer. 2011;104:1372–6.

81. Wong DD, de Boer WB, Platten MA, Jo VY, Cibas ES, Kumarasinghe MP. HER2 testing in malignant effusions of metastatic gastric carcinoma: is it feasible? Diagn Cytopathol. 2015;43:80–5.

82. Yoo KH, Kim NK, Kwon WI, Lee C, Kim SY, Jang J, Ahn J, Kang M, Jang H, Kim ST, Ahn S, Jang KT, Park YS, Park WY, Lee J, Heo JS, Park JO. Genomic alterations in biliary tract cancer using targeted sequencing. Transl Oncol. 2016;9:173–8.

83. Golan T, Atias D, Barshack I, Avivi C, Goldstein RS, Berger R. Ascites-derived pancreatic ductal adenocarcinoma primary cell cultures as a platform for personalised medicine. Br J Cancer. 2014;110:2269–76.

84. Lee JY, Kim SY, Park C, Kim NK, Jang J, Park K, Yi JH, Hong M, Ahn T, Rath O, Schueler J, Kim ST, Do IG, Lee S, Park SH, Ji YI, Kim D, Park JO, Park YS, Kang WK, Kim KM, Park WY, Lim HY, Lee J. Patient-derived cell models as preclinical tools for genome-directed targeted therapy. Oncotarget. 2015;6:25619–30.

85. Fushida S, Oyama K, Kinoshita J, Yagi Y, Okamoto K, Tajima H, Ninomiya I, Fujimura T, Ohta T. VEGF is a target molecule for peritoneal metastasis and malignant ascites in gastric cancer: prognostic significance of VEGF in ascites and efficacy of anti-VEGF monoclonal antibody. Onco Targets Ther. 2013;6:1445–51.

86. Ha SY, Lee J, Jang J, Hong JY, Do IG, Park SH, Park JO, Choi MG, Sohn TS, Bae JM, Kim S, Kim M, Kim S, Park CK, Kang WK, Kim KM. HER2-positive gastric cancer with concomitant MET and/or EGFR overexpression: a distinct subset of patients for dual inhibition therapy. Int J Cancer. 2015;136:1629–35.

87. Park S, Lee J, Do IG, Jang J, Rho K, Ahn S, Maruja L, Kim SJ, Kim KM, Mao M, Oh E, Kim YJ, Kim J, Choi YL. Aberrant CDK4 amplification in refractory rhabdomyosarcoma as identified by genomic profiling. Sci Rep. 2014;4:3623.

88. Sakaizawa K, Ashida A, Uhara H, Okuyama R. Detection of BRAFV600K mutant tumor-derived DNA in the pleural effusion from a patient with metastatic melanoma. Clin Chem Lab Med. 2017;55:e92–5.

# Appendix A:
# Immunohistochemistry

The previous chapters provided an overview regarding the very broad differential diagnosis of serous effusions. As discussed elsewhere in this book, relevant clinical data may greatly facilitate the diagnostic work-up, especially in the event of disease recurrence. Age and gender should be taken into consideration and complement the morphological findings in establishing a differential. Nevertheless, even when provided with all available data, cytopathologists often need to resort to ancillary methods in order to provide a diagnosis. Among these methods, immunohistochemistry has absolute supremacy at present, reducing considerably the previously central role of electron microscopy and histochemistry in this setting. Flow cytometry has a central role in the diagnosis of hematological malignancy, but may be considered as complementary to immunohistochemistry, as it is an antibody-based technique.

Whereas molecular biology is becoming more and more part of pathology practice, its diagnostic role is largely limited to diseases in which pathognomonic genomic changes have been defined, i.e., soft tissue tumors and hematological cancers. In the more common setting of metastatic carcinoma, the role of molecular biology to date is mainly within the setting of predictive studies and targeted therapy.

As immunohistochemistry is used on a daily basis by most cytopathologists, this appendix has the aim of detailing the authors' suggested panels for the most common differential diagnostic settings. The extent of the panel used and the choice of antibodies clearly depend on multiple factors, including the possible diagnoses considered by the cytopathologist, personal experience, local laboratory preferences, economy, etc. In many cases, the use of three to four antibodies is sufficient. We nevertheless hope that these lists will help in directing the choice of markers in a judicious manner. Antibodies are graded as excellent (denoting near-100% sensitivity or specificity), good, or fair, in terms of sensitivity and specificity, whereas those performing poorly in our opinion are discussed in the relevant chapters, but omitted here. Markers for which data is inconclusive are listed as such. Less frequent/rare tumors are discussed in the relevant chapters. Naturally, poorly differentiated tumors, especially with single-lying nondescript cells, would require, as in other organs, a broader panel, including carcinoma, melanoma, sarcoma, and lymphoma/leukemia markers.

**Table A1** Reactive mesothelial proliferation vs. malignant mesothelioma

| Marker | Target cells | Sensitivity | Specificity | Recommended |
|---|---|---|---|---|
| **EMA** | Mesothelioma | Excellent | Excellent[a] | Yes |
| **Desmin** | Reactive mesothelium | Excellent | Excellent[b] | Yes |
| **BAP1** | Reactive mesothelium | Good | Excellent[c] | Yes |
| **p53** | Mesothelioma | Fair | Good[d] | Optional |
| **Glut-1** | Mesothelioma | Good | Undecided | Pending |

[a]Weak, usually focal cytoplasmic staining may be seen in reactive mesothelium, but is easy to distinguish from the thick brush-like membrane pattern in mesothelioma
[b]Mesotheliomas stain negatively or focally (usually <5% of cells)
[c]25–60% of malignant mesotheliomas are reported to have loss of BAP1
[d]Reactive mesothelial cells occasionally positive

© Springer International Publishing AG, part of Springer Nature 2018
B. Davidson et al. (eds.), *Serous Effusions*, https://doi.org/10.1007/978-3-319-76478-8

**Table A2** Reactive mesothelial proliferation vs. metastatic adenocarcinoma

| Marker | Target cells | Sensitivity | Specificity | Recommended |
|---|---|---|---|---|
| **Calretinin** | Reactive mesothelium | Excellent | Good[a] | Yes |
| **Desmin** | Reactive mesothelium | Excellent | Excellent | Yes |
| **WT1** | Reactive mesothelium | Excellent | Variable[b] | Depends on differential |
| **D2-40/Podoplanin** | Reactive mesothelium | Excellent | Variable[c] | Depends on differential |
| **Ber-EP4** | Adenocarcinoma | Excellent | Excellent | Yes |
| **MOC-31** | Adenocarcinoma | Excellent | Excellent | Yes[d] |
| **B72.3** | Adenocarcinoma | Excellent | Excellent | Yes |
| **BG-8** | Adenocarcinoma | Good | Excellent | Yes |
| **EMA** | Adenocarcinoma | Excellent | Excellent[e] | Yes |
| **CEA** | Adenocarcinoma | Variable[f] | Excellent | Yes |
| **CDX2** | Adenocarcinoma | Variable[g] | Good | Depends on differential |
| **Claudin-4** | Adenocarcinoma | Excellent | Excellent | Yes |

[a]Focal staining seen in some serous Müllerian carcinomas
[b]Not useful for differentiating reactive mesothelium from serous adnexal/peritoneal carcinoma
[c]Inconclusive data regarding the differentiation from serous adnexal/peritoneal carcinoma
[d]It is generally sufficient to use either Ber-EP4 or MOC-31, and data is inconclusive as to which of these two antibodies performs better
[e]Weak, usually focal cytoplasmic staining may be seen in reactive mesothelium, but is easy to distinguish from the strong combined membrane and cytoplasmic pattern in adenocarcinoma
[f]Excellent for gastrointestinal carcinomas, good for breast and lung adenocarcinoma, and not useful for serous adnexal/peritoneal carcinoma
[g]Excellent for gastrointestinal carcinomas, less relevant for the majority of other carcinomas

**Table A3** Malignant mesothelioma vs. metastatic non-serous adenocarcinoma

| Marker | Target cells | Sensitivity | Specificity | Recommended |
|---|---|---|---|---|
| **Calretinin** | Mesothelioma | Excellent | Good[a] | Yes |
| **WT1** | Mesothelioma | Excellent | Good[b] | Yes |
| **D2-40/Podoplanin** | Mesothelioma | Excellent | Good[c] | Yes |
| **EMA** | Both tumors[d] | Excellent | Good[e] | Yes |
| **Ber-EP4** | Adenocarcinoma | Excellent | Good[f] | Yes |
| **MOC-31** | Adenocarcinoma | Excellent | Good[f] | Yes[g] |
| **Claudin-4** | Adenocarcinoma | Excellent | Excellent | Yes |
| **B72.3** | Adenocarcinoma | Good | Excellent | Yes |
| **BG-8** | Adenocarcinoma | Good | Good | Yes |
| **CEA** | Adenocarcinoma | Variable[h] | Excellent | Yes |
| **CDX-2** | Adenocarcinoma | Variable[i] | Excellent | Depends on differential |
| **ER** | Adenocarcinoma | Variable[j] | Excellent | Depends on differential |

[a]Focal staining seen in some serous Müllerian carcinomas, but most other adenocarcinomas are negative
[b]Not useful for differentiating malignant mesothelioma from serous adnexal/peritoneal carcinoma, but most other adenocarcinomas are negative
[c]Inconclusive data regarding the differentiation from serous Müllerian carcinoma; the majority of other carcinomas stain focally or negatively
[d]Thick brush-like membrane pattern in mesothelioma vs. strong combined membrane and cytoplasmic pattern in adenocarcinoma
[e]Thick brush-like membrane pattern mimicking mesothelioma may be infrequently seen in adenocarcinoma
[f]Staining is seen fairly often in epithelioid mesothelioma, but is generally focal, although exceptions do occur
[g]It is generally sufficient to use either Ber-EP4 or MOC-31, and data is inconclusive as to which of these two antibodies performs better
[h]Excellent for gastrointestinal carcinomas, good for breast and lung adenocarcinoma, and not useful for serous ovarian/peritoneal carcinoma
[i]Excellent for gastrointestinal carcinomas, less relevant for the majority of other carcinomas
[j]Positive in many breast and female genital carcinomas, may be occasionally expressed in other adenocarcinomas

**Table A4** Malignant mesothelioma vs. serous adenocarcinoma (AC)

| Marker | Target cells | Sensitivity | Specificity | Recommended |
|---|---|---|---|---|
| **Calretinin** | Mesothelioma | Excellent | Good[a] | Yes |
| **EMA** | Both tumors[b] | Excellent | Good[c] | Yes |
| **Ber-EP4** | Serous AC | Excellent | Good[d] | Yes |
| **MOC-31** | Serous AC | Excellent | Good[d] | Yes[e] |
| **B72.3** | Serous AC | Excellent | Excellent | Yes |
| **BG-8** | Serous AC | Good | Good | Yes |
| **MUC4** | Serous AC | Excellent | Excellent | Yes |
| **PAX2** | Serous AC | Moderate | Excellent | Yes |
| **PAX8** | Serous AC | Excellent | Excellent | Yes |
| **Claudin-4** | Serous AC | Excellent | Excellent | Yes |

[a]Focal staining seen in some serous Müllerian carcinomas
[b]Thick brush-like membrane pattern in mesothelioma vs. strong combined membrane and cytoplasmic pattern in adenocarcinoma
[c]Thick brush-like membrane pattern mimicking mesothelioma may be infrequently seen in serous carcinoma
[d]Staining is seen fairly often in epithelioid mesothelioma, but is generally focal, although exceptions do occur
[e]It is generally sufficient to use either Ber-EP4 or MOC-31, and data is inconclusive as to which of these two antibodies performs better

**Table A5** Malignant mesothelioma vs. lung adenocarcinoma (AC)

| Marker | Target cells | Sensitivity | Specificity | Recommended |
|---|---|---|---|---|
| **Calretinin** | Mesothelioma | Excellent | Excellent | Yes |
| **WT1** | Mesothelioma | Excellent | Excellent | Yes |
| **D2-40/Podoplanin** | Mesothelioma | Excellent | Excellent | Yes |
| **Cytokeratin 5/6** | Mesothelioma | Excellent | Good | Yes |
| **EMA** | Both tumors[a] | Excellent | Good | Yes |
| **Ber-EP4** | Lung AC | Excellent | Good[b] | Yes |
| **MOC-31** | Lung AC | Excellent | Good[b] | Yes[c] |
| **B72.3** | Lung AC | Good | Excellent | Yes |
| **BG-8** | Lung AC | Good | Good | Yes |
| **CEA** | Lung AC | Good | Excellent | Yes |
| **TTF-1** | Lung AC | Good | Excellent | Yes |
| **Surfactant**[d] | Lung AC | Good | Excellent | Yes |
| **Napsin A** | Lung AC | Good | Excellent | Yes |

[a]Thick brush-like membrane pattern in mesothelioma vs. strong combined membrane and cytoplasmic pattern in adenocarcinoma
[b]Staining is seen fairly often in epithelioid mesothelioma, but is generally focal, although exceptions do occur
[c]It is generally sufficient to use either Ber-EP4 or MOC-31, and data is inconclusive as to which of these two antibodies performs better
[d]Several isoforms

**Table A6** Malignant mesothelioma vs. pulmonary squamous cell carcinoma (Sqcc)

| Marker | Target cells | Sensitivity | Specificity | Recommended |
|---|---|---|---|---|
| **Calretinin** | Mesothelioma | Excellent | Good[a] | Yes |
| **WT1** | Mesothelioma | Excellent | Excellent | Yes |
| **Ber-EP4** | Sqcc | Good | Good[b] | Yes |
| **MOC-31** | Sqcc | Good | Good[b] | Yes[c] |
| **B72.3** | Sqcc | Good | Excellent | Yes |
| **BG-8** | Sqcc | Good | Good | Yes |
| **CEA** | Sqcc | Good | Excellent | Yes |
| **p63** | Sqcc | Excellent | Excellent | Yes |
| **p40** | Sqcc | Excellent | Excellent | Yes |

[a]Focal staining not infrequently observed in Sqcc
[b]Staining is seen fairly often in epithelioid mesothelioma, but is generally focal, although exceptions do occur
[c]It is generally sufficient to use either Ber-EP4 or MOC-31, and data is inconclusive as to which of these two antibodies performs better

**Table A7** Serous Müllerian vs. pulmonary vs. breast adenocarcinoma

| Marker | Target cells | Sensitivity | Specificity | Recommended |
|---|---|---|---|---|
| WT1 | Müllerian | Excellent | Excellent | Yes |
| PAX8[a] | Müllerian | Excellent | Excellent | Yes |
| PAX2[a] | Serous AC | Moderate | Excellent | Yes |
| ER | Müllerian + breast | Good | Good | Yes |
| GATA3 | Breast | Excellent | Excellent | Yes |
| GCDFP-15 | Breast | Fair | Good | Yes |
| Mammaglobin | Breast | Good | Good | Yes |
| TTF-1 | Lung | Good | Excellent | Yes |
| Surfactant[b] | Lung | Good | Excellent | Yes |
| Napsin A | Lung | Good | Excellent[a] | Yes |

[a]Reported to stain renal cell carcinoma but appears to be negative in other adenocarcinomas
[b]Several isoforms

# Appendix B: Common Primary Sites for Malignant Effusions

The majority of patients with malignant serous effusions have a known history which helps in the differential diagnosis. Common primary sites for malignant effusions according to sex, age, and the cavity involved are shown in Table B1.

The leading cause of malignant effusions in adults is metastatic carcinoma, and adenocarcinoma is the most common histologic type. On the other hand, malignant effusions in children are almost always caused by hematopoietic malignancies, followed by other small round cell tumors, such as Wilms tumor, neuroblastoma, rhabdomyosarcoma, and Ewing sarcoma. Lung carcinoma and breast carcinoma are the most common causes of malignant effusions in the pleural and pericardial cavities. In the peritoneal cavity, ovarian carcinoma in females and gastrointestinal tract carcinomas in males are the leading causes. Lymphomas/leukemias commonly cause malignant effusions in all cavities also in adults. The incidence of mesothelioma varies and depends on the geographic location and the occupational history of the patient population [1–5].

The presence of an effusion in a cancer patient does not, of course, necessarily mean that the effusion is malignant. Besides, second primary tumors are not rare. For a correct diagnosis of a serous effusion, the clinical and morphologic features should always be evaluated together, and when needed, ancillary tests should be included in the work-up.

**Table B1** The most common primary sites for malignant effusions according to the sex, age, and the cavity involved

| Malignant effusions | Pleural | Peritoneal | Pericardial |
|---|---|---|---|
| **Male—adult** | Lung<br>Lymphoma/leukemia<br>Gastrointestinal tract<br>Pancreas<br>Mesothelioma[a] | Gastrointestinal tract<br>Lymphoma/leukemia<br>Pancreas<br>Genitourinary | Lung<br>Lymphoma/leukemia<br>Gastrointestinal tract |
| **Female—adult** | Breast<br>Lung<br>Ovary<br>Lymphoma/leukemia<br>Gastrointestinal tract<br>Pancreas | Ovary<br>Uterus<br>Breast<br>Gastrointestinal tract<br>Lymphoma/leukemia | Breast<br>Lung<br>Lymphoma/leukemia<br>Gastrointestinal tract |
| **Children** | Lymphoma/leukemia<br>Other small round blue cell tumors | Lymphoma/leukemia<br>Other small round blue cell tumors | Lymphoma/leukemia<br>Other small round blue cell tumors |

[a]The incidence of mesothelioma varies according to the geographic location and occupational profile of the patient population

# References

1. DeMay RM, editor. The art & science of cytopathology. Chicago: ASCP Press; 1996. p. 257–325.
2. Roberts ME, Neville E, Berrisford RG, Antunes G, Ali NJ. BTS Pleural Disease Guideline Group. Management of a malignant pleural effusion: British Thoracic Society pleural disease guideline 2010. Thorax. 2010;65(Suppl 2):ii32–40.
3. American Thoracic Society. Management of malignant pleural effusions. Am J Respir Crit Care Med. 2000;162:1987–2001.
4. Maisch B, Ristic A, Pankuweit S. Evaluation and management of pericardial effusion in patients with neoplastic disease. Prog Cardiovasc Dis. 2010;53:157–63.
5. Hallman JR, Geisinger KR. Cytology of fluids from pleural, peritoneal and pericardial cavities in children. A comprehensive survey. Acta Cytol. 1994;38:209–17.

# Index

Printed by Printforce, the Netherlands